Ventricular
Function and
Blood Flow in
Congenital Heart
Disease

To my wife Rani, without whose love and support this book would not be possible and will always be the better part of me

To my children Arielle and Benjamin, for always keeping me young and energetic

To my brother Bobby, who taught me that being a true seeker of truth and understanding is not just a dream and

To my mother Sylvia, who helped me become who I am today

Ventricular Function and Blood Flow in Congenital Heart Disease

EDITED BY

Mark A. Fogel, MD, FACC, FAAP

Associate Professor of Pediatrics and Radiology
Director of Cardiac MRI
The Children's Hospital of Philadelphia
The University of Pennsylvania School of Medicine Philadelphia, Pennsylvania

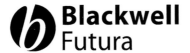
Blackwell
Futura

© 2005 by Blackwell Publishing
Blackwell Futura is an imprint of Blackwell Publishing

Blackwell Publishing, Inc., 350 Main Street, Malden, Massachusetts 02148-5018, USA
Blackwell Publishing Ltd, 9600 Garsington Road, Oxford OX4 2DQ, UK
Blackwell Science Asia Pty Ltd, 550 Swanston Street, Carlton, Victoria 3053, Australia

First published 2005

ISBN-13: 978-1-4051-2211-5
ISBN-10: 1-4051-2211-0

Library of Congress Cataloging-in-Publication Data

Ventricular function and blood flow in congenital heart disease / edited by Mark A. Fogel.
    p. ; cm.
  Includes bibliographical references and index.
  ISBN-13: 978-1-4051-2211-5
  ISBN-10: 1-4051-2211-0
  1. Congenital heart disease in children–Pathophysiology.   2. Heart–Ventricles.
  [DNLM: 1. Heart Defects, Congenital.   2. Ventricular Function. WG 220 V4665 2005]
    I. Fogel, Mark A.

  RJ426.C64V46 2005
  618.92′12043–dc22

                        2004018315

A catalogue record for this title is available from the British Library

Acquisitions: Steve Korn
Production: Fiona Pattison
Set in 9/12 pt Photina by TechBooks
Printed and bound in India by Gopsons Papers Ltd., Noida

For further information on Blackwell Publishing, visit our website:
www.blackwellfutura.com

The publisher's policy is to use permanent paper from mills that operate a sustainable forestry
policy, and which has been manufactured from pulp processed using acid-free and elementary
chlorine-free practices. Furthermore, the publisher ensures that the text paper and cover board
used have met acceptable environmental accreditation standards.

Notice: The indications and dosages of all drugs in this book have been recommended in the
medical literature and conform to the practices of the general community. The medications
described do not necessarily have specific approval by the Food and Drug Administration for use
in the diseases and dosages for which they are recommended. The package insert for each drug
should be consulted for use and dosage as approved by the FDA. Because standards for usage
change, it is advisable to keep abreast of revised recommendations, particularly those concerning
new drugs.

Contents

List of Contributors

Lee Benson, MD, FRCP(C), FSCAI

The Department of Pediatrics, Division of Cardiology, The Hospital for Sick Children, The University of Toronto School of Medicine, Toronto, Canada

Robert C. Brasch

Professor of Radiology and Pediatrics, University of California, California 94143, USA

Martin Charron, MD

Director Nuclear Medicine, Children's Hospital of Philadelphia, and Associate Professor of Radiology, University of Pennsylvania, PA, 19104-4399, USA

Michael Cheung, MB, ChB, MRCP (UK)

The Department of Pediatrics, Division of Cardiology, The Hospital for Sick Children, The University of Toronto School of Medicine, Toronto, Canada

Meryl S. Cohen, MD

Assistant Professor of Pediatrics, Director, Non-Invasive Cardiovascular Laboratory, University of Pennsylvania School of Medicine, The Children's Hospital of Philadelphia, Philadelphia, Pennsylvania, USA

Steven Colan, MD

Professor of Pediatrics, Harvard Medical School, Director, Division of Noninvasive Cadiology, Boston, MA, USA

Debra Dodd, MD

Associate Professor of Pediatrics, Division of Pediatric Cardiology, Vanderbilt University Medical Center, Nashville, TN 37232, USA

Stanford Ewing, MD FAAP FRCP(C)

Clinical Assistant Professor, University of Pennsylvania, Division of Cardiology, 34th St. and Civic Center Blvd, Philadelphia, PA 19104, USA

Mark A. Fogel, MD, FACC, FAAP

Associate Professor of Pediatrics and Radiology, Director of Cardiac MRI, The Children's Hospital of Philadelphia, The University of Pennsylvania School of Medicine, 34th St. and Civic Center Blvd, Philadelphia, PA 19104, USA

Thomas P. Graham Jr, MD

Director of Pediatric Cardiology, Ann & Monroe Carell Professor of Pediatrics, TN 37232, USA

Brian D. Hanna, MD, PhD

Clinical Associate Professor of Pediatrics, University of Pennsylvania School of Medicine, The Children's Hospital of Philadelphia, Philadelphia, PA 19104, USA

Amy H. Schultz, MD

Instructor, Department of Pediatrics, University of Pennsylvania School of Medicine, Division of Cardiology, Children's Hospital of Philadelphia, Philadelphia, PA, USA

Julien I.E. Hoffman, MD, FRCP (London)

Professor of Pediatrics (Emeritus), Department of Pediatrics, Senior Member of the Cardiovascular Research Institute, University of California, San Francisco, California 94143, USA

Ann Kavanaugh-McHugh, MD

Assistant Professor of Pediatrics, Vanderbilt University Medical Center, TN 37232, USA

Hiroumi Kitajima, MS

Wallace H. Coulter Department of Biomedical Engine, Georgia Institute of Technology and Emory University School of Medicine, Atlanta, Georgia, USA

Bruce Y. Lee, MD

Division of General Internal Medicine, University of Pennsylvania, 1125 Blockley Hall, 423 Guardion Street, Philadelphia, PA 19104, USA

Stephen Paridon, MD

Associate Professor of Pediatrics, Medical Director, Exercise Physiology Laboratory, The Children's Hospital of Philadelphia, The University of Pennsylvania School of Medicine, 34th St. and Civic Center Blvd, Philadelphia, PA 19104, USA

Andrew Redington, MD, FRCP(C) (UK)

Head, Division of Cardiology, University Avenue, Toronto, Ontario, M5G 1X8, Canada

Jack Rychik, MD

Associate Professor Pediatrics, The Children's Hospital of
Philadelphia, Philadelphia, PA 19104, USA

Theresa Ann Tacy, MD

University of California, San Francisco, USA

Ajit P. Yoganathan, PhD

Regents' Professor, Wallace H. Coulter Department of
Biomedical Engine, Georgia Institute of Technology and
Emory University School of Medicine, Atlanta, GA 30332-0,
USA

Foreword

Though flattered by Dr Fogel's invitation, it is awkward for a surgeon to preface a book written by such an eminent panel of bioengineers, physiologists, cardiologists, and clinical investigators.

Having accepted the task, however, I have found it very refreshing and most enjoyable to glance through the various chapters of this book of applied physiology to congenital heart diseases. It reminds me of the intellectual pleasure I experienced as a junior trainee when I read Abraham Rudolph's book on congenital diseases of the heart.

Major advances in invasive and noninvasive methods of investigation of the cardiovascular system have contributed greatly to the understanding of the physiopathology of treated and untreated congenital malformations of the cardiovascular system. The impact of these innovations on the management of congenital heart diseases is highlighted throughout this book. It is pleasing to note that a chapter (Chapter 3) has been dedicated to history and physical examination, which, in an age of high technology and multidisciplinary team approach, are too often forgotten or underestimated. It is a reminder that our first duty is to improve quality of life and longevity. The emphasis on exercise performance (Chapters 10 and 18) is most appropriate in that context.

A book on the physiological approach to the management of congenital heart defects is rational and timely. The following are just a few examples.

A better understanding of right ventricular physiology has helped to elucidate the arcanes of low cardiac output syndrome after repair of tetralogy of Fallot. A more accurate assessment of ventricular function in volume or pressure overload situations has contributed to the refinement of indications and timing for intervention.

The evolution of strategies to palliate univentricular hearts, from the Norwood operation to the variety of Fontan procedures, has been an exhibition of applied physiology to clinical practice. Mathematical modeling has been helpful in optimizing the flow dynamics of some of these procedures. The marriage of magnetic resonance imaging and computational fluid dynamics could potentially open the field of virtual reality, of tailor-made surgical and interventional procedures.

The understanding and prevention of late attrition of the Fontan circulation remains an outstanding research question for the cardiovascular physiologist. A comprehensive approach to the problem must, however, include a thorough investigation of the systemic venous and the lymphatic circulations, which have not been given the attention they deserve in the literature.

Surgical successes of the past fifty years have created a new population of patients: adults with operated congenital heart disease. They now represent a new spectrum of research questions for the cardiovascular physiologist. Longitudinal follow-up studies using noninvasive methods of investigation are mandatory in order to provide these patients with evidence-based treatment. There is today no scientific consensus with regard to the management of lesions as common as residual/recurrrent mild to moderate coarctation of the aorta or pulmonary valve regurgitation late after repair of tetralogy of Fallot.

Because of my lifelong interest in cardiovascular physiology I am probably biased in my acclamation of this book. It is my belief that physiology is, and will remain, the hub of all sciences dealing with congenital heart defects. Clinical results will continue to be assessed by physiological measurements. Future advances in pharmacology, electrophysiology, interventional and surgical procedures, as well as in basic sciences such as cellular and molecular biology, gene therapy, etc, will inevitably be translated into physiological improvements.

Dr Fogel and his coauthors must be congratulated for their tour de force. This book will attract a wide audience, from trainees to practitioners and scientists.

Marc R de Leval MD FRCS
Professor of Cardiothoracic Surgery
Great Ormond Street Hospital for
Children NHS Trust, London, UK

Preface

Congenital heart disease is one of the major causes of morbidity and mortality in pediatrics. In addition, because of major advances over the past 50 years, more and more of these children are growing into adulthood and require medical attention and follow-up. It is therefore incumbent, not only on the pediatrician, pediatric cardiologist, cardiac surgeon, or cardiac anesthesiologist to familiarize themselves with all the nuances of this branch of pediatrics, but the family practitioner, internist, adult cardiologist, and intensivist also need to have a working knowledge of this as well.

To understand congenital heart disease is to also understand that it is one of the more technical disciplines within pediatrics and medicine in general. This is based on the continued evolution of diagnosis and management grounded on advances in technology. With the advent of advanced imaging techniques, invasive monitoring, and many other breakthroughs, our knowledge of this field is vastly different now than it was just 10 years ago. But congenital heart disease is not just technical in that respect; complex anatomy, physiology, hemodynamics, ventricular function, and blood flow along with their interactions with each other form an intricate web of connections and associations that need to be deciphered. Basic principles need to be applied so that any one of the varied types of congenital heart disease that present to the practitioner can be analyzed and a reasonable plan of action can be implemented. In addition, precise definitions must always be used to assure correct communication of what is truly going on in the patient.

Within congenital heart disease, ventricular function and blood flow is a discipline that is very exacting and yet so misunderstood and misused. There may be two fundamental reasons for this:

- As individuals who work in this field, we borrow a lot from our adult colleagues when its applicability may not be wholly appropriate.
- What we learn as pediatric residents, cardiology fellows, and as an attending on this subject is gleaned from multiple sources, which are not totally devoted to this topic (e.g., a short chapter in a textbook). As such, all the nuances are not totally explained.

It would have been instructive and much more efficient, I thought, to have had thorough summaries of all the aspects of ventricular function and blood flow in one place that is devoted solely to congenital heart disease. The idea for this textbook is to allow the trainee, practitioner, and the researcher to have a repository of information to base their fundamental understanding, practice, and experiments on.

Any text on this subject must be organized in a logical way for the reader to get a complete understanding of the issues involved. Towards that end, the textbook is divided into three major sections. The first involves familiarizing the reader with the minimum tools needed to understand ventricular function and blood flow in this book and elsewhere, and hence, the Overview section with its Basics of the Discipline chapters. This section also includes a lengthy "justification" for the need for such a textbook as those unfamiliar with the discipline may require. The next section discusses the various techniques and technology used in evaluating how well the heart pumps and the way blood flows. Specifically, these chapters focus on these techniques and technologies as they relate to pediatrics. Finally, the third and largest section deals with broad categories of congenital heart disease on this subject. Although there are many ways to organize and categorize congenital heart disease, I thought it best to sort it both "physiologically" (i.e., Pressure Overload Lesions, Volume Overload Lesions) as well as "anatomically" (e.g., The Right Ventricle in a Dual Chambered Circulation). There are also additional chapters on special topics such as the intensive care unit and pharmacology.

Because of space and time constraints, this textbook cannot be encyclopedic. Indeed, issues related to molecular biology, genetics, etc have not been explored. I have endeavored to make the format of this textbook a "core curriculum" with references to the high quality publications on the parts of this discipline, which are not covered here. My hope is that this textbook will not only be used as a learning tool and reference, but will also act as a springboard to further study of ventricular function and blood flow in congenital heart disease. It is also my hope that this textbook will excite the reader about this fascinating field and will spur future advances, which may one day impact patients.

Mark Fogel

Acknowledgments

Any project of this magnitude can never be done by one individual alone. I would first thank Steve Korn of Blackwell-Futura, who was willing to give a project like this a shot and whose enormous help in organizing this textbook, advice, and persistence has paid off. There are many other people in Blackwell-Futura who contributed many long and hard hours who I would thank such as Katrina Chandler, Fiona Pattison, Manjari Mohan. This book would not be possible without the long list of my colleagues and contributors who did such wonderful and thorough work on their topics—I owe them a debt of gratitude. I had much help on the administrative side from Roseanne Lovelick and Stacey Casper and I thank them for all their efforts.

I would also thank some of the people who inspired me through the years:

- Paul Weinberg, Alvin Chin, Gerald Barber, and Henry Wagner have been my teachers in pediatric cardiology and have contributed much to my understanding of the field. Henry Wagner especially stands out as a "true gentleman cardiologist" as well as being an outstanding clinician. Charlie Kleinman was the division chief of pediatric cardiology when I was a resident at Yale who was there for me when I needed someone the most.

- All pediatric cardiologists work closely with our cardiothoracic surgical colleagues and our symbiotic relationship always seems to lead to a better understanding of the field in which we work. Working with the likes of Bill Norwood, Marshall Jacobs, and Tom Spray, I have learned not only to think through a problem but also the importance of "thinking outside the box" as the saying goes.

- I could not have had a better pediatric residency than I did at Yale and although I thank the entire attending staff during my years there, Tom Dolan, Paul McCarthy, and George Lister stand out as extraordinary physicians. I also owe a debt of gratitude to my fellow pediatric residents who were there for me always and whose friendship I will always treasure.

- Finally, no medical student who has gone through the program at Upstate Medical Center in Syracuse, NY, in the 80s can ever publish a scholarly textbook without the mention of Robert Rohner, who not only was one of the best teachers ever but also instilled the love of medicine in us all and taught us to be proud of who we are.

Ultimately, however, I want to thank you, the reader, whose interest in reading or purchasing this textbook is the spark which gave this project its life in the first place.

PART I
Overview

CHAPTER 1

Pediatric Congenital and Acquired Heart Disease as It Relates to Ventricular Function and Blood Flow

Mark A. Fogel, MD, FACC, FAAP

Introduction

Any textbook on congenital heart disease (CHD) must start with a basis from which any future discussion will arise. Definitions are important, especially in a textbook on ventricular function and blood flow, where the exact anatomy and physiology need to be known to understand the altered loading conditions of the heart and the flow abnormalities that occur. To that end, we will use the definition of CHD proposed by Mitchell *et al.* [1], which is a "gross structural abnormality of the heart or intrathoracic great vessels, that is actually or potentially of functional significance." Therefore, this textbook focuses on lesions which have an impact on physiology, and will not deal with those lesions which are clinically insignificant such as a persistent fifth aortic arch [2].

One of the reasons why this textbook is necessary is that CHD is a fairly common lesion. Hoffman and Kaplan [3] recently reported the results of a survey of the literature and found the incidence of moderate to severe forms of CHD to be 6/1000 live births, rising to 19/1000 live births if potentially serious bicuspid aortic valves are included. All forms of CHD represent 75/1000 live births including such lesions as tiny as muscular ventricular septal defects. In addition, the New England Infant Cardiac Program [4] reported that 3/1000 live births need cardiac catheterization, surgery, or will die with CHD in early infancy (excluding premature infants with patent ductus arteriosus). This number rises to 5/1000 live births who will need some kind of specialized facilities during their lifetime.

Not only is CHD a common lesion, but with improvements in diagnosis and treatment of CHD along with a greater understanding of the anatomy and physiology, patients are living longer [5–7]. This represents a growing population seen by adult cardiologists and internists. In 1980, there were an estimated 300 000 adults with CHD while in the year 2000, this rose to approximately 1 million. In 2020, the number is anticipated to be 1.4 million.

This textbook is meant for physicians and other clinical care givers, as well as clinician scientists and researchers, who address the needs of this burgeoning population. It is through a greater understanding of this important aspect of the disease process that improvements in care will come. There is no comprehensive place for ventricular function and blood flow in CHD that individuals can turn to for learning about these processes; this book is meant for that purpose.

Pediatrics and CHD: The need for a special textbook

The question may rightfully arise: why should there be a "carve-out" for pediatrics and CHD with regards to ventricular function and blood flow? After all, the principles of myocardial contraction and fluid flow would appear to be universal. There are a number of issues, however, which set the pediatric acquired and CHD apart from the rest of the field:
- Age related changes
- Unique anatomy and physiology of CHD

- Technical challenges
- The fetal environment

Age related changes
As is fairly obvious, as children grow and develop, so does their cardiovascular system. It is not obvious, however, what changes are induced during this development or that these changes are linear. Indeed, children's growth is not linear and growth spurts at various stages do occur [8].

One specific example is the amount of contribution by each cavae to systemic venous return, which was studied by Salim *et al.* [9]. In their study, they demonstrated that in normal children, the caval contributions to systemic venous return vary with age, from a low of 45% in the inferior vena cava in approximately 2.2-year-olds to a high of 65% in 6.6-year-olds, which is the adult value [10,11]. This bit of trivia, however, matters when it comes to the Fontan procedure [12] for single ventricle repair, where there is a total cavo-pulmonary connection created. Much of the literature dedicated to evaluating the physiology and fluid mechanics of this flow [10,11,13–15] is predicated on the knowledge of the relative caval contributions to pulmonary flow, systemic venous return and the amount of blood flow to each lung. Surgeons have even tried to alter the Fontan procedure to account for this flow discrepancy [16] and a study published in 1999 [17] confirmed in Fontan patients of nearly two years of age what Salim *et al.* had demonstrated in healthy children.

Further, it is not clear how these growth related changes are impacted by the presence of CHD. For example, Salim *et al.* [9] delineated how the caval contribution of systemic venous return changes in healthy children and although the Fontan study [17] confirmed this in patients of nearly two years of age, it is unclear how this relative flow changes with patient's age. CHD in turn, may impact on growth—for example, a patient in congestive heart failure may fail to thrive—which can make the age related changes to caval contributions disease specific as well as individualized to a given patient. As you can tell, this can get very complex.

To account for age and size as well, clinicians and researchers who take care of or study children with CHD index their findings to age and/or size. For example, cardiac output is always put in terms of liters/minute/meter^2 and drug doses are portioned out on the basis of either weight or body surface area and age.

Unique anatomy and physiology of CHD
Another difficulty in studying CHD arises because of the varied anatomy, which can become very complex. This differs from the adult without CHD where, for example, the left ventricle is always on the left side of the circulation and the pulmonary veins always connect to the left atrium. Indeed, one takes for granted in the adult without CHD that there are two pumping chambers for the two circulations! In pediatric cardiology, none of this can be taken for granted.

Moreover, the physiology of CHD is much different from disease processes in the adult. For example, shunt flow (whether that be left to right or right to left) and mixing lesions figure prominently in CHD. Regurgitant and stenotic lesions (which is more common in the adult population than shunt lesions), whether that be from the atrioventricular or semilunar valves, also play a major role in CHD physiology.

Ventricular function

A comprehensive study of ventricular function in CHD is difficult to achieve because of the variety of right and left ventricles (right and left ventricle defined by the unique morphological features of each)! The following questions need to be asked in CHD before a discussion of ventricular function can be entertained (the right ventricle will be used as an example although a parallel construction of the left ventricle can be made as well).
- Is the right ventricle a pulmonary pumping chamber as in the normal case, or is it a systemic ventricle in a dual-chamber circulation as in transposition of the great arteries after an atrial inversion operation (i.e. Senning or Mustard procedure) [18–22]?
- Is the right ventricle shaped in a right handed geometry (D-looped) as in normals or shaped in a left handed geometry (L-loop) as in the so-called corrected transposition (transposition of the great arteries {S,L,L} [23,24]?
- Is the right ventricle in a dual-chambered circulation (systemic or pulmonary pumping chamber) or is it in a single ventricle physiology as in hypoplastic left heart syndrome [25]?

These ventricles, unfortunately, are not comparable. Is the normal ejection fraction for a D-looped right ventricle the same for an ʟ-looped ventricle? To assess ventricular performance of a systemic right ventricle, is it fair to compare it to a systemic left ventricle [26]? To what standard can we hold a single right, or for that matter, even a single left ventricle? How should a pulmonary pumping left ventricle perform [27]?

With all these categories, issues can still get even more complex. Is a heart with dextrocardia expected to have comparable ventricular performance to a heart in a different position in the chest (which can have any of the above configurations) such as situs inversus totalis, isolated levocardia, or ectopia cordis [28,29]? How can the heart of thoracopagus conjoined twins who share a fused heart (e.g. three pumping chambers and three atria) be assessed [30,31]?

Only once these questions are put into perspective (which are unique to CHD) can questions concerning whether the ventricle is pressure and/or volume loaded be addressed. Even that, however, is not so simple. Is the volume load from atrioventricular or semilunar valve regurgitation, is it from shunt flow, or do all of these play a role? If it is from shunt flow, at what level is it (e.g. one of the major determinants of shunt flow at atrial level is relative ventricular compliance while at the great artery level, it is relative systemic and pulmonary resistances)? With a large ventricular septal defect (left ventricular volume load in the usual case), how is regional wall performance measured when a substantial portion of the septal wall is missing?

Another factor in assessing ventricular function in CHD is whether the heart is in its native state or has undergone an intervention. Both cardiothoracic surgery and interventional catheterization play an important role in CHD as the reader will see in many places in this textbook. The intervention may cause a change in myocardial performance or the loading conditions of the heart not normally seen in the native state of the disease [32]. For example, a heart undergoing cardiopulmonary bypass and circulatory arrest with its attendant ischemic time may alter myocardial contractility. Balloon angioplasty of a stenotic aortic valve may change the lesion from a pressure loaded one to a volume loaded one if the intervention causes aortic insufficiency in the process. A patient with single ventricle undergoing staged Fontan reconstruction will undergo volume unloading and change coronary blood flow [32].

All this information must be interpreted in light of the milieu in which the heart is pumping. For example, the amount of circulating red blood cells is an important determinant of the amount of shunt flow; it is known that an increase in the amount of circulating red blood cells that can decrease the amount of left to right shunt in a patient with a ventricular septal defect [33].

In summary, the assessment of ventricular function in CHD must be stratified in a number of ways to be meaningful. This includes whether or not the ventricle is a right or left ventricle, whether it is a systemic or pulmonary pumping chamber, whether it is in a ᴅ- or ʟ-looped configuration, whether it is in a dual chambered circulation or single ventricle physiology, the location in the chest, whether it is volume loaded and/or pressure loaded, and whether the heart is in its native state or has undergone an intervention.

Blood flow

The wide variety of blood vessels, surgical reconstructions and shunt physiology in CHD makes the study of blood flow just as difficult to study in a comprehensive fashion as ventricular function. A substantial amount of adult literature is devoted to blood flow as it relates to arterial compliance and atherosclerosis, and indeed, the study of blood flow in CHD has its parallels with noncompliant materials used in surgical reconstructions [34]. There are, however, so many more avenues of investigation that just like the study of ventricular function, categories must be made to come to some semblance of understanding.

There is, of course, the obvious distinction between the systemic, pulmonary and coronary circulations that must be dealt with. In CHD, however, these circulations may interact in different ways. The circulations may all originate from the same great vessel, as in truncus arteriosus [35] with all the attendant implications for altered flow and pressure. The circulations may abnormally connect in the microcirculation, such as with arteriovenous fistulae on the coronary (rare), systemic [36] and pulmonic [37,38] sides of the circulation which result in either a left to right shunt with potentially congestive heart failure or a right to left shunt with cyanosis. In either case, the interaction between the circulations can become very complex and the alterations to flow profiles and other parameters of blood flow need to be addressed.

Aside from the potential complex interactions, which may occur in CHD, lesions within each circulation can make things even more complex. An example that typifies a lesion on the systemic circulation side is coarctation of the aorta, where a narrowing of the aorta usually in the proximal descending aorta causes obstruction to flow. This obstruction causes marked hemodynamic and fluid mechanical changes to parameters such as blood pressure, velocity, pressure pulse contour, and vascular impedance [39]. The increased blood velocity and turbulence seen in typical coarctation of the aorta is one of the most widely known fluid dynamic changes in CHD.

Coarctation of the aorta, however, has multiple variations on the theme. Its position along the aorta (can occur anywhere from the transverse arch to the abdominal aorta), the character of the obstruction (discrete, long segment narrowing) and the interaction of the obstruction with branches of the aorta, all play a role in the complex flow in this lesion. In addition, it can be associated with other lesions such as
• Bicuspid aortic valve which may cause no problem or may be stenotic, regurgitant or both,
• Ventricular septal defect with shunting across the lesion.
Finally, collaterals to circumvent the obstruction may develop (dilating intercostal arteries and causing the classic "rib-notching" seen on X-ray), even to the point of carrying nearly all the cardiac output to the rest of the body with very little pressure gradient measured across the lesion. All these associated abnormalities must be taken into account when figuring out the complex blood flow changes induced by this lesion.

A classic example where understanding blood flow phenomenon (fluid dynamics) can make the difference in obtaining the correct diagnosis or not is supravalvar aortic stenosis which can be iatrogenic (e.g. created inadvertently by surgery) or found in cases of Williams Syndrome. Besides the obstruction to left ventricular outflow and the gradient, patients with this lesion tend to have higher blood pressures in the right arm than in the left arm which might make one think that clinically, there is aortic obstruction between the innominate and left subclavian arteries. This finding, however, is due to a "streaming" effect, where the high velocity jet caused by the obstruction "shoots blood" preferentially into the innominate artery, increasing the blood pressure of the right arm [40]. As can be seen, understanding flow phenomenon such as this (called the Coanda effect) is important in the differential diagnosis of physical findings.

On the pulmonary side, just as on the systemic side, there are many lesions that can occur such as valvar pulmonic stenosis, pulmonary atresia (in, for example, pulmonary atresia with intact ventricular septum), branch pulmonary artery hypoplasia (may occur in tetralogy of Fallot), or massive branch pulmonary artery dilation (may occur in tetralogy of Fallot with absent pulmonary valve leaflets). As one might expect in these lesions, there are significant flow disturbances, which need to be addressed.

For example, in patients with pulmonary atresia and intact ventricular septum, the pulmonary arteries are fed retrograde through the patent ductus arteriosus. In tetralogy of Fallot with absent pulmonary valve leaflets [41], not only is there a massive dilation of the pulmonary arteries, but there is also a simultaneous mixture of pulmonary annular regurgitation and stenosis. Altered primary and secondary flow profiles along with its implications for cardiovascular energetics are important factors to tease out for the long-term health of the cardiovascular system.

Surgical and catheter interventions play an important role in CHD and these iatrogenic situations require an understanding of the blood flow characteristics they induce to improve the design and implementation of these therapies. They include interventions on the systemic side such as balloon angioplasty of a coarctation [42], aortic root replacement in a patient with a dilated aorta in Marfan's syndrome or a left ventricle to descending aortic conduit [43] (which is not used much anymore because of its complications). On the pulmonary side, structures such as a right ventricle to pulmonary artery conduit (to repair tetralogy of Fallot with a coronary crossing the right ventricular outflow tract), a left ventricle to pulmonary artery conduit (to repair a patient with inverted ventricles and severe pulmonary stenosis), or a unifocalization procedure (to repair tetralogy of Fallot with pulmonary atresia) are just some of the many examples of varied surgical interventions [44]. This applies to blood flow phenomenon even within the heart, such as creating baffles to switch the atria in transposition of the great arteries (Senning [45] or Mustard [46] procedure) or creating intracardiac pathways from ventricle to great artery as in a Rastelli procedure for transposition of the great arteries with a ventricular septal defect and pulmonic stenosis [44].

Understanding surgical reconstructions are important in that the geometry of the surgical creations or the biomaterials used can impact blood flow phenomenon and alter cardiovascular energetics. An area where this has been vigorously studied is in the Fontan reconstruction for single ventricle repair. Computation fluid dynamic models have been created, alterations in the geometry of the systemic venous pathway have been suggested, and *in vivo* velocity profiles have been imaged, all to minimize energy losses and optimize blood flow efficiency [47–52]. Examples of these studies include:
• A suggestion that angling the superior vena cava flow toward the left pulmonary artery would send less blood to the lung which accommodates less flow [53],
• A demonstration that changing where the superior vena cava is connected to the right pulmonary artery (in relation to where the inferior vena cava baffle is placed) can change the power loss incurred [49] and,
• An estimation of the contribution of respiratory versus cardiac driving forces to passive flow into the lungs [51].
There is a special chapter on single ventricles in this textbook for further reading.

Shunt flow (i.e. a "short circuit" of blood between two circulations) is common in CHD and may cause flow disturbances, which may impact the well being of the cardiovascular system. A classic example is a ventricular septal defect, which allows blood to cross from left to right ventricles and into the pulmonary circulation. This increased flow, which may or may not be accompanied by a significant rise in pulmonary pressures, may cause altered velocity profiles in the pulmonary circulation. This flow may be so large that high-output congestive heart failure may occur in infancy and need to be treated medically with diuretics and digoxin or surgically with closure of the defect. Alternatively, pulmonary hypertension and subsequent obstructive pulmonary vascular disease may lead to Eisenmenger's Syndrome [54], which may be devastating. Understanding the fluid mechanics in this situation may be the key to early diagnosis, unlocking the potential cure or the preventative measures needed.

Technical challenges

Besides needing to deal with age related changes and the unique anatomy and physiology of CHD (which has its own technical challenges and special requirements), it is no secret that smaller individuals require different and most of the time smaller instruments and more precise measures than larger individuals. This has posed technical challenges to anyone who is involved with the care of children or in research to push the field forward.

A classic example is cardiac catheterization. Obviously, with the smaller blood vessels of children, smaller catheters are required to navigate the intravascular space. This is fairly complex and no easy feat; besides the problem of physically creating smaller catheters, techniques were developed to ensure that these smaller catheters do not thrombose. In addition, transducers must be responsive to smaller absolute changes in pressure since infants and children generate smaller pressures and pressure changes than adults do. Furthermore, different methods of catheter manipulation are needed for various types of congenital heart disease (e.g. manipulating the catheter into the pulmonary arteries in transposition of the great arteries). This is very important in CHD since the extent of hemodynamic and angiographic data needed to be obtained from a cardiac catheterization in children with CHD is significantly more than what is required to evaluate adults with structurally normal hearts. This includes obtaining data in various conditions (e.g. before and after balloon occlusion of an atrial septal defect, during administration of oxygen and nitric oxide in a patient with pulmonary hypertension, etc.). Finally, magnification for smaller structures is important in addition to various angled view that were developed to highlight the salient points of the anatomy and physiology. All of these issues present technical challenges to studying ventricular function and fluid mechanics in CHD.

There are also technical challenges from a cardiac catheterization interventional point of view, which can of course affect ventricular function and fluid mechanics. These usually take the form of either specialized devices for specific lesions in CHD (which, as mentioned above, need to be small) or smaller devices and/or catheters, which are modified from the adult world. For example, much work is being done on closure devices for atrial septal defects and to a lesser extent, ventricular septal defects. Balloon valvuloplasty and angioplasty play an important role in diseases such as pulmonary valve stenosis or coarctation of the aorta. Stents can be routinely placed in stenotic pulmonary arteries in patients with tetralogy of Fallot. Research is being done on a combination of catheter and surgical interventions to reconstruct lesions such as single ventricles into the Fontan circulation.

Another example of a field that has many technical challenges in children is cardiac magnetic resonance imaging (MRI), where many tradeoffs are made to make imaging quicker and simpler. For example, spatial resolution can be increased at the cost of temporal resolution and visa versa. This is a particularly important point in children since they require greater spatial resolution because of size as well as greater temporal resolution because of higher heart rates. Therefore, the tradeoffs that can be performed in adults can only be taken advantage to a limited degree in children. Furthermore, children less than 7–9 years of age usually require sedation, which make sequences designed for breath-holding useless. Since this is the mainstay of adult cardiac MRI, "work-arounds" have been developed. Modifications or new approaches to imaging infants and children with cardiac MRI, therefore, have been developed to successfully image the small patient.

The fetal environment

With the advent of better imaging and other diagnostic techniques along with the ability to treat the unborn child, understanding ventricular function and blood flow in the presence of the unique anatomy and physiology of CHD in the fetal environment becomes even more important.

The fetal environment is a matchless place in the world of cardiology. The extent to which fetal life differs from the post-natal environment is beyond the scope of this chapter and textbook, although there are many other excellent textbooks devoted to this topic, which can be used for more information. However, a few highlights of how the fetal environment affects ventricular function and blood flow are in order.

The fetal heart is under a number of limitations when compared to the postnatal state including myocyte immaturity, decreased ventricular compliance, ventricular sensitivity to increasing afterload, and the constraint the chest wall, pericardium, and

specifically the collapsed lung places on the fetal ventricle, limiting cardiac expansion [55]. For these reasons, the fetal ventricle has limited cardiac reserves. Obviously, this has implications for fetal ventricular function.

Similarly, fetal fluid mechanics are a special case. In addition to the patent ductus arteriosus supplying blood antegrade to the body, there is little flow to the branch pulmonary arteries because of the collapsed lungs. There are streaming effects where highly oxygenated blood is directed from the inferior vena cava through the patent foramen ovale into the left side of the heart and then out to the brain. Less oxygenated blood is directed from the superior vena cava into the right ventricle and through the pulmonary artery and patent ductus arteriosus to the lower half of the body.

Conclusion

There are many reasons for a separate textbook for CHD in ventricular function and blood flow; the unique situations that occur with CHD (different from adult pathology) demands a collection of essays which focus on this topic to lay the foundation for improved surgical and medical management of CHD.

References

1. Mitchell SC, Korones SB, Berendes HW. Congenital heart disease in 56,109 births. Incidence and natural history. Circulation 1971; 43:323–332.
2. Van Praagh R, Van Praagh S. Persistent fifth arterial arch in man: Congenital double-lumen aortic arch. Am J Cardiol 1969; 24:279–282.
3. Hoffman JIE, Kaplan S. The incidence of congenital heart disease. J Am Coll Cardiol 2002; 39:1890–1900.
4. Fyler DC, Buckley LP, Hellenbrand WE, et al. Report of the New England regional infant cardiac program. Pediatrics 1980; 65(suppl):376–460.
5. Bricker ME, Hillis LD, Lange RA. Congenital heart disease in adults [part 1]. N Engl J Med 2000; 342:256–263.
6. Bricker ME, Hillis LD, Lange RA. Congenital heart disease in adults [part 2]. N Engl J Med 2000; 342:334–342.
7. Perloff JK. Congenital heart disease in adults: A new cardiovascular subspecialty. Circulation 1991; 84:1881–1890.

8. Hamill PV, Drizd TA, Johnson CL, *et al.* Physical growth: National Center of Health Statistics percentiles. Am J Clin Nutr 1979; 32:607–629.

9. Salim MA, DiSessa TG, Arheart KL, *et al.* Contribution of superior vena caval flow to total cardiac output in children. A Doppler echocardiographic study. Circulation 1995; 92:1860–1865.

10. de Laval MR, Dubini G, Migliavacca F, *et al.* Use of computational fluid dynamics in the design of surgical procedures: Application to the study of competitive flows in cavopulmonary connections. J Thorac Cardiovasc Surg 1996; 111:502–513.

11. Lardo AC, Webber SA, del Nido PJ, *et al.* Does the right lung receive preferential blood flow in Fontan repair? Comparison of total cavopulmonary and atriopulmonary connections: An in vitro flow study. Circulation 1995; 92:I–I123.

12. Fontan F, Baudet E. Surgical repair of tricuspid atresia. Thorax 1971; 26:240–248.

13. de Laval MR, Kilner P, Gewillig M, Bull C. Total cavopulmonary connection: A logical alternative to atriopulmonary connection for complex Fontan operations. J Thorac Cardiovasc Surg 1988; 96:682–695.

14. Sharma S, Goudy S, Walker P, *et al.* In vitro flow experiments for determination of optimal geometry of total cavopulmonary connection for surgical repair of children with functional single ventricle. J Am Coll Cardiol 1996; 27:1264–1269.

15. Fogel MA, Weinberg PM, Hoydu A, *et al.* The nature of flow in the systemic venous pathway in Fontan patients utilizing magnetic resonance blood tagging. J Thorac Cardiovasc Surg 1997; 114:1032–1041.

16. Laks H, Ardehali A, Grant PW, *et al.* Modification of the Fontan procedure. Superior vena cava to left pulmonary artery connection and inferior vena cava to right pulmonary artery connection with adjustable atrial septal defect. Circulation 1995; 91:2943–2947.

17. Fogel MA, Weinberg PM, Rychik J, *et al.* Caval contribution to flow in the branch pulmonary arteries of Fontan patients using a novel application of magnetic resonance presaturation pulse. Circulation 1999; 99:1215–1221.

18. Fogel MA, Weinberg PM, Fellows KE, *et al.* A Study in ventricular–ventricular interaction: Single right ventricles compared with systemic right ventricles in a dual chambered circulation. Circulation 1995; 92(2):219–230.

19. Mustard WT. Successful two-stage correction of transposition of the great vessels. Surgery 1964; 55:469.

20. Senning A. Surgical correction of transposition of the great vessels. Surgery 1959; 45:966.

21. Quaegebeur JM, Rohmer J, Brom AG, *et al.* Revival of the Senning operation in the treatment of transposition of the great ateries. Thorax 1977; 32:517.

22. Fogel MA, Weinberg PM, Rychik J, *et al.* Caval contribution to flow in the branch pulmonary arteries of Fontan patients using a novel application of magnetic resonance presaturation pulse. Circulation 1999; 99:1215–1221.

23. Van Praagh R. What is congenitally corrected transposition? N Engl J Med 1970; 282:1097–1098.

24. Friedberg DZ, Nadas AS. Clinical profile of patients with congenitally corrected transposition of the great arteries. A study of 60 cases. N Engl J Med 1970; 282:1053–1059.

25. Fogel MA, Weinberg PM, Fellows KE, *et al.* A Study in ventricular–ventricular interaction: Single right ventricles compared with systemic right ventricles in a dual chambered circulation. Circulation 1995; 92(2):219–230.

26. Fogel MA, Gupta KB, Weinberg PW, *et al.* Regional wall motion and strain analysis across stages of Fontan reconstruction by magnetic resonance tagging. Am J Physiol Heart Circ Physiol 1995; 269:H1132–H1152.

27. Fogel MA, Gupta K, Baxter MS, *et al.* Biomechanics of the deconditioned left ventricle. Am J Physiol Heart Circ Physiol 1996; 40(3):H1193–H1206.

28. Gutgesell HP. Cardiac malposition and heterotaxy. In: Garson A, Bricker JT, Fisher DJ, Neish SR, eds., The Science and Practice of Pediatric Cardiology. Williams & Wilkins, Baltimore, MD, pp. 1539–1561, 1997.

29. Hornberger LK, Colan SD, Lock JE, *et al.* Outcome of patients with ectopia cordis and significant intracardiac defects. Circulation 1996; 94 (suppl II):II-32–II-37.

30. Gerlis LM, Seo J-W, Yen Ho S, *et al.* Morphology of the cardiovascular system in conjoined twins: Spatial and sequential arrangement in 36 cases. Teratology 1993; 47:91–108.

31. Joffe HS, Rose A, Gersh BJ, *et al.* Figure-of-eight circulation in thoracopagus conjoined twins with a shared heart. Eur J Cardiol 1977; 6:157–166.

32. Fogel MA, Rychik J, Vetter J, *et al.* Effect of volume unloading surgery on coronary flow dynamics in patients with aortic atresia. J Thorac Cardiovasc Surg 1997; 113:718–727.

33. Lister G, Hellenbrand WE, Kleinman CS, *et al.* Physiologic effects of increasing hemoglobin concentration in left-to-right shunting in infants with ventricular septal defects. N Engl J Med 1982; 306:502–206.

34. Fogel MA, Weinberg PM, Hoydu A, *et al.* Effect of surgical reconstruction on flow profiles in the aorta using magnetic resonance blood tagging. Ann Thorac Surg 1997; 63:1691–1700.

35. Van Praagh R, Van Praagh S. The anatomy of common aorticopulmonary trunk (truncus arteriosus communis) and its embryologic implication. Am J Cardiol 1965; 16:406–425.

36. Knudson RP, Alden ER. Symptomatic arteriovenous malformation in infants less than 6 months of age. Pediatrics 1979; 64:238–241.

37. Barbe T, Losay J, Grimon G, *et al*. Pulmonary arteriovenous shunting in children with liver disease. J Pediatr 1995; 126:571–579.

38. Shah MJ, Rychik J, Fogel MA, *et al*. Pulmonary AV malformations after superior cavo-pulmonary connection: Resolution after inclusion of hepatic veins in the pulmonary circulation. Ann Thorac Surg 1997; 63:960–963.

39. Nichols WW, O'Rourke MF (eds). McDonald's Blood Flow in Arteries: Theoretical, Experimental and Clinical Principles. Arnold Publishing Co, London, UK, pp. 405–414, 1998.

40. Goldstein RE, Epstein SE. Mechanism of elevated innominate artery pressures in supravalvar aortic stenosis. Circulation 1970; 52:23–30.

41. Pinsky WW, Nihill MR, Mullins CE *et al*. The absent pulmonary valve syndrome: Consideration of management. Circulation 1978; 57:159–62.

42. Rao PS, Galal O, Smith PA, *et al*. Five- to nine-year follow-up results of balloon angioplasty of native aortic coarctation in infants and children. J Am Coll Cardiol 1996; 27:462–470.

43. Frommelt PC, Rocchini AP, Bove EL. Natural history of apical left ventricular to aortic conduits in pediatric patients. Circulation 1991; 84:III213–218.

44. Fogel MA, Hubbard A, Weinberg PM. A simplified approach for assessment of intracardiac baffles and extracardiac conduits in congenital heart surgery with two- and three-dimensional magnetic resonance imaging. Am Heart J 2001; 142(6):1028–1036.

45. Senning A. Surgical correction of transposition of the great vessels. Surgery 1959; 45:966–980.

46. Mustard WT. Successful two-stage correction of transposition of the great vessels. Surgery. 1964; 55:469–472.

47. de Laval MR, Dubini G, Migliavacca F, *et al*. Use of computational fluid dynamics in the design of surgical procedures: Application to the study of competitive flows in cavopulmonary connections. J Thorac Cardiovasc Surg 1996; 111:502–513.

48. de Laval MR, Kilner P, Gewillig M, *et al*. Total cavopulmonary connection: A logical alternative to atriopulmonary connection for complex Fontan operations. J Thorac Cardiovasc Surg 1988; 96:682–695.

49. Sharma S, Goudy S, Walker P, *et al*. In vitro flow experiments for determination of optimal geometry of total cavopulmonary connection for surgical repair of children with functional single ventricle. J Am Coll Cardiol 1996; 27:1264–1269.

50. Lardo AC, Webber SA, del Nido PJ, *et al*. Does the right lung receive preferential blood flow in Fontan repair? Comparison of total cavopulmonary and atriopulmonary connections: An in vitro flow study. Circulation 1995; 92:I-123.

51. Fogel MA, Weinberg PM, Hoydu A, *et al*. The nature of flow in the systemic venous pathway in Fontan patients utilizing magnetic resonance blood tagging. J Thorac Cardiovasc Surg 1997; 114:1032–1041.

52. Fogel MA, Weinberg PM, Rychik J, *et al*. Caval contribution to flow in the branch pulmonary arteries of Fontan patients using a novel application of magnetic resonance presaturation pulse. Circulation 1999; 99:1215–1221.

53. Laks H, Ardehali A, Grant PW, *et al*. Modification of the Fontan procedure. Superior vena cava to left pulmonary artery connection and inferior vena cava to right pulmonary artery connection with adjustable atrial septal defect. Circulation 1995; 91:2943–2947.

54. Wood P. The Eisenmenger syndrome. Br J Med 1958; 2:701–708.

55. Grant DA, Walker AM. Pleural and pericardial pressures limit fetal right ventricular output. Circulation 1996; 94:555–561.

CHAPTER 2

Ventricular Function—The Basics of the Discipline

Mark A. Fogel, MD, FACC, FAAP

Introduction

Ventricular function is one of the most important disciplines within the cardiovascular field; obviously, getting blood to the lungs and the body is the primary purpose of the heart. Yet ventricular function is also misunderstood by many health care workers and the term is abused by most individuals who are not aware of the nuances. Although a whole textbook can be written on this topic alone, the purpose of this chapter is to familiarize the reader with the basics of the study of ventricular function to be used as a springboard for its application to specific lesions in congenital heart disease.

The study of ventricular function can be stratified into three separate divisions and it is helpful to keep this in mind when reviewing these principles:
• The molecular and chemical basis of myocardial contraction. (Although there is a brief mention of this area of study, it is not the focus of this chapter. The reader is referred to other textbooks wherein this subject is well covered.)
• Studies of isolated myocyte contraction and relaxation.
• Studies of whole heart contraction *in vivo* and *in vitro*.
In addition, it is also important to keep in mind that to a large extent other organ systems, which depend upon blood flow, monitor only the amount of blood delivered and respond accordingly if the blood supply is compromised. These organ systems are unaware, for the most part, of the *way* in which the heart achieves this blood delivery (e.g., increasing ejection fraction with aortic insufficiency) or even the state of well being of the myocardium. The cardiac response

is a complex interaction between the external signals received and its internal compensatory responses to these. It is the difference between the heart being viewed as a "black box" versus an intricate muscular pump that varies multiple parameters to achieve an adequate blood supply.

The cardiac cycle

Although the reader is probably familiar with the cardiac cycle (Fig. 2.1), which is divided artificially into systole and diastole, a brief review is in order. These two broad divisions are convenient to study ventricular function, but it should be noted that they are intimately interconnected. For example, the twisting of the myocardium in systole stores potential energy and is released in diastole in the form of elastic recoil. This recoil is part of what has been termed the "sucking" action of the heart during diastole, actively pulling blood into the ventricle [1,2].

During systole, the process of pressure generation begins when calcium ions allow interaction between actin and myosin fibers. When the pressure in the ventricle exceeds atrial pressure, which occurs in the left ventricle (LV) before the right ventricle (RV), closure of the atrioventricular valve occurs (actually, this does not occur immediately when the ventricular pressure exceeds atrial pressure because of the inertia of the blood) and isovolumic contraction begins. As the name implies, no change in volume occurs in this phase of contraction as both atrioventricular and semilunar valves are closed; only more and more myofibers are recruited and pressure increases. Once the pressure in the ventricle exceeds aortic (for

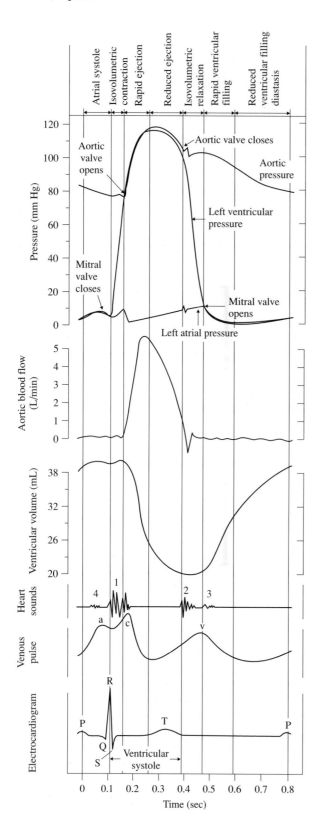

Figure 2.1 Mechanical events in the cardiac cycle. Pressures in the aorta, left ventricle, and left atrium are recorded along with aortic blood flow, ventricular volume, heart sounds, venous pulse, and electrocardiogram along with the names of the components of each wave or sound. Note (although not clearly shown here) that the mitral valve closure occurs after the crossover point of atrial and ventricular pressures. From Berne and Levy [4] with permission.

the LV) or pulmonary (for the RV) pressures, the semilunar valve opens and a phase of rapid ejection begins. The ventricular pressure rises, peaks, and subsequently begins to fall as calcium is taken up by the cytoplasmic reticullum and myofibers begin to enter the relaxed state. As this occurs, the rate of ejection decreases.

When the pressure in the aorta (for the LV) or the pulmonary artery (for the RV) exceeds ventricular pressure, the semilunar valve closes. During this period, ventricular pressure exceeds atrial pressure and as a result both semilunar and atrioventricular valves are closed, resulting in isovolumic relaxation. Eventually, atrial pressure exceeds ventricular pressure and the atrioventricular valve opens, resulting in a phase of rapid ventricular filling, which accounts for most of ventricular filling [3]. As the pressures in both atria and ventricle equalize, the rate of filling slows considerably; this part of the cycle is called diastasis. Finally, atrial systole occurs, causing a transient increase in pressure and forcing blood into the ventricle prior to ventricular systole. This phase is important especially when the compliance of the ventricle is poor [3]. The pressure, flow, volume, ECG, and heart sounds as they relate to the cardiac cycle are represented graphically in Fig. 2.1.

There is debate as to what parts of the cardiac cycle to consider the beginning and ending of systole and diastole; this is more of a debate over which definition has greater utility than the other. Opinions exist as to whether, in the definition of systole, that part of the cycle should begin at isolvolumic contraction (physiological systole) or the close of the mitral valve (cardiological systole). Similarly, in the definition for the end of systole (and therefore, beginning of diastole), there is debate about whether it should be immediately after peak ejection (the end of physiological systole, as LV pressure falls) or the closure of the aortic valve (cardiological diastole). In either case, it appears as just a matter of semantics as long as the various components of the entire cycle are understood individually and as a whole.

The ventricular pressure–volume loop relates intracardiac pressure changes as a function of volume changes during the cardiac cycle (Fig. 2.2), essentially removing the time axis from the pressure and volume curves of the ventricle shown in Fig. 2.1. As will be shown later, this graph is a convenient method to understand the four major determinants of myocardial oxygen demand, which in turn

underlay a good portion of the assessment of ventricular function. As can be seen during the beginning of systole, energy of contraction is used to increase ventricular pressure to the level of the great vessel diastolic pressure without change in ventricular volume while atrioventricular valve is closed (nearly verticle line on the right of the curve)—known as isovolumic contraction. When ventricular pressure exceeds great vessel pressure, the semilunar valve opens, ventricular shortening begins, and ventricular volume begins falling (nearly horizontal line at the top of the curve). When ventricular pressure falls below great vessel pressure as myocardial fibers relax, the semilunar valve closes, cardiac ejection stops, and ventricular pressure rapidly declines prior to the atrioventricular valve opening (nearly verticle line on the left of the curve)—known as isovolumic relaxation. With the opening of the atrioventricular valve as the atrial pressure exceeds ventricular pressure, ventricular volume begins to increase and the pressure–volume loop becomes complete. The area subtended by the closed loop gives a measure of energy (pressure–volume energy) used by the heart to pump blood out to the body—this is what is termed as stroke work.

Myocardial mechanics and the great relationships

A basic understanding of ventricular function requires knowledge of the way muscle fibers work. Models of muscle contraction are important in the analysis of the way the heart muscles contract [5]. The two-element model does not take into account diastolic stretch (Fig. 2.3a) and so the three-element Maxwell model (Fig. 2.3b) was created as a theoretical construct, which postulates that the sarcomere consists of

• a contractile element (CE) in series with an undamped, nonlinear series elastic element (SE) and
• a nonlinear parallel elastic element (PE) which is in parallel with both the CE and SE.

In the Voight model (Fig. 2.3c), the CE and PE are in parallel with each other, and this CE–PE unit is in series with the SE. One can think of the CE as the energy generating unit for force/velocity development and the elastic elements as springs that stretch when a force is applied to them and return to their unstretched state when the force is removed. They are "lumped" parameters of elasticity in muscle. At rest,

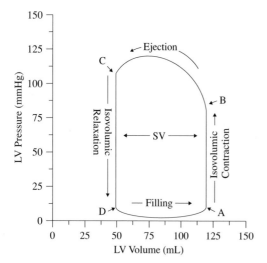

Figure 2.2 Pressure–volume loop. This is created by removing the time axis from the pressure and volume curves shown in Fig. 2.1. The direction in time of the cycle is shown by the arrows (see text for details). A = beginning of isovolumic contraction, B = end of isovolumic contraction, C = end of systolic ejection, D = end of isovolumic relaxation, and LV = left ventricle.

the CE is freely extensible and does not contribute to stress; the element that resists stretching of the muscle in this state is the PE. Once the muscle is excited, the CE begins to shorten and pulls on the SE:

• If there is no load present to resist this pull, the SE will move unstretched with the same velocity as the CE, developing force as a function of the shortening properties of the CE and the compliance of the SE.
• If a submaximal load is present, force is developed as the CE stretches the SE until the force equals the load, and then the load is lifted—this is isotonic contraction. Muscle shortening then occurs at a fixed length of the SE, which reflects shortening of the CE alone.
• If a maximal load is present, force is developed by CE contraction as the SE is stretched as far as possible on its compliance curve. There will be no load lifted and no change in fiber length—this is isometric contraction.

Following contraction, the elastic energy stored in the SE may lead to CE reextension. The force opposing hyperextension is provided by the PE.

It is useful at this point to define preload, afterload, and contractility for the isolated muscle preparation, which will have its parallels in the intact heart:

• *Preload:* The stretching force a muscle is subjected to in the relaxed state or conversely the muscle force which resists this stretch.
• *Afterload:* The force which resists muscle shortening in the active state of contraction or conversely the force developed by muscle during contraction.
• *Contractility:* The intensity of the force of contraction which is independent of preload and afterload.

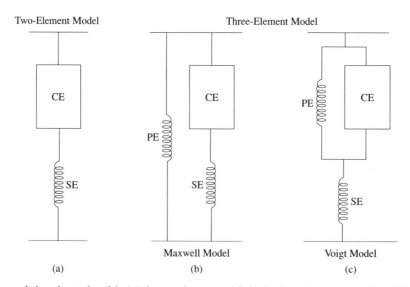

Figure 2.3 Myocardial mechanical models. (a) The two-element model, (b) the three-element Maxwell model, and (c) the three-element Voight model. CE = contractile element, PE = parallel element, and SE = series elastic element. From Yang *et al.* [6] with permission.

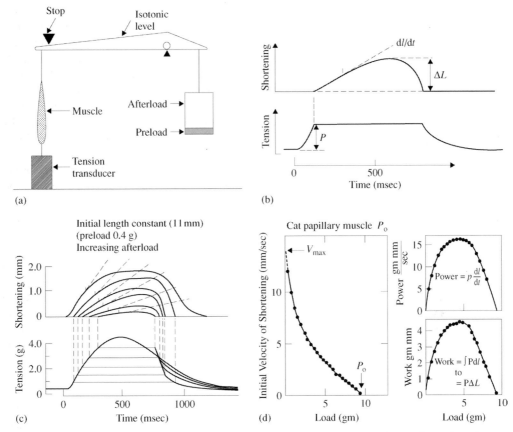

Figure 2.4 Experiments utilizing afterloaded contractions isotonically to derive the force–velocity relationship. (a) A papillary muscle in a bath of Krebs–Ringers solution and with stimulating electrodes is attached at one end to a lever and at the other end to a tension transducer. (b) Tracings of tension (bottom) and shortening (top) over time after the onset of contraction as measured by the transducer during afterloaded isotonic contraction. Maximum velocity is reached at the onset of contraction and is represented by the tangent to the curve designated by the dashed line dl/dt. ΔL is the maximum change in length and P is the pressure developed. (c) Force–displacement curves (bottom figure shows tension curve and top figure shows shortening curve) at a constant preload and with increasing afterload. As the afterload is increased, the tension generated becomes greater, equaling the force of the afterload; however, the velocity and extent of fiber shortening decreases. Dashed lines on the shortening curve represent maximum velocity and dashed lines between the shortening and tension curves represent simultaneous readings. (d) By taking out the time factor in these two curves (see Fig. 2.4c) the force–velocity relationship is generated. Work (energy) and power (first time derivative of work) versus load shown to the right (bottom and top, respectively). From Braunwald *et al.* [7] with permission.

An appreciation of studies of isolated muscle preparations can help conceptualize how muscle contracts in the intact heart (Fig. 2.4a). The classic example is of muscle attached at one end to a lever and at the other end to a tension transducer to measure contraction parameters such as velocity of shortening [7,8]. The fulcrum of the lever is toward the right. At the other end of the lever is a small weight that stretches the muscle at rest to a length consistent with its tension–length relation. This small weight

is the "preload" and a "stop" is placed to prevent any further muscle stretching and so that if any weight is added above the preload will not be sensed until contraction begins. This added weight to the preload therefore represents "afterload."

With this experimental set up, one of the best known relationships in cardiac mechanics was shown: the force–velocity relationship. Figure 2.4b shows the tracings of tension and shortening over time after the onset of contraction as measured by the

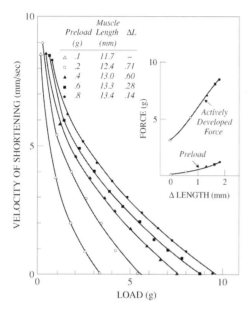

Figure 2.5 Effects of increasing preload on the force–velocity relationship. Several initial muscle lengths are shown. With increasing preload, V_{max} is little changed although P_0 increases. The inset shows the active and passively developed force for each initial muscle length. From Sonnenblick [11] with permission.

transducer in the muscle preparation during afterloaded isotonic contraction. Tension increases isometrically and then plateaus with the onset of contraction after the force equals the load, and subsequent shortening begins. Maximum velocity occurs shortly after contraction begins. In Fig. 2.4c, the changes to these curves with increasing afterload are shown. As the afterload is increased, the tension generated becomes greater, equaling the force of the afterload; however, the velocity and extent of fiber shortening decreases. By taking out the time factor in these two curves, the force–velocity relationship is generated (see Fig. 2.4d). Note the inverse curvilinear relationship—as load is increased, the velocity of shortening decreases. The extrapolation of the curves back to zero load, which cannot be measured directly, is the maximum velocity the muscle can attain with a given preload, termed V_{max} [9,10]. At the other extreme, if the afterload is maximal, there is no shortening and all the energy goes into tension development, termed P_0. To summarize, the force–velocity relationship describes an inverse correlation between the velocity of fiber shortening and the tension generated.

The logical next step is to alter the initial muscle length by altering "preload" with the resulting curves shown in Fig. 2.5. Increasing the initial muscle length shifts the curve characteristically to the right, thereby increasing the velocity of fiber shortening at any given afterload. Interestingly, however, V_{max} is little changed by this maneuver. In the intact heart, this capacity to increase the force of contraction as a function of preload is one of the major principles of cardiac function and is termed the Frank–Starling law or Starling's law of the Heart.

In 1895, Frank reported that the greater the initial left ventricular volume, the greater the rate of rise of pressure, the greater the maximum pressure reached, and the faster the rate of relaxation occurred. Frank, therefore, described both increased inotropy as well as lusitropy with increased initial left ventricular volume. In 1918, Starling proposed that the larger the volume of the heart, the greater the energy of its contraction. Together, their law describes a fundamental property of the myocardium, based upon the ultrastructure of thick and thin myofilaments within the sarcomeres [12]. With increasing end-diastolic length, the degree of overlap of the filaments changes [13], which has been put forward to account for most of the effect observed. Yet, it has been shown that even at 80% of maximum length, only 10% of the maximum force is developed. "Length-dependent activation" is another favored explanation, where an increase in calcium sensitivity (enhanced excitation–contraction coupling) of the myocytes occurs with initial sarcomere increase in length.

Dovetailing with Starling's law of the heart is the resting length–tension relationship (Fig. 2.6, lower curve). Increasing the initial muscle length not only increases the force of contraction when the muscle is stimulated, but in the relaxed state, this stretch produces increased tension (represented by PE in the muscle model). As a progressive increase in stretch is produced, the tension increases only slightly at first but then rises more markedly with increased lengthening in an exponential fashion (this is equivalent to the end-diastolic pressure–volume relationship discussed later in this chapter). The stiffness of the resting muscle is represented by dP/dL (the change in tension with respect to the change in length) with larger values indicating greater stiffness. Things that tend to increase muscle stiffness include marked tachycardia (presumably because relaxation is not

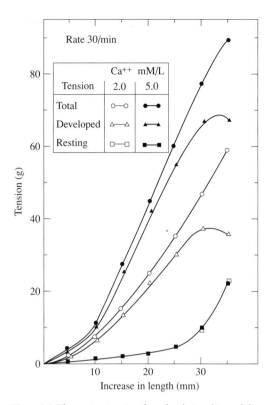

Figure 2.6 The resting tension–length relationship and the effect of increasing calcium on rest and developed tension. Calcium was infused at 2 and 5 mM/L. The resting tension–length relationship (filled and open squares on lower curve) did not change; however, the developed tension increased. From Braunwald [14] with permission.

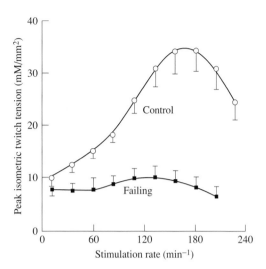

Figure 2.7 The force–frequency relationship in both normal individuals and patients with congestive heart failure due to mitral insufficiency. The curves represent steady state isometric tension (Y-axis) versus stimulation frequency (X-axis). From Mulieri *et al.* [15] with permission.

completed at end-diastole), aging (as an adult), as well as ischemia.

Increasing the frequency of muscle activation can also increase the force of contraction in isolated muscle preparations and this phenomenon has been termed the Bowditch or Treppe effect or the force–frequency relationship (Fig. 2.7). This model is used as one of the explanations for postextrasystolic potentiation, where the beat after a premature depolarization is more forceful than a normal heartbeat (the premature beat is actually less forceful than a normal heartbeat). When this was studied with constant preload in the isovolumically beating heart, the increase in the force of the postextrasystolic beat was directly related exponentially to the degree of prematurity of the previous beat. This relationship is thought to be due to increased myocardial calcium (which increases tension development, Fig. 2.6) at higher heart rates [16]. In the intact heart *in vivo*,

this effect is augmented by increased filling (preload) with subsequent increased force of contraction via the Frank–Starling law. The effect of postextrasystolic potentiation can be maintained when pairs of stimuli are delivered ("paired electrical stimulation") [17].

The uncoupling of the force–frequency relationship takes place in a few different situations: On either ends of the frequency spectrum, which is at decreased heart rates or at extremely rapid stimulation, a negative effect is noted [15]. The proposed mechanism of this fall off of force during rapid stimulation is that an increase in sodium and calcium ions entering the myocardium overwhelms the ability of the myocyte pumps to perform their function. In addition, when the heart rate is too rapid, there is decreased time for diastolic filling, which also impairs the force–frequency relationship. Furthermore, diseased hearts demonstrate differing responses to increased stimulation; in severe mitral regurgitation, there is hardly any response to increased heart rates (Fig. 2.7), while in patients with cardiomyopathy, an increased heart rate produced decreased twitch tension [18].

Another directly proportional relationship involving ventricular force generation is the Anrep effect or homeometric autoregulation. When aortic pressure is elevated abruptly, an increase in ventricular force is noted within 1–2 min and because this effect is independent of muscle length, it represents a true increase in contractility. There is speculation that the mechanism of action is an increase in wall tension, which is sensed by myocardial stretch receptors, with resulting increase in cytosolic sodium and then an increase in cytosolic calcium by the sodium–calcium exchange pump.

In the intact heart, cardiac volumes and pressure are analogous to muscle length and tension in individual cardiac muscle fibers. Because of the three-dimensional nature of the intact ventricle, the concept of wall stress was introduced, which measures pressure exerted on a cross-sectional area. It is a major factor in determining myocardial oxygen demand and in its simplest form, is described by another great relationship called Laplace's law. This law states that average circumferential wall stress (σ) is proportional to interventricular pressure (P) and internal radius (R) and inversely proportional to wall thickness (H): $\sigma = PR/2H$ (see Fig. 2.8). Therefore, the greater the radius or pressure, the greater the wall stress and increase in myocardial oxygen demand. The reader must be cognizant that there are three major simplifying assumptions made in this law: (a) The ventricle is a sphere with uniform radius and wall thickness, (b) the ventricle is in static equilibrium (i.e., it is not moving), and (c) the wall is thin ($H/R < 0.1$) so that stress may be considered constant throughout the wall.

It follows from Laplace's law that with hypertrophy, wall thickness increases to normalize σ when pressure (as with, e.g., aortic stenosis) or radius (as with, e.g., mitral insufficiency) increases. In the failing heart, the radius, for example, increases insufficiently for the heart to normalize σ.

Wall stress can be described geometrically in three different ways in the intact ventricle. Circumferential wall stress is the pressure exerted per unit cross-sectional area around the circumference of the ventricle, while meridional wall stress is along the long axis of the ventricle. Finally, radial wall stress is the pressure exerted per unit cross-sectional area in the radial direction outward from the centroid of the ventricular cavity (Fig. 2.8). Calculation of wall stress is an inexact science and makes geometric assumptions about the ventricle [20,21]. Circumferential σ_c and meridional σ_m wall stress can be approximated

as follows:

$$\sigma_c = \left(\frac{Pb}{H}\right)\left(1 - \frac{H}{2b}\right)\left(1 - \frac{Hb}{2a^2}\right)$$

$$\sigma_m = \frac{PR}{2H(1 + H/2R))}$$

where a and b are the major and minor semiaxes and P, R, and H are pressure, radius, and wall thickness, respectively.

Related to wall stress is the concept of ventricular compliance, which is defined simply as the change in ventricular volume as a function of the change in ventricular pressure (dV/dP). This is, of course, the inverse of the slope of the various parts of the pressure–volume loops described earlier. Chamber stiffness is the reciprocal of compliance, and therefore defined as dP/dV. Both terms express how the volume and pressure change with respect to each other as a function of the mechanical properties of the ventricle. With increased compliance, the ventricle can hold more blood volume at a given pressure, and with decreased compliance, the reverse is true. (See Table 2.1 for a list of great relationships.)

Determinants of myocardial oxygen consumption

Myocardial oxygen consumption is directly proportional to the amount of cardiac energy utilization and as such, is a major consideration in the assessment of ventricular performance. Now that the great relationships have been defined, the four major determinants of oxygen uptake by the myocardium can be discussed rigorously: preload, afterload, contractility, and heart rate. All together, these determinants account for 80% of myocardial oxygen consumption. The additional two minor determinants of myocardial oxygen consumption, basal metabolic activity ($\sim$20% of oxygen consumption) and electrical activation ($<$1% of oxygen consumption), will not be discussed. The parameters used to assess ventricular performance by various invasive and noninvasive modalities all in some way touch on one of these four major concepts.

Preload
Preload can now be defined as the wall stress at end-diastole, which represents the maximal resting length of the sarcomere. Wall stress is difficult to measure precisely *in vivo* since complex ventricular geometry, especially in congenital heart disease,

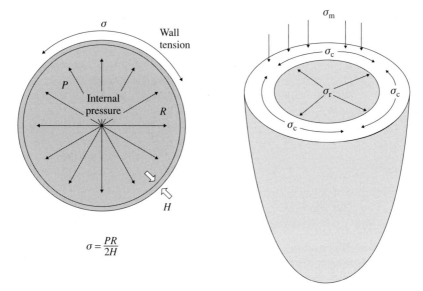

Figure 2.8 Laplace's law and the wall stress. The wall stress developed (σ) is directly proportional to the internal pressure (P) and the radius (R) and is inversely proportional to the wall thickness (H). The three types of wall stress shown are circumferential σ_c, meridional σ_m, and radial σ_r. From Grossman [19] with permission.

Table 2.1 The Great Relationships.

Relationship	Explanation
Force–velocity	Inverse correlation between the velocity of fiber shortening and the tension generated
Starling's law of the heart	The capacity to increase the force of contraction as a function of preload—the greater the initial left ventricular volume, the greater the inotropy and lusitropy
Resting tension–length	Increasing the initial muscle length increases resting tension
Force–frequency	Increasing heart rate increases the force of contraction
Homeometric autoregulation	When afterload is increased abruptly, the force of contraction also increases
Laplace's law	Wall stress is directly proportional to pressure and radius and inversely proportional to wall thickness ($\sigma = PR/2H$)
End-diastolic pressure–volume	The relationship between pressure and volume as the ventricle is filled in a fully relaxed state ($\text{EDP} = P_o + \beta V^\alpha$)
End-systolic pressure–volume	At any given level of contractility, if the loading conditions are varied, the end-systolic pressure and volume will fall on a straight line

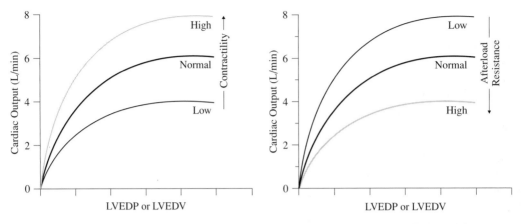

Figure 2.9 Frank–Starling curves relating cardiac output with end-diastolic pressure/volume and effects of altering contractility and afterload. With increasing afterload, at the same end-diastolic pressure/volume, the cardiac output decreases. With decreasing contractility, a similar phenomenon is noted. LVEDP = left ventricular end-diastolic pressure and LVEDV = left ventricular end-diastolic volume.

makes the simplifications of the wall stress formulas inapplicable. In addition, it is also known that stress is related to strain (deformation of the myocardial wall) by either a constant (in the case of Hookean relationship) or more complex relationships, and it has been demonstrated that strain is not homogenous throughout the ventricle [22–24]. The implication is that wall stress is also not homogeneous.

The amount of preload, besides being a major determinant of myocardial oxygen consumption, is a major component of how much ventricular ejection occurs via the Frank–Starling relationship. With increasing preload, more ejection occurs given the same end-systolic pressure/volume (Fig. 2.9). The increase in the amount of preload that an individual can attain is called the preload reserve, and with volume loading, it has been demonstrated that stroke volume can increase 13–31% [25].

Control of preload is a function of a number of factors. Systemic venous return to the heart is a major determinant of the amount of preload a ventricle is under and can change cardiac output substantially. Maneuvers that alter venous return, such as positive pressure ventilation, change in posture, or changes in blood volume, all influence the amount of preload. In addition, structural diseases such as ventricular septal defect, patent ductus arteriosus, anomalous pulmonary venous connection, or arteriovenous fistulae all increase ventricular volume and hence preload. When peripheral vascular resistance is decreased by pharmaceutical agents or by exercise, increased venous return also occurs.

However agents that cause venodilation may actually decrease venous return, preload, and hence cardiac output, even if the agent decreases peripheral vascular resistance.

Total blood volume also affects preload, although small changes are easily tolerated by the body. Dehydration will decrease total blood volume and therefore preload, while congestive heart failure and salt/water retension will increase total blood volume and preload. There are a number of controls on total blood volume including the kidneys and the brain. One of the controls of total blood volume, however, is in the atria, where volume sensors are located and release atrial natriuretic peptide (ANP) in response to stretch as well as hormones such as angiotensin II [26].

Total blood volume, however, is only part of the story as the distribution of this volume is extremely important for ventricular performance. For example, the decrease in intrathoracic pressure during inspiration increases venous return to the heart, increases preload, and causes the P_2 component of the S_2 to be delayed because the right ventricle needs to pump more blood out to the lungs. With positive pressure ventilation, however, the increase in intrathoracic pressure decreases venous return to the heart with decreased intrathoracic blood volume. Other factors that control the distribution of blood volume are as follows:

• *Venous tone:* The venous system acts as a reservoir for blood by the relaxation of smooth muscle in the walls of the veins, which can cause a decrease in venous return, and therefore, preload. This can be accomplished by a number of neuro-humeral mechanisms or by medication. An increase in venous tone shifts this reservoir into the heart and can occur with exercise, hypotension, or being anxious. A mechanical increase in venous tone outside the venous system can occur with the contraction of skeletal muscle—squatting on physical examination increases venous return to the heart, increases ventricular volume, and may elicit the click of mitral valve prolapse.

• *Body position:* When an individual is upright, blood tends to pool in the lower extremities, decreasing venous return to the heart and preload via gravity. When an individual becomes supine, is weightless, or if the legs are placed in water, there is little pooling of blood in the lower extremities and venous return is increased.

The following are the mechanical factors that affect the amount of preload placed on the ventricle:

• Pericardial pressure is an external influence on preload. An increase in pericardial pressure, such as with a pericardial effusion or constrictive pericarditis, will impede cardiac filling by "pushing" on the ventricle and not allowing expansion. This, in turn, will decrease the flexibility of the heart to use the Frank–Starling mechanism to alter cardiac output and may actually decrease cardiac output in severe cases.

• Decreased ventricular compliance, as in ventricular hypertrophy or myocardial infarction, will decrease the amount of preload the ventricle can accept. Drugs such as beta blockers increase ventricular compliance and increase preload.

• Atrial contraction at end-diastole augments ventricular filling by mechanically pushing blood into the ventricle in excess of what it can accept with passive filling alone, acting as a booster pump [27,28]. This abruptly elevates ventricular end-diastolic pressure and volume. Loss of this function, whether it be because of lack of coordination between atria and ventricle such as in atrioventricular dissociation (third-degree atrioventricular block, e.g.) or because of loss of rhythm as in atrial fibrillation may cause a marked decrease in cardiac output. This is especially important in patients with compromised ventricular performance or in patients with decreased ventricular compliance.

• Tachycardia decreases the amount of time the ventricle can fill with blood during diastole. With excessive tachycardia, the ventricular filling may be impaired and preload will suffer as a result with ultimately a decrease in cardiac output ensuing. This is the uncoupling of the force–frequency relationship mentioned earlier in this chapter.

During exercise, decreased peripheral vascular resistance is present and preload reserve is utilized. There is an increase in ventricular volume and preload, which augments tachycardia and stoke volume to increase cardiac output [29]. However, with increased exercise and tachycardia, ventricular end-diastolic volume decreases because of the mechanical mechanism described above and cardiac output is maintained by a decrease in end-systolic volume.

Changes in preload also appear to be important in maintaining the balance of cardiac output between both ventricles. Both the lungs and the systemic venous system (as mentioned earlier) act as reservoirs for blood and balancing the cardiac outputs between right and left ventricle, which utilizes changes in these reservoirs, is a function of changing the preload of each ventricle. This occurs on a beat-to-beat basis and acts over all changing physiologic conditions from normal respiration to extreme exercise.

Afterload

Similar to preload, afterload may also be defined in terms of wall stress; that is, afterload is the wall stress acting on the myocardium after the onset of contraction. It is one of the key determinants to cardiac output (Fig. 2.9). It is important to understand that during systole, the ventricular cavity radius decreases (R goes down) and the heart thickens (H goes up) with only a relatively small rise in aortic pressure (Fig. 2.2), and therefore, by Laplace's law, wall stress decreases. Essentially, the heart unloads itself throughout systole with a continually decreasing wall stress. Unlike preload and contractility (see below) which are directly proportional to myocardial fiber shortening, afterload is inversely proportional to it—as afterload increases, cardiac output decreases (Fig. 2.9).

Afterload can be thought of as comprising of and controlled by three components that are interrelated:

• Peak arterial pressure is one component which can be elevated in disease states such as coarctation of the aorta, branch pulmonary artery stenosis in Allageille's syndrome, or in essential hypertension. Pressure is in the numerator of Laplace's law so it is directly proportional to wall stress during systole. In addition, it is the product of cardiac output and peripheral vascular resistance, which is another component mentioned below.

• Arterial compliance is another component, defined similar to ventricular compliance; it is the change in arterial diameter or volume as a function of the change in arterial pressure. Arterial compliance may be decreased, for example, in the elderly where aortic stiffening is noted or may be iatrogenically decreased when noncompliant materials are used to reconstruct the aorta as in the Norwood Stage I procedure for hypoplastic left heart syndrome [30]. Arterial compliance is inversely proportional to afterload. It is related to peak pressure—at a given cardiac output and peripheral vascular resistance (see below), a decrease in arterial compliance will increase peak pressure.

• One of the most important components is systemic/pulmonary peripheral vascular resistance, which may be elevated, for example, in essential hypertension, by neurohumeral mechanisms or after cardiopulmonary bypass. Peripheral vascular resistance is directly proportional to afterload. It is also related to peak pressure—at a given cardiac output and arterial compliance, an increase in systemic/pulmonary peripheral vascular resistance will increase peak pressure.

Related to both aortic compliance and systemic/pulmonary peripheral vascular resistance is the concept of arterial impedance. In it's most simplest form, "instantaneous resistance" is calculated by an analysis of the relationship between pulsatile flow and pressure waves in the arterial system. It is based on the theories of Fourier analysis where flow and pressure waves are decomposed into their basic components and provides a measure of resistance at different flow rates and pressures. Unlike aortic compliance and systemic/pulmonary peripheral vascular resistance, which are "static" measures, arterial impedance relates instantaneous pressure and flow and is "dynamic" across the entire cardiac cycle. It is the most comprehensive description of the intrinsic properties of the arterial tree as it pertains to understanding the influence of afterload on ventricular performance.

These afterload parameters are interrelated to each other by feedback mechanisms. For example, when afterload is increased by increasing peripheral vascular resistance and elevating peak pressure, cardiac output and myocardial fiber shortening are decreased. By decreasing cardiac output, pressure decreases reducing afterload somewhat.

To complicate matters further, feedback mechanisms are not restricted to afterload parameters, and in fact, feedback loops exist between afterload and the other three determinants of myocardial oxygen uptake. One feedback loop that has already been discussed is the Anrep effect, where an abrupt increase in afterload is offset by an increase in contractility. Another feedback loop occurs when a substantive amount of preload reserve exists—an elevation in afterload is met by an increase in end-diastolic volume and preload. By this method, stroke volume is maintained in the normal heart since less myocardial shortening is needed when end-diastolic volume is larger (i.e., less shortening is needed for a given stroke volume in larger hearts than in smaller ones). The cost to this compensatory mechanism is increased wall stress by Laplace's law, increasing afterload further. In summary, in a normal heart, cardiac output and stroke volume are maintained with increased afterload with compensatory increases in end-diastolic pressure and volume at the cost of increased wall stress and work of the heart (see below). In diseased hearts, however, with little preload reserve, this compensatory mechanism is not available and stroke volume falls [31,32].

There is a complex interplay between the ability of the heart to pump out blood and the arterial system into which it is pumping, termed as ventriculoarterial coupling, where afterload plays an important role. Simplistically, in the heart, as the pressure and afterload increase, cardiac output decreases in an inverse relationship. However, in the arterial system, as cardiac output increases, pressure increases as well in a direct relationship. Where these two relationships meet, depending upon the state of the ventricle and arterial tree, determines the "equilibrium" cardiac output and pressure, which can be described in the pressure–volume plane. To fully understand the relationship between ventricle and cardiovascular tree, the concept of "elastance" needs to be brought into play (more about this later in the chapter).

Contractility

This term is abused by many clinicians to mean any change in ventricular performance; however, in the study of ventricular function, it has a specific meaning. Similar to the contractility in isolated cardiac muscle, contractility in the intact heart is rigorously defined as the intensity of the force of contraction that is independent of preload and afterload, which essentially equates to the intrinsic strength of the muscle. Other terms for contractility are "contractile" or "inotropic" state. It is directly proportional to cardiac output—as contractility increases, cardiac output increases as well (Fig. 2.9).

Contractility is mediated on a cellular level by either one or all of the following mechanisms: The affinity of myofilaments for calcium, the amount of intracellular calcium released, or the alteration in the number of myofilaments participating in contraction. Calcium plays a key role in contraction by interacting with troponin, which allows actin and myosin to interact with each other and generate force (Fig. 2.6). The more sensitive troponin is to interacting with calcium or the more available calcium is in the cell, the greater the number of actin–myosin interactions.

The regulation of contractility *in vivo* is performed in numerous ways:
• Circulating catecholamines can stimulate β-adrenergic receptors on the myocardium and increase the force of contraction.
• Sympathetic nerve stimulation is a quicker mechanism of action than circulating catecholamines and probably represents the major determinant of myocardial contractility.
• The force–frequency relationship, as noted previously, relates how heart rate mediates the force of contraction independent of preload and afterload and operates by manipulation of intracellular calcium.
• Exogenous pharmaceutical agents play an important role in changing contractility, especially in disease states. These agents can either potentiate contractility, such as digoxin, phosphodiesterase inhibitors, caffeine, and other sympathomimetic agents, or can depress contractility, such as general anesthetics and barbiturates.
• Decreased oxygen delivery to the myocardium, such as with ischemic heart disease or an anoxic insult of other kinds (e.g. traumatic birth), may depress myocardial contractility.

The search for the ideal measure of contractility has been an elusive goal for years. Nevertheless, there are a number of ways that can demonstrate a change in contractility, and it is useful to review two of the most significant methods here.

The force–velocity relationship was described earlier relating the force of contraction with the velocity of muscle shortening and measures of maximal velocity at no load (V_{max}) and maximal force at

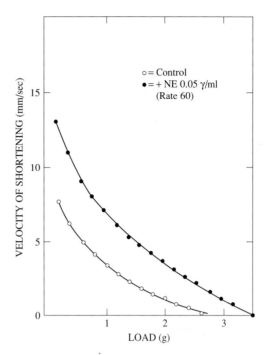

Figure 2.10 Force–velocity relationship with increasing contractility. After norepinephrine (NE) administration, at any given load, velocity is increased and both V_{max} and P_0 increase. From Braunwald *et al.* [7] with permission.

isometric contraction (P_0) were noted. With increased contractility, as demonstrated with the administration of norepinephrine, both V_{max} and P_0 increase along with a shift of the force–velocity curve upward and to the right [33,34] (Fig. 2.10). When this occurs, there is an increased velocity and extent of wall shortening with the duration of contraction decreasing the duration of relaxation increasing (with heart rate held constant).

It is necessary to introduce another two relationships not previously mentioned in the "Myocardial Mechanics and the Great Relationships" section, but certainly qualify—they are called the end-systolic and end-diastolic pressure–volume relationship (ESPVR and EDPVR, respectively). The concept is introduced at this point since it is a key variable in the measure of contractility and it would be understood less well prior to an extended discussion of contractility.

At end-diastole, the ventricle is in a state of complete relaxation. Experimentally, if the ventricle was empty at that point, there would be no pressure, and as it is filled with blood, there is initially little resistance to as the ventricle expands to a certain point.

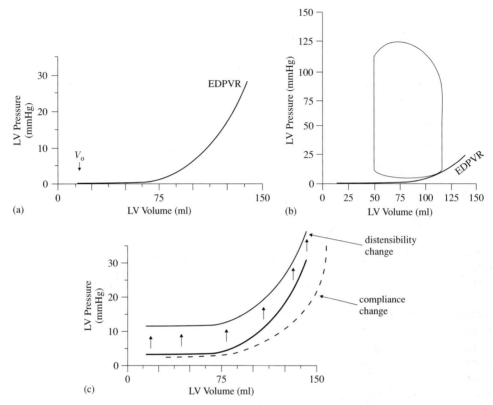

Figure 2.11 End-diastolic pressure–volume relationship (EDPVR) and changes in compliance and distensibility. Three pressure–volume graphs are shown. (a) The nonlinear pressure–volume relationship. (b) This graph demonstrates that the EDPVR defines the lower bound of where the pressure–volume loop may fall. (c) A distinction is made between compliance and distensibility changes. When there is a change in compliance, by its definition, the shape of the EDPVR is changed (slope of the tangent line to this curve changes—solid versus dashed lines). When there is a change in distensibility, the curve is shifted without change in shape so that at any given volume the pressure is increased (in this example) or decreased (not shown). V_0 = unstressed volume.

Up to that point, the volume increases, but pressure does not change. This volume it termed as V_0, or the maximal volume at which pressure is still 0 mm Hg (unstressed volume). As the volume increases, resistance to filling of the ventricle increases, indicating that the pressure is becoming higher and higher. A typical relationship between pressure and volume in the ventricle at end-diastole is shown in Fig. 2.11a. Quantitative analysis of such curves has shown that pressure–volume relationship is a nonlinear function and may be described by

$$EDP = P_0 + \beta V^\alpha$$

where EDP is the end-diastolic pressure, V is the ventricular volume, P_0 is the pressure at the lowest volume (close to 0), and α and β are constants that are used to specify the curvature of the line. Both α and β are determined by the mechanical properties of the muscle as well as the structural features of the ventricle. This relationship between pressure and volume as the ventricle is filled at end-diastole is termed the end-diastolic pressure–volume relationship (EDPVR) and defines the lower bound of where the pressure–volume loop can fall (Fig. 2.11b).

Chamber stiffness, as described earlier, is the slope of the EDPVR at a given point and since the curve is nonlinear, chamber stiffness will vary with volume—stiffness is greatest at high volumes and smallest at low volumes. Compliance is the reciprocal of stiffness and just the reverse is true.

In examining the pressure–volume loop (Fig. 2.2) at end-systole, it is noted that the muscles are in their maximally activated state. If attention is focused at the volume and pressure at that point, which is

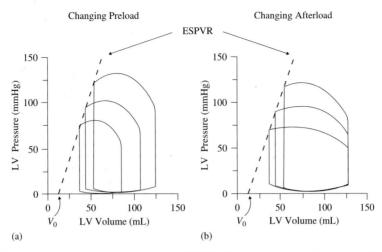

Figure 2.12 End-systolic pressure–volume relationship (ESPVR). Whether changing (a) preload or (b) afterload , a linear relationship exists to all generated end-systolic pressure–volume points at a given level of contractility. V_0 = unstressed volume.

inscribed in the upper-left corner of the loop, varying the loading conditions of the ventricle at a given level of contractility will vary the points at where the end-systolic volume and pressure meet. Varying the loading conditions can be performed by vena caval occlusion, volume expansion, or administration of vasoconstrictors or vasolidators that are not inotropic, such as phenylepherine or nitroglycerin. If these points are then plotted simultaneously on the pressure–volume graph, a linear relationship, that is the ESPVR, is generated and has been shown to be reasonably linear over a wide range of conditions (Fig. 2.12). The linearity of this relationship is derived from experimental data. As a general rule of thumb as found in the canine left ventricle, for a given afterload, the myocardium will shorten to the same final length regardless of the end-diastolic volume (preload) [35] and thus the ESPVR, for a given afterload, is independent of preload. Similarly, if afterload is varied and contractility is constant, all the end-systolic pressure–volume points will vary but will lie on a straight line [35,36].

Examples of different pressure–volume loops are shown in Fig. 2.12. Figure 2.12b shows three pressure–volume loops that have the same end-diastolic volume but different aortic pressures. This was done by changing peripheral vascular resistance without modifying anything about the way the ventricle works and keeping contractility constant. The upper-left corner of each loop falls on the ESPVR. Figure 2.12a shows three different loops that have

different end-diastolic volumes and different aortic pressures. Here the loops were obtained by changing end-diastolic volumes without modifying anything about the heart or the arterial system and keeping contractility constant. The upper-left corner of each loop again falls on the ESPVR.

Because of the linearity of the ESPVR, it can be expressed as a simple equation:

$$P_{es} = E_{es}(V_{es} - V_0) \quad \text{or} \quad E_{es} = \frac{P_{es}}{V_{es} - V_0}$$

where P_{es} and V_{es} are pressure and volume at end-systole, respectively, V_0 is the x intercept of this line (the volume at which no pressure may be detected), and E_{es} is the slope of the line termed end-systolic elastance. E_{es} stands for end-systolic elastance and gives the change in pressure for a given change in volume. Elastance means nearly the same thing as stiffness; the higher the elastance, the stiffer the wall of the chamber. Because we originally defined E_{es} at a given state of contractility but varied the loading conditions, E_{es} is an independent measure of contractility.

Technically, what is really being sought is the peak value of the ratio of pressure and volume, which is actually obtained, on average, 8 msec prior to the end of ejection. The pressure and volume at this point have been called the "corner" values and slope of the line created by these corner values by varying loading conditions is termed E_{max} [35] and is a more true measure of contractility than is E_{es}.

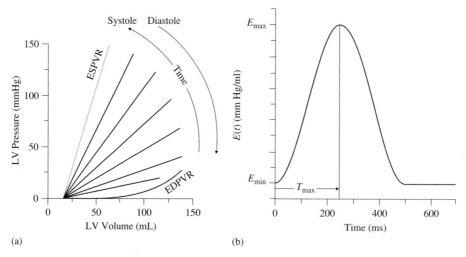

Figure 2.13 Time varying elastance ($E(t)$). If each time point in the cardiac cycle generates a systolic and diastolic pressure–volume relationship by altering preload and afterload, multiple linear relationships similar to the ESPVR and EDPVR are generated. A number of these relationships are shown in (a) (counterclockwise: systole; clockwise: diastole). EDPVR is the notable exception of nonlinearity. If the slopes of these lines are plotted against time, the curve shown in (b) is generated. E_{max} and E_{min} are the maximum and minimum slopes to these lines, respectively, and the time to E_{max} is designated at T_{max}.

Not only can pressure–volume relationships be developed for just two points in the cardiac cycle (end-diastole and end-systole), but this can be performed at any point during the cardiac cycle. To explain, at each point during the cardiac cycle, there exists a pressure–volume relationship similar to the ESPVR and EDPVR. It has been demonstrated experimentally that there is a relatively smooth transition from the EDPVR to the ESPVR and back during the cardiac cycle, as shown in Fig. 2.13a. In general, these relations are linear and they all intersect close to V_0. The one exception is the EDPVR where there are significant nonlinearities at higher volumes. Since the instantaneous pressure–volume relationships are reasonably linear and intersect at V_0, the time course of the slope change can be plotted to characterize the change in the ventricular mechanical properties. A representative curve of the instantaneous elastance throughout a cardiac cycle is shown in Fig. 20.13b. E_{max} is the maximum slope obtained and the minimum slope, E_{min}, is the slope of the EDPVR in the low volume range. This is referred to as time varying elastance, $E(t)$, which relates instantaneous pressure with volume throughout the cardiac cycle:

$$P(t) = E(t)[V(t) - V_0]$$

where V_0 and $E(t)$ are as defined above and $V(t)$ is the time varying volume.

The effect of increased contractility on the ESPVR is that the line rotates counterclockwise resulting in a higher E_{max} and a steeper slope (Fig. 2.14). This implies a more complete end-systolic emptying at a given pressure. With decreased contractility, just the opposite is true, that is, the ESPVR is rotated clockwise with E_{max} smaller and the slope more shallow.

Figure 2.15 demonstrates various pressure–volume curves in diseases that volume overload (mitral regurgitation) and volume underload (mitral stenosis) the left ventricle. In addition, pressure overload of the left ventricle (aortic stenosis) and a combination of both volume and pressure overload (aortic stenosis in combination with aortic insufficiency) are plotted. In theory, each one of these loops can have different E_{max} values or the same, depending on V_0 and the slope it creates with the corner point.

Heart rate

One of the major determinants of myocardial oxygen consumption, heart rate, has been discussed in the previous sections, including the force–frequency relationship. There are a few other issues, however, which should be noted.

In the normal heart in conscious patients, as physiologic tachycardia increases, increased venous return to the heart augments ventricular diastolic filling and increased cardiac output is the result;

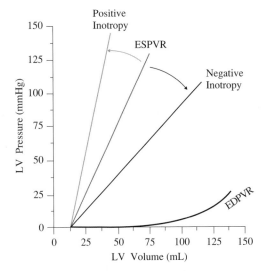

Figure 2.14 The effect of contractility on the ESPVR. Increasing contractility (positive inotropy) rotates the line counterclockwise and as a result has a steeper slope implying a more complete end-systolic emptying at a given pressure. With decreased contractility (negative inotropy), just the opposite is true—the ESPVR is rotated clockwise with a resulting smaller slope.

indeed, tachycardia is an important mechanism in increasing cardiac output during exercise [38]. During exercise, there is potentiation of systolic and diastolic function to accommodate the increased

venous return, despite the decreased diastolic filling time. However, if the heart rate of a subject at rest is artificially increased by pacing, for example, there is a minimal effect on cardiac output as compensatory mechanisms come into play to stabilize cardiac output despite the force–frequency relationship [39].

In anesthetized dogs, where sympathetic drive is blunted and the ventricle is artificially paced, tachycardia elevated V_{max} and shifted the force–velocity relationship upward and to the right. In addition, by increasing the frequency of contraction, the rate of stroke work production (i.e., the rate of change of the area subtended by the pressure–volume loop— stroke power) is increased for any given level of end-diastolic pressure [40]. It can be readily seen, since cardiac output is directly proportional and linearly related to heart rate, that at a constant stroke volume, the ability to alter heart rate is critical to altering cardiac output. Heart rate is mostly a function of the slope of the Phase 4 depolarization of the sinoatrial node, which in turn can be affected by temperature, thyroid status, acetylcholine (negatively related), and norepinephrine (positively related).

It should be remembered, however, that excess tachycardia will decrease diastolic filling time and at a certain point will actually decrease cardiac output [40].

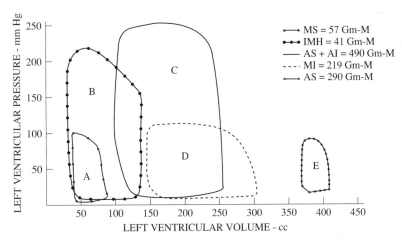

Figure 2.15 Various pressure–volume curves in disease states. A: mitral stenosis (MS, note small loop and volumes); B: aortic stenosis (AS, note high pressures); C: aortic stenosis and insufficiency (AS+AI, note the high pressures and increased volume when compared to isolated aortic stenosis); D: mitral insufficiency (MI, note normal pressures and increased volumes); and E: primary cardiomyopathy, note high volumes and small loop). From Dodge *et al.* [37] with permission.

Diastolic function

The discussion up to this point has mostly centered on the systolic function of the heart. Although it is clear that this has been the focus of studies into ventricular function for a long time, the increasing importance of diastolic function or the "lusitropic" state of the heart has been noted. Indeed, "diastolic" heart failure (congestive heart failure in the presence of a normal ejection fraction) has become the study of many investigations in the adult literature. It is convenient to divide the study of diastole into four phases:

• In the isovolumic relaxation phase (first phase), where there is no ventricular filling and just a decrease in pressure at constant volume, there is ATP usage for calcium uptake by the sarcoplasmic reticulum. This is, in fact, an active and energy-consuming process with some estimates that this diastolic phase consumes up to 15% of the total cardiac energetics. If this process is impaired, such as in myocardial ischemia, hypothyroidism, or congestive heart failure, there is a delayed uptake of cytosolic calcium, which in turn allows continued interaction of actin and myosin bridges [41].

• In the second phase, early diastolic filling, the atrioventricular valve opens and there is rapid filling of the ventricle.

• In diastasis or the third phase of diastole, there is only a small amount of blood that enters the ventricle, accounting for about 5% of ventricular filling.

• Finally, the last phase of diastole is atrial systole, also called the "atrial boost" phase or "presystole," where atrial contraction forces blood into a distended ventricle, accounting for approximately 15% of ventricular filling.

Besides the active role of calcium uptake by the sarcoplasmic reticulum, a major factor that determines diastolic function is the mechanical properties of the ventricle. The EDPVR, chamber compliance and stiffness have already been discussed. Other useful concepts in discussion of the mechanical properties of the ventricle are listed below:

• *Stress:* The amount of force exerted per unit cross-sectional area.

• *Strain:* The amount of change in dimension or shape of the ventricular cavity or wall with the application of a stress, usually expressed as a percentage from the unstressed dimensions.

• *Elastic modulus:* The proportionality term between stress and strain.

• *Specific compliance:* In an effort to correct for ventricles of different sizes and starting volumes, the compliance is divided by the starting volume (i.e., $dV/(dP \times V)$).

• *Volume elasticity (volume stiffness):* The reciprocal of specific compliance.

In examining the EDPVR further (Fig. 2.11), the curvelinear nature of the relationship is noted, where there is a "shallow" portion at low volumes (where large changes in volume are accompanied by only small changes in pressure) and a "steep" portion at high volumes (where large changes in pressure are accompanied by only small changes in volume). The study by Diamond *et al.* [42] in dogs, subsequently confirmed in man [43], concluded that the pressure–volume relationship was linear up to a pressure of approximately 2.5 mm Hg. Above this pressure, dP/dV became linearly related to P, making the pressure–volume curve exponential; as the volume increases, the instantaneous compliance (dV/dP) decreases and the chamber stiffness (dP/dV) increases. Therefore, the ventricular compliance may change with different diastolic loading conditions. Mathematically, this translates to

$$\frac{dP}{dV} = aP + b$$

which after integration and rearrangement becomes

$$P = \frac{e^{-aC}e^{aV}}{a} - \frac{b}{a}$$

where a is the slope of dP/dV on P (the so called volume elastic constant), b is the Y intercept, and C is a constant of integration. For example, a patient with a large shunt across a ventricular septal defect with left ventricular volume loading will have decreased left ventricular compliance, while a patient with partial or total anomalous pulmonary venous connection to the right side of the heart will have increased left ventricular compliance. In addition, as the ventricle fills during diastole, its compliance changes and becomes stiffer and hence the need for the "atrial boost" at the end of diastole to fill the ventricle.

Although a ventricle may move along a particular diastolic pressure–volume curve during the course of filling, the curve itself may change in two different ways (Fig. 2.11). Distensibility is the amount of pressure required to fill a ventricle at a given volume. A change in "distensibility" occurs when the curve is "shifted" without changing shape, which leaves compliance unchanged. For example, if a diastolic pressure–volume curve is shifted upward without changing shape, although the compliance is the same, the distensibility is decreased since a greater pressure is required to fill the ventricle at the same volume. If the shape of the curve itself is changed, then by definition, the compliance changes (the slope of the tangent to the curve, see Fig. 2.11). One or both of these mechanisms (changing compliance or distensibility) can be in play at a given time and these mechanisms do not always change in the same direction. In the example above, if the curve is shifted upward, the distensibility will be decreased; however, if the curve "flattens out" at the same time, the compliance will actually increase.

The major drawback of using pressure–volume relationships and the concept of compliance and stiffness is that conceptually they lack a normalization for chamber size and wall thickness. Nevertheless, these concepts are rooted in the study of ventricular function and have added to our knowledge of diastole. In addition, differences have been found between adult normal individuals and those with heart disease [44].

It was Mirsky and Parmley who suggested using stress–strain rather than pressure–volume relationship to assess diastolic mechanics [45]. This concept appeared to be more intellectually satisfying since it describes parameters of the ventricular wall rather than intracavity parameters. Stress (σ) and strain (ε) and the elastic modulus (E), the term that relates the two, have been defined earlier. In an ideal Hookean relationship, the relationship between σ and ε is constant and E is termed Young's modulus. However, papillary muscle experiments have demonstrated E not to be constant but rather a function of the forced developed and the length from which the muscle was stretch; E appears to linearly increase with stress:

$$\frac{dx}{dy} = E = k\sigma + c$$

which after integration and rearrangement becomes

$$\sigma = \frac{e^{-k\varepsilon}e^{k\varepsilon}}{k} - \frac{c}{k}$$

and since strain is zero when stress is zero, this becomes

$$\sigma = \frac{c}{k}\left(e^{k\varepsilon} - 1\right)$$

where k is the slope of $d\sigma/d\varepsilon$ or E on σ (and is termed the elastic constant) and c is the Y intercept. Note the similarity between the above equations and

the ones for the pressure–volume relationship. E is termed the "tangential modulus of elasticity"—it is a variable slope—and σ grows exponentially to linear increments of ε implying that the muscle gets much stiffer as it is stretched to greater and greater lengths.

If one takes the stress–strain formulas above and combines them with the formula for Laplace's law, the following complex equation for the pressure–volume relationship can be obtained [46]:

$$P = a\eta\,(2 + \eta)$$
$$\times \left[\exp\left(b\,(2 + \eta)\sqrt[3]{\left(\frac{3\pi^2}{32}\right)(V - V_0)}\right) - 1\right]$$

where η is $H/R = \sqrt[3]{(4p/3V)}$ and the other symbols are as described earlier in this chapter. This complex formula demonstrates the fine interaction between all the concepts discussed (stress–strain, pressure–volume, and Laplace's law) and reveals that the pressure–volume relationship depends on three things: the elastic properties of the myocardium a and b, the wall thickness H, and the ventricular equilibrium volume V_0.

Another concept in diastolic filling is the "diastolic suction" effect, also termed elastic recoil [47–49]. As the ventricle contracts in systole, it stores potential energy in the elastic elements of the myocardium as the ventricle twists [50]. When the ventricle is allowed to relax as the cytosolic calcium is taken up by the sarcoplasmic reticulum, negative pressure is generated as the elastic elements begin to return to their relaxed state and as the ventricle untwists (Fig. 2.16). These restoring forces are inhomogeneous around the ventricular wall [50], making this a very complex process. The strength of this mechanism has been demonstrated to be inversely related to end-systolic volume and enhances diastolic filling. Another method by which diastolic suction may work is the movement of the atrioventricular valve ring, which moves toward the ventricular apex during systole, enlarging the atria and causing negative pressure to develop in the atria suctioning blood from the pulmonary venous system [51].

There are other factors that can also influence diastolic function. Pericardial constraint obviously can restrict how easily the ventricle can expand to accept the volume being presented to it by the atria. This is especially important in the fetus [52,53]. In addition, compression of the heart by external

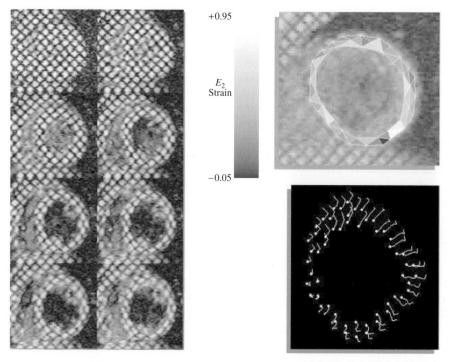

$+0.95$

E_2
Strain

-0.05

Figure 2.16 Diastolic strain and wall motion. Using magnetic resonance imaging and spatial modulation of magnetization, the myocardium is divided into "cubes of magnetization" and regional diastolic strain can be visualized and quantified. (Left): Raw images of six phases of diastole of a normal infant are shown. (Upper right): Quantitative strain mapped onto a grayscale and superimposed onto the anatomic image (E_2 or circumferential lengthening strain). (Lower right): Diastolic untwisting is visualized by tracking the "cubes of magnetization" through diastole; dots represent the starting position at end-systole and tails represent the subsequent motion in diastole.

factors such as tumor or increased intrathoracic pressure by, for example, tension pneumothorax, can also restrict ventricular expansion. When ventricular–ventricular interaction occurs, volume loading of the contralateral ventricle can alter the ipsilateral ventricle's performance as may be seen with paradoxical septal wall motion in a volume loaded right ventricle. Factors intrinsic to the myocardium, such as ventricular hypertrophy or fibrosis also alter stress–strain and pressure–volume relationships.

Other indices of diastolic performance

At this point, it is useful to describe some of the indices of diastolic ventricular performance other than the ones described above. They are organized into the following groups: (a) isovolumic relaxation, (b) early ventricular filling, (c) diastasis, and (d) atrial contraction. One of the most discussed measures of diastolic relaxation is τ or the constant of isovolumic relaxation. During pressure decay at the time

of isovolumic relaxation, the pressure–time curve may be fitted to a formula for the section of it from $-dP/dT_{max}$ (or dP/dT_{min}) to the opening of the mitral valve (Fig. 2.17):

$$P(t) = P_0 e^{-t/\tau} + P_B$$

where P_0 is the pressure at dP/dT_{min}, t is the time, τ is the time constant of isovolumic relaxation, and P_B is the asymptote (the theoretical pressure to which the ventricle would relax if the ventricle were held at a constant end-systolic volume and allowed to relax completely). A simplifying assumption is that P_B is 0. τ is, therefore, the time required for the pressure to drop to $1/e$ from dP/dT_{min} and is usually calculated by differentiating both sides of the equation and then performing a linear-least-squares fit to the equation:

$$\frac{dP}{dT} = -\left(\frac{1}{\tau}\right)(P(t) - P_B)$$

(normal values: 37–67 msec)

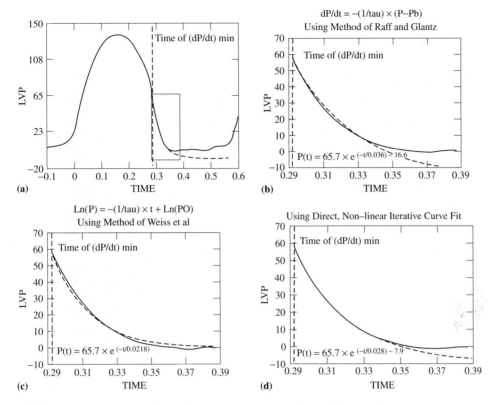

Figure 2.17 The constant of isovolumic relaxation (τ). During isovolumic relaxation, the pressure–time curve may be fitted to an exponential decay curve using a constant τ, which is a measure of diastolic relaxation. (a) Left ventricular pressure (LVP) time curve over one cardiac cycle. The boxed region is the area of interest for fitting the pressure–time curve during isovolumic relaxation.) (b, c, and d) Various ways to fit this decay curve to derive τ. From Colan [54] with permission.

By using a simplifying assumption that P_B is 0, τ can be derived by fitting a curve to the form:

$$\ln P = \ln P - \frac{\tau}{T} \quad \text{(normal values: 28–45 msec)}$$

τ has some unique advantages as a measure of ventricular relaxation. It is independent of changes in ventricular volume, end-diastolic pressure, stroke volume, end-systolic fiber length, and heart rate in isovolumically contracting dog hearts and in isolated contracting left ventricles on right heart bypass. τ is, however, affected by other conditions. It is increased by conditions that slow and/or cause asynchronous ventricular relaxation, ischemia, myocardial depression, propranalol administration, or phenylephrine administration (increasing afterload), while it is shortened by sympathetic stimulation and, in some cases, with increasing heart rate.

Following are the other measures of diastolic relaxation:

- $-dP/dT_{max}$ (the maximum rate of pressure fall) itself has been suggested as a measure of isovolumic relaxation but is strongly influenced by aortic pressure at the time of aortic valve closure—it is not a good measure.
- The time interval between aortic valve closure and mitral valve opening (isovolumic relaxation).
- Peak rate of ventricular wall thinning during isovolumic relaxation and during ventricular filling, which may be measured by echocardiography or MRI.
- Peak filling rate (PFR) and the time to peak filling rate (TPFR): In early diastolic filling, the PFR represents the integration of left atrial pressure, ventricular wall thickness, preload, the elastic properties of the ventricle, and extrinsic factors acting on the ventricle. It is decreased in conditions such as hypovolemia and hypertrophic cardiomyopathy. TPFR varies inversely with PFR, and both of these may be

measured by angiography, echocardiography, MRI, or nuclear scans.
• Regional E_1 and E_2 diastolic strain and "untwist" has been measured using myocardial tagging via MRI (Fig. 2.16) [50].
• Echocardiography measures (can also be measured by velocity mapping of the atrio-ventricular valve by MRI): Transmitral flow velocities on Doppler spectral recording have been used for many years now to try to assess ventricular diastolic performance. Measures are divided into diastolic time intervals, velocity/acceleration parameters, and Doppler area fractions. Examples of some of the many parameters in the literature include the following:
• Diastolic time intervals include isovolumic relaxation time (time between aortic valve closure to the beginning of mitral inflow and needs either a phonocardiogram or continuous wave Doppler of aortic and mitral flow), acceleration time (time between the beginning of diastolic inflow to peak E wave), deceleration time (time from peak E to when the velocity returns to baseline), and duration of early diastolic flow (beginning of diastolic flow to when the E wave returns to baseline).
• Velocity/acceleration: Peak E and A waves, the ratio of the E and A waves, and deceleration slopes of each wave.
• Doppler area fractions: This is the area under the curve of various parts of Doppler transmitral flow.
Besides transmitral flow, other measures of diastolic function include pulmonary venous flow patterns, which has been studied in single ventricle patients [55], color M-mode Doppler echocardiography [56], and Doppler tissue imaging [57].

Other parameters in ventricular function

This chapter has described many parameters of ventricular function including pressures and volumes. Parameters already mentioned include end-diastolic pressure, end-diastolic volume, end-systolic volume, ESPVR, EDPVR, elastance, E_{max}, and V_{max}. Nevertheless, there are a number of other ventricular function parameters that should be mentioned here for the sake of completeness.

Cardiac index is the integrated result of all the determinants of myocardial oxygen consumption, which makes it both useful and not useful at the same time. As the heart's primary function is to deliver oxygenated blood to the tissues, it indeed provides useful information about the pumping ability of the heart. At the same time, however, because it is critically dependent on preload and afterload, it does not describe intrinsically how well the heart is pumping. In addition, cardiac index can be altered by pharmacologic manipulation; indeed, two people can have the same cardiac index of 4.5 L/(min m^2) yet if one is on no medication and the other is on dopamine, dobutamine, and epinephrine together, their hearts' intrinsic pumping ability are not the same.

Cardiac index is the product of stroke volume and heart rate or the change in pressure divided by resistance and by body surface area (BSA). Another way this can be measured is by the arteriovenous oxygen difference (AVO_2) (difference between systemic mixed venous and arterial oxygen content), which indicates whether the cardiac index is satisfying the metabolic needs of the body. The normal AVO_2 difference is approximately 40 mL O_2 per liter in adults, and as cardiac output declines, this rises as oxygen extraction by the tissues increase. This can readily be seen by the Fick equation:

$$AVO_2 \text{ difference} = \frac{\text{Total } O_2 \text{ consumption}}{\text{cardiac output}}$$

There are other parameters which are linked to cardiac index and are considered ejection-phase parameters. The most well known of these are as follows:
• *Ejection fraction (EF)*: This parameter indexes stroke volume to the end-diastolic volume (EDV) (SV/EDV). It has widespread use [58] but is a very insensitive measure of ventricular function. It is dependent on preload, afterload, heart rate, and contractility. Global EF can be normal with hypokinesis of impaired regional walls of the myocardium compensated for by hyperkinesis in other regions.
• *Ventricular stroke work index (VSWI)*: The product of stroke volume and mean systolic pressure divided by BSA. Similar to cardiac index and EF, it is a function of preload, afterload, heart rate, and contractility.

• *Contractility index*: Indexing the VSWI to EDV to remove its dependence on preload (VSWI/EDV).

• *Ventricular power*: Power is work per unit time and the common parameter used to measure this is VSWI divided the systolic ejection period.

• *Double product*: Also known as the "index of cardiac effort," it is the product of peak left ventricular pressure and heart rate.

• *Triple product*: Also known as the "tension–time index (TTI)" and the "pressure per time minute," it is the product of the mean left ventricular ejection or mean aortic systolic pressure, the systolic ejection period per beat, and the heart rate.

• *Contractile element work (CEW) index*: This index is thought to be a measure of the work performed by the contractile element in fiber shortening and the stretching in the series elastic element. To calculate this index, first obtain the mean systolic volume by adding end-systolic and end-diastolic volumes and then dividing by 2 and the body surface area. Further divide this by 9.6 (a constant related to the stiffness of the series elastic element (SE)) and then add the result to the stroke volume index. The CEW index is the product of this number, the mean left ventricular systolic pressure, and 1.33 (conversion factor).

• *Circumferential fiber shortening velocity (V_{CF})*: This is the velocity of shortening at the equator of the left ventricle (measured as the difference in circumferences per unit time) divided by the left ventricular instantaneous circumference. Peak V_{CF} is the instantaneous measure and is sensitive to changes in contractility, afterload, and heart rate but is relatively independent to preload. Mean V_{CF} is the circumference difference between end-diastole and end-systole divided by the product of the circumference at end-diastole and the ejection time. This too is sensitive to changes in contractility, afterload, and heart rate but is relatively independent to preload. It is thought to be more sensitive to contractility because the time factor is added.

Peak dP/dT is the maximum rate of rise of ventricular pressure and is an isovolumic measure of ventricular function. It usually occurs before opening of the aortic valve and is therefore independent of afterload. It is, however, dependent on preload and contractility with changes in preload causing modest alterations in peak dP/dT. This measure also does not take into account wall thickness. Since peak

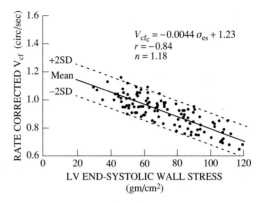

Figure 2.18 The inverse linear relationship between end-systolic wall stress and the velocity of circumferential fiber shortening. From Colan [54] with permission.

dP/dT, as a measure of contractility, depends upon being an isovolumic measure, if mitral regurgitation is present, this whole concept gets called into question. In addition, since peak dP/dT in the right ventricle occurs after the pulmonary valve opens, it becomes dependent on afterload on the right side of the heart.

In an attempt to obtain a measure of contractility independent of preload and heart rate and taking afterload into consideration, Colan *et al.* developed the left ventricular end-systolic wall stress–velocity of fiber shortening relation [59]. By echocardiography/phonocardiography/carotid pulse tracing, they measured fractional shortening indexed to heart rate (velocity of fiber shortening) and end-systolic wall stress in 78 normal individuals. Afterload was increased in 25 patients with methoxamine infusion and in 8 patients after increasing preload with dextran. Contractility was enhanced in 7 patients with dobutamine. They found an inverse linear correlation between the two parameters ($r = -0.84$) with narrow confidence intervals in normal individuals (Fig. 2.18). Any values falling outside the range were considered increased or decreased contractility.

Ventriculo–arterial coupling

No discussion of ventricular function is complete without a discussion of "ventriculo–arterial coupling" (the interaction between the intrinsic ventricular performance and the arterial tree). With the

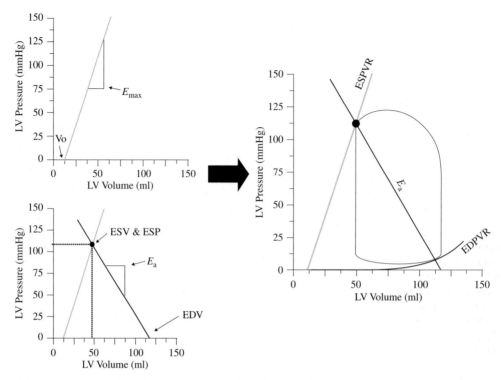

Figure 2.19 Ventriculo–arterial coupling (plotting ventricular and arterial elastance on the same pressure–volume graph). In the upper-left graph, the ESPVR is plotted as demonstrated previously. In the lower-left graph, the arterial elastance relationship (E_a) is plotted on the same graph as is E_{max}. E_a is defined as the slope of the line plotted in the pressure–volume plane from end-diastole to end-systole (end-systolic pressure (ESP)/stroke volume). The ESPVR and the E_a line intersect at one point, which is the equilibrium point for both the intrinsic properties of the arterial tree and ventricular performance (end-systolic volume (ESV) and ESP). This may be more clearly seen in the graph on the right, which overlays the ventricular pressure–volume loop and the EDPVR onto the plots of ESPVR and E_a.

concept of "elastance" (discussed earlier), we can combine the two interacting systems to determine some elementary parameters of ventricular function by using the pressure–volume diagram. This will allow combining the determinants of myocardial oxygen consumption (preload, afterload, contractility and heart rate) on the diagram so that such important variables as cardiac output (stroke volume) and arterial pressure can be determined from ventricular and vascular properties.

Similar to the pressure–volume loops and E_{max}, the arterial system also undergoes a related pressure–volume cycle and an "effective arterial elastance" can be calculated (designated as E_a). Similar to E_{max} units of pressure/volume, E_a is defined as the pressure at end-systole divided by the stroke volume and as such, represents the slope of the line drawn from the pressure–volume coordinate at end-diastole to the one at end-systole (Fig. 2.19). Because

systemic vascular resistance (SVR) is the pressure (P) difference in the aorta and right atrium divided by cardiac output (CO) and CO is the product of stroke volume (SV) and heart rate (HR), it can be easily demonstrated that E_a is a function of and directly proportional to heart rate and systemic vascular resistance:

$$SVR = P/CO \qquad CO = SV \times HR$$
$$SVR = P/(SV \times HR)$$

Since $E_a = P/SV$ (assumes central venous pressure is zero and mean systolic pressure is similar to end-systolic pressure in the ventricle), we can solve for

$$E_a = P/SV = SVR \times HR$$

Since the E_a line represents the pressure–volume cycle in the arterial tree, it can also be plotted on the same pressure–volume diagram as the ESPVR

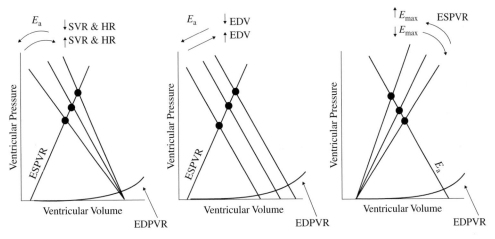

Figure 2.20 Alterations in systemic vascular resistance (SVR), heart rate (HR), end-diastolic volume (EDV), and contractility on ventriculo–arterial coupling. Since E_a is a function of SVR, HR, and EDV, alterations in these parameters will shift the E_a line and the equilibrium point between the intrinsic properties of the arterial tree and the ventricle. The graph on the left demonstrates how the E_a line rotates clockwise with increasing SVR and HR, while the graph in the middle demonstrates how the E_a line is shifted in parallel to the right with increasing EDV keeping SVR and HR constant. The graph on the right demonstrates how the ESPVR rotates counterclockwise with increasing contractility (increasing E_{max}). In all the graphs, the reverse relationship also holds in the opposite direction. In addition, for all graphs, new equilibrium points are reached when the lines are shifted or rotated.

(determined by E_{max} and V_0) and EDPVR (Fig. 2.19); it starts at EDV, has a slope of $-E_a$, and intersects with the ESPVR at one point. This is one way to represent SVR on the pressure–volume diagram as a measure of afterload. This intersection point determines end-systolic pressure and volume. If EDPVR is also drawn on the same diagram, it is then possible to form an approximate pressure–volume loop:
• End systole is the intersection point between ESPVR and E_a.
• Isovolumic relaxation is represented by a verticle line dropped from the intersection point between ESPVR and E_a to EDPVR.
• Diastolic filling is represented by the points along the EDPVR between the isovolumic relaxation and the intersection of EDPVR with E_a.
• Isovolumic contraction is represented by a verticle line drawn from the intersection of EDPVR with E_a to the *pressure value* at the intersection point between ESPVR and E_a.
• Finally, systolic ejection is represented by a horizontal line between the end of isovolumic contraction (see above point) to end-systole (see first point in this list).

When the slope of the arterial elastance line is changed by altering SVR, HR, or shifted in parallel

by altering EDV, the intersection point between this line and ESPVR changes (Fig. 2.20). Increasing SVR or HR will rotate the E_a line clockwise and increasing EDV will shift the E_a line to the right. Similarly, by altering the slope of the ESPVR line by changing contractility, the intersection point between ESPVR and the E_a line again changes (Fig. 2.20, increasing contractility rotates ESPVR counterclockwise). These alterations in the intersection points represent a new equilibrium state between the arterial and ventricular system and the resulting mean arterial pressure and stroke volume reflect this change.

Conclusion

This chapter just scrapes the surface of the essentials of ventricular function and is the bare minimum necessary to understand this topic. Application to congenital heart disease is even more complex and the reader is suggested many good reviews of this topic and of ventricular function in general in other publications [60,61].

References

1. Suga H, Goto Y, Nozawa T, *et al.* Ventricular suction under zero source pressure for filling. Am J Physiol 1986; 251:H47.

2. Hori M, Yellin EL, Sonnenblick EH. Left ventricular suction as a mechanism of ventricular filling. Jpn Circ J 1982; 46:124.

3. Ohno M, Cheng CP, Little WC. Mechanism of altered patterns of left ventricular filling during the development of congestive heart failure. Circulation 1994; 89:2241.

4. Berne RM, Levy MN. Cardiovascular Physiology, 3rd edn. CV Mosby Co, St Louis, 1977.

5. Parmley WW, Sonnenblick EH. Series elasticity: In relation to contractile element velocity and proposed muscle models. Circ Res 1967; 20:112.

6. Yang SS, Bentivoglio LG, Maranhao V, et al. From Cardiac Catheterization to Hemodynamic Parameters, 3rd edn. FA Davis, Philadelphia, PA, 1988.

7. Braunwald E, Ross J Jr, Sonnenblick EH. Mechanisms of Contraction of the Normal and Failing Heart, 2nd edn., Little, Brown and Co., Boston, 1976.

8. Sonnenblick EH. Implications of muscle mechanics in the heart. Fed Proc 1962; 21:975.

9. Sonnenblick EH. Force-velocity relations in mammalian heart muscle. Am J Physiol 1962; 202:931.

10. Brutsaert DL, Sonnenblick EH. Force-velocity length-time rations of the contractile elements in heart muscle of the cat. Circ Res 1969; 24:137.

11. Sonnenblick EH. Series elastic and contractile elements in heart muscle. Changes in muscle length. Am J Physiol 1964; 207:1330.

12. Lakatta EG. Starling's law of the heart is explained by an intimate interaction of muscle length and myofilament calcium activation. J Am Coll Cardiol 1987; 10:1157.

13. Noble NIM, Pollack GH. Molecular mechanisms of contraction. Circ Res 1977; 40:333.

14. Braunwald EA. Heart Disease, 4th edn. WB Saunders, Philadelphia, PA, 1992.

15. Mulieri LA, Leavitt BJ, Martin BJ. Myocardial force-frequency defect in mitral regurgitation heart failure is reversed by forskolin. Circulation 1993; 88:2700.

16. Yue DT, Burkhoff D, Franz MR, et al. Postextrasystolic potential of the isolated canine left ventricle: Relationship to mechanical restitution. Circ Res 1985; 56:340.

17. Frommer PL, Robinson BF, Braunwald E. Paired electrical stimulation. A comparison of the effects on performance of the failing and nonfailing heart. Am J Cardiol 1966; 18:738.

18. Hasenfuss G, Reinecke H, Studer R, et al. Relation between myocardial function and expression of sarcoplasmic reticulum Ca^{2+}-ATPase in failing and non-failing human heart. Circ Res 1994; 75:434.

19. Grossman W. Pressure measurement. In: Grossman W, Baim DS, eds., Cardiac Catheterization and Angiography, 4th edn. Lea and Febiger, Philadelphia, PA, 1990.

20. Regen DM. Calculation of left ventricular wall stress. Circ Res 1990; 67:245.

21. Regen DM, Anversa P, Capasso JM. Segmental calculation of left ventricular wall stresses. Am J Physiol 1993; 264:H1411.

22. Fogel MA, Weinberg PM, Fellows KE, et al. A study in ventricular–ventricular interaction: Single right ventricles compared with systemic right ventricles in a dual chambered circulation. Circulation 1995; 92(2):219.

23. Fogel MA, Gupta KB, Weinberg PW, et al. Regional wall motion and strain analysis across stages of Fontan reconstruction by magnetic resonance tagging. Am J Physiol 1995; 269(38):H1132.

24. Fogel MA, Gupta K, Baxter MS, et al. Biomechanics of the deconditioned left ventricle. Am J Physiol 1996; 40(3):H1193.

25. Lee JD, Tajimi T, Pattrita J, et al. Preload reserve and mechanisms of afterload mismatch in the normal conscience dog. Am J Physiol 1986; 19:H464.

26. Focaccio A, Volpe M, Ambrosio G, et al. Angiotensin II directly stimulates release of atrial natriuretic factor in isolated rabbit hearts. Circulation 1993; 87:192.

27. Hoit BD, Shao Y, Gabel M, et al. In vivo assessment of left atrial contractile performance in normal and pathological conditions using a time-varying elastance model. Circulation 1994; 89:1829.

28. Braunwald E, Frahm CJ. Studies on Starling's law of the heart: IV. Observations on hemodynamic functions of left atrium in man. Circulation 1961; 24:633.

29. Higginbotham MB, Morris KG, Williams RS, et al. Regulation of stroke volume during submaximal and maximal upright exercise in normal man. Circ Res 1986; 58:281.

30. Fogel MA, Weinberg PM, Hoydu A, et al. Effect of surgical reconstruction on flow profiles in the aorta using magnetic resonance blood tagging. Ann Thorac Surg 1997; 63:1691.

31. Ross J Jr. Afterload mismatch and preload reserve: A conceptual framework for the analysis of ventricular function. Prog Cardiovasc Dis 1976; 18:255.

32. Ross J Jr, Braunwald E. The study of left ventricular function in man by increasing resistance to ventricular ejection with angiotensin. Circulation 1964; 19:739

33. Sonnenblick EH, Skelton CL. Reconsideration of the ultrastructural basis of the cardiac tension-length relation. Circ Res 1974; 35:517.

34. Ford LE. Mechanical manifestations of activation in cardiac muscle. Cric Res 1991; 68:621.

35. Suga H, Sagawa K, Shoukas AA. Load independence of instantaneous pressure-volume ratio of the canine left ventricle and effects of epinephrine and heart rate on the ratio. Circ Res 1973; 32:314.

36. Taylor RR, Covell JW, Ross J Jr. Volume-tension diagrams of ejecting and isovolumic contractions in the left ventricle. Am J Physiol 1969; 216:1097.

37. Dodge HT *et al.* Usefulness and limitations of radiographic methods for determining left ventricular volume. Am J Cardiol 1966; 18:10.

38. Higginbotham MB, Morris KG, Williams RS, *et al.* Regulation of stroke volume during submaximal and maximal upright exercise in normal man. Circ Res 1985; 58:281.

39. Vatner SF, Braunwald E. Cardiovascular control mechanisms in the conscience state. N Engl J Med 1975; 293:970.

40. Mitchell JH, Wallace AG, Skinner NS. Intrinsic effects of heart rate on left ventricular performance. Am J Physiol 1963; 205:41.

41. Cory CR, Grange RW, Houston ME. Role of sarcoplasmic reticulum in loss of load-sensitive relaxation in pressure overload cardiac hypertrophy. Am J Physiol 1994; 266:H68.

42. Diamond G, Forrester JS, Hargis J, *et al.* Diastolic pressure-volume relationship in the canine left ventricle. Cir Res 1971; 29:267.

43. Gaasch WH, Battle WE, Oboler AA, *et al.* Left ventricular stress and compliance in man. With special reference to normalized ventricular function curves. Circulation 1972; 45:746.

44. Fester A, Samet P. Passive elasticity of the human left ventricle. The "parallel elastic element." Circulation 1974; 50:609.

45. Mirsky I, Parmley WW. Assessment of passive elastic stiffness for isolated heart muscle in the intact heart. Circ Res 1973; 33:233.

46. Glantz SA, Kernoff RS. Muscle stiffness determined from canine left ventricular pressure-volume curves. Circ Res 1975; 37:787.

47. Hansen DE, Daughters, GT, Alderman EL, *et al.* Effect of acute human allograft rejection on left ventricular systolic torsion and diastolic recoil measured by intramyocardial markers. Circulation 1987; 76:998.

48. Hori M, Yellin EL, Sonnenblick EH. Left ventricular diastolic suction as a mechanism of ventricular filling. Jpn Circ J 1982; 46:124.

49. Nikolic S, Yellin EL, Tamura K, *et al.* Passive properties of the canine left ventricle: diastolic stiffness and restoring forces. Circ Res 1988; 62:1210.

50. Fogel MA, Weinberg PM, Hubbard A, *et al.* Diastolic biomechanics in normal infants utilizing MRI tissue tagging. Circulation 2000; 102:218.

51. Grossman W, McLaurin LP. Diastolic properties of the left ventricle. Ann Int Med 1976; 84:316.

52. Grant DA. Ventricular constraint in the fetus and newborn. Can J Cardiol 1999; 15:95.

53. Grant DA, Maloney JE, Tyberg JV, *et al.* Effects of external constraint on the fetal left ventricular function curve. Am Heart J 1992; 123:1601.

54. Colan SD. Assessment of ventricular and myocardial performance. In: Fyler DC, ed., Nadas Pediatric Cardiology. Mosby-Yearbook Co., St. Louis, MO, 1992.

55. Rychik J, Fogel MA, Donofrio MT, *et al.* Comparison of patterns of pulmonary venous blood flow in the functional single ventricle heart after operative aorto-pulmonary shunt versus superior cavo-pulmonary shunt. Am J Cardiol 1997; 80:922.

56. Taktsuji H, Mikami T, Urasawa K, *et al.* A new approach for the evaluation of left ventricular diastolic function: Spatial and temporal analysis of left ventricular filling flow propagation by color M-mode Doppler echocardiography. J Am Coll Cardiol 1996; 27:365.

57. Garcia MJ, Thomas JD, Klein AL. New Doppler echocardiographic applications for the study of diastolic function. J Am Coll Cardiol 1998; 32:865.

58. Fogel MA. Use of ejection fraction (or lack thereof), morbidity/mortality and heart failure drug trials: A review. Int J Cardiol 2002; 84:119.

59. Colan SD, Borow KM, Neuman A. Left ventricular end-systolic wall stress-velocity of fiber shortening relation: A load-independent index of myocardial contractility. J Am Coll Cardiol 1984; 4:715.

60. Graham TP. Ventricular performance in congenital heart disease. Circulation 1991; 84:2259.

61. Gilbert JC, Gantz SA. Determinants of left ventricular filling and of the diastolic pressure-volume relation. Circ Res 1989; 64:827.

CHAPTER 3

Blood Flow—The Basics of the Discipline

Hiroumi Kitajima, MS & Ajit P. Yoganathan, PhD

Introduction

Blood is a multipart medium of suspended cells in plasma. The complexity of blood distinguishes it from most other naturally encountered fluids that are largely uniform such as air or water. The flow of blood is an additionally complex phenomenon because blood travels through intricate, flexible geometries in a pulsatile, or time dependent, manner. Therefore, the science of fluid dynamics used to study aircraft flight or water in a hose must be adapted from classical fluid mechanics to hemodynamics. Toward this end, the material presented in this chapter will cover a summary of the applicable principles that are required to bridge the gap.

Before illustrating the dynamics of blood flow, it is first necessary to describe blood in terms of fluid properties and governing equations. The assumptions imposed on the conservation equations give an application of generalized laws toward specific flow characteristics.

Since blood flow in the human circulation is dictated largely by geometry, it is useful to characterize hemodynamics in terms of its environment. Because the cardiovascular system is primarily a network of vessels, the study of straight pipe flow is a logical beginning. Stenotic flow, or flow through a decreased cross-sectional area, is of interest because such geometries are encountered in atherosclerotic vessels or aortic coarctation. Flow through an orifice is a classically studied phenomenon and applies to communication of pulmonary and systemic blood through a septal defect or to valvular stenoses. Curved pipe flow also deserves discussion because of the tortuous pathways of blood flow. Especially significant is curved flow in the aortic arch.

There are special flow structures associated with flows when a larger vessel separates into two smaller vessels or when two vessels combine. The carotid bifurcation is an area of intense research. Branches are another type of splitting flow but differ from bifurcations because the branching vessel is small compared to the main vessel. End-to-side anastomoses warrant attention because of their wide use in bypass conduits. The modified Blalock–Taussig shunt and the bi-directional Glenn procedure both incorporate an end-to-side anastomosis to compensate for a congenital heart defect. The total cavopulmonary connection, or Fontan procedure, is a unique flow geometry where two end-to-side anastomoses are used to create a junction of two inflows and two outflows.

Note that all properties are given in centimeters-grams-seconds (cm-g-sec), or CGS, units. However, there are two exceptions due to convention in hemodynamics. Pressure is often expressed in millimeters of mercury (mm Hg) and volumetric flow rate is often expressed in liters per minute (L/min). Therefore, pressure must be converted to dynes per square centimeter (1 mm Hg = 133 dyne/cm^2 or g/(cm sec^2) and volumetric flow rate must be converted to cubic centimeters per second (1 L/min = 16.7 cm^3/sec) when used in equations to match the CGS units of other variables. The CGS units indicated for each variable introduced are a matter of convenience to the reader and are not required for the respective equations unless specified.

Fluid properties

Velocity, acceleration, and shear strain rate
When characterizing a fluid and its flow, there are several properties worthy of consideration. The

most intuitive are velocity (u, cm/sec) and transient acceleration (a, cm/sec^2). Transient acceleration is the time rate of change of velocity as shown in Eq. (3.1). Shear strain rate (ε, sec^{-1}) is defined in Eq. (3.2) and is also a velocity gradient, but it is the length rate of change. Shear strain rate is the effect of fluid particles being deformed because of flow. Shear strain rate is of concern in hemodynamics because the stresses it creates can result in hemolysis and platelet activation.

$$a = \frac{\partial u}{\partial t} \tag{3.1}$$

$$\varepsilon = \frac{\partial u}{\partial y} \tag{3.2}$$

Transient and convective acceleration

Transient acceleration is not to be confused with convective acceleration. In transient acceleration, an external force causes velocity at a point in space to increase in time. The heart is responsible for the transient acceleration of blood caused by the force of the ventricles. Conversely, convective acceleration is the acceleration of a particle as it moves along its path. The particle experiences velocity as it moves through the field, but the velocity field does not change. In the narrowing of vessels, the decrease of cross-sectional area is responsible for convective acceleration. This acceleration is caused by the conversion of pressure energy to kinetic energy as the cross-sectional area decreases. Convective acceleration can be evaluated by the Bernoulli equation and will be illustrated in the discussion of conservation equations.

Dynamic viscosity

Also related to the effect of flow on a fluid is its dynamic viscosity (μ, cP or g/(cm sec). Dynamic viscosity is a property that characterizes the frictional resistance of a fluid to flow. Under normal physiologic conditions, blood in large vessels has a constant dynamic viscosity of 3.5 cP [1].

Temperature, density, and pressure

Thermodynamic properties such as temperature, density (ρ, g/cm^3), and pressure (P, dyne/cm^2 or g/(m sec^2) typically play a large role in fluid mechanics. However, blood flow temperature is relatively constant at 37 $^\circ$C as dictated by homeostasis

of the human body. Density varies considerably in gases, but most liquids are incompressible. Blood is no exception, where the density is constant at about 1.06 g/cm^3 [2]. Therefore, effects of temperature and density changes are neglected in hemodynamics.

Pressure, on the other hand, is the most relevant thermodynamic quantity in hemodynamics because it varies greatly and is responsible for flow. Pressure ranges from 120 mm Hg in the aorta to less than 5 mm Hg in the pulmonary veins. The effect of pressure changes on flow is integral to hemodynamics.

Conservation equations

Balance equations

It is necessary to formulate conservation equations to relate the fluid properties to each other. This is done through the balance equations of conserved mass and momentum. The conservation of mass is also known as continuity. The conservation of energy is also customarily considered, but here it is omitted because the focus is on a constant temperature system. The balance equations of mass and momentum for all continuum matter are shown in Eqs. (3.3) and (3.4), respectively. Here, $\frac{D}{Dt}$ is the material derivative, $\vec{T}$ is the stress tensor (dyne/cm^2 or g/(cm sec^2)), and $\vec{f}$ is the body force tensor (cm/sec^2). The material derivative is the sum of transient and convective derivatives.

$$\frac{D\rho}{Dt} + \rho \nabla \cdot \vec{u} = 0 \tag{3.3}$$

$$\rho \frac{D\vec{u}}{Dt} = \nabla \cdot \vec{T} + \rho \vec{f} \tag{3.4}$$

Newtonian fluid

The balance equations can be simplified for an incompressible, Newtonian fluid. A Newtonian fluid is one that has a linear relationship between shear stress (τ, dyne/cm^2 or g/(cm sec^2)) and shear strain rate as shown in Eq. (3.5). The constant of proportionality is the dynamic viscosity. Therefore, it can also be said that a Newtonian fluid has a constant dynamic viscosity over shear strain rates.

$$\tau = -\mu \frac{\partial u}{\partial y} \tag{3.5}$$

Wall shear stress

Wall shear stress (τ_{wall}, dyne/cm^2 or g/(cm sec^2)) is simply the shear stress taken at the wall as shown in Eq. (3.6).

$$\tau_{wall} = -\mu \left. \frac{\partial u}{\partial y}\right|_{y=0} \tag{3.6}$$

Wall shear stress is a concern because it is a measure of the interaction between the viscous fluid and a solid boundary. When wall shear stress becomes significantly high, the material properties of the wall must be taken into consideration in analyzing fluid dynamics. Therefore, it stands to reason that a very high wall shear stress in vessels could cause damage to the endothelial layer. However, Giddens, *et al.* have in fact shown that low or oscillatory wall shear stresses can promote atherosclerosis [3,4].

Navier–Stokes equations

With incompressibility and the constitutive relation between shear stress and shear strain rate of a Newtonian fluid, it is possible to simplify the balance equations (Eqs. 3.3 and 3.4) into the celebrated Navier–Stokes equations as shown in Eqs. (3.7) and (3.8).

$$\nabla \cdot \vec{u} = 0 \tag{3.7}$$

$$\rho \frac{D\vec{u}}{Dt} = -\nabla P + \mu \nabla^2 \vec{u} + \rho \vec{f} \tag{3.8}$$

The Navier–Stokes equations are the basis of analysis for most fluid mechanics. Where it does not apply is dictated by its assumptions of an incompressible, Newtonian fluid.

Non-Newtonian blood

As previously stated, blood in large vessels at normal, physiologic conditions has a constant dynamic viscosity of 3.5 cP. However, due to its complexity, blood is not always Newtonian. Therefore, cases where blood is non-Newtonian must be considered.

Shear strain rate

Figure 3.1 indicates that blood has a variable dynamic viscosity under low shear strain rates. As shear strain rates rise to about 100 sec^{-1}, dynamic viscosity becomes more constant and blood can be considered to behave like a Newtonian fluid. When shear strain rates are lower than 100 sec^{-1}, the dynamic viscosity increases considerably because of the tendency of blood to form rouleaux, or aggregated erythrocytes [5].

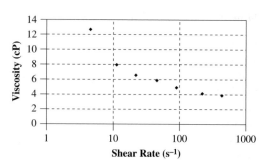

Figure 3.1 Effect of shear strain rate on the dynamic viscosity of whole human blood.

Therefore, blood cannot be considered a Newtonian fluid at low shear strain rates. The Newtonian assumption is only valid where variable dynamic viscosity does not vary.

Vessel diameter

Blood experiences lower shear strain rates in capillaries. Therefore, it would be intuitive to say that dynamic viscosity rises as vessel diameter increases. However, in reality blood cells interact less with each other and with the walls in capillaries. Blood cells tend to line up in the middle of capillaries. Therefore, blood actually behaves similarly to water in such a situation, causing dynamic viscosity to decrease.

In general, if the vessel diameter is greater than 0.5 mm, blood can be considered Newtonian. For vessels with a diameter of less than 0.5 mm, dynamic viscosity decreases with decreasing diameter [6].

Hematocrit

Plasma has a dynamic viscosity of 1.2 cP and a density of 1.02 g/cm^3 [5]. Since water has a dynamic viscosity of 1 cP and a density of 1 g/cm^3, blood cells account for much of the dynamic viscosity of blood. Dynamic viscosity and density rise with increased hematocrit. This is significant because the effects of some congenital heart diseases have been shown to be similar to those observed at high altitude, where hematocrit can rise dramatically. Of course, the reverse is significant as well, where conditions such as anemia can lower hematocrit and subsequently lower blood dynamic viscosity and density [6]. Therefore, the Navier–Stokes equations can still be applied in large vessels of patients with pathologic hematocrit, but different values for dynamic viscosity and density must be assigned.

Flow characterization

Viscous flow

Streamlines

The Navier–Stokes equations can be simplified further by comparing two points on the same streamline. Streamlines are traces of the pathway of a fluid particle moving through smooth and predictable, or laminar flow. The velocity vector is always parallel to a streamline. There is no mass flow through any streamline, and the mass flow rate through any two streamlines is constant.

Generalized Bernoulli equation

With the momentum conservation of the Navier–Stokes equations, it is possible to derive the Bernoulli equation shown in Eq. (3.9). Here, Point 1 represents an upstream location and Point 2 is a downstream location on the same streamline. s is the streamline distance (cm), $R_{viscous}$ is the generalized term for viscous losses (dyne/cm^2 or g/(cm sec^2), g is the gravitational acceleration (9.8×10^2 cm/sec^2), and h is the height (cm). By comparing Eq. (3.9) to the Navier–Stokes momentum equation in Eq. (3.8), it is possible to see the source of each term in the Bernoulli equation.

$$\int_1^2 \rho \frac{\partial u}{\partial t} \partial s + \frac{1}{2}\rho \left(u_2^2 - u_1^2\right)$$
$$= P_1 - P_2 - R_{viscous} - \rho g (h_2 - h_1) \qquad (3.9)$$

The Bernoulli equation is used extensively in noninvasive cardiology to determine pressure drops. Therefore, a more useful form of the Bernoulli equation is to solve for the pressure drop as shown in Eq. (3.10).

$$P_1 - P_2 = \int_1^2 \rho \frac{\partial u}{\partial t} \partial s + \frac{1}{2}\rho \left(u_2^2 - u_1^2\right)$$
$$+ \rho g (h_2 - h_1) + R_{viscous} \qquad (3.10)$$

The terms on the left of Eq. (3.10) represent the pressure change between Points 1 and 2. The first term on the right side is the transient acceleration term. It vanishes when the equation is taken at peak systole and peak diastole because transient acceleration is zero. It is also negligible when it is taken over a region where the transient acceleration and deceleration energies cancel. The second term on the right side is a measure of the kinetic energy, or convective acceleration, of the fluid. The third term on the right side represents the hydrostatic pressure difference. The final term represents the irreversible viscous loss of mechanical energy or momentum.

In order for the Bernoulli equation to be applicable to viscous flow, a generalized viscous term is included to account for the additional losses. Because the integral of the Navier–Stokes momentum equation is taken to obtain the Bernoulli equation, it must be taken at two points on the same streamline to remain valid.

Inviscid flow

Simplified Bernoulli equation

If some additional assumptions are made, a very applicable version of the Bernoulli equation can be derived. If transient acceleration/deceleration, hydrostatic forces, and viscous losses are negligible, the Bernoulli equation reduces to the inviscid form shown in Eq. (3.11).

$$P_1 - P_2 = \frac{1}{2}\rho \left(u_2^2 - u_1^2\right) \qquad (3.11)$$

In addition, if Point 2 is taken in an area of high velocity downstream such that the velocity at Point 1 is comparably small, Eq. (3.12) is obtained. In this case, u must be in m/sec, P must be in mm Hg, and ρ must be approximately 1 g/cm^3.

$$P_1 - P_2 \approx 4u_2^2 \qquad (3.12)$$

Equation (3.12) is particularly useful to calculate pressure drop across a stenosis or across a valve. u_2 is commonly measured by Doppler echocardiography but can be determined by magnetic resonance imaging as well.

Turbulent flow

It is possible to characterize a flow based on its viscous forces. In laminar flow, viscous forces dominate and the fluid travels in predictable paths. However, as velocity increases, a point can be reached when predictable flow breaks down into motion with a random component. This is known as turbulence. It is only possible to characterize a turbulent flow by its mean flow ($\bar{u}$, cm/sec) and a fluctuating component (u', cm/sec). This can be seen in Eq. (3.13). Figure 3.2 depicts the concept of turbulent fluctuations by examining the difference in interrogating a velocity at a single point over time.

$$u = \bar{u} + u' \qquad (3.13)$$

As one can see, the turbulent velocity trace has a mean value but it also has a random fluctuating

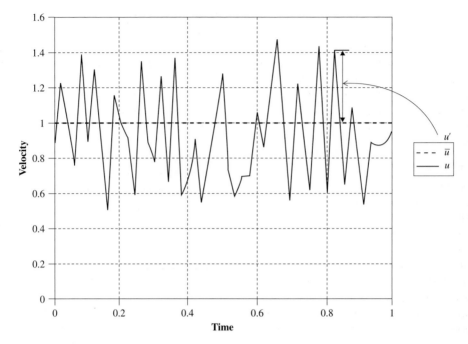

Figure 3.2 Representation of turbulent flow as expressed by mean and fluctuating components.

component that makes turbulent flow inherently unsteady.

Reynolds number

The characteristic parameter for the transition from laminar to turbulent flow is the Reynolds number (Re_x), which is a dimensionless ratio of inertial to viscous forces. This is expressed in Eq. (3.14) where u is a characteristic velocity (cm/sec) and x is a characteristic length (cm).

$$Re_x = \frac{\rho u x}{\mu} \tag{3.14}$$

Lower Reynolds numbers indicate laminar flow whereas higher Reynolds numbers characterize turbulent flow. There is a transition phase from laminar to turbulent flow where eddies begin to appear. The critical Reynolds number depends on the geometry of the flow since a characteristic length defines the Reynolds number.

Turbulent shear stress

In turbulent flows, inertial forces outweigh viscous forces. Therefore, viscous shear stresses are no longer the dominant stresses. Rather, it is more important to consider turbulent shear stresses ($\tau_{turbulent}$, dyne/cm^2 or g/(cm sec^2)), which are also known as

Reynolds shear stresses. They arise from the velocity fluctuations in inertial terms of momentum conservation. Turbulent shear stresses act on length scales of the same order as that of the smallest turbulent fluctuations. They are the product of the density and the time average of the product of the velocity fluctuations ($\overline{u'v'}$, cm^2/sec^2) as in Eq. (3.15).

$$\tau_{turbulent} = -\rho\overline{u'v'} \tag{3.15}$$

Turbulence intensity

A useful, dimensionless means of quantifying turbulence is by turbulence intensity (I). Turbulence intensity estimates the amount of energy in turbulent fluctuations. It is expressed as the percentage ratio of the root-mean-square of velocity fluctuations (u_{RMS}, cm/sec) to the mean velocity ($\bar{u}$, cm/sec) at a point as formulated in Eqs. (3.16) and (3.17).

$$u_{RMS} = \sqrt{\overline{u'^2}} \tag{3.16}$$

$$I = \frac{u_{RMS}}{\bar{u}} \times 100\% \tag{3.17}$$

Hemolysis/platelet activation

If the Reynolds number is sufficiently large, turbulent shear stresses can become elevated. If the stresses cause excessive shear to cell membranes, they can cause hemolysis or platelet activation. This is of particular concern downstream of a stenotic region or valve prosthesis because the high ejection velocities can contribute to Reynolds shear stresses. However, if the turbulent shear stresses act on length scales much larger than the diameter of a blood cell, the cell may not experience the shear stress because they tend to rotate the entire cell rather than shearing the cell wall.

Pulsatile flow

Steady, oscillatory, and pulsatile flow
Steady flow does not change with time. However, blood flow is typically dependent on time and therefore is unsteady. There are a few types of unsteadiness. Oscillatory flow simply implies that there is a periodicity in the flow. However, pulsatile flow as characterized in the arteries, exhibits an oscillatory flow with a net forward flow motion.

Thus far, all analyses in this chapter have been on steady flow. However, as Fig. 3.3 exhibits, aortic flow rate varies considerably over a cardiac cycle in a pulsatile flow. Unsteadiness is not limited to the aorta as it also appears in most other parts of the circulatory system except the capillaries. Indeed, steady flow is actually the exception in cardiovascular fluid mechanics.

Womersley number
The Womersley number (α) is used as a measure of pulsatility in a flow. Like the Reynolds number, the Womersley number is a dimensionless measure of the ratio between inertial and viscous forces. It can also be thought of as the ratio of the local acceleration to the viscous forces. Equation (3.18) is a definition of the Womersley number in terms of the vessel diameter (d, cm), density, frequency related to heart rate (ω, sec^{-1}), and dynamic viscosity. The Womersley number ranges from 10^{-3} in capillaries to 18.0 in the ascending aorta in the human circulation [7]. The Womersley number is also a parameter used to predict turbulence in a flow. In pulsatile flow, higher Reynolds numbers can exist without turbulence [6].

$$\alpha = \frac{d}{2}\sqrt{\frac{\rho\omega}{\mu}} \tag{3.18}$$

Flow morphologies

Boundary layer flow
The flow over a flat plate is a geometry of considerable interest in fluid mechanics. In a steady unidirectional freestream flow over an infinite flat plate aligned in the flow direction, there is a predictable boundary layer around the plate. The perpendicular distance it takes for the velocity to assume 99% of the freestream value is the thickness of the boundary layer. This is shown in Fig. 3.4.

No slip condition
To understand boundary layers, it is first necessary to study the boundary conditions associated with such

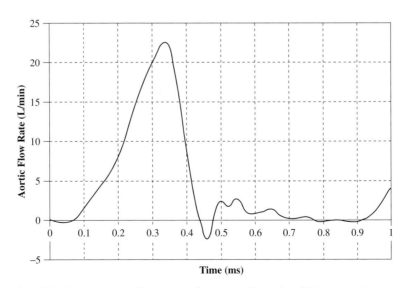

Figure 3.3 Changes in aortic flow rate over human cardiac cycle at 60 beats per min.

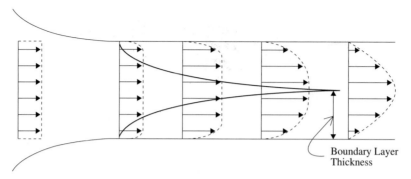

Figure 3.4 Entrance effect in steady, laminar, straight pipe flow.

a flow. There are two boundary conditions associated with flow over a flat plate. First, the velocity is zero at the surface of the plate and second, the velocity is equal to the freestream value at an infinite distance from the plate. The zero velocity constraint on the plate is called the no slip condition.

Straight pipe flow

Entrance flow

In cardiovascular studies, flow over a flat plate is not encountered. But by circularizing the flat plate into a pipe, the principles of boundary layer flow are still applicable. Because of the vascular nature of the circulatory system, pipe flow is of keen interest. However, rather than considering all of the factors of distensible, semi-permeable, curved, and branched walls, it is first useful to approximate vessels as a straight, rigid, circular pipe.

Freestream flow is a steady, uniform, and parallel flow without obstruction as depicted on the left side of Fig. 3.4. When a freestream flow encounters a straight pipe with circular cross section, an entrance flow phenomenon in the form of boundary layers is observed on the inner wall because of shear stresses encountered between the fluid and the walls.

Fully developed flow

Eventually, the boundary layers reach each other and the flow assumes a parabolic velocity profile. The velocity profile is a result of a balance between viscous forces by the wall and inertial forces of the fluid. When the velocity profile in pipe flow is parabolic, it is called fully developed flow because the velocity pro-

file no longer changes so long as the geometry of the pipe is unchanged and flow is steady.

Entrance length The length of the pipe required for a fully developed flow is referred to as the entrance length. Entrance length depends on whether the flow is laminar or turbulent. It should be noted that the entrance length for arteries is about 3 m [7]. Therefore, blood flow is not likely to be fully developed at any point in the body. Nevertheless, *in vitro* experiments frequently use a fully developed flow assumption because the true velocity profile is unknown and because the velocity profile, while not perfectly parabolic, is 90% parabolic 10 diameters downstream of entrance flow [7].

Laminar velocity profile The laminar velocity profile in fully developed flow is a function of the maximum velocity at the centerline (u_{max}, cm/sec), the radial location (r, cm), and the radius of the vessel (R, cm) as shown in Eq. (3.19).

$$\frac{u}{u_{max}} = 1 - \left(\frac{r}{R}\right)^2 \qquad (3.19)$$

The maximum velocity can be shown to be approximately equal to twice the average velocity across the cross section.

Turbulent velocity profile When turbulent flow develops, it can no longer be assumed that the fully developed flow in a pipe is parabolic in profile. Since turbulence induces radial velocity fluctuations, the centerline velocity decreases and the velocity profile becomes more uniform. The velocity gradient at the wall, and therefore also the wall shear stress, increases because of the resulting flattened profile. If turbulent flow exists, the velocity profile must be determined by the empirical formula in Eq. (3.20) [8].

$$\frac{u}{u_{max}} = \left(1 - \frac{r}{R}\right)^{\frac{1}{n}} \qquad (3.20)$$

Here, $n = 6$ when $Re = 4 \times 10^3$, $n = 7$ when $Re = 100 \times 10^3$, and $n = 10$ when $Re = 3240 \times 10^3$ [8]. Therefore, the velocity profile becomes flatter as Reynolds number increases.

Flow rate
Velocity profiles are significant in blood flow because they can be used to calculate volumetric flow rate (Q, cm^3/sec). Equation (3.21) defines volumetric flow rate over an area (A, cm^2).

$$Q = \int_{section} u \, dA \qquad (3.21)$$

Note that Eq. (3.21) can be applied to a cross section of any shape so long as the velocity profile across the area is known. Equation (3.22) specifically applies to a pipe taken at a circular cross section, where $r = 0$ (cm) at the center of the pipe and $r = R$ (cm) at the pipe wall.

$$Q = 2\pi \int_0^R ur \, dr \qquad (3.22)$$

The calculation of volumetric flow rate makes it possible to derive a relation between pressure and flow in a straight pipe.

Cardiac output Volumetric flow rate makes it possible to calculate the volume of blood pumped in one cardiac cycle (CC, sec), or the stroke volume (SV, cm^3), as shown in Eq. (3.23). With the stroke volume, cardiac output (CO, cm^3/sec) can be computed by taking the product of the stroke volume and the frequency related to heart rate (ω, sec^{-1}), as in Eq. (3.24), assuming a constant heart rate.

Convenient points of measurement for stroke volume are adjacent to heart valves where the cross-sectional areas can be assessed. Doppler echocardiography is used to obtain velocity and cross-sectional area to noninvasively compute the cardiac output.

$$SV = \int_0^{CC} Q \, dt \qquad (3.23)$$

$$CO = SV \times \omega \qquad (3.24)$$

More generally, cardiac output can be calculated at any point in the circulatory system before major branching such as the aorta or the main pulmonary artery. For a pipe, the cross-sectional area and the average velocity across the cross section are required for volumetric flow rate. If the velocity profile is uniform, the uniform velocity is the average velocity. The average velocity can be simply found in the case of a parabolic profile as well. However, in clinical practice, determination of an average velocity is more difficult because the velocity profile is not known. The estimation of the average velocity normally causes errors with *in vitro* cardiac output calculations.

Poiseuille flow
When a flow becomes fully developed, the velocity profile no longer changes. Therefore, as a particle moves down a pipe with fully developed steady flow, it no longer experiences transient or convective acceleration. Poiseuille flow describes how a pressure gradient can cause flow. Poiseuille's Law is derived from the Navier–Stokes equations, where material acceleration and body forces are neglected. Equation (3.25) relates the higher upstream and lower downstream pressure (P_1 and P_2, $dyne/cm^2$ or $g/(cm\,sec^2)$) to viscosity, downstream distance (x, cm), volumetric flow rate, and diameter (d, cm).

$$P_1 - P_2 = \frac{128\mu x Q}{\pi d^4} \qquad (3.25)$$

The assumptions of Poiseuille flow are as follows:
1 Incompressible, Newtonian fluid
2 Steady, laminar flow
3 Straight pipe with constant circular cross section
4 Fully developed velocity profile
5 No body forces
6 No slip condition
7 Rigid walls

For the Reynolds number or Womersley number in a straight pipe flow, the characteristic velocity is the average velocity and the characteristic length is taken as the diameter. In pipe flow, a Reynolds number over 2300 usually indicates turbulence [9]. In the ascending aorta where flow is unsteady, the critical peak flow Reynolds number for transition has been found to be about 8000 [9]. Therefore, under normal physiologic flow conditions, turbulence is not encountered in the human circulation. However, if it does exist, turbulence is more likely encountered in deceleration because flow acceleration is more stable than flow deceleration [9].

Another noteworthy consideration is that Poiseuille flow is based on a rigid pipe model. Having distensible vessels causes errors of roughly 10% in the Poiseuille equation [6]. Therefore, care must be taken to realize that the Poiseuille equation is more appropriate for arterial flow and that venous flow measurements must be considered to have greater error because they have six times greater distensibility. For most cardiovascular flows, especially those in smaller vessels, the Poiseuille equation overestimates flow rate [6].

Stenotic flow

A stenosis, where the cross-sectional area decreases abnormally along a short distance, is sometimes observed in cardiovascular flows. This is seen particularly in congenital heart disease with aortic coarctation, tricuspid valve stenosis, and pulmonary artery stenosis. With such conditions, flow parameters change dramatically.

Geometry
Throat Figure 3.5 shows the various components of a stenosis. The local minimum in cross-sectional area is referred to as the throat. The size and smoothness of the throat determine the degree of stenosis. In gradual stenotic flows, the cross-sectional area can decrease smoothly to reach a minimum and then increase again slowly. In such a flow, fluid properties do not change radically. On the other hand, the cross-sectional area can change more suddenly. Subsequently, there would be more pronounced flow disruption, which contributes greatly to viscous losses.

Vena contracta Although the vessel diameter at the throat is a minimum, it is often not the site where flow parameters are the minimum or maximum. When inertial forces are substantial, fluid has difficulty turning sharp corners. The fluid cannot turn to meet the boundary wall; rather, it continues to converge past the throat. In such a case, the effective minimum area is further downstream. The location of effective minimum area is known as the vena contracta.

Jet flow Downstream of a major stenosis, there is a region of high velocity that is described as jet flow. Jet flow is characterized by a diminishing potential core that shears with and entrains a slower fluid. For jet flow, the characteristic length for Reynolds number or Womersley number is the throat diameter. The characteristic velocity is the centerline velocity at the throat. Transition in a steady jet occurs at a Reynolds number of approximately 1000 and fully turbulent flow appears at 3000 [9].

Stenotic valve flow Blood traveling through a pathological valve can exhibit stenotic flow. The high pressure difference across the valve creates a large jet. The jet causes an increase in velocity and a compensating decrease in pressure across the valve. In normal valves, the ejection phase comprises the time when the valve is open to fluid passing though it. The closed phase is when there is no fluid passage because the valve is closed. In leaking valves the closed phase may still pass fluid because of regurgitant jets that push fluid backward through the valve. Stenotic valves have a decreased valve area that amplifies convective acceleration and pressure drop. Since the valve is the throat, the valve area is a determinant in the extent of the stenosis.

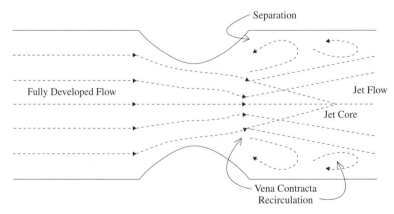

Figure 3.5 Flow structure as fully developed, steady, laminar flow encounters a stenosis.

Flow structures

Separation Thus far, boundary layers have developed while attached to the boundary wall. However, the boundary layer may separate past a stenosis because of a reversal of flow at the boundary surface. Figure 3.5 illustrates flow separation downstream of a stenosis. The inertial force of the fluid causes separation downstream of a stenosis.

Separation is created by an adverse pressure gradient that causes the flow to turn back on itself. An adverse pressure gradient is a pressure gradient against the direction of flow. Adverse pressure gradients can be geometric or temporal. Geometric adverse pressure gradients are usually present where the cross-sectional area increases, causing velocity to decrease by necessity of the continuity equation. An example of a temporal adverse pressure gradient is present when the pulsatility of blood flow causes the velocity to decrease in the cardiac cycle. The decrease in velocity causes an adverse pressure gradient.

Vorticity When the velocity direction is shifted such as in boundary layer separation, rotational flow becomes an issue. Vorticity can be described as the amount of flow rotation with respect to an axis at the point of interrogation. An example of vortex regions in hemodynamics would be the near-wall flow downstream of a stenosis, as shown in Fig. 3.5. In the cardiovascular system, vorticity can be encountered downstream of a valve or the right ventricular outflow tract.

Recirculation Vorticity creates a region of recirculating flow that can cause high particle residence times and oscillatory shear stresses. Recirculatory Flow is shown in Fig. 3.5 where flow separation and rotational flow appears. Such effects are known to be correlated with pathological wall shear stresses and atherosclerosis.

Flow parameters

Valve Area The conservation of mass can be used to provide an approximation of valve area. Consider a generalized control volume that has one inflow at Point 1 and one outflow at Point 2 as shown in Fig. 3.6. The conservation of mass simplifies greatly as shown in Eq. (3.26). Here A is the cross-sectional area (cm^2). Points 1 and 2 must be taken along a volume that has no other inflows or outflows.

$$A_1 u_1 = A_2 u_2 \tag{3.26}$$

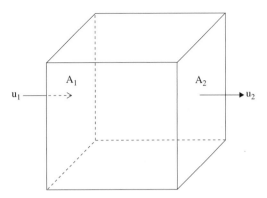

Figure 3.6 Control volume approach to determine conservation of mass for incompressible flow.

Let Point 1 be a velocity upstream and Point 2 be the vena contracta. By rewriting the simplified continuity equation integrated over systole as in Eq. (3.27), the cross-sectional area at vena contracta can be determined.

$$A_2 = \int_{systole} \frac{u_1(t)}{u_2(t)} A_1 dt \tag{3.27}$$

Regurgitant flow rate In heart valve insufficiency, it is important to quantify the regurgitant flow. Regurgitant flow rate is a measure of retrograde flow in the cardiac cycle. It is equal to the sum of the backward flow rate while the valve is closing and the leakage flow rate while the valve is closed. Regurgitant jets are small orifice flows and can be analyzed in many of the same ways to determine retrograde flow rates.

Pressure recovery In steady pipe flow with decreasing cross section, velocity increases and pressure decreases in accordance with the Bernoulli equation. When the cross-sectional area of the pipe increases again past the throat, some of the velocity and pressure is restored. However, viscous losses in the stenosis prevent the velocity and, more severely, the pressure from achieving their original values at the same cross-sectional area. The pressure increase from the throat to the point of restored cross-sectional area is called pressure recovery. By comparing the recovered pressure to the pressure drop across the stenosis, it is possible to compute the percentage of pressure energy that is lost and recovered with the stenosis. In general, flow with smaller or smoother stenoses have superior pressure recovery.

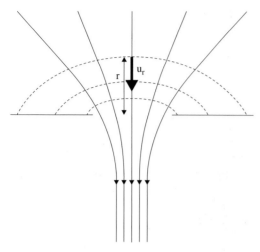

Figure 3.7 Flow through an orifice with proximal isovelocity surface area variables and isovelocity contours.

Proximal isovelocity surface area The proximal isovelocity surface area (PISA) technique may be utilized to measure volumetric flow rates through septal defects, fenestrations, and regurgitant valves. If an orifice is circular, there is a series of concentric hemispheric isovelocity contours upstream of the flow as the fluid accelerates toward the orifice as indicated in Fig. 3.7. If a control volume is analyzed that has boundaries coincident with the orifice, streamlines, and the isovelocity contour, the flow rate across the orifice can be calculated. As depicted mathematically in Eq. (3.28), the flow rate is the product of the measured velocity at the contour and the surface area of the hemispheric contour. Here, Q_o is the flow rate at the orifice (cm^3/sec), u_r is the radial velocity perpendicular to the isovelocity surface (cm/sec), and r is the radial distance from the orifice at which the velocity is measured (cm).

$$Q_o = \left(4\pi r^2\right) u_r \tag{3.28}$$

Note that PISA requires the isovelocity contours to be hemispherical around the orifice. Deviations from the hemispherical assumption introduce errors in flow measurements.

Pulmonary to systemic flow ratio The pulmonary to systemic blood flow ratio (Q_p/Q_s) is a measure of the degree of shunting in the heart. The pulmonary flow, which is measured at the tricuspid or pulmonary valves, is normally approximately equal to the systemic flow, which is measured at the mitral or aortic valves [10].

Curved pipe flow

In curved pipe flow, the flow no longer solely depends on downstream distance and radial location. Accordingly, the flow becomes highly three-dimensional. The flow through a curved tube depends on the amount of curvature, the Reynolds number, and the inlet flow profile.

Dean number

The Dean number (*De*) is a useful, dimensionless means of measuring the effects of curvature. It also incorporates the effects of the Reynolds number as indicated in Eq. (3.29). For a given curvature, higher Reynolds numbers are possible before transition to turbulence [7].

$$De = Re\sqrt{\frac{r_{\text{cross-section}}}{r_{\text{curvature}}}} \tag{3.29}$$

Aortic arch

The aortic arch is a good example of curvature in the cardiovascular system. The complexity of flow in the aortic arch can be understood by considering the differences in curved flow between a fully developed and a uniform profile. With a parabolic profile such as in Fig. 3.8, inertial or centrifugal force causes the profile to be shifted toward the outer wall. Since

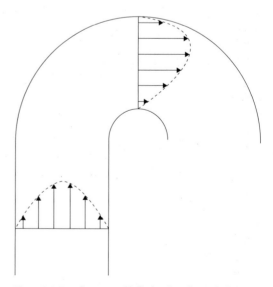

Figure 3.8 Development of fully developed, steady, laminar velocity profile around a curved pipe.

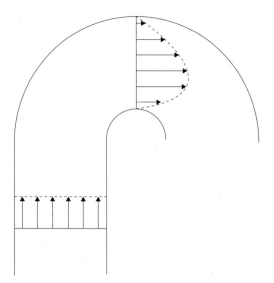

Figure 3.9 Development of flat velocity profile around a curved pipe.

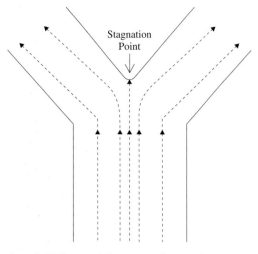

Figure 3.10 Flow in a bifurcation with stagnation point streamline indicated.

the fluid is skewed toward the outer wall, there is a radial flow component that develops in the pipe. Figure 3.9 shows that in a uniform profile, centripetal force causes the profile to be skewed toward the inner wall [7]. However, since the centripetal effect is combined with that observed in a flow with a fully developed profile, the net effect is that there are two counter-rotating helices [7].

The flow profile in the ascending aorta is relatively flat. So, while blood is ascending, it favors the inner wall, but when the blood arrives at the arch the flow profile shifts to the outer wall [6]. Because of such a shift, there is generally a separation region on the inner wall of the descending aorta.

Divided pipe flow

Bifurcations

Bifurcations such as in Fig. 3.10 are present when a larger vessel splits into two vessels of similar cross section [6]. Well-explored examples of bifurcations include the carotid artery and the pulmonary arteries.

Bifurcations create regions of varying wall shear stress. Inner walls have high shear stresses while outer walls have low shear stresses [7]. In bifurcations, the cross-sectional area usually increases at the point of branching [6]. Therefore, the flow decelerates and it is more stable as it branches into other vessels.

However, there are usually vortical regions that develop in the bifurcation. When flow impinges on the wall joining the smaller vessels, usually small vortices form. Near the outer walls, the flow is generally more uniform [6].

Pulsatile flow affects flow structures in bifurcations. The deceleration of diastole creates recirculation in the bifurcation that does not exist during systole.

Branches

Branches are present when there is one major vessel from which a smaller vessel branches off such as the coronary arteries off the ascending aorta or the renal arteries off the descending aorta.

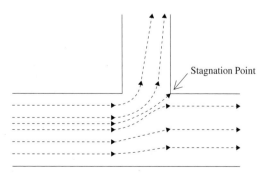

Figure 3.11 Flow in a branch where the stagnation point streamline is indicated.

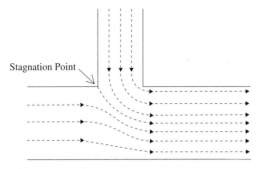

Figure 3.12 Flow in an end-to-side anastomosis with stagnation point streamline indicated.

Branches are more pronounced versions of bifurcations, as illustrated in Fig. 3.11. The outer walls generally have separation and recirculation. There are normally small eddies that form on the outer wall of the main vessel. Branches also have areas of varying wall shear stress. In general, the angle of branching has strong implications on the flow structure [7].

Anastomoses
End-to-side anastomoses such as the one shown in Fig 3.12 are uncommon in the native arterial system since it is a connection where a smaller flow joins a larger vessel. Nevertheless, surgical repairs can create such environments, such as in a coronary artery bypass graft. The coronary bypass is a highly researched end-to-side anastomosis configuration. More applicable to congenital heart disease is the modified Blalock–Taussig shunt, which is a connection between the subclavian artery and the pulmonary artery. The bidirectional Glenn shunt is also an end-to-side anastomosis that involves severing the superior vena cava and reattaching the proximal side to the right pulmonary artery to reroute superior vena caval flow around the right heart. In both the modified Blalock–Taussig and the bidirectional Glenn shunts, flow structure issues are similar to those in bifurcations and branches, where there is varying wall shear stress and disturbed flow. Like branches, the angle of the anastomosis greatly impacts the flow. A smaller angle between the inflows would yield a smoother flow convergence.

Total cavopulmonary connection
An especially complex branching flow is the total cavopulmonary connection (TCPC), where the streams from the superior and inferior vena cavae impinge and exit out to the left and right pulmonary arteries. The TCPC is the center of present research because of its unique configuration of two inflows and two outflows. A flow visualization image of a simplified TCPC geometry is shown in Fig. 3.13. There is energy loss and a highly vortical region associated with the TCPC.

Yoganathan *et al.* have found that there are less energy losses when there is an offset distance between the superior and inferior vena cavae. When there is an offset, the caval flows impinge on opposite walls [11]. Thus, there are stagnation regions at the points of impingement and a vortex in the connection. There are also less energy losses when the connections are flared [12].

Secondary flow Secondary flow within a pipe is radially and tangentially oriented and creates a helical swirling effect. This can be seen qualitatively in Fig. 3.13. The flow is largely secondary downstream of the TCPC. In fact, in curved flows and dividing flows there is also a great deal of secondary flow because of the three-dimensional nature of the vessel.

Energy loss Control volume. Energy loss can be estimated by control volume analysis as shown in Eq. (3.30), which requires that pressures and flow rates are known for each of the inflows and outflows. Here, $\dot{E}_{\text{loss}}$ is the energy loss per unit time (erg/sec or g sec^{3}cm^2/sec^3), n is a direction normal to the control surface (CS), and S is an area corresponding to the control surface (cm^2).

$$\dot{E}_{\text{loss}} = - \oiint_{\text{CS}} \left[P + \frac{1}{2} \rho u_i u_i \right] u_j n_j \mathrm{d}S \qquad (3.30)$$

Such an analysis, while unappealing for *in vivo* applications because of invasive pressure measurements, is useful for *in vitro* experimentation because only four interrogation points are necessary. Therefore, control volume estimation of energy loss can be used to compare relative efficiencies of two TCPC *in vitro* models.

Viscous dissipation. The viscous dissipation method is an alternate form of energy loss analysis that requires whole field velocity information within the studied geometry as shown in Eqs. (3.31)

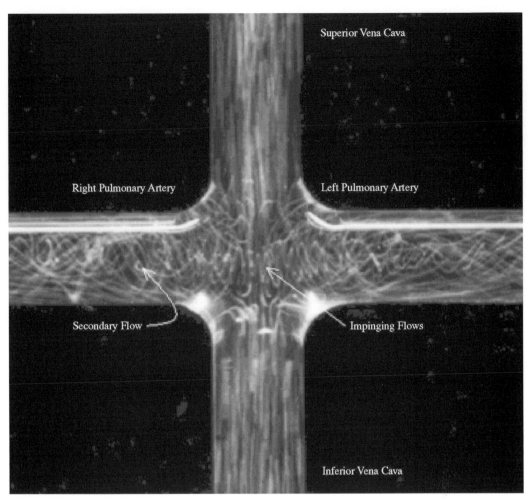

Figure 3.13 40 μm particle flow visualization through a glass model of a simplified total cavopulmonary connection at a cardiac output of 4 L/min. Impinging caval flows and helical secondary flows are shown.

and (3.32). In these equations, ϕ is the dissipation function (sec^{-2}), x is the directional axis (cm), $\dot{E}_{loss}$ is the energy loss per unit time (erg/sec or g sec^{3}cm^2/sec^3), and V is the volume (cm^3) corresponding to the control volume (CV).

$$\phi = \frac{1}{2}\left(\frac{\partial u_i}{\partial x_j} + \frac{\partial u_j}{\partial x_i}\right)^2 \qquad (3.31)$$

$$\dot{E}_{loss} = \mu \iiint_{CV} \phi \, dV \qquad (3.32)$$

Magnetic resonance imaging can provide velocity data over the scanned area to be used in viscous dissipation analysis. This method makes *in vivo* estimation of energy loss a possibility. In addition, particle image velocimetry is an *in vitro* experimentation technique that provides whole field velocity data as well, which makes viscous dissipation analysis possible. Finally computational fluid dynamics (CFD) can yield a full velocity and pressure fields. Therefore, CFD has been a method of verifying *in vivo* estimation and *in vitro* experimentation because of its ability to utilize both energy loss methods.

Conclusion

This chapter presented fluid dynamics in the context of fluid properties, conservation equations, and commonly encountered flow geometries in the cardiovascular system. Analysis included a straight rigid tube with steady flow, and assumptions were relaxed to make additional considerations for pulsatile flow in changing geometries. Qualitative flow concepts such as stagnation, recirculation, and separation were addressed as well as quantitative parameters such as cardiac output, valve area, pressure drop, and energy loss. If a more comprehensive study of fluid mechanics is desired, the reader is encouraged to examine texts by Schlichting or White [8,13]. For supplementary sources on biofluids, references by Fung, Caro, or Nichols are recommended [5,14,15]. The reader is encouraged to explore additional materials that address specific flow regimes as required.

Nomenclature

a	Transient acceleration (cm/sec^2)
A	Area (cm^2)
CC	Cardiac cycle (sec)
CO	Cardiac output (cm^3/sec)
De	Dean number
$\dot{E}_{loss}$	Power loss (erg/sec or g sec^{3}cm^2/sec^3)
$\vec{f}$	Body force (cm/sec^2)
$\vec{g}$	Gravitational acceleration (cm/sec^2)
h	Height (cm)
i, j	Directional index
I	Turbulence intensity
n	Empirical constant, normal direction
P	Pressure (dyne/cm^2 or g/(cm sec^2)
Q	Volumetric flow rate (cm^3/sec)
Q_o	Volumetric flow rate through orifice (cm^3/sec)
Q_p	Pulmonary flow rate (cm^3/sec)
Q_s	Systemic flow rate (cm^3/sec)
r	Radial location (cm)
$r_{cross-section}$	Cross-sectional radius (cm)
$r_{curvature}$	Radius of curvature (cm)
R	Radius (cm)
$R_{viscous}$	Viscous loss (dyne/cm^3 or g/(cm^2 sec^2)
Re	Reynolds number
s	Distance along streamline (cm)
S	Control surface (cm^2)

SV	Stroke volume (cm^3)
t	Time (sec)
$\vec{T}$	Stress (dyne/cm^2 or g/(cm sec^2)
u	Velocity (cm/sec)
$\bar{u}$	Mean velocity (cm/sec)
u'	Fluctuating velocity (cm/sec)
u_{max}	Centerline maximum velocity (cm/sec)
u_r	Radial velocity perpendicular to isovelocity surface (cm/sec)
u_{RMS}	Root-mean-square velocity (cm/sec)
V	Control volume (cm^3)
x, y, z	Cartesian coordinate (cm)
x	Length (cm)
α	Womersley number
ε	Shear strain rate (sec^{-1})
ϕ	Dissipation function (sec^{-2})
μ	Dynamic viscosity (cP or g/(cm sec)
ρ	Density (g/cm^3)
τ	Shear stress (dyne/cm^2 or g/(cm sec^2)
$\tau_{turbulent}$	Turbulent (Reynolds) shear stress (dyne/cm^2 or g/ (cm sec^2)
τ_{wall}	Wall shear stress (dyne/cm^2 or g/ (cm sec^2)
ω	Frequency related to heart rate (sec^{-1})

References

1. Otto CM. Textbook of Clinical Echocardiography, 2nd edn. Saunders, Philadelphia, PA, 2000.
2. Lanzer P, Topol EJ. Panvascular Medicine. Springer, Berlin, New York, 2002.
3. Carabello, BA, Grossman, W. Calculation of stenotic valve orifice area. In: Grossman W, Baim DS, eds., Cardiac Catheterization, Angiography, and Intervention. Williams & Wilkins, Baltimore, MD, p. xvi, 879, 1996.
4. Giddens DP, Zarins CK, Glagov S. The role of fluid mechanics in the localization and detection of atherosclerosis. J Biomech Eng 1993; 115(4B): 588–594.
5. Nichols WW, O'Rourke MF, McDonald, DA. Mcdonald's Blood Flow in Arteries: Theoretic, Experimental and Clinical Principles, 3rd edn. E. Arnold, London, 1990.

6. Weyman AE. Principles of flow. In: Weyman AE, ed., Principles and Practice of Echocardiography. Lea & Febiger, Philadelphia, PA, p. xvii, 1335, 1994.

7. Yoganathan AP, Chatzimavroudis GP, Hemodynamics. In: Lanzer P, Topol EJ, eds., Panvascular Medicine, Springer, Berlin, p. xv, 1941, 2002.

8. Schlichting H. Boundary-Layer Theory, 7th edn. McGraw-Hill, New York, 1979.

9. Yoganathan AP, Travis BR. Fluid dynamics of prosthetic valves. In: Otto CM, ed., Textbook of Clinical Echocardiography. Saunders, Philadelphia, PA, p. xiv, 443, 2000.

10. Chapman JV. Blood flow measurement by Doppler ultrasound. In: Chapman JV, Sutherland GR, eds., The Noninvasive Evaluation of Hemodynamics in Congenital Heart Disease: Doppler Ultrasound Applications in the Adult and Pediatric Patient with Congenital Heart Disease. Kluwer Academic Publishers, Dordrecht, Boston, p. xv, 354, 1990.

11. Ensley AE, Ramuzat A, Healy TM, *et al.* Fluid mechanic assessment of the total cavopulmonary connection using magnetic resonance phase velocity mapping and digital particle image velocimetry. Ann Biomed Eng 2000; 28(10): 1172–1183.

12. Ensley AE, Lynch P, Chatzimavroudis GP, *et al.* Toward designing the optimal total cavopulmonary connection: An in vitro study. Ann Thorac Surg 1999; 68(4): 1384–1390.

13. White FM. Viscous Fluid Flow, 2nd edn. McGraw-Hill, New York, 1991.

14. Fung YC. Biomechanics: Circulation, 2nd edn. Springer, New York, 1997.

15. Caro CG. The Mechanics of the Circulation. Oxford University Press, Oxford, New York, 1978.

Further Reading

Anderson JD. Modern Compressible Flow: With Historical Perspective, 2nd edn. McGraw-Hill, New York, 1990.

Bassiouny HS, White S, Glagov S, *et al.* Anastomotic intimal hyperplasia: Mechanical injury or flow induced. J Vasc Surg 1992; 15(4):708–716; discussion 716–717.

Fifer MA, Grossman W. Measurement of ventricular volumes, ejection fraction, mass, wall stress, and regional wall motion. In: Grossman W, Baim DS, eds., Cardiac Catheterization, Angiography, and Intervention. Williams & Wilkins, Baltimore, MD, 1996.

Gersony WM, Rosenbaum, MS. Single ventricle. In: Gersony WM, Rosenbaum MS, eds., Congenital Heart Disease in Adults. McGraw-Hill, New York, London, p. 300, 2001.

Grossman W. Shunt detection and measurement. In: Grossman W, Baim DS, eds., Cardiac Catheterization, Angiography, and Intervention. Williams & Wilkins, Baltimore, MD, 1996.

Grossman W. Pressure measurement. In: Grossman W, Baim DS, eds., Cardiac Catheterization, Angiography, and Intervention. Williams & Wilkins, Baltimore, MD, 1996.

Grossman W. Clinical measurement of vascular resistance and assessment of vasodilator drugs. In: Grossman W, Baim DS, eds., Cardiac Catheterization, Angiography, and Intervention. Williams & Wilkins, Baltimore, MD, 1996.

Grossman W. Blood flow measurement: The cardiac output. In: Grossman W, Baim DS, eds., Cardiac Catheterization, Angiography, and Intervention. Williams & Wilkins, Baltimore, MD, 1996.

Hatle L, Angelsen B, Physics of blood flow. In: Hatle L, Angelsen, B, eds., Doppler Ultrasound in Cardiology : Physical Principles and Clinical Applications. Lea & Febiger, Philadelphia, PA, p. xiii, 331, 1985.

Huhta J. Doppler ultrasound assessment of blood flow in the chest. In: Huhta J, ed., Pediatric Imaging/Doppler Ultrasound of the Chest: Extracardiac Diagnosis. Lea & Febiger, Philadelphia, PA, p. xiii, 225, 1986.

Keane JF, Lock JE. Hemodynamic evaluation of congenital heart disease. In: Lock JE, Keane JF, Perry SB, eds., Diagnostic and Interventional Catheterization in Congenital Heart Disease. Kluwer Academic Publishers, Boston, MA, p. xix, 377, 2000.

Kenner T. Physiology of circulation. In: Dalla Volta S, Bayés de Luna A, Braunwald E, eds., Cardiology. McGraw-Hill International (UK), London, New York. p. xv, 834, I-38, [8] of plates, 1999.

Linker DT. Practical Echocardiography of Congenital Heart Disease: From Fetus to Adult. Churchill Livingstone, New York, 2001.

Marshall SA, Weyman, AE, Doppler estimation of volumetric flow. In: Weyman AE, ed., Principles and Practice of Echocardiography. Lea & Febiger, Philadelphia, PA, p. xvii, 1335, 1994.

Rudolph AM. Congenital Diseases of the Heart: Clinical-Physiological Considerations, 2nd edn (updated). Futura Publishing Co., Armonk, NY, 2001.

Skjaerpe T, Hegrenaes L, Ihlen H. Cardiac output. In: Hatle L, Angelsen B, eds., Doppler Ultrasound in Cardiology: Physical Principles and Clinical Applications. Lea & Febiger, Philadelphia, PA, p. xiii, 331, 1985.

Snider AR, Serwer GA, Ritter SB. Echocardiography in Pediatric Heart Disease, 2nd edn. Mosby, St. Louis, 1997.

Sugawara M. Blood Flow in the Heart and Large Vessels. Springer-Verlag, Tokyo, 1989.

Thomas JD, Davidoff R, Cape EG. Fluid dynamics of regurgitant jets and their imaging by color doppler. In: Weyman AE, ed., Principles and Practice of Echocardiography, Lea & Febiger, Philadelphia, PA, p. xvii, 1335, 1994.

CHAPTER 4

History and Physical Examination

Amy H. Schultz, MD & Mark A. Fogel, MD

History and physical examination

The history and physical examination (H&P) is the entry point of patients into the evaluative process. A thorough history generates a differential diagnosis and is the context in which all subsequent tests are interpreted. The physical examination can be considered the first diagnostic test applied and has many desirable attributes: it poses essentially no risk, causes minimal discomfort, involves no radiation, is performed quickly, is interpreted immediately and, given that the patient has already presented to the physician for evaluation, adds no cost.

How accurate is H&P for the evaluation of ventricular function and blood flow in congenital heart disease? Experience and skill of the examiner are undoubtedly important. Several studies have examined this question in children presenting to a pediatric cardiologist for evaluation of a heart murmur. Most have demonstrated the sensitivity of H&P for identification of a pathologic murmur to be 92–96% and the specificity to be 93–95% [1,2], although one study found a sensitivity of 68% [3]. Echocardiography has been shown to provide valuable clarification of the diagnosis in patients thought, by a pediatric cardiologist, to have a pathologic murmur [2]. Thus, the current practice of pediatric cardiologists to screen patients with murmurs by H&P with selective use of echocardiography in those with pathologic findings is justified. However, H&P may be less reliable for detecting critical heart disease in the early stage[4,5]. H&P is also used to follow the patient with an established diagnosis over time. Although less objective data exists, it seems that a skillful practitioner can often spare the patient time, discomfort and expense of other tests by effective use of H&P.

Little data is available describing the effectiveness of H&P for the evaluation of ventricular function in patients with congenital heart disease. Most available studies relate H&P to the evaluation of left ventricular dysfunction in adults with ischemic or dilated cardiomyopathy. In this context, H&P is more reliable for evaluation of acute heart failure than chronic heart failure [6,7], suggesting that when ventricular function needs to be evaluated over time, the H&P should be supplemented by imaging studies.

The discussion that follows assumes an understanding of the general principles and techniques of H&P and focuses on aspects particularly relevant to ventricular function and blood flow in congenital heart disease. The reader is referred to more general textbooks of Pediatrics, Cardiology, or physical examination for discussion of more fundamental principles. For the reader who desires a more in depth discussion of physical findings in specific lesions, particular references are highly recommended [8,9].

The history

Many patients with congenital heart disease are asymptomatic and come to attention due to abnormal physical findings noted on a routine examination. However, among those who do have symptoms, historical features tend to cluster into one of the patterns presented below.

History must be solicited and interpreted in the context of the patient's age. When considering the presentation of congenital heart disease, children can be broken down into three age groups: neonates, young infants and those beyond early infancy. The overwhelming majority of complex congenital lesions will be diagnosed in neonates. Lesions which become manifest as pulmonary vascular resistance falls, such as ventricular septal defect (VSD) and atrioventricular canal defect, typically present in neonates or in early infancy. Beyond early infancy, the likelihood of unrecognized congenital heart disease becomes progressively lower with age. In a series of children referred to a pediatric cardiology practice for evaluation of a murmur, the prevalence of pathologic murmur was 57% in children less than 1 year of age and 18% in those over 1 year of age [1]. Lesions such as atrial septal defect (ASD), valvar aortic stenosis (AS), valvar pulmonary stenosis (PS), coarctation, and the rare more complex lesion may surface at this age. Acquired heart disease, including cardiomyopathies, may present at any age.

Heart failure can arise from either ventricular dysfunction or a large left to right shunt, both of which result in similar historical features at a given age. However, a history consistent with heart failure is very different in different age groups. Infants should normally grow rapidly and feeding represents significant exertion in this age group. Therefore, an infant with heart failure takes a long time to feed, pauses due to breathlessness between sucks, may be diaphoretic while feeding, and fails to gain weight. Position does not usually affect dyspnea in infants. Heart failure will lead to dyspnea with exertion and exercise intolerance in toddlers and young children, but these symptoms can be difficult to gauge. The patient rarely voices complaints, so reliance on parental observation is necessary. The patient may self-limit activity or may appear amazingly active despite significant heart disease, since few activities at this age require sustained physical exertion. It is often helpful to have parents compare the child's activity level to that of peers or siblings. The parents may comment on excessive sleeping or poor weight gain. Dyspnea with standard activities such as climbing a flight of stairs provides another useful benchmark. Older children and teenagers are able to provide more subjective reports of dyspnea with exertion, orthopnea, and exercise intolerance. They, too, may self-limit their activities or be reluctant to admit symptoms, so it is helpful to ask how well they keep up with their peers in structured activities such as gym class.

Cardiovascular collapse at several days of age indicates congenital heart disease with ductal-dependent systemic blood flow until proven otherwise and should prompt initiation of prostaglandin therapy. The differential diagnosis would also include sepsis and metabolic disorders, so historical features suggestive of these etiologies should be explored and presumptive therapy for infection should be initiated.

Cyanosis must reflect true arterial desaturation to be attributable to heart disease and therefore should be noted centrally, in the lips and tongue. Peripheral vasoconstriction due to cold exposure can result in a blue discoloration of the extremities without arterial desaturation. Arterial desaturation can be difficult to see [10], so if there is any question of cyanosis, pulse oximetry should be performed. The classic presentation of cyanotic congenital heart disease is cyanosis in the absence of respiratory distress. The presence of respiratory symptoms raises the likelihood of a pulmonary etiology, but exceptions should be noted. Vascular rings can cause stridor or choking and coughing with feeding. In some neonates with critical congenital heart disease, cyanosis and respiratory distress do coexist, the latter resulting from metabolic acidosis or pulmonary congestion. Intermittent cyanosis, especially with agitation, suggests intermittent right to left shunting, such as may occur with Tetralogy of Fallot. Profound cyanosis from the moment of delivery which does not respond to the usual ventilatory maneuvers strongly suggests congenital heart disease with obstruction to pulmonary venous return or Transposition of the Great Arteries with poor mixing of systemic and pulmonary venous return.

Syncope or chest pain. Overall, these are common and usually benign complaints in the pediatric population. However, *syncope during exertion* or true *angina* raises entirely different specters and underscores the importance of defining the circumstances and characteristics of the complaint in detail. Concerning features of syncope include occurrence at the peak of exercise (rather than just after the conclusion of exercise), prolonged loss of consciousness, young age, and absence of vasodepressor triggers and premonitory symptoms. Older children can describe angina as having the characteristic pressure quality and radiation to the arm or neck, while in infants it may be noted merely as unexplained irritability, particularly with or after feeding. The mechanistic differential diagnosis of these two complaints includes inadequate myocardial perfusion or inability to augment cardiac output, such as seen in severe pulmonary hypertension, severe AS, hypertrophic cardiomyopathy, or coronary anomalies. Syncope during exertion can also be caused by exercise-induced arrhythmias.

Other anomalies. A significant fraction of congenital heart disease is associated with another anomaly or syndrome [11]. The two most commonly encountered syndromes are Trisomy 21 and the 22q11 microdeletion syndrome, commonly known as DiGeorge syndrome. Thus, a history of any other congenital anomaly, unexplained developmental delay, or failure to thrive should be elicited.

Family history. At present, a minority of children with congenital heart disease has a recognized family history of it, but this proportion is likely to grow. A familial or genetic contribution is already recognized for a significant fraction of conotruncal anomalies [12], as well as some cases of left heart obstructive lesions [13], arch anomalies [14], ASD [15], and patent ductus arteriosus (PDA) [16]. The family history should be explored for congenital heart disease or other manifestations of syndromes that are inconsistently associated with congenital heart disease. For example, Alagille Syndrome is associated with both liver disease and congenital heart disease; the liver disease may be manifest in other family members without identified congenital heart disease. The expression of congenital heart disease may be less severe in family members; a grandparent may have a bicuspid aortic valve while the grandchild has a more severe left heart obstructive disease. However, a history of murmur in family members without a diagnosis of structural heart disease is likely to represent an innocent murmur.

The physical examination

The cardiovascular physical examination involves making inferences about the anatomy and hemodynamic state of the patient from things that the practitioner can see, feel, or hear. A tremendous variety of anatomic lesions and functional disturbances of the heart exist, most along a continuum of severity. Memorizing all possible patterns of physical findings is not practical. Rather, the practitioner must be able to "derive" potential presentations of a given cardiac lesion from knowledge of cardiac anatomy, pathophysiology, and principles of physical examination. A thorough understanding of the events of the cardiac cycle is therefore *essential*. The cardiac cycle is discussed in detail in Chapter 2 and is shown in Fig. 4.1. The reader is encouraged to inspect this

figure carefully and refer back to it throughout the chapter, paying particular attention to the relative pressures in chambers and vessels, how these pressures vary during the cycle, and the timing of closure of the individual heart valves.

It is also important to note that neonates with severe forms of many lesions have little physiologic reserve. This age group may present in a systemically decompensated state, with more distress and vital sign abnormalities, lacking some of the typical auscultatory findings due to diminished cardiac output.

Inspection and palpation

Inspection should include a general assessment of the nutritional state of the patient, any dysmorphic features, and the presence or absence of distress, particularly respiratory distress. Respiratory distress may be manifest by tachypnea, breathlessness, nasal flaring, grunting, or retractions. A conscious effort should be made to look for central cyanosis of the lips and tongue. Assessment of the jugular venous pulse, discussed in more detail below, yields an estimate of the right atrial pressure. The chest should be inspected for evidence of previous thoracic surgery or for a precordial bulge, consistent with significant cardiomegaly. The apical impulse may be visible. Scoliosis is seen in adolescent and adult patients with congenital heart disease. Finally, the extremities should be inspected for evidence of cyanosis, clubbing, edema, or deformities.

Palpation should be used to assess the location and quality of the apical impulse, abnormal precordial impulses, and thrills. Pulses are palpated in all extremities and the extremities should be assessed for adequacy of perfusion and presence of edema. The size of the liver and spleen are determined, palpating from the lower quadrants upwards to the costal margin so that a very inferiorly displaced edge will not be missed. In infants and small children, very gentle pressure with the side of the index finger parallel to the costal margin can be used, allowing the abdominal respiratory motion to bring the edge of the organ back and forth across the examiner's finger. This technique is often more successful than firmer palpation, which tends to induce crying and tensing of the abdominal muscles. Percussion is a useful adjunct in assessing liver and spleen size. Both palpation and percussion can be used to assess for ascites.

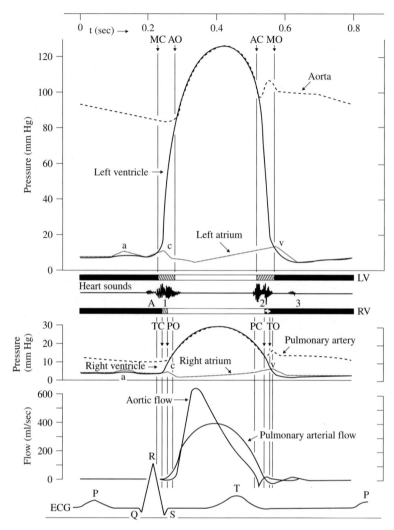

Figure 4.1 The events of the cardiac cycle. Downward from top: pressure in aorta, LV, and LA; duration of LV diastole (heavy shading), isometric periods (diagonal shading) and systole (unshaded); heart sounds ($1 = S_1$, $2 = S_2$, $3 = S_3$, $A = S_4$); pressure in pulmonary artery, RV, and RA; blood flow in aorta and pulmonary artery; and electrocardiogram. Valvular opening and closure are indicated by *AO* and *AC*, respectively, for aortic valve; *MO* and *MC* for mitral valve; *PO* and *PC* for pulmonic valve; and *TO* and *TC* for tricuspid valve. Reprinted from Milnor [35] with permission from Elsevier.

Inspection of the jugular venous pulse

Inspection of the jugular venous pulse provides information about mean atrial pressure and disturbances of atrial hemodynamics. It requires practice and is most useful in older children and adults. Small infants have short necks and little ability to cooperate; palpation of the liver is a more straightforward way to assess central venous pressure in this age group.

Perloff [17] recommends positioning the patient supine with the trunk elevated 30 degrees using an adjustable examining table. The examiner stands on the patient's right and turns the patient's head slightly to the right, to avoid compression of the internal jugular vein. The angle of the trunk is adjusted to maximally visualize pulsations in the right internal jugular vein. The average height of the column of blood above the sternal angle in centimeter is noted. Traditionally, 5 cm is added to this height to yield an estimate of mean right atrial pressure in centimeters of blood (Fig. 4.2), which can be multiplied by 0.736 to convert to mm Hg [18]. This method has been shown to underestimate right

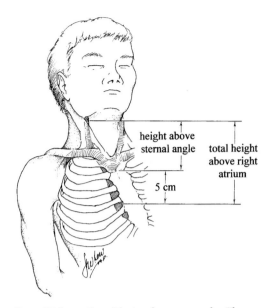

height above
sternal angle   total height
above right
atrium

5 cm

Figure 4.2 Inspection of the jugular venous pulse. The
vertical height of the column of blood in the right internal
jugular vein above the sternal angle is measured. In
adults, the sternal angle is considered to be 5 cm above
the center of the right atrium, regardless of the patient's
position. However, as discussed in the text, the latter
assumption may not be valid in children, in whom a more
qualitative assessment of right atrial pressure is
appropriate. See text for further description.

atrial pressure, particularly in patients with very elevated pressures[19,20], and in smaller children the
sternal angle may not be 5 cm from the center of the
right atrium. A qualitative assessment of mean right
atrial pressure is thus more appropriate in pediatric
practice. McGee suggests considering the central venous pressure to be elevated when the top of the column of blood is more than 3 cm of vertical distance
above the sternal angle [21].

The normal pattern of venous pulsations includes
two peaks in pressure for each cardiac cycle (A and
V waves). The A wave, generated by atrial contraction, occurs just before the carotid pulse, while the V
wave, due to atrial filling against the closed tricuspid
valve during ventricular systole, follows the carotid
pulse. Venous pulsations may be distinguished from
arterial pulsations by their relative rates, simultaneous palpation of the left carotid pulse, or abolishing
venous pulsations by light pressure at the base of the
neck. Amplitude, timing, and consistency of jugular
venous pulsations give insight into tricuspid valve
function, rhythm disturbances, and ventricular

filling. Some of these disorders will be described further below; a more detailed discussion is available in
reference [18].

General principles of auscultation
Auscultation is often viewed as the central part of the
cardiovascular physical exam, and it does play a very
important role. However, the data acquired are most
informative in the context of the entire physical examination. Cardiac auscultation includes the assessment of heart sounds, (Table 4.1) murmurs, clicks,
gallops, snaps, bruits and rubs, with characterization of the location, quality, timing of these sounds,
and their response to maneuvers. Auscultation of
the lung fields seeks evidence of rales or effusions.

The stethoscope should have both a diaphragm
and a bell; two sizes of each are helpful in pediatric practice. The diaphragm is best for high-pitched
sounds and firmer pressure will amplify sounds. The
bell brings out low-pitched sounds and should be applied to the chest with the minimum pressure that
results in a circumferential seal. Usually, the weight
of the head of the stethoscope alone provides sufficient pressure. As more pressure is applied, the very
low-pitched sounds may be lost.

Multiple locations on the chest are auscul-
tated. Traditionally, an area is designated where
sounds referable to each heart valve are best heard
(Fig. 4.3a). In the case of *situs inversus*, these positions are located in the mirror image. Additional
important areas where murmurs may radiate or be
best heard are the right and left infraclavicular areas, the axillae, the neck, and the back. Veasy has
suggested that the location of structures other than
valves should be kept in mind, as murmurs may
arise between or within chambers or great vessels
(Fig. 4.3b) [22]. Although individual approaches
vary, a systematic assessment of each area should be
performed. The examiner should listen consciously
with the diaphragm to S_1 and S_2, note the regularity
and rate of the heart rhythm, seek out murmurs in
systole and then in diastole, and listen for gallops,
clicks, snaps, and rubs. Then the examiner switches
to the bell and listens specifically for low frequency
sounds at the left lower sternal border and apex, such
as diastolic inflow sounds and gallops. In small infants, this process is usually carried out with the patient supine or semi-recumbent in the parents' arms.
In older patients, auscultation should be performed
in the supine, sitting, and standing positions.

Table 4.1 Abbreviations Used to Designate Heart Sounds.

Abbreviation	Description	Corresponding event
S_1	First heart sound	Atrioventricular valve closure
T_1	Tricuspid component of S_1	Tricuspid valve closure
M_1	Mitral component of S_1	Mitral valve closure
S_2	Second heart sound	Semilunar valve closure
P_2	Pulmonic component of S_2	Pulmonic valve closure
A_2	Aortic component of S_2	Aortic valve closure
S_3	Third heart sound; gallop	Passive filling of the ventricle in early diastole, especially in the setting of ventricular dysfunction
S_4	Fourth heart sound; presystolic gallop	Atrial contraction against a noncompliant ventricle

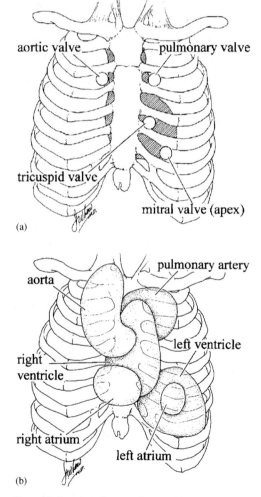

(a)

(b)

Figure 4.3 Locations for auscultation. (a) Sites corresponding to the four heart valves. (b) Sites corresponding to other cardiac structures, after Veasy [22].

The two components (M_1 and T_1) of S_1 are usually heard as one sound, but in some patients S_1 can be heard to split in the tricuspid area [8]. Characterization of S_2 is of *utmost* importance in the physical diagnosis of congenital heart disease, particularly the timing of the A_2 and P_2 components and the loudness of P_2 [1,8]. Normally, the time between A_2 and P_2 varies with the respiratory cycle. During inspiration, P_2 follows A_2 by about 60 msec and two components are heard separately at the left upper sternal border. With expiration, P_2 follows A_2 by only about 30 msec and the two are perceived as a single sound [8]. This pattern is termed physiologic splitting. It results from an interplay between altered ventricular preload and an increase in the pulmonary "hangout" interval (the time between the onset of right ventricular pressure fall and P_2), which is felt to be due to decreased impedance of the pulmonary vascular bed with inspiration [23]. In addition, a loud P_2 indicates pulmonary hypertension [8]. Several abnormalities of S_2 with particular relevance to congenital heart disease are summarized in Table 4.2; for more detailed lists, see other references [8,24,25].

Murmurs, which are created by turbulent blood flow, are challenging to characterize. Fortunately, classification by (1) timing in the cardiac cycle and (2) contour of the murmur reduces this problem to a manageable number of possibilities (Fig. 4.4). When information about pitch, location and pattern of radiation are added, a specific diagnosis or a narrowed differential diagnosis can be formulated. The first step is to assign the murmur to a phase of the cardiac cycle, namely systole (between S_1 and S_2), diastole (following S_2), or both (termed continuous).

Table 4.2 Abnormalities of the Second Heart Sound Most Relevant to Congenital Heart Disease.

Wide splitting	Narrow splitting or single S_2	Reversed splitting	Single S_2
Early A$_2$	**Delayed A$_2$**	**Delayed A$_2$**	**Only one semilunar valve present or audible**
Ventricular septal defect	Moderate aortic stenosis	Complete LBBB	Pulmonary atresia
Mitral regurgitation		RV paced or ectopic beats	Aortic atresia
		Severe aortic stenosis	Post-surgical: pulmonary transannular patch
		Dilation of the aortic root	Anteroposterior position of semilunar valves: D-TGA
		Patent ductus arteriosus	
Delayed P$_2$	**Early P$_2$**		
Complete RBBB	Primary pulmonary hypertension		
LV ectopic or paced beats	Eisenmenger syndrome		
Pulmonary stenosis with intact ventricular septum	Pulmonary hypertension secondary to pulmonary venous obstruction or left atrial hypertension		
Atrial septal defect			
Unexplained expiratory splitting in a normal subject			

Adapted from Shaver JH and O'Toole JD [24,25]. LV, left ventricle; RV, right ventricle; LBBB, left bundle branch block; RBBB, right bundle branch block; D-TGA, D-transposition of the great arteries.

When the heart rate is slow, systole is shorter than diastole. When the heart rate is fast, simultaneous palpation of a central pulse and auscultation is helpful; systolic murmurs coincide with the pulse. Two particular points should be made about continuous murmurs. First, murmurs that extend from systole into diastole, but do not persist through all of diastole are classified as continuous. As put by one author, "The term 'continuous' is best applied to the uninterrupted progress of the murmur through the second heart sound, rather than to persistence of a murmur throughout all of the cardiac cycle" [26]. Second, multiple murmurs in different phases of the cardiac cycle may occur in a single patient. The presence of both a systolic and a separate diastolic murmur (Fig. 4.5) does *not* constitute a continuous murmur.

Systolic murmurs can be classified into one of two contours, although some loud systolic murmurs become difficult to distinguish. A crescendo–decrescendo murmur, also termed a systolic ejection murmur, arises from turbulence produced during ejection of blood from the heart. They generally fade before the end of systole, and thus do not obscure S_2. Holosystolic murmurs, also called pan-systolic murmurs or in some cases systolic regurgitant murmurs, have a flat contour because the pressure gradient which gives rise to them is relatively constant throughout systole. These murmurs usually arise from atrioventricular valve regurgitation or VSDs and typically obscure S_2. It should be noted that there are exceptions to these generalizations. For example a small muscular VSD may produce a crescendo–decrescendo murmur.

Likewise, diastolic murmurs can be classified into one of two types: diastolic regurgitant murmurs and diastolic inflow murmurs. Diastolic regurgitant murmurs are decrescendo in contour and arise from regurgitation across semilunar valves. Diastolic inflow murmurs (also called diastolic rumbles) result from turbulent inflow across atrioventricular valves and may have variable contours. The inflow across atrioventricular valves can be turbulent for

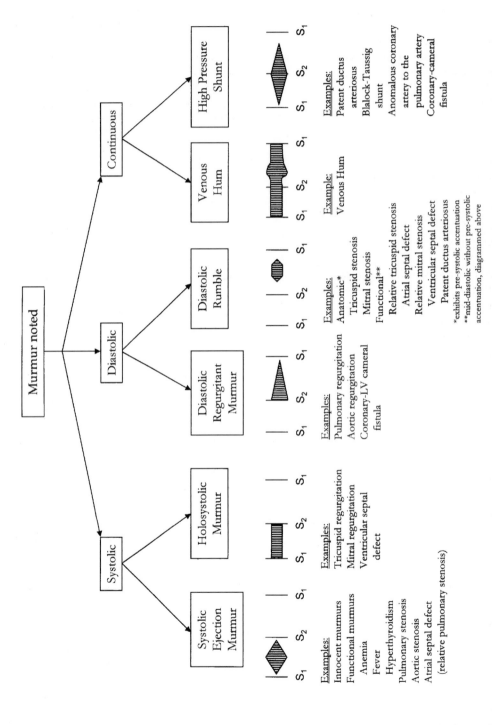

Figure 4.4 Differential diagnosis of cardiac murmurs. Contours and timing with respect to S_1 and S_2 of each type of murmur are shown diagrammatically. Representative, although not comprehensive, examples of lesions generating these murmurs are listed at the bottom.

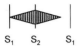   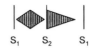

(a) Continuous Murmur   (b) To-and-fro murmur

Figure 4.5 The true continuous murmur versus the to-and-fro murmur. A true continuous murmur continues without interruption through S_2 while a to-and-fro murmur consists of separate systolic ejection and diastolic regurgitant murmurs, and thus for a brief period around S_2, no murmur is present.

one of two reasons: first, there is an increased amount of flow across a normal valve; second, the valve itself is stenotic. The former generates a mid-diastolic murmur while the latter leads to a diastolic murmur with presystolic accentuation. Diastolic inflow murmurs are easily missed; they are low pitched and therefore best heard with the bell.

Continuous murmurs arise when a pressure gradient exists in a given direction irrespective of the phase of the cardiac cycle. This situation can arise in the normal venous system, in the abnormal arterial system, or in connections between the high-pressure arterial system and a low-pressure lumen. Continuous murmurs are not generally subclassified by contour, but an examination of contour is helpful in the distinction between a continuous murmur and the combination of a systolic ejection murmur and a diastolic regurgitant murmur ("to-and-fro" murmur, Fig. 4.5).

The remaining characteristics of a murmur (pitch, quality, location of greatest intensity, radiation, and variation of the murmur with various maneuvers) tend to coalesce into a profile. The pitch is determined by the pressure gradient that generates the murmur, with high-pressure gradients resulting in high-pitched murmurs. The quality is described by a number of adjectives (vibratory, harsh, blowing, etc.) best learned by experience. Location of greatest intensity should be compared with the named valve locations and knowledge of the underlying anatomy. In general, murmurs radiate along the known trajectory of blood flow. Finally, the profile of the murmur should be combined with the rest of the auscultatory findings into a cohesive hypothesis.

The physical examination in the evaluation of ventricular function

Abnormal ventricular hemodynamics can result from systolic dysfunction, diastolic dysfunction, or excessive volume load despite a fundamentally normal myocardium. The physical examination identifies their final common pathway, congestive heart failure (CHF), and may not identify mild degrees of dysfunction or volume load that do not lead to CHF. Resting tachycardia, tachypnea, evidence of elevated filling pressures and gallop rhythm are the core clinical signs of CHF; some other findings may help distinguish one etiology from another. Peripheral edema is present in older children with ventricular dysfunction, while pure volume load from an intracardiac shunt rarely causes peripheral edema in infants. If present, edema is first manifested in the eyelids in infants. Longstanding ventricular dilation can result in a precordial bulge. Signs specific to right versus left ventricular dysfunction or volume load are discussed below.

Gallops are generated by abnormal filling of either ventricle [8]. An S_3 gallop follows S_2 during the passive filling phase of diastole and usually indicates ventricular dysfunction. Classically, an S_3 was associated with ventricular systolic dysfunction, but a study of adult patients with CHF in the setting of normal or decreased systolic function showed a similar prevalence of S_3, about 30–40% [27]. An S_4 gallop or presystolic gallop is generated by the force of atrial contraction and occurs just before S_1. It becomes audible when the ventricle is noncompliant, either due to generalized myocardial dysfunction or ventricular hypertrophy. S_1 may be soft if ventricular contractility is depressed.

Right ventricular dysfunction or volume load
Physical findings: Resting tachycardia is present. There may be evidence of tachypnea and increased respiratory effort. Inspection of the neck veins demonstrates an elevated jugular venous pressure. Palpation and percussion may reveal a right ventricular heave at the left lower sternal border, hepatomegaly, and in severe right-sided heart failure, ascites. Right ventricular systolic dysfunction may lead to tricuspid regurgitation, manifested by a holosystolic murmur.

Left ventricular dysfunction or volume load
Physical findings: Resting tachycardia, tachypnea, and increased respiratory effort are present. Left-sided CHF can lead to secondary pulmonary hypertension and right-sided CHF, with corresponding manifestations. Palpation demonstrates a diffuse, laterally displaced apical impulse or an

inappropriately quiet apical area if there is ventricular dilation and systolic dysfunction. Diastolic dysfunction on the basis of hypertrophy may lead to a normally placed but excessively forceful impulse. Volume load results in a generally hyperdynamic precordium. On auscultation, rales are consistent with systolic dysfunction, but can be absent in chronic CHF and are rarely heard in infants with large volume loads. LV systolic dysfunction can lead to mitral regurgitation, with its corresponding holosystolic murmur.

The physical examination in the evaluation of blood flow

Physical examination can detect evidence of many types of disturbed blood flow in addition to evidence of normal blood flow:

• Normal blood flow: innocent murmurs and the physiologic S_3
• Insufficient peripheral blood flow due to low systemic cardiac output states
• Pulmonary arterial hypertension
• Obstruction to blood flow within the heart or great vessels
• Regurgitation of blood flow within the heart or great vessels
• Ineffective pulmonary blood flow: left to right shunting
• Blood flow bypassing the lungs: right to left shunting
• Complex congenital heart disease

Most of the lesions described below exist on a continuum of severity and an individual patient will fall along a continuum of physical findings. In general, the full spectrum of physical findings as well as evidence of systemic decompensation will be present in patients with the most severe lesions.

Normal blood flow: Innocent murmurs and the physiologic S_3

Innocent murmurs are nearly ubiquitous in childhood. These murmurs are best identified by their characteristic features and "the company that they keep" [8]. The history and the remainder of the cardiovascular physical examination should be normal. These murmurs will be accentuated by increased venous return and anything that augments cardiac output, including fever, anemia, exercise, and beta adrenergic agonists. Some authors have made the point that "innocent" murmurs which are augmented by noncardiac pathology such as thyrotoxicosis or severe anemia are not truly innocent and have instead termed them "functional" murmurs [8]. The practitioner will usually be tipped off to the underlying pathology by abnormal history, vital signs, or general physical examination, excessive precordial activity, unusual intensity of the murmur, hyperdynamic pulses, or accompanying gallops.

Physical findings: The patient appears generally healthy, well nourished, and without increased respiratory effort or central cyanosis. The vital signs and growth parameters are normal. In newborns it is often helpful to include a pulse oximetry reading, to rule out minor arterial desaturation, which may not be visible. The jugular venous pulse is normal. The apical impulse is appropriately placed and normal in quality. The rest of the precordium is quiet. The liver is not enlarged, and symmetric, full pulses should be easily palpable in all four extremities with no delay between the radial and femoral pulses. The extremities are warm to touch with brisk capillary refill and no evidence of clubbing or edema. On auscultation, the rhythm has an appropriate rate and is regular, with the exception of variation consistent with sinus arrhythmia. S_2 is physiologically split and P_2 is of normal intensity. There are no clicks, snaps, or rubs. A soft S_3 can be normal in childhood in the absence of any other concerning features, but a loud S_3 or any S_4 should be considered pathologic. Characteristic features of innocent murmurs are present and there are no concerning features [1]. A murmur must be either systolic ejection or continuous to be considered innocent. Overwhelmingly, innocent murmurs are grade I or II; a grade III deserves a hard second thought as to whether it is innocent, and any murmur of grade IV or greater should be considered pathologic. No diastolic murmurs should be considered innocent. The quality should be vibratory or blowing, not harsh. More detail on specific types of innocent murmurs is given in Table 4.3.

Low systemic cardiac output states

There are diverse causes of low systemic cardiac output, but all result in inadequate tissue perfusion, with certain physical findings common to all etiologies.

Physical findings: The patient with an acute low systemic cardiac output state generally appears unwell, limp or lethargic and may demonstrate respiratory distress. Pallor or peripheral duskiness is noted.

Table 4.3 Typical Features of Innocent Murmurs.

Murmur	Type	Maximal location	Radiation	Other comments
Peripheral PS (PPS)	Blowing or vibratory SEM	Pulmonic area	Axillae and back; typically louder in these locations	Common in newborns; usually disappears by 6 months of age, certainly by 18 months; Consider Williams Syndrome, Alagille Syndrome, or Congenital Rubella Syndrome in patients outside of typical age range
Still's murmur	"Twanging" or vibratory SEM	Left lower sternal border	Little radiation	Common in school aged children; Described as sounding like a "plucked string"
Innocent pulmonic ejection murmur (a.k.a. basal ejection murmur)	Blowing or vibratory SEM	Pulmonic area	Little radiation	
Supraclavicular arterial bruit	Very short, early SEM	Left supraclavicular area	Little radiation	Can be accompanied by a thrill (grade IV); Softer with hyperextension of shoulders; Softer below clavicle; Disappears with compression of the subclavian artery
Continuous venous hum	Low-pitched, continuous	Right infraclavicular area	Also heard at the base	Louder in diastole and inspiration; Only heard with patient upright; Disappears supine and with manipulation of head position
Mammary soufflé	Continuous, relatively high-pitched, usually systolic component predominates	Second right or left intercostal space	Little radiation	Only heard during the third trimester of pregnancy or lactation; Can be brought out or abolished by varying pressure of stethoscope; Sometimes only systolic component heard

Patients with chronic low systemic cardiac output states often appear ruddy due to compensatory polycythemia. The heart rate and respiratory rate are generally elevated, the latter as a consequence of elevated left heart filling pressures, elevated pulmonary blood flow, or as a compensatory mechanism for metabolic acidosis due to inadequate tissue perfusion. The blood pressure is generally low, although in infants it may be preserved until just prior to circulatory collapse. Core temperature can be elevated in postoperative low cardiac output states. Neonates with inadequate cardiac output may become hypothermic. The hallmarks of a low systemic cardiac output state are cool extremities and thready peripheral pulses.

Pulmonary artery hypertension

The importance of recognizing the findings associated with pulmonary artery hypertension cannot be overemphasized. While there are diverse causes of pulmonary hypertension, certain physical findings are consistent and others are common secondary effects of decompensated pulmonary hypertension. These findings are emphasized in the discussion that follows.

Physical findings: Tachypnea and increased respiratory effort are noted in circumstances that lead to pulmonary edema. The patient may appear malnourished, which will be reflected in growth parameters. In patients with marginal compensation, a resting tachycardia is often present. If a septal defect or PDA is present, right to left shunting may result, reflected in low pulse oximetry values and possibly cyanosis and clubbing. Elevated right heart filling pressures may be evident from inspection of the jugular veins. A right ventricular impulse may be visible and is easily palpated along the left lower sternal border. Hepatomegaly with or without ascites is palpable in the presence of right heart failure.

The hallmark physical finding in pulmonary hypertension is a loud P_2 [8]. With severe pulmonary hypertension, P_2 becomes palpable in the pulmonic area. The loudness of P_2 is determined by the rate of change of the pressure gradient between the pulmonary artery and the right ventricle (RV). An elevated pulmonary artery pressure results in a higher gradient. In addition, the timing of P_2 relative to A_2 is altered. As the impedance of the pulmonary vascular bed increases, the pulmonary hangout time decreases [28], P_2 occurs earlier and is more coincident with A_2, and S_2 is perceived as narrowly

split or single. However, a single S_2 is not mandatory in pulmonary hypertension. If other factors affect the relative timing of A_2 and P_2, S_2 may still be split (even widely) in the presence of pulmonary hypertension [8]. For example, in the presence of a large VSD, pulmonary artery pressure will be elevated, but A_2 will occur relatively early, due to shortened LV ejection time and the discrepancy in the volume of blood being ejected through the aorta and pulmonary artery. The result is a widely split S_2 with a loud P_2. S_3 or S_4 gallops may be heard with RV dysfunction or noncompliance, respectively.

Obstruction of blood flow within the heart or vascular system

Obstruction of pulmonary veins

Occlusion of one pulmonary vein is usually well tolerated, but obstruction of multiple pulmonary veins causes pulmonary edema. If the obstruction is sufficient to cause pulmonary hypertension, the corresponding signs will be present.

Physical findings: Pulmonary venous obstruction results in pulmonary edema leading to tachypnea, increased work of breathing, and if severe, respiratory distress and decreased systemic saturation. Chronic pulmonary venous obstruction also causes failure to thrive, with low weight for height. Usually, no murmur corresponding to flow across the obstructed veins is audible. Rales may be present due to pulmonary alveolar edema.

Obstruction of blood flow from atrium to ventricle

Blood flows from the atrium to the ventricle during diastole, at low pressures. Thus, the hallmark finding in this category of obstruction is the diastolic rumble. The murmur can be augmented by increasing the heart rate.

Tricuspid stenosis

Physical findings: Inspection of the jugular venous pulse demonstrates prominent A-waves, as the hypertrophied right atrium (RA) contracts against a stenotic tricuspid valve. The estimate of the mean jugular venous pressure may be elevated. The liver may be engorged or pulsatile. On auscultation, an opening snap may be present, introducing a diastolic rumble, which is loudest at the left lower sternal border or xiphoid area and best heard with the bell. The murmur is accentuated with right atrial contraction (pre-[ventricular] systolic accentuation), but since right atrial systole occurs before left atrial systole, it may be perceived to fade before S_1, resulting in a diamond-shaped contour [15]. Inspiration makes the murmur more prominent. These findings will be largely obscured if the patient is in atrial fibrillation.

Mitral stenosis
Physical findings: Moderate to severe disease will result in tachypnea, increased work of breathing or respiratory distress and failure to thrive. On auscultation, a narrowly split or single S_2 with a loud P_2 is heard in moderate to severe mitral stenosis, due to secondary pulmonary hypertension. Thickened mitral valve leaflets secondary to rheumatic heart disease may generate an opening snap, which is heard between the left lower sternal border and the apex. The diastolic rumble is best heard at the apex with the bell and is accentuated as the mitral leaflets start to close, just prior to S_1 [8]. In infants, especially when tachycardic and in respiratory distress, and in patients with atrial fibrillation, the murmur may be difficult to appreciate [9].

Obstruction of blood flow from ventricle to great artery

Outflow obstruction affects the ejection of blood, resulting in a systolic ejection murmur and can occur at the valvar, subvalvar, or supravalvar level. The discussion that follows focuses on general principles of outflow obstruction, rather than subtle differences in physical findings.

Right Ventricular Outflow Tract Obstruction Lesions in this category include double chambered RV, tetralogy of Fallot, valvar PS, and supravalvar PS. A pressure load to the RV is generally well tolerated for long periods of time. Signs of right heart dysfunction may be present, although these are uncommon in children.

Physical findings: These patients usually appear well, without growth failure or respiratory distress. Cyanosis or arterial desaturation as measured by pulse oximetry may be present if there is a coexisting ASD plus severe RV hypertrophy or a VSD. A palpable RV impulse is present at the left lower sternal border. A thrill may be palpable along the left sternal border in the case of subvalvar obstruction, or in the pulmonic area in the case of valvar PS.

The hallmark auscultatory finding is a harsh systolic ejection murmur, loudest in the pulmonic area

and radiating to the lung fields. The murmur may be loudest along the lower left sternal border if the obstruction is intracavitary. Generally, the murmur lengthens as the obstruction becomes more severe, and as a result may obscure A_2 [8]. Valvar PS results in a systolic ejection click loudest in the pulmonic area that diminishes with inspiration and increases in expiration. In valvar and subvalvar stenosis, P_2 becomes softer and more delayed relative to A_2 in proportion to the severity of obstruction. In patients over 2 years of age with valvar PS, a murmur of grade III or less, accompanied by a normal intensity P_2, usually indicates a gradient at catheterization of 50 mm Hg or less. In the first Natural History Study, this combination of findings was present in only 11% of patients with a gradient of 50–79 mm Hg and 1% of patients with a gradient exceeding 80 mm Hg [29].

Left Ventricular Outflow Tract Obstruction Lesions in this category include subaortic membrane, hypertrophic obstructive cardiomyopathy (HOCM), valvar AS and supravalvar AS. Signs of LV dysfunction may develop in severe obstruction.

Physical findings: By and large, these patients appear well, without evidence of growth failure or respiratory distress, except for those patients with LV dysfunction. In these patients, tachypnea and tachycardia are present, particularly in the neonate with critical valvar AS and ductal closure. The apical impulse is normally located, but is more forceful and sustained than normal when the left ventricle (LV) is significantly hypertrophied, and an S_4 may be palpable.

In any form of LV outflow tract obstruction, LV ejection is prolonged by increasing severity of obstruction, delaying A_2 [9]. S_2 can therefore be narrowly split, single, or paradoxically split (A_2 *follows* P_2) although the latter two findings are uncommon in children with even severe valvar AS [30]. An S_4 may be audible in patients with significant LV hypertrophy. A harsh systolic ejection murmur is present in variable locations along the LV outflow tract, depending on the lesion. In valvar AS, the murmur is typically loudest in the aortic area or the left upper sternal border, but frequently also well heard at the apex. The murmur is transmitted into the neck. Supravalvar AS results in a murmur that is maximal higher up the right sternal border or in the neck, while the murmur of subvalvar obstruction is loudest more inferiorly along the left sternal border.

Particular features of valvar AS include a thrill in the suprasternal notch or aortic area, which is transmitted into the carotid arteries. A thrill is very common (78%) in children with gradients less than 25 mm Hg, but becomes almost universal with increasing severity, such that the absence of a thrill essentially rules out a gradient of 50 mm Hg or more [30]. The classic pulse associated with severe valvar AS is *pulsus parvus et tardus*—low amplitude and occurring later than normal, relative to the cardiac cycle. A systolic ejection click that does not vary with respiration is heard at the apex, unless the aortic valve leaflets are immobile. A_2 is often prominent in mild valvar AS; one can think of this as the inverse of the click. Most patients with valvar AS, across a wide range of severity, have murmur of grade III to IV. A murmur of only grade I to II is a fairly reliable indicator that the gradient is less than 25 mm Hg, while a grade V or VI murmur usually accompanies a gradient of greater than 50 mm Hg, and most frequently greater than 80 mm Hg [30].

Hypertrophic obstructive cardiomyopathy also has characteristic features. The apical impulse and pulses may be bifid (*pulsus bisferiens*). The pulses also typically rise very briskly. The gradient and the murmur of HOCM are augmented by decreasing systemic vascular resistance, increasing contractility, or decreasing preload. The easiest maneuvers to perform at the bedside are those which decrease preload, namely upright posture and the strain phase of the Valsalva maneuver. The inverse is also true: the murmur diminishes when venous return increases, immediately after squatting and when supine. Pharmacologic manipulation of afterload has also been described, but most clinicians do not use these techniques in the office.

Obstruction to blood flow within the pulmonary or systemic arterial systems

Like obstruction to blood flow from the ventricles to the great arteries, obstruction within the arterial system is manifested when blood is ejected into it, and thus is associated with a systolic ejection murmur.

Pulmonary artery stenosis

Pulmonary artery stenosis can occur as multiple, discrete branch stenoses or diffuse hypoplasia of the peripheral pulmonary arteries. Facial dysmorphisms typical of Williams, Alagille, or Congenital Rubella Syndromes may be present. Otherwise, vital signs, inspection, and palpation/percussion are the same as in RV outflow tract lesions.

Physical findings: While the systolic pulmonary artery pressure proximal to the stenosis is elevated, the diastolic pulmonary artery pressure is normal in these conditions. Thus, S_2 is usually normal. The maximal location of the systolic ejection murmur and its radiation varies with the location of the stenoses. In general, the murmur is well heard in the pulmonic area with wide radiation into the axillae and back. In peripheral PS the murmur usually has a blowing quality, while with discrete branch pulmonary artery stenoses the murmur is harsher.

Coarctation

Physical findings: These patients are generally well appearing, except for the neonate with critical coarctation and ductal constriction who will have respiratory distress, tachycardia, and poor perfusion. The hallmark finding is a gradient between the upper and lower extremity systolic blood pressures. The right upper extremity blood pressure is more reliable than the left, as the left subclavian artery can be involved in the coarctation. Lower extremity blood pressure may not be measurable if the coarctation is severe, while extensive collaterals can minimize the blood pressure discrepancy. Upper extremity hypertension is typical, but may be absent in newborns. The femoral pulses are weak and delayed relative to the radial pulses, or absent. The apical impulse is forceful but not displaced. Hepatomegaly may be present in the neonate with critical coarctation and ductal constriction.

On auscultation, S_2 is generally normal. A harsh systolic ejection murmur originating from the coarctation is best heard anteriorly at the left upper sternal border and radiates to the left back, inferior to the scapula. If the obstruction is severe, the murmur may extend into diastole (qualifying as continuous). In addition, soft continuous murmurs originating from collateral flow to the distal aorta may be heard in the back. An S_3 will be heard in the presence of secondary LV dysfunction, while an S_4 may result from compensatory LV hypertrophy.

Regurgitation of blood flow in the heart or great vessels

Regurgitation across the atrioventricular valves is a systolic event, while regurgitation across the semilunar valves is a diastolic event. Regurgitation of either type results in a volume load to the involved ventricle and findings of ventricular volume load proportional to the degree of regurgitation. The regurgitant volume must move forward again, and if the regurgitant fraction is large, findings of relative valvar "stenosis" of the same valve will result.

Regurgitation of atrioventricular valves

During systole, there is a continuous pressure gradient, which is relatively constant in magnitude from the ventricle to the atrium (Fig. 4.1), resulting in a holosystolic murmur. Assuming generally normal hemodynamics, the LV pressure significantly exceeds the RV pressure, while the atrial pressures are close to equal. Thus, the greater pressure gradient in the left heart results in the mitral regurgitation murmur having a higher pitch than the tricuspid regurgitation murmur. These murmurs also differ in their location, as described below.

Tricuspid regurgitation

Physical findings: Inspection of the jugular venous pulse demonstrates prominent V-waves and possibly an elevated mean pressure. A precordial bulge may be present if there is marked cardiomegaly. The RV impulse is prominent. The liver may be enlarged and pulsatile in significant disease. A low pitched, harsh, holosystolic murmur is present at the left lower sternal border. If RV hypertension coexists with tricuspid regurgitation, the pitch of the murmur will be higher. If the etiology of regurgitation is Ebstein's anomaly, multiple systolic clicks may be heard.

Mitral regurgitation

Physical findings: Severe mitral regurgitation can cause left atrial hypertension and CHF. In this scenario, tachypnea, tachycardia, and growth failure will be present. Weight can be low for height in moderate mitral regurgitation without overt CHF. Marked cardiomegaly results in a precordial bulge. If left heart failure results in pulmonary hypertension or right heart failure, corresponding signs are present. The apical impulse is laterally displaced and hyperdynamic. The murmur of mitral regurgitation is a high-pitched, blowing holosystolic murmur at the apex, radiating to the left axilla. An S_3 may be present in severe mitral regurgitation.

Regurgitation of semilunar valves

During diastole, there is a pressure gradient from the great artery to the ventricle, but its magnitude declines as the pressure falls in the great artery and rises in the ventricle (Fig. 4.1). Thus, the murmur of semilunar valve regurgitation has a decrescendo contour. Assuming generally normal hemodynamics, the aortic pressure significantly exceeds the pulmonary artery pressure, while the ventricular diastolic pressures are close to equal. Thus, the greater pressure gradient results in the aortic regurgitation murmur having a higher pitch than the pulmonary regurgitation murmur.

Pulmonary regurgitation The volume load on the RV is generally well tolerated for long periods of time. Longstanding, moderate to severe pulmonary regurgitation can result in RV dilation and dysfunction and the accompanying physical findings.

Physical findings: The patient appears generally well, with normal vital signs. An RV impulse is palpable at the left lower sternal border. On auscultation, S_2 is single if the pulmonary valve is completely incompetent. The relatively low-pitched diastolic decrescendo murmur at the left lower sternal border is heard most easily with the patient sitting up and leaning forward. The increased volume of blood ejected from the RV usually generates a pulmonary ejection murmur. These two murmurs together are called a "to and fro" murmur. If pulmonary hypertension is present, the murmur of pulmonary regurgitation will be high pitched.

Aortic regurgitation Aortic regurgitation imposes a volume load on the LV and results in low diastolic blood pressure and, more importantly, low coronary perfusion pressure. Aortic regurgitation is not as well tolerated as pulmonary regurgitation, especially when acute in onset. Left-sided CHF can result, with corresponding physical findings.

Physical findings: Patients are generally well appearing unless the onset is acute or the regurgitation is severe, leading to CHF. In these circumstances, tachycardia and tachypnea are present. The diastolic blood pressure is low in patients with greater than mild regurgitation. Manifestations of wide pulse pressure include bounding peripheral pulses with diastolic collapse (waterhammer pulse), visible pulsations of the carotids (Corrigan pulse), or movement of the earlobes with each heartbeat. The latter two findings occur in severe aortic regurgitation. The apical impulse is laterally displaced and prominent. Auscultation may reveal an ejection click if regurgitation is due to a bicuspid aortic valve and A_2 may be soft in severe regurgitation. The characteristic high-pitched,

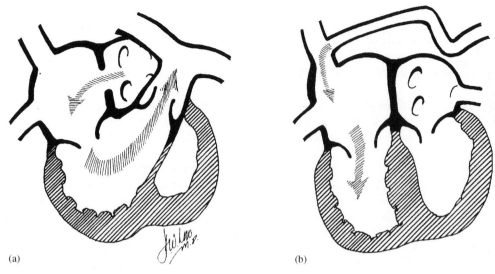

Figure 4.6 Atrial-level left to right shunting. (a) ASD and (b) PAPVR both result in an increased volume of blood passing through the RA, tricuspid valve, RV, and pulmonary arteries.

blowing, diastolic decrescendo murmur at the left lower sternal border is best heard with the patient sitting up and leaning forward, in fixed expiration. An additional murmur is present in some patients: the Austin Flint murmur, described by Dr. Flint as a "presystolic blubbering" at the apex [26]. It results from the regurgitant jet pushing the anterior mitral valve leaflet closed while the force of atrial contraction ejects blood through the mitral valve into the LV. Finally, as the ventricle ejects the forward plus the regurgitant stroke volume, an aortic systolic ejection murmur is frequently generated, which in combination with the diastolic regurgitant murmur, is heard as a "to and fro" murmur.

Left to right shunting

Left to right shunts cause oxygenated blood to be returned to the pulmonary vascular bed instead of continuing to the systemic circulation. Pulmonary blood flow is increased, causing various degrees of pulmonary vascular congestion and left atrial hypertension. The shunt can occur at the atrial, ventricular, or the great vessel level. Each level of shunt has a characteristic pattern of physical findings and will be discussed separately.

Atrial-level shunting

Atrial-level shunting due to an ASD or its physiologic equivalent partial anomalous pulmonary

venous return (PAPVR) results in an increased volume of blood traversing the right heart, pulmonary arteries, and left atrium (LA) (Fig. 4.6). There is no significant pressure load on the RV. Generally, ASD or PAPVR does not cause CHF in childhood. In the rare infant with CHF, a concomitant left-sided obstructive lesion exacerbating the left to right shunt should be sought.

Physical findings: Children with these lesions appear generally well with normal vital signs. Uncommonly, there may be mild elevation of the jugular venous pulse or a prominence of the left precordium due to significant RV volume overload. An RV impulse is often palpable. Rarely, there may be hepatomegaly consistent with elevated right-sided filling pressures.

The hallmark of an atrial level shunt is fixed splitting of the second heart sound in both inspiration and expiration. This has been explained by the lack of alteration of RV preload with the respiratory cycle, since RV preload is supplied by both systemic and pulmonary venous return [8]. In addition, a frequently unimpressive systolic ejection murmur may be heard in the pulmonary position due to the increased volume of blood ejected from the RV to the pulmonary arteries. When the amount of atrial level shunting is particularly large, a mid-diastolic rumble of relative tricuspid stenosis can be heard in the tricuspid position. Flow across the ASD itself is silent.

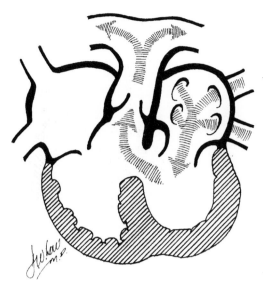

Figure 4.7 Ventricular-level left to right shunting. An increased volume of blood passes through the pulmonary arteries, LA, and LV.

Ventricular-level shunting

A VSD results in an increased volume of blood traversing the left heart and pulmonary arteries (Fig. 4.7). Large defects result in equalization of the right and left ventricular pressures, leading to findings of RV pressure overload and pulmonary hypertension. CHF is common in unrestrictive VSDs in infancy as the pulmonary vascular resistance falls.

Physical findings: A patient with a small VSD appears generally well with normal vital signs. When a large shunt is present, the patient may appear wasted and demonstrate increased respiratory effort, tachypnea and mild tachycardia, and low weight for height. Cardiac motion may be visible in the precordium and a precordial bulge may be present in the setting of longstanding volume load. A large VSD in a neonate whose pulmonary vascular resistance has not yet fallen may result in mild desaturation on pulse oximetry (low to mid 90s) due to bidirectional shunting at the VSD.

A large VSD leads to a hyperdynamic precordium with a laterally displaced LV impulse and findings of pulmonary hypertension. The liver is frequently enlarged. In the case of a restrictive VSD, a thrill may be palpable along the left sternal border while the findings of pressure and volume overload are absent.

The auscultatory findings of a VSD are very variable, depending on its size. S_2 is often widely split in the presence of a large VSD and P_2 is loud due to pulmonary hypertension. When a large, unrestrictive VSD is present with relatively high pulmonary vascular resistance, there will be little shunt and no pressure gradient across the defect, generating little murmur. As pulmonary vascular resistance falls, a pulmonary ejection murmur may be generated from the increased volume of blood passing across the RV outflow tract. In addition, as a pressure gradient develops across the VSD, a holosystolic murmur is generated, with the pitch proportional to the pressure gradient. These murmurs tend to obscure S_2, are loudest along the left sternal border, and radiate to the back. A lumen of small muscular VSD may be obliterated during systole as the muscle fibers shorten and thicken, resulting in a blowing, less than holosystolic murmur at the left lower sternal border, which does not obscure S_2. In the presence of a large shunt, a mid-diastolic rumble of relative mitral stenosis can be heard at the apex. Finally, a large volume load can result in a gallop at the apex, best heard with the bell.

Great vessel-level shunting

Multiple types of communications can result in shunting at this level with somewhat varying manifestations (Table 4.4). Great vessel level shunting results in a volume load to the left heart and in most circumstances, the pulmonary arteries carry increased flow (Fig. 4.8). If the communication is unrestrictive, it will cause pulmonary hypertension, a pressure load to the right heart and CHF in early infancy, with the attendant physical findings.

Physical findings: In the presence of significant diastolic runoff, diastolic blood pressure is low. A PDA, which is restrictive to pressure but still has a large flow across it, may have a palpable thrill in the left infraclavicular area.

The hallmark physical finding of most, although not all, shunts at the great vessel level is a continuous murmur (Table 4.4). The murmur arises because a continuous pressure gradient exists between the systemic artery and the pulmonary artery or cardiac chamber. The pitch is proportional to the pressure gradient. A mid-diastolic rumble of relative mitral stenosis due to left atrial volume load may be heard at the apex if the shunt is large. It may be difficult to separate this murmur from the diastolic component of the continuous murmur.

Table 4.4 Great Vessel Level Shunts.

Lesion	Arterial source	Distal termination	Murmur timing	Location	Other physical findings or comments
Patent ductus arteriosus	Aorta	Pulmonary artery	Continuous	Under left clavicle or 1st or 2nd left intercostal space	Continuum of size exists; No findings in tiny ("silent") PDAs; Multiple systolic ejection clicks can be heard in larger PDAs (inconsistent)
Aortopulmonary window	Aorta	Pulmonary artery	Predominantly systolic (crescendo–decrescendo) in large defect; continuous in rare small defects	3rd or 4th left intercostal space	Usually unrestrictive; Frequently confused with a VSD murmur; Systolic ejection click may be present
Anomalous left coronary	Aorta via right coronary artery	Pulmonary artery via retrograde flow in left coronary from collaterals	Continuous	2nd left intercostal space	Presentation with continuous murmur rare; more commonly poor collateralization leads to LV dysfunction in infancy; Murmur louder in diastole
Coronary–cameral fistula to atrium	Aorta via coronary artery	Atrium	Continuous	Along right or left sternal border	Loudest in systole; Rarely sufficient volume load to cause CHF
Coronary–cameral fistula to right ventricle	Aorta via coronary artery	Right ventricle	Continuous	Left lower sternal border	Loudest in diastole; Rarely sufficient volume load to cause CHF
Coronary–cameral fistula to left ventricle	Aorta via coronary artery	Left ventricle	Diastolic decrescendo	Left lower sternal border	Mimics aortic insufficiency; rarely sufficient volume load to cause CHF
Blalock–Taussig shunt	Innominate artery or aorta	Pulmonary artery	Continuous	Variable; typically under right clavicle	Usually used in patients with single ventricle physiology; designed to be restrictive to pressure; Typical $Q_P:Q_S$ 1–2:1
Major aorto–pulmonary collaterals	Aorta, typically multiple separate vessels	Segmental pulmonary arteries	Continuous	Scattered over back	Often very soft; typically present in tetralogy of Fallot with pulmonary atresia

$Q_P:Q_S$, pulmonary to systemic flow ratio.

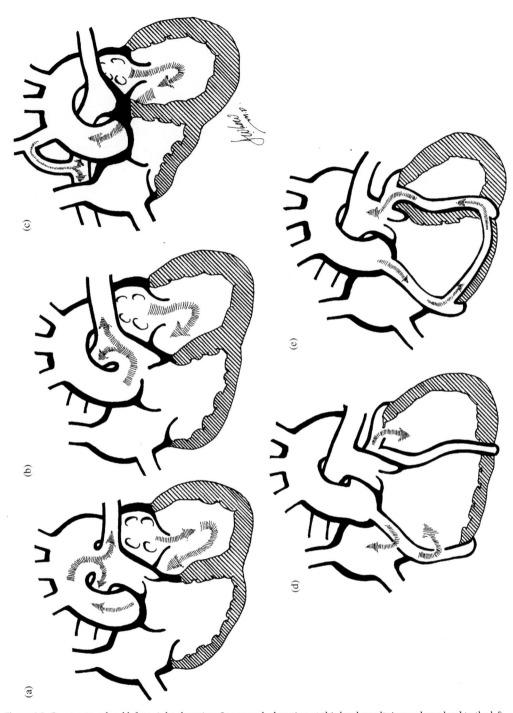

Figure 4.8 Great artery-level left to right shunting. In general, shunting at this level results in a volume load to the left atrium, left ventricle, and pulmonary arteries. Schematics are shown for (a) PDA, (b) aortopulmonary window, (c) Blalock–Taussig shunt, (d) coronary cameral fistulae, and (e) anomalous left coronary artery arising from the pulmonary artery.

Right to left shunting

In a series circulation, a right to left shunt results in desaturated blood being returned to the systemic circulation without being oxygenated in the lungs. Thus, the hallmark of a right to left shunt is arterial desaturation, which when visible is termed cyanosis. A pure right to left shunt *reduces* the volume load to the pulmonary circulation and consequently, does not result in CHF. Right to left shunting can occur at multiple anatomic levels and for multiple reasons.

Physical findings: The most important vital sign for detection of right to left shunting is pulse oximetry. It should be noted where the reading was obtained and what fraction of inspired oxygen the patient was receiving. Normal values for infants and children are 97% and above in room air [31]. Newborns achieve saturations in this range fairly consistently by 2 h of life [32], with mean pulse oximetry readings on admission to the newborn nursery (2.7 ± 1.3 h of life) of 97% [33]. A large, fixed, right to left shunt will result in arterial desaturation, which responds minimally to increased inspired oxygen. Small amounts of right to left shunting may not result in a detectable drop in arterial saturation as measured by pulse oximetry.

If the amount of right to left shunting is sufficient, cyanosis will be noted. The appearance of cyanosis is related to the concentration of deoxyhemoglobin and is therefore more evident in the presence of polycythemia. Central cyanosis has been reported to be apparent to the careful observer when the absolute level of deoxyhemoglobin is at least 1.5 g/dL [34]. This amount corresponds to an oxyhemoglobin saturation of 88% at a hemoglobin of 12 g/dL or 90% at a hemoglobin of 15 g/dL. However, other studies have documented physical examination to be unreliable in detecting cyanosis until desaturation is profound, even when the observation is deliberate as part of a study. In a study of neonates, patients with arterial oxygen saturation of 85–89% by arterial blood gas analysis were rated as cyanotic in the lips only approximately 55% of the time [10]. This percentage increased to approximately 70% at an arterial saturation of 75–79% and exceeded 90% only at a saturation of less than 75%. There was also a significant rate of false positives, with 28% of neonates with a saturation over 90% rated as cyanotic. The reliability of physical examination would likely be even poorer outside of a study.

In contrast to the pulmonary causes of arterial desaturation, right to left shunting does not cause respiratory distress unless desaturation is profound. With longstanding cyanosis, digital clubbing develops. Early clubbing is manifested by loss of the angle between the cuticle and the nailbed; advanced clubbing also features rounding of the soft tissues of the distal phalanx (Fig. 4.9).

Differential cyanosis refers to differences in arterial oxygenation in different parts of the body, most commonly comparing the right arm to the lower extremities. This phenomenon occurs when: (1) one ventricle supplies the circulation proximal to the ductus arteriosus; (2) the other ventricle supplies at least some blood to the circulation distal to the ductus arteriosus; and (3) the ventricles contain blood with differing oxygen saturations. Usual differential cyanosis results in higher right arm saturation than leg saturation. Examples of this scenario include persistent pulmonary hypertension of the newborn, interrupted aortic arch, and PDA with Eisenmenger syndrome. Reverse differential cyanosis (leg saturation higher than right arm saturation) occurs in transposition physiology with a PDA, and is more pronounced if coarctation is present. Deoxygenated RV blood passes to the aorta and the proximal arch vessels, while oxygenated LV blood is ejected into the pulmonary artery and some shunts across the ductus arteriosus to the descending aorta. Either of these patterns may be altered by abnormal aortic arch branching patterns, particularly when a subclavian artery arises aberrantly from the descending aorta.

Complex lesions with both right to left and left to right shunting

Many forms of complex congenital heart disease are compatible with life only when right to left and left to right shunts coexist and patients therefore have findings of both cyanosis and volume load. In addition, they may be associated with septal defects, valve abnormalities, surgically constructed shunts, or pulmonary hypertension. The physical diagnostician must combine components of the principles outlined above to be able to interpret the physical findings in these patients.

Acknowledgment

The author gratefully acknowledges artistic contributions to this chapter from David W. Low, M.D., Associate Professor of Surgery, University of Pennsylvania School of Medicine.

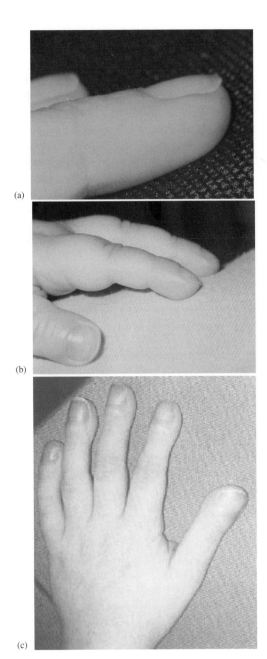

(a)

(b)

(c)

Figure 4.9 Digital clubbing. (a) Normal; note the angle between the cuticle and the nailbed. (b) Clubbing is still quite subtle in a 7-month old cyanotic since birth (arterial saturation 70%); note the loss of the angle between the cuticle and the nailbed. (c) More advanced clubbing in an older cyanotic patient; note the rounding of the tips of the fingers.

References

1. McCrindle BW, Shaffer KM, Kan JS, *et al.* Cardinal clinical signs in the differentiation of heart murmurs in children. Arch Pediatr Adolesc Med 1996; 150:169–174.
2. Geva T, Hegesh J, Frand M. Reappraisal of the approach to the child with heart murmurs: Is echocardiography mandatory? Int J Cardiol 1988; 19:107–113.
3. Klewer SE, Samson RA, Donnerstein RL, *et al.* Comparison of accuracy of diagnosis of congenital heart disease by history and physical examination versus echocardiography. Am J Cardiol 2002; 89:1329–1331.
4. Abu-Harb M, Hey E, Wren C. Death in infancy from unrecognised congenital heart disease. Arch Dis Child 1994; 71:3–7.
5. Ainsworth SB, Wyllie JP, Wren C. Prevalence and clinical significance of cardiac murmurs in neonates. Arch Dis Child Fetal Neonatal Ed 1999; 80:F43–45.
6. Stevenson LW, Perloff JK. The limited reliability of physical signs for estimating hemodynamics in chronic heart failure. JAMA 1989; 261:884–888.
7. Butman SM, Ewy GA, Standen JR, *et al.* Bedside cardiovascular examination in patients with severe chronic heart failure: Importance of rest or inducible jugular venous distension. J Am Coll Cardiol 1993; 22:968–974.
8. Shaver JA, Leonard, JJ, Leon DF. Auscultation of the Heart. Examination of the Heart. American Heart Association, 1990.
9. Perloff JK. The Clinical Recognition of Congenital Heart Disease. WB Saunders, Philadelphia, PA, p. 785, 1994.
10. Goldman HI, Maralit A, Sun S, *et al.* Neonatal cyanosis and arterial oxygen saturation. J Pediatr 1973; 82:319–324.
11. Goldmuntz E. The epidemiology and genetics of congenital heart disease. Clin Perinatol 2001; 28:1–10.
12. Goldmuntz E, Clark BJ, Mitchell LE, *et al.* Frequency of 22q11 deletions in patients with conotruncal defects. J Am Coll Cardiol 1998; 32:492–498.
13. Gerboni S, Sabatino G, Mingarelli R, *et al.* Coarctation of the aorta, interrupted aortic arch, and hypoplastic left heart syndrome in three generations. J Med Genet 1993; 30:328–329.
14. McElhinney DB, Clark BJ, Weinberg PM, *et al.* Association of chromosome 22q11 deletion with isolated anomalies of aortic arch laterality and branching. J Am Coll Cardiol 2001; 37:2114–2119.
15. Schott JJ, Benson DW, Basson CT, *et al.* Congenital heart disease caused by mutations in the transcription factor NKX2-5. Science 1998; 281:108–111.
16. Mani A, Meraji SM, Houshyar R, *et al.* Finding genetic contributions to sporadic disease: A recessive

locus at 12q24 commonly contributes to patent ductus arteriosus. Proc Nat Acad Sci USA 2002; 99:15054–15059.

17. Perloff JK. The jugular venous pulse and third heart sound in patients with heart failure. New Engl J Med 2001; 345:612–614.

18. Crawford MH. Inspection and Palpation of the Venous and Arterial Pulses. Examination of the Heart. American Heart Association, 1990.

19. Davison R, Cannon R. Estimation of central venous pressure by examination of jugular veins. Am Heart J 1974; 87:279–282.

20. Stein JH, Neumann A, Marcus RH. Comparison of estimates of right atrial pressure by physical examination and echocardiography in patients with congestive heart failure and reasons for discrepancies. Am J Cardiol 1997; 80:1615–1618.

21. McGee SR. Physical examination of venous pressure: a critical review. Am Heart J 1998; 136: 10–8.

22. Veasy LG. History and physical examination. In: Emmanouilides GC, Riemenschneider, T. A., Allen, H. D., Gutgesell, H P, eds., Heart Disease in Infants, Children, and Adolescents, Vol. 1. Williams and Wilkins, Baltimore, pp. 131–146, 1995.

23. Curtiss EI, Matthews RG, Shaver JA. Mechanism of normal splitting of the second heart sound. Circulation 1975; 51:157–164.

24. Shaver JA, O'Toole JD. The second heart sound: Newer concepts. Part I: Normal and wide physiological splitting. Mod Concepts Cardiovasc Dis 1977; 46: 7–12.

25. Shaver JA, O'Toole JD. The second heart sound: Newer concepts. Part II: Paradoxical splitting and narrow physiological splitting. Mod Concepts Cardiovasc Dis 1977; 46:13–16.

26. Perloff JK. Physical Examination of the Heart and Circulation. WB Saunders, Philadelphia, p. 291, 1990.

27. Thomas JT, Kelly RF, Thomas SJ, et al. Utility of history, physical examination, electrocardiogram, and chest radiograph for differentiating normal from decreased systolic function in patients with heart failure. Am J Med 2002; 112:437–45.

28. Shaver JA, Nadolny RA, O'Toole JD, et al. Sound pressure correlates of the second heart sound. An intracardiac sound study. Circulation 1974; 49:316–325.

29. Ellison RC, Freedom RM, Keane JF, et al. Indirect assessment of severity in pulmonary stenosis. Circulation 1977; 56 (suppl I):I14–I20.

30. Wagner HR, Weidman WH, Ellison RC et al. Indirect assessment of severity in aortic stenosis. Circulation 1977; 56 (suppl I):I20–I23.

31. Poets CF, Southall DP. Noninvasive monitoring of oxygenation in infants and children: Practical considerations and areas of concern. Pediatrics 1994; 93:737–746.

32. Reddy VK, Holzman IR, Wedgwood JF. Pulse oximetry saturations in the first 6 hours of life in normal term infants. Clin Pediatr 1999; 38:87–92.

33. Levesque BM, Pollack P, Griffin B, et al. Pulse oximetry: What's normal in the newborn nursery? Pediatr Pulmonol 2000; 30:406–412.

34. Goss GA, Hayes JA, Burdon JG. Deoxyhaemoglobin concentrations in the detection of central cyanosis. Thorax 1988; 43:212–213.

35. Milnor WR. The heart as a pump. In: Mountcastle VB, ed., Medical Physiology. Mosby, St. Louis, MO, pp. 986–1006, 1980.

CHAPTER 5

Plain Radiographic Examination of the Heart and Chest

Julien I.E. Hoffman & Robert C. Brasch

Before the ascent of echocardiography, the main noninvasive diagnostic method for congenital heart disease was the plain chest X-ray taken in four projections, sometimes accompanied by barium swallow and even fluoroscopy. Today fluoroscopy is not used for diagnosis, except perhaps to evaluate prosthetic valve function, the barium swallow is restricted to diagnosing vascular rings and slings, and only one or two projections are used for the X-ray [1,2]. The radiation dose for a frontal and lateral chest X-ray is only about 10–30 mSv [1].

The major use of the chest X-ray is to examine the lungs that are not resolved on the echocardiographic study; at the same time, heart size and shape, the position of the aorta and pulmonary artery, the size of the thymus, and even abdominal situs can be evaluated. The bony thorax is well shown and may show abnormalities relevant to the diagnosis of heart disease.

Technical issues

The patient must not be rotated and inspiration should be deep enough for the diaphragm to be at the level of the eight or ninth rib posteriorly. Too shallow a breath makes the heart appear too wide and the lung fields too dense, with at times the false appearance of pulmonary edema or increased pulmonary vascularity. Too deep a breath, and the heart is narrow, with hyperlucent lung fields that suggest pulmonary underperfusion. If there is a lordotic view, with clavicles above the lung apex, the right ventricular apex is elevated and simulates right ventricular hypertrophy. Pulmonary vascular markings are also influenced by the degree of penetration and the kilovoltage used. An overpenetrated film (thoracic spine very prominent) makes the lung fields dark and suggests underperfusion, whereas an underpenetrated film (spine not resolvable) exaggerates pulmonary vascular markings. Some of the potential problems from variable exposure factors are mimimized by the use of computed radiography with its normalization of appearance on the video monitor.

Bony thorax

Rib and vertebral anomalies and scoliosis are quite common when there is associated congenital heart disease. Straight back syndrome and pectus excavatum are associated with innocent murmurs but also with mitral valve prolapse and Marfan's syndrome. Rib notching may be seen with coarctation of the aorta generally in children beyond the age of 4 years (Fig. 5.1). A narrow anterior–posterior chest diameter distorts the heart shape and size.

Situs problems

The position of the liver, the gastric air bubble, the cardiac apex, and the aortic arch give information about whole body and atrial situs, and therefore, abnormalities may indicate one of the heterotaxies. Of more importance is the anatomy of the major bronchi [3]. Normally, the left bronchus is long and does not bifurcate until it is crossed by the pulmonary artery to the left lower lobe; the right bronchus, by contrast, is short and bifurcates before being crossed by the artery to the right lower lobe. In mirror image

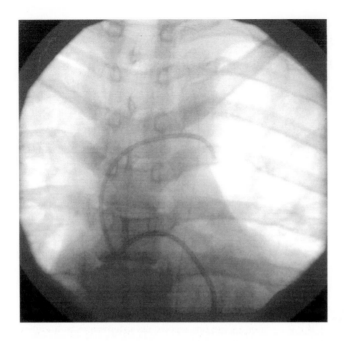

Figure 5.1 Marked rib notching in an adult patient with coarctation of the aorta.

dextrocardia (complete situs inversus) these patterns are reversed. In right-sided isomerism (typically with asplenia) there are two similar right bronchi and bilateral minor fissures in the lungs, and in left-sided isomerism (typically with polysplenia) there two similar left bronchi and no minor fissures.

Thymus

This organ is typically involuted during periods of stress and thus very small in neonates with complete D-transposition of the great arteries, leading to the classical narrow mediastinal shadow in this lesion (Fig. 5.2).

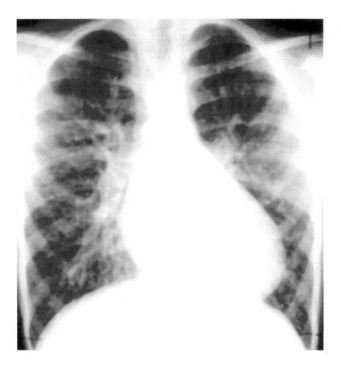

Figure 5.2 Classical frontal view of D-transposition of the great arteries. The mediastinum is narrow because the thymus is tiny and the aorta is in front of the pulmonary artery. The pulmonary vascularity is increased.

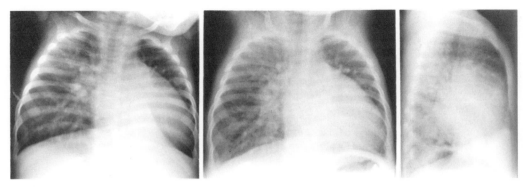

Figure 5.3 Frontal view showing collapsed left lower lobe in a child with a large ventricular septal defect.

Lung fields

Parenchymal disease, including consolidation and lobar lung collapse, is important to detect before cardiac catheterization; massive collapse may explain cardiac malposition (Fig. 5.3).

Pulmonary edema is shown by blurred hilar vessels, blurring of the peripheral vascular markings, and blurring of the interface between the right atrium and the lung. The fissures are prominent and there may also be horizontal Kerley B lines at the lung bases, representing interstitial edema of the interlobular septa (Figs. 5.4 and 5.5).

Pulmonary oligemia, as a result of decreased lung perfusion, is a feature of many forms of cyanotic congenital heart disease with decreased pulmonary blood flow. It is suggested by dark lung fields and small, sparse vascular markings, but special effort must be made to be sure that the X-ray technique is optimal (Fig. 5.6). Another decreased vascular pattern is seen in those with severe pulmonary vascular disease (Eisenmenger's syndrome). Normally, the smaller pulmonary arteries can be seen two-thirds of the way to the edge of the thorax. In severe pulmonary vascular disease, however, the peripheral

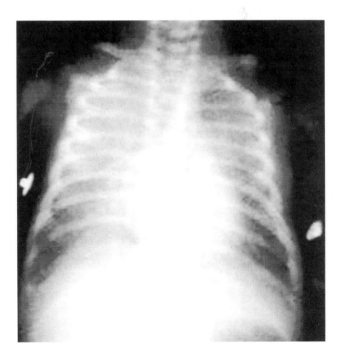

Figure 5.4 A neonate with obstructed pulmonary venous drainage due to total anomalous pulmonary venous connection below the diaphragm. The heart is small and the right heart border is blurred by the pulmonary edema that is evident throughout most of the lungs.

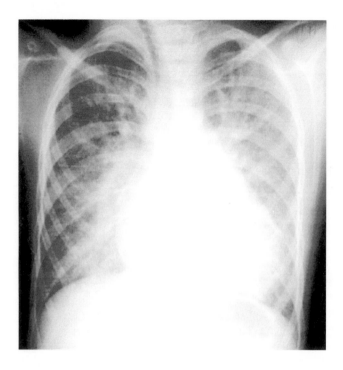

Figure 5.5 Frontal view of a child with a large atrioventricular septal defect and pulmonary edema due to congestive heart failure. The heart borders are obscured by the edema, the horizontal fissure is well shown, and the upper pulmonary veins are dilated. The cardiac silhouette is enlarged.

pulmonary arteries are sparse and pruned, which with the enlarged central pulmonary artery gives rise to the "tree in winter" pattern. Finally, it is possible to have regional oligemia if blood flow is reduced or absent to a portion of the lung because of congenital stenosis or absence of a branch pulmonary artery or because that artery is occluded by thrombus or embolus.

Pulmonary venous hypertension is associated with obstructed (total) anomalous pulmonary venous connection or to a high left atrial pressure from left ventricular failure, hypoplastic left heart syndrome

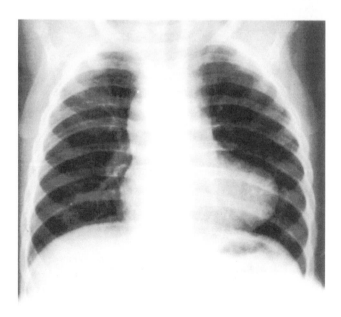

Figure 5.6 Tetralogy of Fallot showing uptilted cardiac apex ("sheep's nose") due to right ventricular hypertrophy; dark lung fields devoid of vascular markings due to pulmonary underperfusion; and a right aortic arch with a right-sided indentation on the tracheal air column.

with inadequate left atrial to right atrial communication, or to cor triatriatum or mitral stenosis. Acutely it shows a fuzzy pattern throughout the lung fields because of the edema of the interlobar septa as well as the other features of pulmonary edema. Small pleural effusions may occur, but are uncommon in children. If the venous hypertension is more chronic, there can be redistribution of blood flow with engorged veins in the apices of the lungs in older children and adults (Fig. 5.5). Normally, when erect, blood flow to the lung apices is minimal because of gravity, and flow increases progressively toward the lung bases [4]. In pulmonary venous hypertension, however, because of the predominantly basilar edema, alveolar hypoxia, and vasoconstriction, blood is diverted to the apices, so that the upper pulmonary veins become more prominent than usual and are wider than the lower pulmonary veins. This mechanism obviously does not apply to infants who are supine most of the day and have a smaller thoracic size.

Pulmonary plethora occurs when pulmonary flow is twice as much as normal or more because of a left to right shunt, and is manifest by generalized enlargement of the pulmonary arteries out to the lung periphery, often seen especially well in the artery to the right lower lobe (Fig. 5.7). The changes occur because the increased flow dilates the pulmonary arteries, and not because of the increased flow *per se*. This dilatation is more marked if pressure is also increased, as in a large patent ductus arteriosus or ventricular septal defect as opposed to a large atrial septal defect. On the other hand, we have seen children who developed large left to right shunts after surgery without enlarged pulmonary arteries because their arteries did not dilate. As a rule, pulmonary plethora is associated with an increased heart size and an enlarged main pulmonary artery segment as long as the great arteries are not malposed. This is in contrast to the changes in isolated pulmonary venous hypertension due to obstruction at or before the level of the left atrium (for example, cor triatriatum, total anomalous pulmonary venous connection) in which the heart is often small. Enlarged pulmonary arteries are also seen with extracardiac shunts such as the great vein of Galen malformations and with high output states, as in anemia.

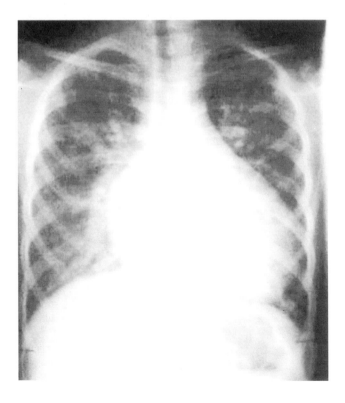

Figure 5.7 Same patient as shown in Fig. 5.5, after treatment of congestive heart failure. The heart is still enlarged but the pulmonary edema has disappeared. The enlarged pulmonary arterial markings, especially to the right lower lobe, are well shown.

Bronchial vascular markings

In severe pulmonary atresia the lungs are supplied by tortuous collaterals from the aorta and by enlarged bronchial arteries. Therefore, the central pulmonary arterial segment is missing, and the tortuous bronchial arteries, frequently seen end-on, show up throughout the lung fields.

Heart and central great arteries

The heart size and shape are well shown radiographically, but the characteristic shapes described in the literature are better seen in older children and may be absent in neonates. The normal left-sided aortic arch and the main pulmonary artery can usually be seen with the trachea bowed slightly to the right side. With a right-sided aortic arch, seen most often in tetralogy of Fallot (Fig. 5.6) and truncus arteriosus, the trachea is pushed to the left. In complete D-transposition of the great arteries the mediastinal stalk is narrow because the thymus is small from stress-related involution and the aorta and pulmonary artery are often one in front of the other (Fig. 5.2). On the other hand, in L-transposition of the great arteries the aorta appears as a straight segment on the left-hand border, in distinction to the curved segment of a normal pulmonary artery. This pulmonary arterial segment will be enlarged if there is a large left-to-right shunt, with poststenotic dilatation in valvar pulmonic stenosis (with the dilatation often extending into the left main pulmonary artery), and in idiopathic dilatation of the main pulmonary artery. In tetralogy of Fallot the main pulmonary arterial segment is absent, and this with the rounded right ventricle and elevated cardiac apex gives the classical "coeur-en-sabot" appearance (Fig. 5.6). In truncus arteriosus the hilar pulmonary arteries may be misplaced and the typical main pulmonary arterial segment is absent.

Interpreting individual chamber size, shape, and pressure is difficult and subject to errors. For example, with a narrow antero–posterior chest diameter the heart is widened in the usual frontal view, but because it is smaller than normal in the lateral view the heart volume is normal. In general, ventricular hypertrophy changes size minimally, and an enlarged mediastinal shadow, if not due to a pericardial effusion, is usually due to chamber dilatation. A dilated right atrium may show an enlarged rounded right heart border, as in Ebstein's anomaly (Fig. 5.8). A hypertrophied right ventricle rotates the heart and lifts up the apex from the diaphragm (Fig. 5.6); with right ventricular dialataion, the heart shadow in the lateral view extends two third of the distance up the sternum as compared to the one third seen normally.

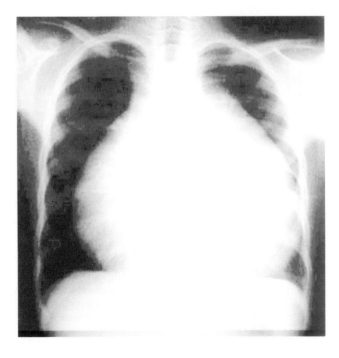

Figure 5.8 Hugely dilated heart, and especially the right atrium, in a patient with Ebstein's anomaly.

An enlarged left atrium may show up as double density on frontal view, as a bulge on the left heart border between the pulmonary artery segment and the apex, or by elevating the left main bronchus and widening the carina. An enlarged left ventricle rotates the heart counterclockwise so that the aortic arch is more prominent, and on the lateral view the cardiac shadow extends well posterior to the inferior vena cava. All these changes are less well shown in neonates than in older children and adults, and all are considerably less specific than is the echocardiogram.

Tracheoesophageal problems

This is one group of lesions for which a barium swallow is very helpful. In investigating stridor, a double aortic arch or a right arch with a constricting left ductus or ligamentum arteriosus makes a double indentation on each side of the esophagus on the frontal view and a posterior esophageal indentation on lateral view. An aberrant right subclavian artery produces a posterior esophageal indentation on lateral view that on frontal view is oblique, passing upward from left to right. With a pulmonary artery sling, there is an anterior esophageal indentation. Occasionally a carotid or innominate artery compresses the trachea anteriorly and an indentation may be seen on the tracheal air shadow.

References

1. Amplatz K. Plain film diagnosis of congenital heart disease. In: Moller JH, Hoffman JIE, eds., Pediatric Cardiovascular Disease. Churchill Livingstone, New York, pp. 143–155, 2000.
2. Reidy JE. The chest radiograph. In: Anderson RH, Baker EJ, Macartney FJ, et al., eds., Paediatric Cardiology. Churchill Livingstone, London, pp. 285–293, 2002.
3. Anderson RH. Nomenclature and classification: Sequential segmental analysis. In: Moller JH, Hoffman JIE, eds., Pediatric Cardiovascular Disease. Churchill Livingstone, New York, pp. 263–274, 2000.
4. West JB. Ventilation/Blood Flow and Gas Exchange, 3rd edn. Blackwell, Oxford, pp. 17–33, 1977.

CHAPTER 6

Cardiac Catheterization

Julien I.E. Hoffman

Cardiac catheterization

The history of cardiac catheterization is described fully by Mueller and Sanborn [1] and only the highlights will be mentioned here. In 1929 Werner Forsmann, a German urologist, passed a urological catheter from an arm vein into his right atrium [2], a daring demonstration that led to his dismissal from his hospital. In the next one and a half decades about 300 right atrial catheterizations were done by radiologists who realized that they could produce better angiocardiograms by injecting into the right atrium rather than through a peripheral vein. At one medical meeting a young European cardiologist suggested that this technique could be used to measure cardiac output by the Fick principle, but the senior cardiologist present dismissed his proposal as being too dangerous! It was not until the 1940s that Andre Cournand and Dickinson Richards introduced cardiac catheterization for diagnostic purposes [3], and in 1946 both of them and Forsmann received the Nobel Prize for this seminal advance. In 1950 Zimmerman *et al.* [4] performed retrograde catheterization of the left heart.

Cardiac catheterization with angiocardiography began to be used extensively for anatomic diagnosis and physiologic assessment. It was gradually adapted for children, but it was not until the mid 1950s that it was applied to infants and by the end of that decade to premature infants. In 1966 Miller and Rashkind developed balloon atrial septostomy to palliate neonates with transposition of the great arteries, thus ushering in the era of interventional cardiology [5]. This was soon followed by techniques for closing a patent ductus arteriosus [6] and an atrial septal defect [7] with clumsy devices that were nevertheless precursors of what we use today. In 1977 Andreas Gruntzig adapted the Dotter and Judkins method of using increasing catheter sizes to dilate stenotic peripheral arteries [8] by developing an effective balloon catheter, and introduced percutaneous transluminal coronary artery dilatation (PTCA) for coronary stenosis [9]. In 1982 Kan used a balloon to open a stenotic pulmonary valve [10] and Park introduced blade atrial septostomy [11]. Stents began to be used in 1989 because of the unsatisfactory response to dilating stenotic vessels [12]. From then on interventional techniques proliferated and were applied to an increasing number of lesions [13].

Cardiac catheterization may be used for diagnosis or for treatment. It is seldom needed to make anatomic diagnoses that can usually be made accurately by noninvasive imaging techniques, but is used to obtain functional information about pressures and flows that can today be only approximated by these other tests. In particular, it is used to evaluate pulmonary vascular resistance, to define lesions of peripheral pulmonary arteries, and to evaluate complex anatomy, especially in the single ventricle group. It may be needed to evaluate problems immediately after surgery when transthoracic echocardiography may be inadequate because of dressings or air in the mediastinum, and can even be used in patients on ECMO (extracorporeal membrane oxygenation) [14]. In the treatment mode it is used to close abnormal communications like a patent ductus arteriosus, atrial septal defect, or an arteriovenous fistula; dilate narrowed structures like a small foramen ovale, a stenotic valve, coarctation of the aorta, peripheral pulmonary arterial stenosis, or narrowed coronary (and other) arteries; or to ablate abnormal tracts or foci that start or maintain arrhythmias.

The catheterization laboratory

This should be big enough to hold present and future equipment comfortably, including anesthesia equipment, and to allow access of doctors and technicians to the patient. A biplane fluoroscopy unit with the ability to angulate the tubes is essential, especially for small sick infants with complex lesions. Measurements and angiograms are inspected as they are produced, and stored, preferably digitally for compactness and ease of retrieval. There are many systems available. Bridges and Freed [15] and Qureshi [16] describe the main requirements.

Preliminaries

Sick patients should be evaluated for dehydration, acid–base and blood gas status, electrolytes, and hemoglobin concentration, and appropriate measures taken to restore normal values as far as can be done before the catheterization. Decisions about intubation, use of prostaglandins, and inotropic support need to be made. It is essential to take a personal and family history of abnormal bleeding or clotting and, if needed, to do coagulation tests; von Willebrand disease occurs in 1% of the population. A hematocrit over 60% should be lowered by a combination of phlebotomy and fluid infusion before the catheterization [13] to avoid problems from hyperviscosity that could be made more severe by dehydration that might occur during the study. Girls of child-bearing age should be assessed for pregnancy to avoid radiating an embryo. If a child has an acute illness, a planned cardiac catheterization should be deferred. Pulmonary infiltrations on chest X-ray, unless known to be chronic, should lead to postponement of the study because of the risk of altering pulmonary vascular resistance.

Sedation and anesthesia

In many centers cardiac catheterization is done under general anesthesia. The arguments in favor of general anesthesia are that the patient is immobile and unaware of the discomforts of the study, airway control is guaranteed, and a trained observer is dedicated to watching the patient's vital signs. The disadvantages are the increased time needed for induction and recovery, the very slight risk of death that any general anesthetic incurs, the need to accommodate another person in the crowded environment around the patient, and possible cardiovascular depression from the anesthetic that changes the physiologic information; in addition, exercise testing during the study is not possible.

Other centers use sedation, the specific agents varying widely [13,15,17–20]. We, for example, give children 2 mg/kg diphenhydramine hydrochloride (Benadryl) by mouth (p.o.) about an hour before they come to the cardiac catheterization suite, and once there they are given 0.5 mg/kg p.o. midazolam (Versed). After an intravenous line has been placed, they are given 2 mg/kg i.v. pentobarbital (Nembutal). In some children, 0.1 mg/kg methadone p.o. is given. Another frequently used combination is meperidine (Demerol) 1.5–2.0 mg/kg, promethazine (Phenergan) 1.0 mg/kg, and chlorpromazine (Thorazine) 1.0 mg/kg given intramuscularly 30–45 min before the study. Ketamine is often used as the sole or supplementary sedative, in a dose of 0.5–1.0 mg/kg i.v. over 30–60 sec or 2 mg/kg intramuscularly [21]. Small infants may be given chloral hydrate 80 mg/kg p.o. None of these agents is completely without effect on the circulation, although ketamine or propofol [19] may cause the least changes. Chlorpromazine should be avoided if it is critical to measure an accurate pulmonary vascular resistance because it can act as a pulmonary (and systemic) vasodilator. Whether or not an anesthesiologist is needed for any of these combinations depends upon the decision of the cardiologist and the policy of the hospital concerning conscious sedation.

General monitoring

The room should be heated to 80–85°F (26.7–29.4°C), and small children should be placed on a warming device and their body temperature be monitored. Respiration is monitored by inspection, often difficult with small infants covered by drapes, and with occasional blood gas measurements. Blood pressure is measured continuously via an arterial line or intermittently by cuff. The electrocardiogram is monitored continuously for heart rate, arrhythmias, and changes in ST segments. Arterial oxygen saturation is measured continuously by a pulse oximeter, with occasional checks by blood gases. In small children, blood removal must be monitored and excessive removal of blood corrected by infusing packed cells.

Vascular access

Vascular access is done under local anesthesia with lidocaine, and because this injection itself is painful, a lidocaine cream that produces surface anesthesia is applied prior to the injection [22]. Usually the vessels are entered percutaneously, and it is rare to have to cut down on the vein or artery [16]. Venous access is usually from the femoral vein, but may occasionally have to be from a brachial, axillary, subclavian, or jugular vein if the femoral veins are occluded [13,15]. The umbilical vein can be used in the first week after birth, but manipulation from it is difficult [15]. The hepatic vein is rarely entered by a transhepatic approach [23]. Details of the techniques are described in several publications [15,16]. Arterial access is usually through the femoral artery, but if needed for special purposes (coronary artery catheterization, critical aortic stenosis in infants) could be from a brachial or carotid artery. If the femoral artery is difficult to find, especially if it is behind the femoral vein, then an ultrasound device on a needle tip is useful for localizing arterial blood flow [24]. Anticoagulation is usually not needed unless an arterial catheter is inserted for more than 30 min, and then 50 units/kg heparin is given. If it is, assess coagulation by measuring activated clotting times every 30–60 min.

Catheters are chosen according to the patient's size. Any catheter smaller than a 5F tends to give overdamped pressure tracings. Catheter–manometer systems should be checked before the study for damping characteristics, realizing that little air bubbles form in the catheter and transducer continuously and degrade catheter performance during the study; frequent flushing is needed. Short and wide catheters may be underdamped, and especially in the right ventricle may produce exaggerated systolic pressures due to catheter fling. The highest fidelity tracings come from micromanometer-tipped catheters, but these are stiff and expensive. They can sometimes be used by connecting the tip of the micromanometer to the hub of the catheter that is in the vessel [25]. Specialized catheters are available for various purposes.

Transseptal puncture

This was adapted by Mullins [26] for children without a patent atrial septum who either needed an atrial opening to be created or required anterograde access to the left atrium and ventricle. A long sheath over a dilator is introduced over a thin guide wire and advanced to the superior vena cava. Then the guide wire is removed and replaced with the long needle that remains inside the dilator, and the assembly is rotated until the tip faces left and posteriorly, withdrawn into the right atrium and then advanced until the tip catches on the upper rim of the fossa ovalis. The needle is advanced through the septum, and its position verified by blood sampling, pressures and, if needed, a small injection of contrast medium. If satisfactory, then the dilator is passed over the needle into the left atrium, the needle is withdrawn, the sheath is aspirated and flushed, and the chosen catheter is advanced through the sheath to its desired destination.

Risks and complications of cardiac catheterization

In well-equipped laboratories and with well-trained experienced operators, the risks and complications are very low, although as judged by troponin I release minor myocardial damage is frequent [27,28]. Arrhythmias are probably the commonest major complications [29]. Occasional supraventricular and ventricular ectopic beats are common and indicate the need for caution when manipulating the catheter in a particular area. Short episodes of supraventricular or ventricular tachycardia are usually self-limited, but on occasion need to be terminated by appropriate intravenous drugs or even countershock. Ventricular fibrillation is rare except in very ill patients. Atrioventricular block, including complete block, may occur rarely, and is usually self-limited. Cardiac perforation sometimes occurs; if through the ventricle (the right ventricular outflow tract is the most likely) there is usually little bleeding and little risk of pericardial tamponade, but atrial perforation is more serious. Repeated echocardiographic checks to make sure that bleeding does not continue are usually all that are needed. Hypotension may occur, sometimes of unknown (possible neurogenic) origin but often related to bleeding or dehydration with inadequate fluid replacement. Occasionally adolescents may have a typical syncopal spell while lying on the table. Hypercyanotic (tetralogy) spells are seldom seen today, and decreased consciousness due to strokes or seizures is rare. Sepsis can occur but is rare. Sometimes there may be allergic reactions to latex or to the injected contrast material, and treatment for anaphylactic shock should be at hand.

Vascular complications are common, and usually minor, and include bleeding and loss of the arterial pulse [29]. Arterial pulse loss is quite common, particularly with prolonged arterial catheterization, many changes of arterial sheaths, and use of over-large sheaths. If the limb circulation seems adequate, observation for 2 h may show resolution of spasm or minor clots, but if the pulse loss persists or the limb appears threatened, clot lysis with urokinase, streptokinase, or tPA is used. Streptokinase is given as a loading dose of 1000 units/kg, and then an infusion of 1000–3000 units/(kg h) for up to 48 h, the dose depending on the arterial response and the fibrinogen level, which should not fall below 1 g/L; results are good [30]. tPA is given at 0.5 mg/(kg h) for 6–8 h, checking to make sure that fibrinogen does not fall below 1 g/L [31]. We start tPA by infusing at 0.1 mg/(kg h), and increase by 0.1 mg/(kg h) every 2 h if the pulse remains absent. If the patient remains pulseless after 2 h at 0.2 mg/(kg h), a fibrinogen level is drawn and if the level is >1 g/L (100 mg/dL), the infusion may be increased to 0.3 mg/(kg h). If fibrinogen is <100 mg/dL but >50 mg/dL we monitor carefully for bleeding and pain, and take vital signs every 2 h. If fibrinogen is <50 mg/dL stop the infusion. Doses >0.3 mg/(kg h) should be used with caution to a maximum dose of 0.5 mg/(kg h); the maximum duration of infusion should be 8 h with a maximum total 8 h dose not to exceed 100 mg. Whatever lysis is used, the groin dressing(s) should be exposed and checked frequently because of the risk of bleeding. Complete or partial restoration of the pulse is achieved in about 85% of children, but bleeding complications are common. Attempts should be made to restore the pulse because occasionally an occluded femoral artery leads to deficient limb growth on that side. Rarely there are late occurrences of an arteriovenous fistula or a pseudoaneurysm that require vascular surgical repair.

Death from cardiac catheterization is rare, and usually occurs in a moribund infant who dies during but not because of the catheterization. With improved techniques and care, the death rate has fallen from about 10% to under 0.5%, and serious nonfatal complications occur in only about 2% [29,32–36]. Complications of interventional catheterization are similar to those described above, but a little more frequent [37].

Measuring cardiac output

Principle

This is done by indicator dilution methods. Let an organ have a constant flow of F (mL/min) through it, and let steady state concentrations (in mg/mL) of an indicator in artery and vein be C_a and C_v, respectively. Since concentration (C, mg/mL) is a quantity (Q, mg) divided by volume (V, mL), then $Q = CV$. Volume per minute equals flow, so that $F = V/\text{min}$. Then each minute $Q_a = FC_a$ mg of indicator enters and $Q_v = FC_v$ mg leaves the organ. The difference $Q_a - Q_v = Q_x$ represents the amount of indicator taken up by (Q_x is positive) or removed from the organ (Q_x is negative). Therefore, $Q_x = Q_a - Q_v = F(C_a - C_v)$, so that $F = Q_x/(C_a - C_v)$. If we can measure Q_x, C_a, and C_v, then we can calculate flow per minute through the organ. For cardiac output by the Fick method, the organ is the lung, Q_x is oxygen consumption, and C_a and C_v are the oxygen contents of pulmonary artery and vein, respectively. (Note that in cardiology, we use Q to mean flow and not quantity.)

For pulmonary flow (Q_p, mL/min), the relevant oxygen contents (mL/L) are in pulmonary veins (C_{pv}) and pulmonary arteries (C_{pa}). For systemic flow (Q_s, mL/min), the relevant oxygen contents are in the aorta (C_{pa}) and mixed venous blood (C_{mv}). Because in the absence of shunts $C_{pv} = C_{ao}$ and $C_{pa} = C_{mv}$, pulmonary and systemic flows are the same (see Table 6.1). If C_{pa} exceeds C_{mv}, then there is a left-to-right shunt, calculated as the difference between systemic and pulmonary flows (Table 6.1). If C_{pv} exceeds C_{ao}, there is a right-to-left shunt, calculated as the difference between systemic and pulmonary flows (Table 6.1). Bidirectional shunts are more complicated. We define effective pulmonary blood flow (Q_{ep}, mL/min) as the amount of deoxygenated venous blood that is oxygenated in the lungs, and calculate it by dividing oxygen consumption by $C_{pv} - C_{mv}$. Pulmonary and systemic flows are calculated as described above. The difference between pulmonary and effective pulmonary flows is the left-to-right shunt, and the difference between systemic and effective pulmonary flows is the right-to-left shunt (Table 6.1). Note that effective pulmonary flow equals systemic and pulmonary flows with no shunts, is the same as systemic flow in a pure left-to-right shunt, and is the same as pulmonary flow in a pure right-to-left shunt.

Table 6.1 Examples of Flow Calculations.

	No shunt	Left-to-right shunt	Right-to-left shunt	Bidirectional shunt
VO_2 (mL/min)	240	240	240	240
C_{pv} (mL/L)	200	200	200	200
C_{ao} (mL/L)	200	200	180	180
C_{pa} (mL/L)	160	180	120	160
C_{mv} (mL/L)	160	160	120	120
Q_p (L/min)	6.0	12.0	3.0	6.0
Q_s (L/min)	6.0	6.0	4.0	4.0
Q_{ep} (L/min)	6.0	6.0	3.0	3.0
Q_{lr} (L/min)	–	6.0	–	3.0
Q_{rl} (L/min)	–	–	1.0	1.0

Practical issues

1 Oxygen consumption must be measured accurately [38,39]. Even though there are tables relating oxygen consumption to age and size [40–43], the variability is too large for accurate estimates.

2 Oxygen content of blood in milliliter per liter is [oxygen carrying capacity of blood (13.6 mL O_2/ (g Hb L blood)) multiplied by percent oxygen saturation (SaO_2)] + dissolved oxygen (mL/L). Dissolved oxygen in milliliter per liter is 0.03 mL O_2/(L mm Hg) partial pressure of oxygen. At a nominal arterial partial pressure of 100 mm Hg and an oxygen saturation of 100% there will be 3 mL/L of dissolved oxygen, a tiny fraction of the oxygen carried by hemoglobin (13.6 × 15 × 1 = 204 mL/L). When breathing 100% oxygen, however, dissolved oxygen could be 0.03 × 600 = 18 mL/L, and this could materially affect the calculation. For example, with a Q_{O_2} of 240 mL/min, a pulmonary venous saturation of 100%, and a pulmonary arterial saturation of 95%, the arteriovenous difference of oxygen content would be 10.2 mL/L if we ignore dissolved oxygen, and Q_p would be 23.5 L/min. However, if we include dissolved oxygen the arteriovenous difference of oxygen content would be ~22 mL/L and Q_p would be ~11 L/min.

3 A small arteriovenous difference in oxygen content across the lung, as in a large left-to-right shunt, can lead to large errors. If the true difference is 5%, the 1% error of the method could easily lead to errors of 20% or more in calculated flows. Thus if Q_{O_2} was 240 mL/min, pulmonary venous saturation was 95%, then C_{pv} would be 13.6 × 15 × 0.95 = 193.8 mL/L + dissolved oxygen = ~197 mL/L breathing room air. If pulmonary arterial saturation was 90%,

then C_{pa} would be ~187 mL/L and Q_p would be 24 L/min. Consider, however, that if the 95% and 90% measurements were really 94% and 91%, the calculated Q_p would be ~34 L/min, or if they were 96% and 89% the calculated Q_p would be ~17 L/min.

4 If there are left-to-right shunts at more than one level (ASD and VSD, ASD and PDA, VSD and PDA, or at all three levels) the contribution that each level makes can be assessed by calculating Q_p successively from oxygen contents in each relevant chamber or vessel as if it were the pulmonary artery. Thus ASD flow is calculated from the difference between Q_s and Q_p(ASD) derived from the difference in oxygen contents in pulmonary vein and right atrium; with perfect mixing, the right atrial and pulmonary oxygen contents would be the same. The flow is then calculated through the VSD by calculating a new Q_p(VSD) derived from the difference in oxygen contents in pulmonary vein and right ventricle. Since Q_p(VSD) is made up of both left-to-right shunts, the difference between Q_p(VSD) and Q_p(ASD) is the flow through the VSD. Similarly, flow through the ductus is the difference between Q_p(PDA) and Q_p(VSD). Note that because mixing may be incomplete, saturations in right atrium or ventricle might not be representative of the shunts; that is why we usually use pulmonary arterial oxygen content to measure left-to-right shunts because of the belief that this represents the best mixed right-sided oxygen content. For this reason, a left-to-right shunt can be calculated only if saturation in the right atrium is 8% greater than that in systemic vein, 5% greater in the right ventricle than that in the right atrium, or 2% greater in pulmonary artery than that in the right ventricle. Second, because each level of shunting reduces the

Table 6.2 Examples of Flow Calculations with Shunts at Three Levels.

	Left-to-right shunt through ASD	Add left-to-right shunt through VSD	Add left-to-right shunt through PDA
VO_2 (mL/min)	240	240	240
C_{pv} (mL/L)	200	200	200
C_{ao} (mL/L)	200	200	200
C_{pa} (mL/L)	170	180	190
C_{rv} (mL/L)	170	180	180
C_{ra} (mL/L)	170	170	170
C_{mv} (mL/L)	160	120	120
Q_p (L/min)	8.0	12.0	24.0
Q_s (L/min)	6.0	6.0	6.0
Q_p(ASD) (L/min)	2.0	2.0	2.0
Q_p(VSD) (L/min)		4.0	4.0
Q_p(PDA) (L/min)			12.0

arteriovenous difference of oxygen content across the lung, the same increase in oxygen saturation at each site gives larger calculated shunts at the more distal sites (Table 6.2). Obviously, the calculation of the third shunt through the PDA is fairly inaccurate.

5 Because calculating both Q_p and Q_s require measurement of oxygen consumption, their ratio does not require this measurement. Because in room air oxygen content and saturation are almost proportional (content $= 13.6 \times$ Hb concentration $\times$ saturation + dissolved oxygen), the Q_p/Q_s ratio can be calculated easily as

$$\frac{Q_p}{Q_s} = \frac{Sat_{Ao} - Sat_{MV}}{Sat_{PV} - Sat_{PA}}.$$

This ratio gives a rough idea of shunt size because in people with no heart failure Q_s is relatively constant. Nevertheless, because Q_s can change with heart failure, anemia, hypoxemia, anxiety, or exercise, the ratio should not be used for critical clinical decisions relative to shunt size.

6 To allow for differences in flows due to differences in body size, we use the fact that cardiac output at rest is approximately proportional to body surface area, with resting output being 3.5 L/min per square meter body surface area (the cardiac index). A pulmonary blood flow of 3.5 L/min is excessive for a newborn infant with a body surface area of 0.25 m^2 but is markedly reduced for an adult with a body surface area of 2 m^2. Therefore, we convert absolute flows to flows/m^2; the easiest way to do this being to index oxygen consumption. If indexing

is done after calculating cardiac output, divide the calculated output by the body surface area

7 *Unsteady concentrations.* If we use an exogenous indicator by injecting indocyanine green or cold saline, then input and output concentrations are not steady, but as long as flow is steady we can use the Kety–Schmidt method. In any small time period the amount of indicator accumulating in the organ is dQ_x, and in this time interval flow is calculated as

$$F \, dt = \frac{dQ_x}{(C_a - C_v)},$$

so that $dQ_x = F \, dt(C_a - C_v)$. Over u minutes we integrate both sides of the equation to give

$$Q_x(u) = F \int_0^u (C_a - C_v) \, dt$$

and so

$$F = \frac{Q_x(u)}{\int_0^u (C_a - C_v) \, dt}$$

where $Q_x(u)$ is the quantity of indicator accumulating in u minutes and $\int_0^u (C_a - C_v) \, dt$ is the integrated difference over the period. For a bolus injection of dye or cold saline, $Q_x(u)$ is the total amount of dye or negative heat injected and $\int_0^u (C_a - C_v) \, dt$ is the area under the arterial curve of indicator (dye concentration or temperature). For dye, C_v is zero prior to recirculation, but for cold saline the temperature of the incoming venous blood must be accounted for. Details of these techniques and their inaccuracies are found in standard texts [44].

Calculating vascular resistance

In electricity, Ohm's law states that

$$\text{Resistance} = \frac{\text{Voltage drop (V)}}{\text{Current (A)}}$$

The equivalent in the circulation is

$$\text{Resistance} = \frac{\text{Pressue drop (mm Hg)}}{\text{Flow (L/min)}}$$

This yields Wood units of $\text{mm Hg}/(\text{L min})$. To convert these to the strictly correct resistance units of dyne sec cm^{-5}, multiply Wood units by 80.

For the systemic circulation, the resistance is usually calculated as

Systemic vascular resistance (SVR or R_s)

$$= \frac{\text{Mean}\,P_{ao} - \text{Mean}\,P_{ra}}{Q_s}$$

where P_{ao} is aortic pressure, P_{ra} is right atrial pressure, and Q_s is systemic blood flow. However, because venous critical closing pressure is usually about 10–12 mm Hg and higher than P_{ra} it is more correct to subtract this value. For the pulmonary circulation two resistances have been calculated:

$$\text{Total pulmonary resistance (TPR)} = \frac{\text{Mean}\,P_{pa}}{Q_p}$$

and

Pulmonary vascular resistance (PVR or R_p)

$$= \frac{\text{Mean}\,P_{pa} - \text{Mean}\,P_{pv}}{Q_p}$$

where P_{pa} is pulmonary arterial pressure, P_{pv} is pulmonary venous pressure, and Q_p is pulmonary blood flow.

Pulmonary arterial wedge or left atrial pressures are usually taken as being similar to pulmonary venous pressure. TPR does not take pulmonary venous pressure into account, and because this may introduce serious errors TPR is seldom used these days.

Practical issues

1 Pulmonary arterial wedge pressures are obtained by gently advancing an end hole catheter into a terminal pulmonary artery until it goes no further. Complete occlusion of the artery is checked by slowly withdrawing blood and determining that it is almost 100% saturated, that is, it represents pulmonary venous blood. If the patient is on positive pressure ventilation, the pressure measured is more likely to represent alveolar than left atrial pressure.

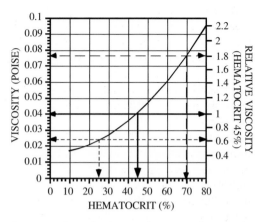

Figure 6.1 Relationship between hematocrit (horizontal axis) and either absolute viscosity (left vertical axis) or relative viscosity (right vertical axis).

2 The viscosity of blood must be considered in all resistance calculations, but especially in the pulmonary circulation. We calculate pulmonary vascular resistance to assess the cross-sectional area of the pulmonary vascular bed. If the resistance is high because viscosity is high, we will then underestimate the cross-sectional area. We should really calculate hindrance that, as its name implies, tells us how much obstruction there is to the blood flow by virtue of vessel cross-sectional area [45,46]:

$$\text{Hindrance} = \frac{\text{Resistance (mm Hg}/(\text{L min}))}{\text{Absolute viscosity (poise)}}$$

The relationship of viscosity to hematocrit is given in Fig. 6.1, and some sample calculations are given in Table 6.3.

It is obvious that although the resistances are the same, the cross-sectional areas that they indicate are quite different. A child having a Fontan procedure would probably do much better with a hindrance of 53.3 than one with a hindrance of 160. Put another way, a child with a hindrance of 160 (last column) would at a normal hematocrit, have a resistance of 6.4 units, and might not be suitable for a single ventricle repair.

Table 6.3 Hindrance Calculations.

Hematocrit %	70	45	25
PVR (mm Hg/(L min))	4	4	4
Absolute viscosity (poise)	0.075	0.04	0.025
Hindrance (mm Hg/ (L min poise))	53.3	100	160

The correction for viscosity is not as exact as implied above for several reasons. Fig. 6.1 shows the effect of hematocrit on viscosity in tubes equal to or bigger than arterioles, but viscosity in capillary size tubes is much lower because of the Fåhraeus–Lindqvist effect where red blood cells form single files, much like bicycle or automobile racers take advantage of the draft. On the other hand, the effect of larger white blood cells and of obstruction at branch points opposes this effect, so that in practice practical corrections can still be made using Fig. 6.1. Another variable is the total red cell or blood volume, because the higher the blood volume the higher the cardiac output (at any given hematocrit), and higher cardiac outputs cause blood vessels to dilate and be recruited, thereby decreasing vascular resistance [47].

3 Interpreting resistance needs care. Normally there is a small pressure gradient of about 5–10 mm Hg across the lung. With a normal cardiac index of 3.5 L/min the normal pulmonary vascular resistance index therefore ranges from 5/3.5 to 10/3.5 units, that is, from 1.4 to 2.9 units/m^2. Were that person to exercise maximally and increase cardiac index to 14 L/min, the pressure gradient across the lung would hardly increase because more pulmonary vessels are recruited and the vessels become wider. Pulmonary vascular resistance drops to about 0.4–0.8 units/m^2. Therefore, if in a patient with a huge left-to-right shunt through a ventricular septal defect the pulmonary vascular resistance is calculated as 2.5 units/m^2, it represents an increased resistance because with that flow the resistance should have been well under 1 unit/m^2. In fact, the easiest way to tell if resistance is abnormal is to measure the pressure gradient across the lung; if it is over 10 mm Hg, then resistance is elevated.

Valve orifice areas

The era of calculating valve orifice areas began in 1951 with the publication by Gorlin and Gorlin [48] who adapted a hydraulic formula for clinical use. They knew that a simple resistance formula was inappropriate because pressure drop and flow through an orifice are not linearly related. They therefore considered the hydraulic analysis of flow through a circular orifice (Fig. 6.2).

In this figure, the streamlines are shown converging at the orifice and continuing to converge for a short distance downstream to provide a minimal

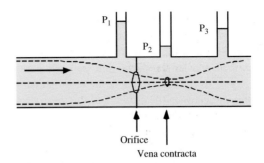

Figure 6.2 Hydraulic principles underlying the Gorlin formula for valve area. The dashed lines indicate the flow streamlines converging at the orifice and then diverging on the other side. P_1, P_2, and P_3 are pressures due to potential energy.

virtual orifice termed the vena contracta; typically this area is about 65% of the actual orifice area. Then the streamlines diverge until they fill the tube again. Because of the law of conservation of matter, each second the same amount of fluid passes the orifice and the entrance to the tube. Because the orifice area is smaller than the proximal tube area, the velocity of flow and kinetic energy must increase; because of the law of conservation of energy, the potential energy (pressure) must decrease as shown by the pressures in side tubes P_1 and P_2. Then as the streamlines widen flow velocity and kinetic energy decreases and potential energy increases, but as shown in side tube P_3 some energy is permanently lost because of turbulence and heat. The relation between the pressure difference $P_1 - P_2$ and the orifice area for any given flow is given by

$$A(\text{cm}^2) = \frac{\text{Flow (mL/min)}}{44.5\sqrt{P_1 - P_2}\,(\text{mm Hg})}$$

where A is the area of the vena contracta.

Gorlin and Gorlin modified this formula to allow for the fact that flow across valves occurred either in systole (aortic and pulmonic valves, first formula) or diastole (mitral and tricuspid valves, second formula) and also introduced empirical constants (K) of 0.85 for the mitral valve and 1 for all other valves.

$$A\,(\text{cm})^2 = \frac{\text{Flow (mL)/systolic second}}{K\,44.5\sqrt{P_1 - P_2}\,(\text{mm Hg})}$$

or

$$A\,(\text{cm})^2 = \frac{\text{Flow (mL)/diastolic second}}{K\,44.5\sqrt{P_1 - P_2}\,(\text{mm Hg})}$$

For the aortic and pulmonary valves, $\sqrt{P_1 - P_2}$ is the square root of the mean systolic pressure difference between the great artery and its respective ventricle, and for the mitral and tricuspid valves $\sqrt{P_1 - P_2}$ is the square root of the mean pressure difference between the atrium and the mean diastolic pressure in the respective ventricle.

What is inaccurate about these formulas is that in practice we measure P_3, not P_2, that is, we measure recovery pressure, not pressure at the vena contracta. Although the difference $P_1 - P_3$ also gets bigger for a given flow as area gets smaller, the relationship is difficult to quantify. Therefore, although the formulas allow us to assess orifice size, the measurement is not very accurate. Dangas and Gorlin [49] provide a discussion of the potential errors.

To do the calculations pressures on each side of the stenosis should be measured with high fidelity and the mean pressure difference in systole or diastole must be calculated. For aortic stenosis a modified formula that is easier to use was proposed by Bache et al. [50]

$$A = \frac{SV\ (mL)/SET\ (sec)}{36.4\sqrt{maximal\ IPG}}$$

where SV is stroke volume, SET is systolic ejection time, and IPG is maximal instantaneous systolic pressure gradient from left ventricle to aorta. An even easier formula that can be used for aortic or pulmonic stenosis (and mitral stenosis) was developed by Iskandrian and colleagues [51,52]:

$$A = \frac{CO\ (L/min)}{\sqrt{\Delta P}\ (mm\ Hg)}$$

where CO is cardiac output and ΔP is the pressure difference across the valve (mean or peak makes little difference). The reason why this simplified formula works well is that flow per systolic second is cardiac output divided by (heart rate × systolic ejection time), and heart rate × systolic ejection time × 44.5 is about 1×10^3

Ventricular function

Ventricular diastolic pressure for evaluating ventricular function can be measured better by cardiac catheterization than by echocardiography. It is, however, not sufficient because it cannot be equated with transmural pressure. The pressure outside the ventricles is not necessarily slightly negative pleural pressure because of pericardial restraint, as de-

scribed by Glantz, Tyberg, and their colleagues [53–55]. Although pericardial pressure is not the same all over the cardiac surface, it can be approximated by right atrial pressure [56,57].

The best method of assessing contractility is probably by obtaining pressure volume loops at different afterloads and calculating E_{max} [58]. Continuous volume measurements are difficult to make in humans, although attempts have been made to use the conductance catheter [59,60]. This technique is difficult to use, and the need for different afterloads adds to the length of the study. Possibly the single beat approximation of Senzaki et al. [61] may solve some of the problems, but at present this remains a research technique.

Endomyocardial biopsy

This may be used to examine cellular infiltrates in the myocardium in transplant rejection or myocarditis, abnormal deposits as in amyloid, and occasionally detecting other forms of myocardial damage and abnormal biochemical composition. A bioptome is passed through a long sheath into the right ventricle [62] or left ventricle [63], the latter being reached through a patent foramen ovale or by transseptal perforation. When in position the bioptome is advanced out of the sheath to take a tissue sample from the septum; usually several samples are taken.

Therapeutic cardiac catheterization.

This is a rapidly changing field, and most of the detailed methods will be given in the chapters dealing with the specific lesions. There are, however, some techniques that are needed in several different types of lesions, and some general principles that need description.

Opening the atrial septum

All pediatric cardiologists need to be able to do a balloon atrial septostomy [5], particularly in the neonates with transposition of the great arteries and a closing ductus arteriosus, but it may be needed in any neonate who needs a large atrial opening for survival. Using a 6F–7F sheath, a Miller–Edwards balloon catheter is advanced into the left atrium and then inflated with diluted contrast medium to 4–6 mL volume. With a jerk of the wrist the balloon is pulled back into the right atrium but not into the inferior vena cava. The process is repeated three to four more times, and tearing of the atrial septum is verified by angiocardiography or echocardiography. This procedure can also be done under echocardiographic control in intensive care or neonatal units [64].

Sometimes the septum is too thick to be torn, especially in patients over 1 month of age. A septal opening can then be made with the Park blade [11]. Using a long sheath, if necessary after transseptal puncture, the blade catheter is pushed into the left atrium and the blade is slowly pushed out of the catheter. It is then drawn carefully back across the atrial septum, the blade is retracted into the catheter, and the process repeated several times. The catheter is then removed and replaced by a balloon catheter to complete the septostomy. Details are provided in other references [11,16]. There are some risks of perforation or air embolism, and the procedure is difficult in those with a very small atrial septum. Alternatives are to do a septostomy by placing a high-pressure balloon in the septal puncture and distending it to rupture the septum, or to use a balloon with blades mounted on the balloon itself [65–67].

Dilating stenotic peripheral pulmonary arteries

Single or multiple peripheral pulmonary arterial stenosis may occur in tetralogy of Fallot with or without pulmonary atresia, in some syndromes (Williams, Alagille, Takayasu, and rubella syndromes, for example), and less often with other forms of congenital heart disease or even as isolated lesions. Because most of these stenoses are in the pulmonary parenchyma, they are not amenable to surgical correction. Early on, these stenoses were dilated with nondistensible balloons capable of accepting high pressures without rupture. Despite reasonable initial dilatation, the stenosis tended to recur [68,69]. Therefore, balloon expandable stents are currently favored [70]. A very stiff wire guide is passed across the stenosis and as far as possible into the distal pulmonary artery, and a long sheath is passed over the wire. The stenosis is not dilated unless it is less than 3 mm in diameter. The stent is mounted on a low-profile balloon that will expand to the needed diameter (not more than 1.5 times

the diameter of the "normal" artery on each side of the stenosis), and the assembly is passed over the guide wire until the stenosis is centered over the stent. The sheath is then withdrawn and the balloon is then blown up. The result is assessed by angiography. If it is necessary to dilate the stent further, a larger balloon can be used to replace the original one, not only at the time of insertion but also years later to allow for growth [71,72]. Occasionally the stenosis cannot be dilated with the usual type of balloon, and then a cutting balloon can be used with success [73].

Dilating stenotic or obstructed veins

The technique used to dilate and stent stenotic pulmonary arteries can be used to dilate stenotic or obstructed veins, for example, superior or inferior vena caval obstruction after the atrial baffle procedure for complete transposition of the great arteries, or thrombosis of the femoral or iliac veins or the inferior vena cava following cardiac catheterization [74]. If the vein is obstructed, it must be pierced first with a stiff guide wire or transseptal needle, after which dilatation and stenting can proceed. In some of these thrombosed veins the occlusion has considerable length, and a series of overlapping stents may need to be implanted. Unless the patient is full sized, the stent should be balloon-dilatable and not self-dilating. Results of these procedures are good, although in general less good for pulmonary vein stenosis [75–78].

Closing abnormal communications

Closure of a patent ductus, atrial septal defect, or some ventricular septal defects will be discussed in chapter 20. On the other hand, occlusion of arteriovenous fistulae, venovenous fistulae after a Glenn procedure, aortopulmonary collaterals in tetralogy of Fallot with pulmonary atresia, or treatment of an aneurysm will be described here. The two common methods are to use coils or balloon occluders. Gianturco coils are 0.025–0.038 in. spring steel coils with attached fibers (Dacron, nylon, or wool) [79], formed into coils from 2 to 15 mm in diameter. First a balloon catheter is used to occlude the vessel, check its diameter, and make sure that closure is not detrimental. Then the coils are loaded into a delivery catheter, and when this is in the correct position the spring wire is pushed out with a standard guide wire. Once it is out of the catheter it forms an irregular ball inside the vessel, obstructs flow, and leads to thrombosis. Several coils may need to be inserted in large vessels. If flow does not cease soon, small pieces of gelfoam may be added through the delivery catheter. Sometimes the vessel to be obstructed is small, distal, and comes off a small, often tortuous feeder vessel that must remain patent; this scenario is most often seen in the central nervous system, but does occur with coronary arteriovenous fistulae. These are best treated with tracker catheters, small flexible 3-F catheters (2.2-F at the tip) that can thread through tortuous small vessels and through which small thin coils can be passed [80]. Often these are Guglielmi platinum coils that may be coated with fibers and once in place can be detached electrolytically [81–84]. These coils are not magnetic and so are not affected by magnetic resonance imaging, and do not alter those images [85]. Whether their nonmagnetic properties are essential for safety in magnetic fields is uncertain [86].

The alternative is to use detachable balloons [87–89]. These come in various sizes. They are introduced through a catheter when its tip is in the correct position, and then inflated with dilute contrast medium to verify position and occlusion. Smaller silicone balloons are filled with isotonic solution before the catheter is detached, larger latex balloons are filled with two silicone monomers that react and solidify. The Grifka–Gianturco vascular occlusion device is a nylon balloon that, once in place, is filled with spring wire until it is tightly apposed to the vessel wall. All these balloons can be retrieved easily before release of the catheter, but are almost impossible to retrieve after release.

Removing foreign bodies

The ends of indwelling polyethylene catheters may be cut loose by the inserting needle, by too tight a suture, or by being cut when removing the suture; these usually end up in the right heart or pulmonary artery. Fragments of broken cardiac catheters or guidewires may embolise, and so may the devices inserted to close atrial septal defects, patent ductus arteriosus, or arteriovenous fistulae [90]. Almost all of these can be removed without the need for open surgery by various devices, including snares, baskets, and endoscopic forceps [13,16,90].

Acknowledgments

I thank Dr Phillip Moore for providing some details about practices in the pediatric cardiac catheterization laboratory in Department of Pediatrics, University of California, San Franciso, CA.

References

1. Mueller RL, Sanborn TA. The history of interventional cardiology: Cardiac catheterization, angioplasty, and related interventions. Am Heart J 1995; 129:146–172.
2. Forsmann W. The catheterization of the right side of the heart. Klin Wochens 1929; 8:2085–2087.
3. Cournand AF, Riley RL, Breed ES, et al. Measurement of cardiac output in man using the technique of catheterization of the right auricle or ventricle. J Clin Invest 1945; 24:106–116.
4. Zimmerman HA, Scott RW, Becker NO. Catheterization of the left side of the heart in man. Circulation 1950; 1:357–359.
5. Rashkind WJ, Miller WW. Creation of an atrial septal defect without thoracotomy. A palliative approach to complete transposition of the great arteries. J Am Med Assoc 1966; 196:991–992.
6. Porstmann W, Wierny L, Warnke H, et al. Catheter closure of patent ductus arteriosus. 62 cases treated without thoracotomy. Radiol Clin North Am 1971; 9:203–218.
7. King TD, Thompson SL, Steiner C, et al. Secundum atrial septal defect. Nonoperative closure during cardiac catheterization. J Am Med Assoc 1976; 235:2506–2509.
8. Dotter CT, Rosch J, Judkins MP. Transluminal dilatation of atherosclerotic stenosis. Surg Gyn and Obstet 1968; 127:794–804.
9. Bollinger A, Schlumpf M. Andreas Gruntzig's balloon catheter for angioplasty of peripheral arteries (PTA) is 25 years old. Vasa 1999; 28:58–64.
10. Kan JS, White RI Jr, Mitchell SE, et al. Percutaneous balloon valvuloplasty: A new method for treating congenital pulmonary-valve stenosis. New Engl J Med 1982; 307:540–542.
11. Park SC, Neches WH, Mullins CE, et al. Blade atrial septostomy: Collaborative study. Circulation 1982; 66:258–266.
12. O'Laughlin MP, Slack MC, Grifka RG, et al. Implantation and intermediate-term follow-up of stents in congenital heart disease. Circulation 1993; 88:605–614.

13. Mullins CE, Nihill MR. Cardiac catheterization hemo-dynamics and intervention. In: Moller JH, Hoffman JIE, eds., Pediatric Cardiovascular Disease. Churchill Livingstone, New York, pp. 203–215, 2000.

14. Booth KL, Roth SJ, Perry SB, et al. Cardiac catheterization of patients supported by extracorporeal membrane oxygenation. J Am Coll Cardiol 2002; 40:1681–1686.

15. Bridges ND, Freed MD. Cardiac catheterization. In: Emmanouilides GC, Riemenschneider TA, Allen HD, et al., eds., Heart Disease in Infants, Children and Adolescents Including the Fetus and Young Adult. Williams & Wilkins, Baltimore, MD, pp. 310–329, 1995.

16. Qureshi SA. Catheterization and angiocardiography. In: Anderson RH, Baker EJ, Macartney FJ, et al., eds., Paediatric Cardiology. Churchill Livingstone, London, pp. 459–511, 2002.

17. Marx GR. Sedation and monitoring for cardiac procedures. In: Emmanouilides GC, Riemenschneider TA, Allen HD, et al., eds., Heart Disease in Infants, Children and Adolescents Including the Fetus and Young Adult. Williams & Wilkins, Baltimore, MD, pp. 147–152, 1995.

18. Donmez A, Kizilkan A, Berksun H, et al. One center's experience with remifentanil infusions for pediatric cardiac catheterization. J Cardiothorac Vascr Anesth 2001; 15:736–739.

19. Gozal D, Rein AJ, Nir A, et al. Propofol does not modify the hemodynamic status of children with intracardiac shunts undergoing cardiac catheterization. Pediatr Cardiol 2001; 22:488–490.

20. Winn CW, Porter AG, Vincent RN. Oral meperidine, atropine, and pentobarbital for pediatric conscious sedation. Pediatr Nurs 2000; 26:500–502, 509.

21. Jobeir A, Galal MO, Bulbul ZR, et al. Use of low-dose ketamine and/or midazolam for pediatric cardiac catheterization. Pediatr Cardiol 2003; 28:236–243.

22. de Waard-van der Spek FB, van den Berg GM, Oranje AP. EMLA cream: an improved local anesthetic. Review of current literature. Pediatr Dermatol 1992; 9:126–131.

23. Johnston TA, Donnelly LF, Frush DP, et al. Transhepatic catheterization using ultrasound-guided access. Pediatr Cardiol 2003; 28:393–396.

24. Cetta F, Graham LC, Eidem BW. Gaining vascular access in pediatric patients: Use of the P.D. access Doppler needle. Cathet Cardiovasc Interven 2000; 51:61–64.

25. Colan SD. Combined fluid-filled and micromanometer-tip catheter system for high-fidelity pressure recordings in infants. Cathet Cardiovasc Diag 1984; 10:619–623.

26. Mullins CE. Transseptal left heart catheterization: experience with a new technique in 520 pediatric and adult patients. Pediatr Cardiol 1983; 4:239–245.

27. Alehan D, Ayabakan C, Celiker A. Cardiac troponin T and myocardial injury during routine cardiac catheterisation in children. Int J Cardiol 2003; 87:223–230.

28. Kannankeril PJ, Pahl E, Wax DF. Usefulness of troponin I as a marker of myocardial injury after pediatric cardiac catheterization. Am J Cardiol 2002; 90:1128–1132.

29. Vitiello R, McCrindle BW, Nykanen D, et al. Complications associated with pediatric cardiac catheterization. J Am Coll Cardiol 1998; 32:1433–1440.

30. Kirk CR, Qureshi SA. Streptokinase in the management of arterial thrombosis in infancy. Int J Cardiol 1989; 25:15–20.

31. Gupta AA, Leaker M, Andrew M, et al. Safety and outcomes of thrombolysis with tissue plasminogen activator for treatment of intravascular thrombosis in children. J Pediatr 2001; 139:682–688.

32. Braunwald E. Cooperative study on cardiac catheterization. Deaths related to cardiac catheterization. Circulation 1968; 37:III17–III26.

33. Cassidy SC, Schmidt KG, Van Hare GF, et al. Complications of pediatric cardiac catheterization: A 3-year study. J Am Coll Cardiol 1992; 19:1285–1293.

34. Cohn HE, Freed MD, Hellenbrand WF, et al. Complications and mortality associated with cardiac catheterization in infants under one year: A prospective study. Pediatr Cardiol 1985; 6:123–131.

35. Porter CJ, Gillette PC, Mullins CE, et al. Cardiac catheterization in the neonate. A comparison of three techniques. J Pediatr 1978; 93:97–101.

36. Stanger P, Heymann MA, Tarnoff H, et al. Complications of cardiac catheterization of neonates, infants, and children. A three-year study. Circulation 1974; 50:595–608.

37. Schroeder VA, Shim D, Spicer RL, et al. Surgical emergencies during pediatric interventional catheterization. J Pediatr 2002; 140:570–575.

38. Lister G, Hoffman JI, Rudolph AM. Oxygen uptake in infants and children: A simple method for measurement. Pediatrics 1974; 53:656–662.

39. Lister G Jr, Hoffman JI, Rudolph AM. Measurement of oxygen consumption: Assessing the accuracy of a method. J Appl Physiol 1977; 43:916–917.

40. Bergstra A, van Dijk RB, Hillege HL, et al. Assumed oxygen consumption based on calculation from dye dilution cardiac output: An improved formula. Eur Heart J 1995; 16:698–703.

41. Fixler DE, Carrell T, Browne R, et al. Oxygen consumption in infants and children during cardiac

catheterization under different sedation regimens. Circulation 1974; 50:788–794.

42. Kendrick AH, West J, Papouchado M, *et al.* Direct Fick cardiac output: Are assumed values of oxygen consumption acceptable? Eur Heart J 1988; 9:337–342.

43. LaFarge CG, Miettinen OS. The estimation of oxygen consumption. Cardiovasc Res 1970; 4:23–30.

44. Bloomfield DA. Dye Curves: The Theory and Practice of Indicator Dilution. University Park Press, Baltimore, MD, 450

45. Cokelet GR. The rheology and tube flow of blood. In: Skalak R, Chien S, eds., Handbook of Bioengineering. Mc-Graw Hill, New York, Ch 14, pp. 1–17, 1987.

46. Fan FC, Chen RYZ, Schuessler GB, *et al.* Effects of hematocrit variations on regional hemodynamics and oxygen transport in the dog. Am J Physiol Heart Circ Physiol 1980; 238 (7):H545–H552.

47. Wardrop CAJ, Holland BH, Jones JG. Red-cell physiology. In: Gluckman PD, Heymann MA, eds., Pediatrics & Perinatology. The Scientific Basis. Edward Arnold, London, pp. 868–876, 1996.

48. Gorlin R, Gorlin SG. Hydraulic formula for calculation of area of stenotic mitral valve, other cardiac valves, and central circulatory shunts. Am Heart J 1951; 41:1–29.

49. Dangas G, Gorlin R. Changing concepts in the determination of valvular stenosis. Prog Cardiovasc Dis 1997; 40:55–64.

50. Bache RJ, Jorgensen CR, Wang Y. Simplified estimation of aortic valve area. Br Heart J 1972; 34:408–411.

51. Hakki AH, Iskandrian AS, Bemis CE, *et al.* A simplified valve formula for the calculation of stenotic cardiac valve areas. Circulation 1981; 63:1050–1055.

52. Hare TW, Hakki AH, Iskandrian AS. Comparison between the Gorlin formula and a simplified formula to measure the severity of pulmonic stenosis. Cathet Cardiovasc Diagn 1983; 9:353–356.

53. Glantz SA, Parmley WW. Factors which affect the diastolic pressure-volume curve. Circ Res 1978; 42:171–180.

54. Smiseth OA, Frais MA, Kingma I, *et al.* Assessment of pericardial constraint: The relation between right ventricular filling pressure and pericardial pressure measured after pericardiocentesis. J Am Coll Cardiol 1986; 7:307–314.

55. Tyberg JV, Belenkie I, Manyari DE, *et al.* Ventricular interaction and venous capacitance modulate left ventricular preload. Can J Cardiol 1996; 12:1058–1064.

56. Smiseth OA, Scott-Douglas NW, Thompson CR, *et al.* Nonuniformity of pericardial surface pressure in dogs. Circulation 1987; 75:1229–1236.

57. Smiseth OA, Thompson CR, Ling H, *et al.* A potential clinical method for calculating transmural left ventricular filling pressure during positive end-expiratory pressure ventilation: An intraoperative study in humans. J Am Coll Cardiol 1996; 27:155–160.

58. Suga H. Cardiac function. In: Moller JH, Hoffman JIE, eds., Pediatric Cardiovascular Medicine. Churchill Livingstone, New York, pp. 65–77, 2000.

59. Baan J, van der Velde ET, de Bruin HG, *et al.* Continuous measurement of left ventricular volume in animals and humans by conductance catheter. Circulation 1984; 70:812–823.

60. Kass DA. Clinical evaluation of left heart function by conductance catheter technique. Eur Heart J 1992; 13(Suppl E):57–64.

61. Senzaki H, Chen CH, Kass DA. Single-beat estimation of end-systolic pressure-volume relation in humans. A new method with the potential for noninvasive application. Circulation 1996; 94:2497–2506.

62. Lurie PR, Fujita M, Neustein HB. Transvascular endomyocardial biopsy in infants and small children: Description of a new technique. Am J Cardiol 1978; 42:453–457.

63. Rios B, Nihill MR, Mullins CE. Left ventricular endomyocardial biopsy in children with the transseptal long sheath technique. Cathet Cardiovasc Diagn 1984; 10:417–423.

64. Zellers TM, Dixon K, Moake L, *et al.* Bedside balloon atrial septostomy is safe, efficacious, and cost-effective compared with septostomy performed in the cardiac catheterization laboratory. Am J Cardiol 2002; 89:613–615.

65. Bergersen LJ, Perry SB, Lock JE. Effect of cutting balloon angioplasty on resistant pulmonary artery stenosis. Am J Cardiol 2003; 91:185–189.

66. Coe JY, Chen RP, Timinsky J, *et al.* A novel method to create atrial septal defect using a cutting balloon in piglets. Am J Cardiol 1996; 78:1323–1326.

67. Rocha-Singh K. The Barath cutting balloon: battling the sword of Damocles. Catheter Cardiovasc Interv 2002; 56:232–233.

68. Kan JS, Marvin WJ Jr, Bass JL, *et al.* Balloon angioplasty–branch pulmonary artery stenosis: Results from the Valvuloplasty and Angioplasty of Congenital Anomalies Registry. Am J Cardiol 1990; 65:798–801.

69. Rothman A, Perry SB, Keane JF, *et al.* Early results and follow-up of balloon angioplasty for branch pulmonary artery stenoses. J Am Coll Cardiol 1990; 15:1109–1117.

70. Qureshi SA, Tynan M, Rosenthal E. Implantation of Palmaz stents in branch pulmonary arteries using Olbert balloons. Cathet Cardiovasc Diagn 1996; 38:92–95.

71. Ing FF, Grifka RG, Nihill MR, *et al.* Repeat dilation of intravascular stents in congenital heart defects. Circulation 1995; 92:893–897.

72. Ing F. Stents: What's available to the pediatric interventional cardiologist? Cathet Cardiovasc Interv 2002; 57:374–386.

73. Rhodes JF, Lane GK, Mesia CI, *et al.* Cutting balloon angioplasty for children with small-vessel pulmonary artery stenoses. Catheter Cardiovasc Interv 2002; 55:73–77.

74. Ing FF, Fagan TE, Grifka RG, *et al.* Reconstruction of stenotic or occluded iliofemoral veins and inferior vena cava using intravascular stents: Re-establishing access for future cardiac catheterization and cardiac surgery. J Am Coll Cardiol 2001; 37:251–257.

75. McMahon CJ, Mullins CE, El Said HG. Intrastent sonotherapy in pulmonary vein restenosis: A new treatment for a recalcitrant problem. Heart 2003; 89:E6.

76. Ungerleider RM, Johnston TA, O'Laughlin MP, *et al.* Intraoperative stents to rehabilitate severely stenotic pulmonary vessels. Ann Thorac Surg 2001; 71:476–481.

77. Vance MS, Bernstein R, Ross BA. Successful stent treatment of pulmonary vein stenosis following atrial fibrillation radiofrequency ablation. J Invasive Cardiol 2002; 14:414–416.

78. Doyle TP, Loyd JE, Robbins IM. Percutaneous pulmonary artery and vein stenting: A novel treatment for mediastinal fibrosis. Am J Respir Crit Care Med 2001; 164:657–660.

79. Wallace S, Gianturco C, Anderson JH, *et al.* Therapeutic vascular occlusion utilizing steel coil technique: Clinical applications. Am J Roentgenol 1976; 127:381–387.

80. Hibbard MD, Holmes DR Jr. The Tracker catheter: A new vascular access system. Cathet Cardiovasc Diagn 1992; 27:309–316.

81. Buheitel G, Ludwig J, Hofbeck M. Transcatheter occlusion of a large coronary arterial fistula with new detachable platinum microcoils. Cardiol Young 2001; 11:571–573.

82. Reidy JF, Qureshi SA. Interlocking detachable platinum coils, a controlled embolization device: Early clinical experience. Cardiovasc Intervent Radiol 1996; 19:85–90.

83. Teitelbaum GP, Reed RA, Larsen D, *et al.* Microcatheter embolization of non-neurologic traumatic vascular lesions. J Vasc Interv Radiol 1993; 4:149–154.

84. Vance MS. Use of platinum microcoils to embolize vascular abnormalities in children with congenital heart disease. Pediatr Cardiol 1998; 19:145–149.

85. Hennemeyer CT, Wicklow K, Feinberg DA, *et al.* In vitro evaluation of platinum Guglielmi detachable coils at 3 T with a porcine model: Safety issues and artifacts. Radiology 2001; 219:732–737.

86. Rutledge JM, Vick GW III, Mullins CE, *et al.* Safety of magnetic resonance imaging immediately following Palmaz stent implant: A report of three cases. Catheter Cardiovasc Interv 2001; 53:519–523.

87. Grifka RG, Mullins CE, Gianturco C, *et al.* New Gianturco-Grifka vascular occlusion device. Initial studies in a canine model. Circulation 1995; 91:1840–1846.

88. Grinnell VS, Mehringer CM, Hieshima GB, *et al.* Transaortic occlusion of collateral arteries to the lung by detachable valved balloons in a patient with tetralogy of Fallot. Circulation 1982; 65:1276–1278.

89. Reidy JF, Jones OD, Tynan MJ, *et al.* Embolisation procedures in congenital heart disease. Br Heart J 1985; 54:184–192.

90. Huggon IC, Qureshi SA, Reidy J, *et al.* Percutaneous transcatheter retrieval of misplaced therapeutic embolisation devices. Br Heart J 1994; 72:470–475.

PART II
Techniques in Assessing Ventricular Function

CHAPTER 7

Echocardiography and Doppler Ultrasound

Jack Rychik, MD

Ultrasound is one of the most commonly used tools in the evaluation of the cardiovascular system. *Echocardiography* is the application of ultrasonic imaging techniques to the heart and the proximal vascular structures. Echocardiography allows for (1) detailed assessment of the architecture and geometry of structures, (2) observation of dynamic movement of these structures through space and time, and (3) the evaluation of blood flow through these structures.

In congenital heart disease, the application of echocardiography has been extremely useful in elucidating the complexities of the structural anomalies [1]. The benefits of applying echocardiography in infants and children with congenital heart disease are many. The *high spatial resolution* of echocardiography allows one to discriminate between very small structures in space—a feature that has provided for assessment of the tiniest of structures in the fetal heart. The *high temporal resolution* of echocardiography allows to reliably track dynamic movement of structures in time—an important feature in subjects in which structures are moving relatively quickly due to rapid heart rates. Equipment *mobility* allows for utilization of echocardiography at the patient bedside, with the potential for repetitive serial evaluations and minimal perturbation of the patient.

The noninvasive nature of echocardiography and its safety profile, in conjunction with these benefits, has made it a ubiquitous tool in the clinical management of congenital heart disease and a major contributor to the overall current excellence in clinical outcomes. However, limitations exist, primarily related to the nature of the energy used to create the image. Image processing is dependant upon quality of the returning ultrasound signal, hence properties such as penetration, scatter, absorption, and reflection play a role. The distance through which the

ultrasound energy must travel and the natural variability in biological tissue density in its path, creates a barrier that degrades the quality of signal return.

This chapter will review the utilization of echocardiography and Doppler techniques in the assessment of ventricular function and blood flow in congenital heart disease.

Fundamental aspects of echocardiography

Ultrasound frequency

Electrical stimulation of piezoelectric crystals results in the emission of ultrasound energy. Multiple piezoelectric crystals are bundled into encasements called transducers. The spectrum of ultrasonic energy used for evaluation of biological tissue ranges from frequencies of 1 to 40 MHz. High-frequency ultrasound energy is generally dissipated quickly and cannot travel long distances; however, spatial resolution at these high frequencies is excellent. Low-frequency ultrasound energy can penetrate deep tissues well, but at the cost of diminished spatial resolution. The relationship between the frequency of ultrasound and the lower limits of spatial resolution is quantifiable and relates to the inability of ultrasound to resolve structures that are smaller than the size of a single wavelength of emitted energy, as described by the formula

$$V = fw,$$

where V is the velocity of ultrasound in biological tissue, which on average is 1540 m/sec, f is the frequency of the emitted energy, and w is the length of the wavelength.

This principle is illustrated in the following clinical example. Oftentimes, precise measurement of a particular structure is critical in the decision-making vis-à-vis choice of surgical strategy. Measurement of the left ventricular outflow tract in a newborn infant with left-sided obstructive disease can play a role in deciding whether the outflow tract is sufficient in size to provide for systemic circulation (plan A), or if permanent support from the right ventricle via a pulmonary artery to aorta anastomosis is necessary (plan B). Let us assume that a cutoff of 4 mm in diameter has been determined to be the critical size, i.e., if the outflow tract is measured to be less than 4 mm, then plan B would be employed. If imaging is performed using a 2 MHz transducer, then the wavelength diameter is 0.77 mm; if imaging is performed using a 10 MHz transducer, the wavelength diameter is 0.15 mm. Hence, if an image of the outflow tract were acquired and a measurement of 4 mm made using the 2 MHz transducer, the margin of error, either plus or minus, could be close to 1 mm—nearly 25% of the entire measurement—with significant potential for either under- or over-estimation of the true diameter. This raises the risk of choosing the wrong surgical strategy to a significant level. Using the higher frequency 10 MHz transducer reduces this risk by reducing the margin of error in spatial resolution to approximately 4% of the measurement (0.15 mm out of 4 mm), thereby making the measurement more reliable. In general, as far as two-dimensional imaging is concerned, higher frequency energy should be used in small subjects in which tiny structures are to be measured but yet penetration is not an issue; similarly lower frequencies are to be used when deep penetration is needed in older children and adults.

Doppler echocardiography

Ultrasound energy emitted toward a moving target is reflected back at a different frequency, depending upon the original emitting frequency, the angle of energy emission, the velocity of the moving target, and the speed of the ultrasound energy in the transmission medium [2]. This relationship was defined mathematically by Christian Johann Doppler in 1842, as

$$F_s = \frac{2 F_i V \cos X}{c}$$

where F_s is the frequency shift, F_i the original emitting frequency, V the velocity of motion of the moving target, cos X the cosine of the angle made

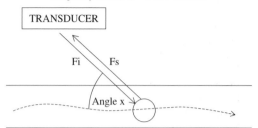

Doppler Principle

Frequency shift (Fs) = 2 Fi V Cos X/c

Figure 7.1 Doppler's equation describing the relationship between the transmitted frequency (F_i), the received frequency shift (F_s), and the vector velocity of flow.

between the line of ultrasound energy emission and the directional line of movement of the target being interrogated, and c the speed of ultrasound energy in the medium (Fig. 7.1).

Since the velocity of movement, of either *blood* or *tissue*, is the unknown parameter of interest, with the variables of frequency emission and received frequency shift known, the equation can be solved in the following manner:

$$V = F_s \frac{c}{2} F_i \cos X$$

The equation, whence observed in this manner, highlights the importance of minimizing the angle formed between the line of the ultrasound beam emission and the line of movement of the target—a parameter that is operator dependant and under operator control. If properly aligned, this angle is $0°$ and hence cos $= 1$, and this variable can then be ignored. Although achieving complete alignment with an angle of $0°$ can be clinically challenging in the patient, it should clearly be the goal and all efforts should be made to maintain alignment at an angle of less than $20°$. This will provide a cos value close to unity. At angles greater than $20°$, the variable becomes significant (a fraction of unity) and angle correctional factors must be incorporated into the equation.

Modes of application of echocardiography

Echocardiography can be clinically applied in the assessment of congenital heart disease in a variety of ways (Table 7.1). *Surface imaging* is the most commonly used. This includes a series of sweeps and views obtained from established, standardized transducer positions [3]. These multiple sweeps

Table 7.1 Echocardiographic Modalities.

Ways in which echocardiography can be applied
  Surface imaging
  Transesophageal echocardiography (TEE)
  Epicardial imaging
  Intracardiac imaging
  Intravascular imaging
  Fetal imaging
Methods for delineation of anatomical structure
  M-mode echocardiography
  Two-dimensional echocardiography
  Three-dimensional echocardiography
Doppler imaging
  Pulsed wave
  Continuous wave
  Color Doppler flow mapping
  Doppler tissue imaging

and views provide for two-dimensional tomographic image slices through the heart and great vessels (see Table 7.2). Although a variety of different approaches and algorithms exist, at The Children's Hospital of Philadelphia we believe strongly in commencing with the subcostal (subxiphoid) approach and its associated sweeps, in particular when imaging an unknown patient for the first time. We believe that the subcostal approach provides for the best means of rapidly establishing the correct anatomical position of structures and allows one to build a correct "working diagnosis" as one continues through the imaging algorithm. This approach prevents ambiguity in the systematic delineation of complex anatomy. No matter where one starts, a rigorous systematic approach that is applied to every patient is suggested, this so that segmental delineation of complex anatomy can reliably and unambiguously take place (i.e., situs, atria, AV valves, ventricles, great arteries). With completion of these multiple surface sweeps, a three-dimensional construct is mentally formed, which provides a dataset of information concerning both cardiac form and function.

Transesophageal echocardiographic (TEE) imaging allows for improved resolution in patients with poor surface windows and enhances the ability to better image posterior structures such as pulmonary veins.

Table 7.2   Suggested Algorithm for Performance of Surface Imaging in the Patient with Congenital Heart Disease.

Sweeps and views	How to acquire
Subcostal (subxyphoid)	
Frontal sweep	Coronal cut sweep starting from posterior (atria) to anterior
Left anterior oblique sweep	30° left oblique from coronal (clockwise rotation of transducer), sweeping from right to left toward apex
Sagittal sweep	90° to coronal, parallel with long axis of the body, sweeping from right to left toward the apex
Right anterior oblique view	30° right oblique from coronal (counter-clockwise rotation of transducer) stationary view
Apical view	
Four chamber view	4th or 5th intercostals space to the left of the mid-axillary line angled cephald
Outflow tract and aorta	Apical position with angling anterior and superiorly
Parasternal	
Long axis view	Aligned along the long axis of the heart at the 3rd or 4th parasternal space
Short axis sweep	At right angles to the long axis starting at the level of the great vessels and sweeping caudad toward the apex
Suprasternal	
Frontal	Suprasternal notch aimed caudad in a coronal plane
Sagittal	Suprasternal notch at 90° to frontal, rotated so as to display the full course of the aortic arch

Performance of the subcostal sweeps and views provides for a complete set of tomographic cuts obtained from all angles, which should allow for a three-dimensional understanding of the anatomy.

It has also revolutionized congenital heart surgery, in that TEE imaging can be performed immediately after separation from bypass but prior to chest closure, thereby allowing for assessment of adequacy of repair and a clearer understanding of post-bypass hemodynamics. The role of TEE in reducing the frequency of residual anomalies and improving overall outcome after surgery for congenital heart disease is well established [4,5]. *Epicardial echocardiography* has similarly been helpful in assessment of post-bypass findings, but requires manipulation by the surgeon within the operative field [6]. Care must be taken not to impair filling of the heart via excessive compression or direct application of the transducer to the structures of interest.

Advances in transducer technology have led to the production of miniaturized probes adapted to catheters through which echocardiographic imaging can take place from within a cardiac chamber or a vessel. *Intracardiac imaging* is currently utilized to monitor placement of occluder devices in the treatment of atrial septal defects [7]. *Intravascular echocardiography* is a technique in which piezoelectric crystals are adapted to a catheter with ultrasound energy emitted from the tip in a radial manner. This provides for a circumferential image with the potential for delineation of the layers of intima and adventitia of a target vessel. This technique has been applied in adults with coronary artery disease and has been helpful in understanding the structural aspects of plaque formation in atherosclerosis.

Cardiac structures can be assessed via echocardiography in a variety of ways, each a measure of complexity greater than the other. *M-mode imaging* is historically one of the earliest developed forms of structural imaging. A single plane slice of image data is displayed against time. Both spatial and temporal resolution in M-mode imaging are of the highest order; however, the scope is limited to just a single thin plane slice of ultrasound interrogation. This modality is best applied when there is interest in obtaining highly resolute linear measures of a chamber cavity or wall thickness during the various phases of the cardiac cycle. Two-dimensional scanning involves generation of a two-dimensional image in a sector area of interest. This is the main form of imaging used to scan anatomy and to aid in directing Doppler echocardiography modalities. Three-dimensional imaging in real time is currently available and is undergoing further investigation

with great potential for application toward congenital heart disease.

Echocardiography in the assessment of ventricular function: Systolic function derived from dimensional changes

Shortening fraction

One of the simplest and most commonly performed assessments of systolic ventricular function is the *percent shortening fraction* (%SF). This involves measurement of the change in ventricular cavity dimension from diastole to systole, by measurement of the degree of apposition of the posterior wall of the left ventricle to the ventricular septum (Fig. 7.2). The %SF is derived from linear measures, which indirectly reflect the volumetric change that occurs during ventricular systole, and hence is related to the ejection fraction. The benefit of this method is in the ease and rapidity with which it can be performed. M-mode is applied at a set designated position across the left ventricular cavity, usually at the level of the tips of the papillary muscles. The M-mode cursor is placed across the left ventricular cavity at the level of the tips of the papillary muscles. The left ventricular cavity is measured at end-diastole (onset of the QRS complex; left ventricle end-diastolic dimension, LVEDD) and at peak systole or the closest point of apposition of the left ventricle posterior wall to the septum (left ventricle end systolic dimension, LVESD). The shortening fraction is then defined as

$$\%SF = \frac{LVEDD - LVESD}{LVEDD} 100$$

The normal range of %SF for the left ventricle is from 28 to 38%. Measures below 28% suggest diminished systolic function, while measures above 38% reflect hyperdynamic function.

There are a number of drawbacks to the use of the %SF. First, it assumes a symmetrically shaped left ventricle (LV) in which the derived measurement of motion at the single slice of ventricular cavity imaged reflects motion of the entire ventricle. Hence in situations of left ventricular dyskinesia, the %SF will not be a true representation of overall LV performance and should not be used. Abnormalities of septal movement in relation to bundle branch block will also provide for values of %SF which may not truly reflect overall ventricular function. Another confounder that may impact upon septal motion

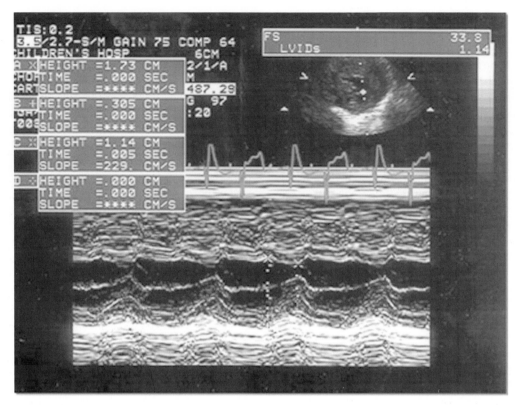

Figure 7.2 M-mode echocardiographic image across the left ventricle in the short axis view. This view allows for precise measurement of the left ventricular cavity at end-diastole (onset of the qrs complex on electrocardiogram) and peak systole (greatest point of septal to posterior wall apposition) and is used to calculate the shortening fraction of the left ventricle.

is right ventricular volume overload. Patients with atrial septal defect have a dilated right ventricle, hence the ventricular septal position at end-diastole may be extended posteriorly and closer to the LV posterior wall at the onset of systole. This may spuriously diminish the %SF value and falsely create an image of diminished overall LV function. Table 7.3 lists the possible conditions in which the %SF may not apply as a valid method for assessing LV systolic function.

As is the case for %SF as well as a number of other methods for assessing LV function, the technique is both preload and afterload dependant. In other words, the %SF value may be influenced by factors other than intrinsic myocardial function. The LVEDD linear measure is influenced by the overall intravascular volume status of the patient and the volume present in the left ventricle at end-diastole. LVEDD may be increased in conditions such as ventricular septal defect or patent ductus arteriosus. LVESD is influenced by the degree of afterload present. Increased systemic vascular resistance may

result in early closure of the aortic valve with increased ventricular volume at end systole, resulting in an elevated LVESD value and hence a lower %SF.

It is therefore important to consider the context within which the %SF is being calculated in order to properly interpret the value obtained. Oftentimes a normal %SF value may reflect abnormal ventricular

Table 7.3 Conditions in Which the Percent Shortening Fraction May Not Reliably Reflect Overall Systolic LV Function.

Conditions
Paradoxical septal wall motion
Abnormally shaped left ventricle
Left ventricular dyskinesia
Right bundle branch block
Right ventricle volume overload
Atrial septal defect
Significant pulmonary insufficiency
Frequent ventricular ectopy

function. A classic example is the situation of an incompetent mitral valve with severe mitral regurgitation. Mitral regurgitation results in increased volume load to the LV and hence LVEDD will be elevated. Also, the incompetent valve adds a venue for low resistance ejection into the compliant left atrial chamber, resulting in overall diminution in ventricular afterload. Under conditions of increased preload and reduced afterload, a normal %SF value may in fact reflect intrinsically diminished myocardial function since these variables should result in a hyperdynamic ventricle with a %SF that exceeds the normal 38%. Another example is that of a patient with frequent premature ventricular contractions or bigeminy. The increased preload of a post-extrasystolic beat may yield normalized preload enhanced values of %SF in a patient with truly diminished myocardial function. Hence the %SF should not be used in patients with frequent ventricular ectopy.

Shortening fraction indexed to afterload: The velocity of circumferential fiber shortening–wall stress relationship

In order to better obtain a noninvasive measure of myocardial function, Colan and colleagues developed a technique that utilizes the principles of ventricular shortening with incorporation of ventricular afterload or wall stress [8]. Since the ventricle shortens only during ejection, one can divide the %SF value by the ejection time to obtain the velocity of circumferential fiber shortening (V_{cf}). Colan and others have argued that the relationship between V_{cf} and wall stress is preload independent, but afterload dependant. Looking at the change in V_{cf} as afterload is altered would provide for way to incorporate afterload into the assessment of ventricular shortening, and hence provide for a more load incorporating measure of ventricular function. Afterload can be assessed by noninvasively measuring the meridional wall stress imposed upon the left ventricle at end-systole. Applying Laplace's law to the LV it was found that the meridional wall stress is directly proportional to the intracavitary pressure and cavity dimensions at end-systole and inversely proportional to the ventricular wall thickness.

The technical aspects of obtaining the measures necessary to calculate the wall stress values are a bit cumbersome and time consuming, but can be mastered with practice. By measuring forearm blood pressure, one obtains systolic and diastolic values, but not end-systolic pressure values. Using a tonometry device, one can obtain a carotid pulse tracing and hence a detailed pulse contour from which the end-systolic blood pressure can be extrapolated by measuring the height from the baseline to the "dicrotic" notch marking. This reflects valve closure. A phonocardiogram-derived signal is linked to the M-mode image of the LV and the end-systolic cavity dimension and posterior wall are measured at the point of aortic closure designated by the first component of the second heart sound. With the measures of LV cavity diameter, wall thickness, and blood pressure all obtained at the same temporal point of end-systole, the meridional end-systolic wall stress can be calculated. The V_{cf} is calculated by obtaining the %SF and then dividing by the ejection time, which may be obtained from the M-mode tracing of the aortic valve opening and closure. The V_{cf} is then corrected for heart rate variability (V_{cfc}) by dividing by the square root of the R–R time interval (Bazett's correction).

Colan found a direct, negative linear relationship between V_{cfc} and wall stress (Fig. 7.3). Intuitively this makes sense, in that as wall stress increases the expected degree of ventricular shortening V_{cfc} will diminish, this in the absence of any change in intrinsic myocardial contractility. For any fixed wall stress, if myocardial contractility is increased, such as by addition of an inotrope, then the V_{cfc} will increase. Similarly, if intrinsic myocardial contractility is diminished at a set wall stress, then V_{cfc} will diminish. By testing normals and adding inotropy, a defined normal relationship has been developed between V_{cfc} and wall stress. Values falling out of the expected range for a particular degree of wall stress indicate abnormal myocardial contractility and define ventricular dysfunction.

Other investigators have questioned the reported linear nature of this relationship, in particular in young infants [9,10]. In order to simplify the technique and to reduce the time it takes to perform the study, some investigators have found the mean blood pressure to be a reliable substitute for the end-systolic blood pressure, which then obviates the need for the carotid pulse tracing [11].

The V_{cfc}–wall stress relationship has been utilized clinically in a variety of disorders. We undertook a study to investigate the effects of the angiotensin converting enzyme inhibitor enalapril on the V_{cfc} – wall

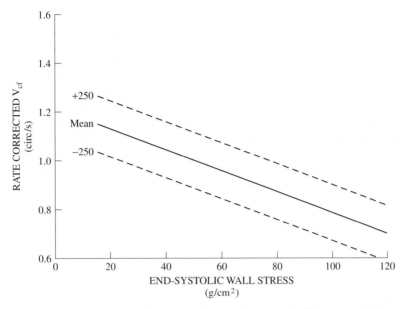

Figure 7.3 Relationship between wall stress on the *x*-axis and V_{cfc} on the *y*-axis. Confidence intervals (two standard deviations) for the expected normal range are displayed. Relationships that fall below the expected range suggest impaired ventricular function, while values above the range suggest a hyperdynamic state, such as during administration of inotropic drugs.

stress relationship in a group of patients who had received anthracycline treatment for childhood cancer [12]. This group was uniquely appropriate for the use of this technique to measure ventricular function since posterior wall thinning, increased wall stress, and myocardial dysfunction are the hallmarks of the disease. Patients were randomized to treatment with Enalapril or placebo. We found that treatment with Enalapril reduced the rate of decline of ventricular performance by reducing end-systolic wall stress in this group of patients.

An important contribution of the V_{cfc}–wall stress relationship concept has been its conveyance of the importance of wall thickness and cavity size in our thinking about the physiology of complex forms of congenital heart disease. We have applied these principles in helping to improve our understanding of patients with single ventricle undergoing superior cavopulmonary operation. Although in a purely quantitative sense, the values obtained may not be clinically useful when comparing between patients with heterogeneously shaped ventricular geometry, observing for changes within individual patients in an investigative protocol can be revealing. Donofrio *et al.* observed nine children undergoing superior cavopulmonary connection before

and early after surgery and measured preload, wall stress, and ventricular function by looking at the traced ventricular end-diastolic areas, wall thickness and cavity areas at end-systole, blood pressure, and fractional area change [13]. End-diastolic areas decreased after surgery and wall thickness increased, while blood pressure remained unchanged, suggesting a decreased preload and decreased afterload. Of note, parameters of systolic function did not change. The authors concluded that although there was no measurable improvement in systolic function, diminished work related to a reduction in loading conditions may result in beneficial long-term effects. Indeed, the clinical course in many children after this type of surgery would support the concept of improved hemodynamics after cavopulmonary connection.

Ejection fraction

While the %SF provides for information concerning the change in linear dimensions in a single plane cut through the short axis of the left ventricle, addition of measurements of the long axis of the left ventricle to the equation can provide for a more multidimensional reflection of volumetric change. The percent *ejection fraction* is the percent change in calculated volume of the LV from diastole to systole (%EF). A variety of formulas exist for calculation of LV volume, which can be used for determination of the %EF [14]. All these formulas essentially assume a particular mathematically defined shape of the left ventricle, which may not necessarily apply when dealing with the left ventricle in a patient with congenital heart disease.

A more precise way to estimate LV volume is to apply the "method-of-discs" or modified Simpson's rule. This principle describes calculating individual areas of discs, which are summed as they are stacked one upon the other, encompassing the volume through the long axis of the heart. This method is very time consuming and open to imprecision via echocardiography, but is much simpler to obtain via computed MRI techniques. Hence, MRI is clearly the superior modality to use when interested in obtaining precise measures of ventricular mass, volume, and change in volume during the cardiac cycle, and is very suited for use in patients with irregularly shaped ventricles.

Automatic border detection

Linear measures of cavity size during various phases of the cardiac cycle are most commonly made using either M-mode images or two-dimensional images. These linear measures are then used to calculate changes in area and volume, albeit based on multiple geometric assumptions. A preferred technique, if possible, would be to directly measure area and area changes without the need for derived calculations and geometric assumptions.

To this end, echocardiographic techniques have been developed to allow for automated border detection (ABD). By modulating the reflective characteristics of the ultrasound signal, a more dramatic distinction between fluid (blood) and tissue (myocardium) border can be achieved with display of real-time changes in the blood–myocardial interface over time. By defining a region of interest on the display screen, the change in area of the blood–myocardial interface over time within the region can be displayed. For example, if the region of interest is designated over the LV cavity in a parasternal short axis plane, quantitation of the area in addition to derivatives such as the rate of area change during phases of the cardiac cycle and percent of area change from maximal to minimal area (a two-dimensional shortening fraction) can be obtained [15].

Although conceptually attractive, the ABD technique has been difficult to use in a routine clinical setting. Creation of the fluid–tissue interface image is very gain dependant and hence prone to subjective factors of border assignment based on image quality. Reproducibility has been questioned, with confounding factors such as respiration significantly affecting the image display. Nonetheless, ABD has been successfully used in experienced hands and in controlled experimental settings to help answer a number of investigational queries [16].

We have used ABD techniques to aid in our understanding of single ventricle physiology. Mahle and colleagues applied ABD techniques to look at the performance of the right ventricle in children with hypoplastic left heart syndrome after Fontan operation [17]. ABD was applied in the short axis to the systemic right ventricle at the level of the tip of the papillary muscle of the RV (Fig. 7.4). Thirty-two children aged 8 ± 3 years were age matched to controls of children with normal hearts in which ABD was applied to the systemic LV. Fractional area change was lower for the systemic RV group than for the normal systemic LV group ($43\% \pm 10$ vs. $55\% \pm 11$, $p < 0.001$). Analysis of the area change waveforms revealed an interesting finding. There appeared to be a much greater percent change in area with atrial contraction for the single RV group than for the normal controls ($32\% \pm 4$ vs. $22\% \pm 4$, $p < 0.001$). This suggests that patients with a single RV after Fontan operation have a much greater reliance upon atrial contraction to achieve ventricular filling than do normals, which is likely related to the differences in compliance between the two types of ventricles. This has implications for the importance of preserving sinus rhythm in these patients and may explain why cardiac output is dramatically altered in the presence of arrhythmia after Fontan operation.

One of the most accurate methods for evaluating load independent ventricular function has been to generate a series of pressure–volume loops and calculate "arterial elastance." By invasively measuring pressure and volume changes one can graph the various loops and determine the slope of the regression generated at end-systole. Senzaki and colleagues modified this concept for use with area changes derived from ABD data. They constructed pressure–area loops and found that area via ABD correlated well with volume assessments [18]. Pressure–area loops were generated using preload reduction via

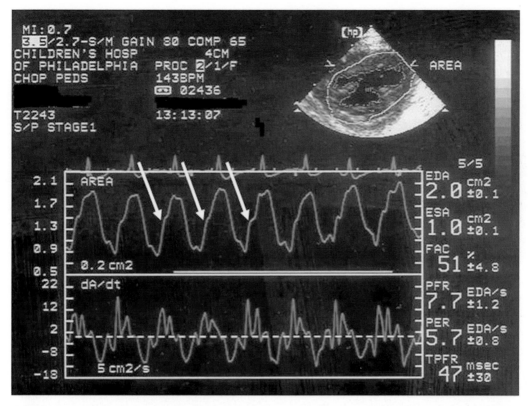

Figure 7.4 Automatic border detection display of changes in area (y-axis) for the right ventricular cavity versus time (x-axis). Top curve reflects absolute changes in area versus time, while the bottom curve is the first derivative of the above curve ($\mathrm{d}A/\mathrm{d}t$). The white arrows point to the inflection in diastolic area change that occurs with atrial contraction as timed by the onset of the "P" wave in the electrocardiogram. Note that this "atrial contraction inflection point" occurs at the mid-course of the increase in diastolic area change, suggesting that a significant amount, oftentimes up to half, of the total area change in diastole is accounted for by atrial contraction. Hence, atrial contraction contributes significantly to the diastolic area change in patients with single right ventricle.

inflow occlusion and contractility augmentation via Dobutamine infusion. They found the results to be highly reproducible. Although perhaps valid in an animal investigational model, such techniques have not yet entered into the mainstream of clinical management of congenital heart disease.

Doppler echocardiography in the assessment of ventricular function: Systolic and diastolic function derived from analysis of blood flow and tissue dynamics

Clinical application of Doppler echocardiography

Doppler echocardiography allows for the generation of spectral display of flow direction and velocity. In addition, the contour and patterns of flow velocity

versus time may be analyzed with considerable information derived. Peak flow velocities, upstroke slopes, downstroke slopes, and a variety of time intervals in both systole and diastole can be measured and may offer information concerning the dynamics of blood flow through the region of interrogation.

One of the most clinically useful pieces of information obtained from Doppler echocardiography is the peak velocity. Velocity data can be converted into pressure gradients. At rest, blood flow velocities within the human heart are typically less than 1.5 m/sec. However, when flow is disturbed such as across an area of narrowing, the peak velocity increases as blood traverses the area of narrowing. In addition, flow proximal to the narrowing exists in a normal "laminar state" in which flow particles within a region are all moving at the same velocity

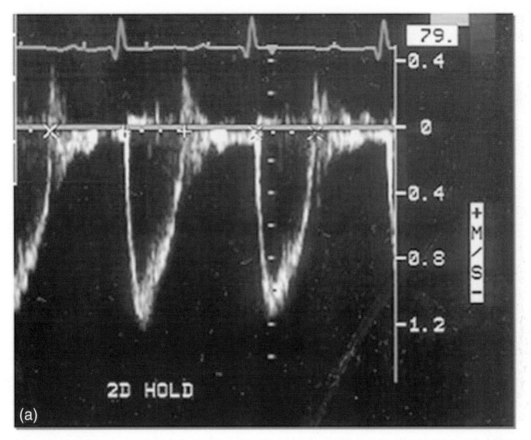

Figure 7.5 (a) Doppler spectral display of pulsed-wave Doppler demonstrating laminar flow. Note the central clearing and smooth contour of the waveform, suggesting a homogeneity in velocities measured in the region at any one point in time. (b) Doppler spectral display of turbulent flow, with high velocity as measured *y* continuous wave Doppler. Note the filled-in spectral envelope and the relatively high velocity, as measured in a child with coarctation of the aorta. Also visible are two peak velocities identified within the region of interrogation (one at 1 m/sec the velocity proximal to the narrowing and one at 3 m/sec, the velocity just distal to the narrowing).

at any given point in time. This is designated as a smooth unfilled envelope on the spectral display (Fig. 7.5). When flow is disturbed as it traverses a narrowing, it becomes nonlaminar or "turbulent" in which the flow particles are moving at different velocities at any one given point in time. This creates the appearance on the spectral display of a filled in envelope.

Measurement of the peak velocity across an area of narrowing can provide for the acquisition of pressure information via the Bernoulli equation. This equation describes the relationship between potential energy, or the pressure difference between two chambers, and kinetic energy or velocity and flow characteristics (Fig. 7.6). The full equation takes into consideration a number of factors including viscosity, frictional, and inertial forces. However, many of these variables can be ignored or incorporated and the equation can be simplified into the following:

Change in pressure or $P_1 - P_2 = 4\left(V_2^2 - V_1^2\right)$

where P_1 and V_1 are the pressure and velocity of flow, respectively, in the proximal chamber and P_2 and V_2 the pressure and flow velocity in the distal chamber (Fig. 7.6). When proximal velocities are low, less than 1 m/sec, then the V_1 variable can be ignored as well, and the equation becomes

Change in pressure or $P_1 - P_2 = 4V_{max}^2$

where V_{max} is the maximal velocity assessed across the area of interest.

This principle is of value in assessing pressure gradients across stenotic valves. One must, however, be

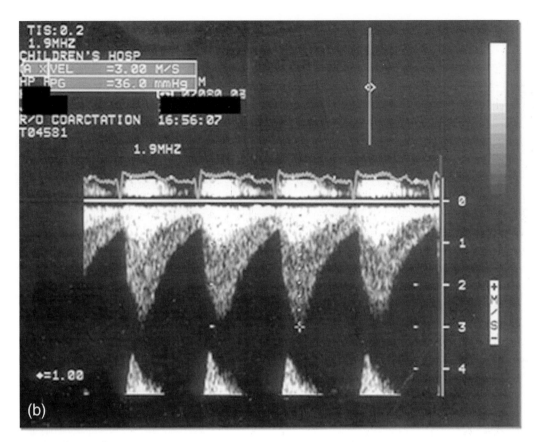

Figure 7.5 Continued

wary of the fact that pressure gradients obtained via Doppler echocardiography may not predict the same pressure gradient obtained via direct cardiac catheterization measures. Doppler techniques will oftentimes overestimate the catheter-derived measure. There are a number of explanations for this.

Bernoulli's Principle

$$P_1 - P_2 = 4 \times (V_2^2 - V_1^2)$$

if $V_1 < 1$ meter/sec, then

Change in Pressure $= 4 \times V{max}^2$

P_1 $\Rightarrow$ V_1 $\Rightarrow$ V_2 $\Rightarrow$ P_2

$\longrightarrow$ *Direction of flow* $\longrightarrow$

Figure 7.6 Illustration of the application of Bernoulli's principle across a region of discrete narrowing. P_1 is the proximal upstream pressure, P_2 the distal downstream pressure, and V_1 and V_2 proximal and distal velocities, respectively.

First, condition under which the data is acquired may be different in that catheterization is typically done under an anesthetic, while echocardiography may be done with simple sedation or without any sedation at all. Second, Doppler echocardiography measures the "peak instantaneous" gradient that occurs within the cardiac cycle, while cardiac catheterization measures a "peak-to-peak" gradient, a pressure difference that may not naturally occur, since the peak pressures achieved in each chamber may be reached at different points in time (Fig. 7.7). Hence, one can argue that Doppler echocardiographically derived gradients are a better reflection of the true physiological pressure load, or afterload, imposed on the heart, than are catheter-derived measures. However, clinical management of congenital lesions that result in pressure gradients has been historically derived from decades of data based on catheter measures. Hence current clinical management decisions are based on these catheter-derived measures.

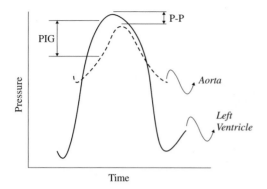

Figure 7.7 Time–pressure curve demonstrating left ventricle (solid curve) and aorta (dashed curve) tracings in a patient with aortic stenosis. P–P is the peak-to-peak pressure difference between left ventricle and aorta; PIG is the peak instantaneous pressure difference. Note that the PIG occurs during the upstroke in ventricular pressure, before peak LV pressure is reached. Also note that the peak pressure in the aorta occurs after peak pressure in the left ventricle is achieved.

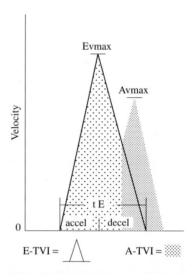

Figure 7.8 Illustration of typical Doppler inflow pattern across the atrioventricular valve. Note the two peaks with overlap of the curves. *A*, late (active) diastolic filling; *E*, early (passive) diastolic filling; TVI, time–velocity integral or area under the Doppler spectral curve.

Doppler spectral patterns of ventricular inflow

Since the 1980s a multitude of investigators have looked toward Doppler-derived inflow patterns across the systemic atrioventricular valve and the pulmonary veins as offering a glimpse at assessing diastolic ventricular performance [19]. The uniqueness in appearance and detail of the typical atrioventricular valve Doppler inflow pattern—two waveforms, often partially fused, with varying peak velocities, time intervals, time–velocity integrals (area under the waveform), and deceleration slopes—lends itself toward a belief that information has to be gained by appropriate analysis (Fig. 7.8). However, 20 years of literature has shown that the confounding factors contributing to the morphology of these waveforms are many. The waveforms are in fact extremely complex readings of flow and are affected by a multitude of variables including age, heart rate, respirations, atrial compliance, ventricular compliance, preload, afterload, and valvar architecture and function. Nonetheless, study of these waveform patterns has allowed for elucidation of a number of mysteries of diastole and provided for a further understanding of the passive and active aspects of this phase of the cardiac cycle. While simple inspection alone can lead to erroneous clinical conclusions, researchers have learned much about cardiac physiology from the detailed systematic analysis of these flow patterns.

Establishing a standard for normative reference values has been an important goal. Schmitz and colleagues published one of the largest series of normal data on left ventricular Doppler inflow parameters [20]. They examined 329 healthy subjects aged 2 months to 39 years. Variables of interest in which centile charts were created included maximal E wave velocity, maximal A wave velocity, E and A time–velocity integrals, the ratios of E/A maximal velocities and E/A time–velocity integrals, as well as the fraction of atrial filling (Figs. 7.9a–7.9g). They also observed the trend in variable changes throughout maturation. Early filling (E wave) time–velocity integral increased throughout maturation to adulthood and both peak atrial (A wave) velocities and the atrial filling fraction decreased from infancy through adolescence, in essence reflecting a shift toward earlier filling with increasing age. The authors also concluded that changes in stroke volume and growth of the mitral annulus, or the "flow-to-gate" relationship, are important modulators of expression of the Doppler inflow pattern.

Pulmonary venous flow patterns have also been studied both from the surface and via transesophageal echocardiography. Pulmonary venous flow patterns differ from atrioventricular valve inflow patterns in that there is typically flow in both systole and diastole, with a small amount of flow

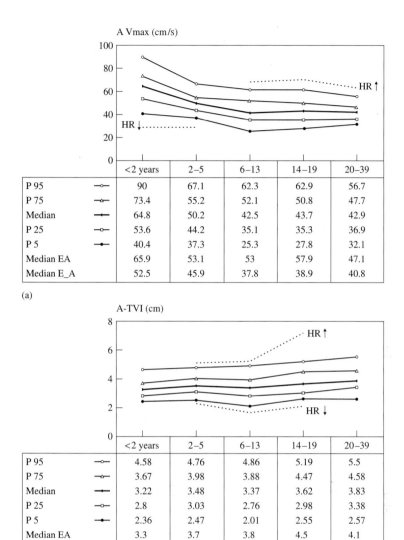

Figure 7.9 Normative data for inflow parameters across the mitral valve in children and young adults. Values are given for various age groups. Data spread is displayed for each category of age grouping via percentile as follows: P95, 95th%; P75, 75th%, median; P25, 25th%; and P5, 5th%. (a) A wave maximal velocity (V_{max}). (b) A wave time–velocity integral (TVI). (c) Percent atrial fractional flow (AFF), defined as the percent of diastolic flow occurring during the atrial contraction phase. (d) E wave maximal velocity. (e) E wave time–velocity integral. (f) E wave to A wave maximal velocity ratio. (g) E wave to A wave time–velocity integral ratio. From Schmitz *et al.* [20] with permission.

reversal during atrial contraction (Fig. 7.10). Abdurrahman and colleagues reported on the pulmonary venous flow patterns of 68 normal children [21]. They found that during the first year of life, systolic phase velocities exceeded diastolic velocities, but that afterward there was great variability. Atrial reversal velocities were less than systolic and diastolic, increased with age, and were relatively independent of heart rate. Of interest, the pulmonary venous atrial reversal velocities did not correlate with the A wave of mitral inflow. Investigators have looked at the characteristics of the pulmonary venous atrial reversal waveform and compared it to the mitral A wave inflow as a gauge of left atrial pressure in adults [22]. If the duration of pulmonary venous atrial reversal is greater than the A wave duration of mitral

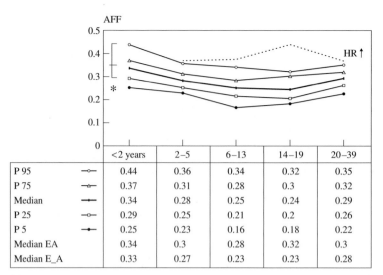

AFF

		<2 years	2–5	6–13	14–19	20–39
P 95	—○—	0.44	0.36	0.34	0.32	0.35
P 75	—△—	0.37	0.31	0.28	0.3	0.32
Median	—+—	0.34	0.28	0.25	0.24	0.29
P 25	—□—	0.29	0.25	0.21	0.2	0.26
P 5	—●—	0.25	0.23	0.16	0.18	0.22
Median EA		0.34	0.3	0.28	0.32	0.3
Median E_A		0.33	0.27	0.23	0.23	0.28

(c)

E Vmax (cm/s)

		<2 years	2–5	6–13	14–19	20–39
P 95	—○—	106	104	108	102	92.6
P 75	—△—	98.7	95.2	94.6	91	77.8
Median	—+—	85.4	89.2	87.8	85.5	66.9
P 25	—□—	77.1	83.7	78.9	78.4	62.5
P 5	—●—	52.9	72.6	70.8	71.4	53.3
Median EA		86.2	88.9	86.8	83.5	69.9
Median E_A		78.6	90.2	88	87.2	70.8

(d)

E-TVI (cm)

		<2 years	2–5	6–13	14–19	20–39
P 95	—○—	10.03	11.3	13.7	14.2	12.5
P 75	—△—	7.73	9.86	11.5	12.4	11.35
Median	—+—	6.52	8.88	10.2	11.4	9.59
P 25	—□—	5.44	8.06	9.16	10.5	8.48
P 5	—●—	3.58	6.44	6.65	8.78	6.98
Median EA		6.6	8.8	9.8	10.9	9.7
Median E_A		6.9	9.2	10.6	11.7	9.9

(e)

Figure 7.9 Continued

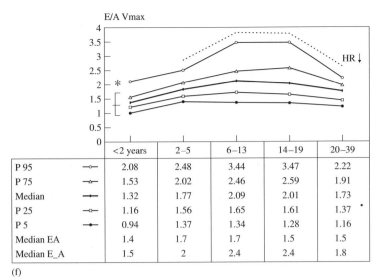

E/A Vmax

		<2 years	2–5	6–13	14–19	20–39
P 95	—○—	2.08	2.48	3.44	3.47	2.22
P 75	—△—	1.53	2.02	2.46	2.59	1.91
Median	—•—	1.32	1.77	2.09	2.01	1.73
P 25	—□—	1.16	1.56	1.65	1.61	1.37
P 5	—•—	0.94	1.37	1.34	1.28	1.16
Median EA		1.4	1.7	1.7	1.5	1.5
Median E_A		1.5	2	2.4	2.4	1.8

(f)

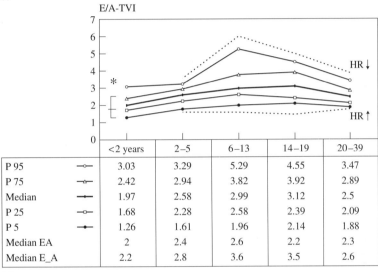

E/A-TVI

		<2 years	2–5	6–13	14–19	20–39
P 95	—○—	3.03	3.29	5.29	4.55	3.47
P 75	—△—	2.42	2.94	3.82	3.92	2.89
Median	—•—	1.97	2.58	2.99	3.12	2.5
P 25	—□—	1.68	2.28	2.58	2.39	2.09
P 5	—•—	1.26	1.61	1.96	2.14	1.88
Median EA		2	2.4	2.6	2.2	2.3
Median E_A		2.2	2.8	3.6	3.5	2.6

(g)

Figure 7.9 Continued

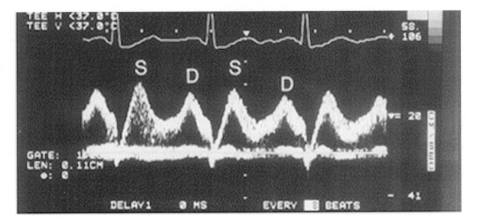

Figure 7.10 Typical Doppler flow pattern across the proximal aspect of the left lower pulmonary vein. Note a prominent S wave (ventricular systole) and a prominent D wave ventricular diastole). Oftentimes there may be a small amount of atrial reversal just prior to the S wave.

inflow (ratio < 0.9), this suggests an elevated LV end-diastolic pressure > 15 mm Hg. Such studies in children are, however, lacking.

The ratio of pulmonary venous systolic to diastolic flow parameters vary in different forms of congenital heart disease. Ito and colleagues looked at pulmonary venous flow patterns in children with unrepaired ventricular septal defect and found a marked increase in diastolic flow in comparison to systolic flow [23]. At The Children's Hospital of Philadelphia, we observed patients with single ventricle and compared their pulmonary venous flow patterns on TEE evaluation as they progressed through the stages of surgical reconstruction [24]. Patients with aortopulmonary shunt physiology had relatively equal flow during both systolic and diastolic phases, with very little atrial flow reversal seen. After superior cavopulmonary connection, overall time–velocity integral for a full cardiac cycle diminished (as overall pulmonary blood flow diminished). Most striking was the finding of marked diminution in pulmonary venous diastolic phase flow relative to systolic phase flow with the systolic to diastolic wave time velocity integral ratio increasing from 1.4 to 2.4 ($p < 0.001$) (Fig. 7.11). This finding highlights the importance of systolic factors in driving blood across the pulmonary vascular bed in patients with single ventricle and Fontan physiology. Since there is no ventricular pump propelling blood forward, the impetus for forward blood flow in the pulmonary veins of the single ventricle must relate to factors such as atrial

compliance and pressure gradient created by descent of the atrioventricular valve toward the apex in systole. An additional finding in our study was the unique pulmonary venous flow pattern seen in children with junctional rhythm after hemi-Fontan. In the absence of atrial contraction, there was a markedly increased atrial reversal velocity, which exceeded either systolic or diastolic wave velocities. The timing of the reversal was consistent with onset of the "qrs" signal on electrocardiogram and likely signified the effect of atrioventricular valve closure on an inadequately emptied left atrium with transmission of the force of valve closure back into the pulmonary veins.

Diastolic inflow patterns have been used to study the long-term effects of Fontan physiology on the ventricle. A number of investigators have demonstrated diminished early diastolic filling in comparison to late atrial filling, suggesting abnormalities of compliance and/or relaxation [25,26].

The myocardial performance index (Tei index): A measure of global ventricular performance

Doppler echocardiography can provide for spectral display of either blood or tissue dynamics over time. Recently, a technique has been described that utilizes variables derived from the time intervals of blood flow across the atrioventricular valves and across the respective ventricular semilunar valves. Tei *et al.* described a global "myocardial performance index," which is the ratio of the sum of the isovolumic

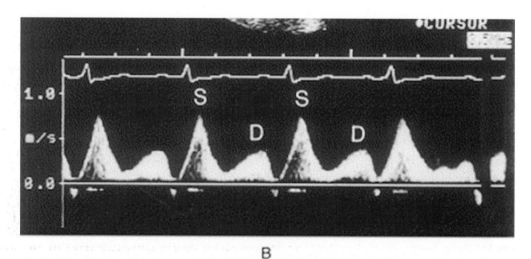

B

Figure 7.11 Doppler flow pattern in the pulmonary vein of a patient following superior cavopulmonary connection (hemi-Fontan). Note the shift in flow toward systole and a diminution in flow during diastole.

ejection and relaxation time intervals to the ventricular ejection time, all derived from Doppler spectral signals of blood flow [27].

The technique is straightforward to perform. From the apical view the Doppler sample cursor is placed at the inlet of the atrioventricular valve and a series of spectral inflow waveforms are displayed. The time interval between cessation of flow (closure of the atrioventricular valve) and the commencement of flow at the next cycle (opening of the atrioventricular valve) is recorded (time a). This time interval is a summation of the time for isovolumic contraction, ventricular ejection, and isovolumic relaxation. Excluded is the time of inflow across the atrioventricular valve. The Doppler sample cursor is then placed in the outflow tracts at the level of the semilunar valve and a spectral display of ejection is obtained. The time interval from commencement of flow to cessation of flow is measured and is the ventricular ejection time (time b). By subtracting time b from time a, one obtains the summed total time interval for isovolumic activity of the ventricle, both isovolumic contraction and relaxation. In dividing this value by the ejection time, one creates a ratio of the time intervals of "isovolumic" activity (no change in ventricular volume) to "dynamic volumic" activity (ventricular volume change) (Fig. 7.12). Hence

$(a - b)/b$, or the MPI, is a global measure of both systolic and diastolic ventricular function.

The MPI is derived from time intervals of blood flow; it is independent of the geometry and architecture of the ventricle. Therefore, the MPI can be applied to the evaluation of either the right or the left ventricle, or to the ventricles of indeterminate or complex shape, as is commonly seen in congenital heart disease. In addition, it is simple to perform, quick, and reproducible—factors that make it clinically attractive for use in the infant and child. Conceptually, the greater the MPI value the greater the amount of time spent in isovolumic activity for any given amount of time of ejection. An elevated MPI value suggests a greater "inefficiency of time" utilized per cardiac cycle and a poorer global myocardial performance. The MPI has been correlated with other invasive catheter-derived indices of ventricular performance in both the human and an animal model [29,30].

Normal values for both the RV and the LV have been generated. Eidem and colleagues studied 152 normal children aged 3–18 years and found the RV MPI to be 0.32 ± 0.03 and the LV MPI to be 0.35 ± 0.03 [28]. They then studied patients with Ebstein's anomaly and found elevation in both the RV and the LV as well as a correlation between the degree of

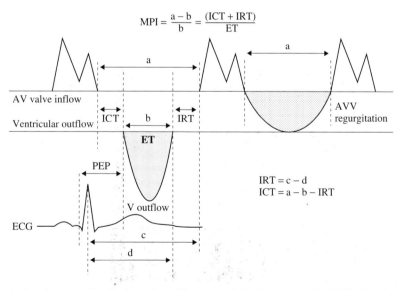

Figure 7.12 Illustration demonstrating the derivation of the myocardial performance index (MPI). AV valve inflow is displayed in the top tracing. Time a is the time from cessation of AV inflow to onset of AV inflow of the next beat. Time b is the ejection time derived from measuring the time from onset to cessation of flow across the semi-lunar valve. ICT is the isovolumic contraction time; IRT is the isovolumic relaxation time. From Eidem *et al.* [28] with permission.

elevated MPI for the RV and other abnormal measures of ventricular performance.

The MPI has been applied in a variety of clinical settings. At The Children's Hospital of Philadelphia we studied 35 asymptomatic patients with hypoplastic left heart syndrome and functionally single right ventricle after Fontan operation [17]. The MPI was significantly higher at 0.41 ± 0.12 for the single ventricle patients versus age-matched controls at 0.30 ± 0.05, $p < 0.001$. The MPI has been used in an attempt to detect acute cellular rejection after heart transplantation. Burgess *et al.* found no change in the calculated MPI value after transplantation; however, there was an increase in the isovolumic relaxation times in the rejection group, suggesting that assessment of the independent variables used to calculate the MPI might be useful indicators [31].

Although reproducibility of the MPI has been demonstrated, the question of whether the index is load dependant continues to be debated in the literature. Eidem and colleagues studied the RV MPI in separate groups of patients with atrial septal defect and pulmonic stenosis lesions, which result in increased RV preload and afterload, respectively [32]. They found no significant difference between the MPI values of normal controls and the MPI values for the groups of atrial septal defect and pulmonic stenosis. They then looked at the right ventricle of patients with corrected transposition of the great arteries and left atrioventricular valve regurgitation and found elevated values (0.72 ± 0.17) in comparison to normal, suggesting that the MPI was elevated only in the presence of altered myocardial function. In contradistinction, Moller and colleagues examined 50 healthy volunteers and observed for changes in the MPI during Valsalva maneuver, passive leg lifting, and administration of nitroglycerin. They found significant changes based on these manipulations of preload [33].

While no conclusive statement can be made concerning the load independence of the MPI, we have found the technique to be useful when observing for changes in myocardial function within a single patient when observing for a response to therapeutic maneuvers. Caution should be exercised when comparing values between different patients.

Doppler tissue imaging

Doppler echocardiography techniques can be applied to the analysis of myocardial tissue dynamics.

Adjusting the ultrasound system settings to that of a low wall filter and minimum gain will enhance the high amplitude low velocity signals of myocardial tissue. Blood flow velocities within the heart are typically 100–150 cm/sec at rest, while myocardial velocities are in the range of 5–20 cm/sec. Hence, not only can the flow of blood be evaluated, but the movement of various regions of myocardium through space and time can be assessed, with identifiable and expected Doppler spectral patterns suggestive of health or disease.

One of the first studies looking at the use of Doppler tissue imaging in the pediatric population was published from data at our institution in 1996. We utilized color-encoded myocardial velocity mapping to direct a sample gate onto the left ventricular free wall beneath the mitral annulus in the apical view and onto the posterior wall of the left ventricle in the parasternal short axis view [34]. Spectral displays of myocardial velocity versus time were generated and distinct differences were noted between the patterns of movement between the two sites. The typical annular signal includes a single systolic wave as well as an early diastolic wave (E_a) and a late diastolic wave (A_a) during atrial contraction (Fig. 7.13). Time intervals between systole and diastole can also be observed with measurements made of the isovolumic contraction and relaxation times.

Annular myocardial tissue velocities are of particular interest since they can be compared to blood inflow patterns and analyzed in a similar manner, with the hope of improving our understanding of ventricular function. Harada *et al.* compared the Doppler spectral velocities of mitral blood inflow to mitral

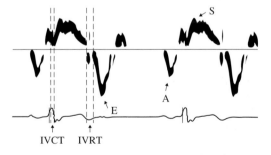

Figure 7.13 Doppler tissue imaging spectral display taken from the atrioventricular basal portion of the left ventricle. A, atrial contraction wave; E, early diastole wave; S, systolic wave. From Weidemann *et al.* [35] with permission.

tissue annular motion in children with elevated left ventricular preload due to ventricular septal defect or patent ductus arteriosus [36]. They found that mitral blood inflow velocities were affected by the left atrial pressures and the degree of preload as measured by the pulmonary-to-systemic flow ratio at cardiac catheterization, while mitral annular velocities were not. They concluded that tissue velocities may be a better reflector of myocardial function and less affected by alterations in preload conditions.

Frommelt and colleagues looked at tricuspid annular motion via Doppler tissue imaging in 141 normal infants and children [37]. A pattern similar to that seen in the mitral annulus was noted, in the presence of a single systolic wave and two diastolic waves. By separate data analysis of infants (<1 year of age) versus children (<1 year of age) differences in tissue–velocity patterns were noted. Infants had decreased early diastolic annular velocities (E_a) and prolonged isovolumic relaxation (interval between A_a and systolic wave) in comparison to the older group, suggesting delayed relaxation. Watanabe and colleagues also looked at tricuspid annular velocities with the intent of describing changes that may be seen in patients with right ventricular pathology [38]. They studied 71 children with congenital heart disease and performed conventional blood flow Doppler of tricuspid inflow, Doppler tissue imaging of the tricuspid annulus, and cardiac catheterization for hemodynamics. The ratio of late to early diastolic tricuspid annular velocities (A_a/E_a) correlated significantly with the ratio of right ventricle to left ventricle pressure and to the right ventricular end-diastolic pressure. Indices of tricuspid blood inflow velocities did not correlate with these measures. These findings further suggest that tissue velocity assessment may be superior to blood flow assessment in offering noninvasive data on ventricular performance. Studies defining the normal range of values for Doppler tissue imaging in children at various regions within the myocardium have been published by Kapusta and colleagues and by Swaminathan and colleagues [39,40] (Table 7.4).

Investigational work looking at myocardial tissue velocities in noncongenital heart disease has been performed. Fyfe and colleagues found a reduction in tricuspid annular velocities in pediatric heart transplant recipients [41]. Kapusta and colleagues found Doppler tissue imaging to be helpful in the detection of subclinical cardiac affects in cancer patients

treated with anthracyclines [42]. These studies suggest that subtle functional changes may be able to be detected much sooner using Doppler tissue imaging than with other more conventional imaging techniques. Recently, Rein and colleagues utilized an innovative technique of applying simultaneous Doppler tissue imaging at various regions throughout the heart. Analysis of the time of onset of tissue motion at the various sites allows for determination of the origin of electrical activity driving the tissue movement. In the absence of an electrocardiogram, such as in the case of fetal arrhythmia, this technique allows for the precise diagnosis of complex fetal arrhythmias [43].

The application of Doppler tissue imaging is still in its infancy as more study is needed in looking at regional myocardial tissue dynamics in various forms of congenital heart disease. A large multicenter study looking at annular velocities in patients with single ventricle after Fontan operation is currently underway.

Myocardial strain analysis

Assessment of myocardial tissue velocities has added new understanding to the evaluation of myocardial function. Individual tissue velocities alone can be influenced by heart motion within the chest and translational movements relative to the transducer-extrinsic variables that may mask the true, intrinsic myocardial dynamics and affect the measured function. In order to reduce the effects of these parameters, one can measure relative velocities at different points within a defined region of myocardium, thereby eliminating these influences since they would theoretically affect both sites similarly.

Current technologies allow for the analysis of ultrasonically determined strain rate and strain [35]. By measuring tissue velocity at point a and at point b and knowing the distance between the two allows for the calculation of the *strain rate* of the myocardial tissue subtended by the two points of reference.

$$\text{Strain rate} = \frac{V_b - V_a}{L}$$

where V_b is velocity at point b, V_a is velocity at point a, and L is the distance between the two points.

Strain occurs in three dimensions within the heart: radially, longitudinally, and circumferentially. Circumferential strain is difficult to measure with

Table 7.4

	Peak systolic velocity (S)	Peak early diastolic velocity (De)	Peak late diastolic velocity (Da)	De/Da ratio	De/S ratio
RVAW	−2.3 (−0.7 to −4.2)	3.2 (1.2 to 6.0)	1.0 (0.2 to 2.4)	3.0 (1.1 to 10.8)	−1.4 (−0.6 to −3.0)
IVSR	−2.1 (−0.9 to −3.5)	3.6 (1.5 to 6.4)	1.5 (0.6 to 2.9)	2.5 (0.7 to 7.9)	−1.6 (−0.8 to −5.9)
IVSL	−3.2 (−2.1 to −4.5)	4.9 (3.0 to 8.4)	1.9 (0.8 to 3.5)	2.6 (1.1 to 7.4)	−1.5 (−0.8 to −3.2)
LVPWen	3.9 (2.4 to 5.8)	−9.8 (−5.3 to −15.0)	−1.2 (−0.4 to −3.2)	8.3 (2.3 to 27.0)	−2.4 (−1.6 to −3.7)
LVPWepi	2.2 (1.1 to 3.5)	−3.7 (−1.8 to −6.7)	−0.7 (−0.2 to −2.4)	5.6 (1.0 to 19.0)	−1.8 (−0.8 to −3.6)

Median (and their 5th–95th percentile) of peak myocardial velocities (cm/s) obtained from apical four-chamber view ($n = 160$)

	S	De	Da	De/Da ratio	De/S ratio
RVW basal	12.8 (10.7 to 16.5)	−16.2 (−12.6 to −21.1)	−8.6 (−5.5 to −12.1)	1.8[a] (1.3 to 3.0)	−1.3[a] (−1.0 to −1.6)
mid	10.9 (8.6 to 13.7)	−13.9 (−9.4 to −17.7)	−7.1 (−4.7 to −10.0)	1.9[a,b] (1.3 to 3.0)	−1.2[a] (−0.9 to −1.6)
apical	8.0 (5.7 to 10.8)	−10.8 (−7.0 to −14.3)	−5.3 (−3.6 to −7.8)	2.0[b] (1.2 to 3.2)	−1.4[b] (−0.9 to −1.9)
IVS basal	8.1 (6.5 to 9.8)	−14.3 (−11.2 to −18.5)	−5.8 (−4.4 to −7.9)	2.5[a] (1.7 to 3.6)	−1.8[a] (−1.5 to −2.2)
mid	6.1 (4.7 to 7.5)	−13.0 (−9.2 to −16.2)	−4.9 (−3.5 to −6.5)	2.7[b] (1.8 to 3.8)	−2.1[b] (−1.4 to −2.8)
apical	4.6 (3.1 to 6.4)	−9.0 (−5.9 to −12.7)	−3.7 (−2.4 to −5.0)	2.5[a] (1.6 to 3.8)	−2.0[b] (−1.3 to −3.0)
LVW basal	9.7 (6.3 to 13.5)	−17.6 (−13.0 to −23.0)	−5.5 (−3.8 to −8.0)	3.3[a] (2.1 to 4.7)	−1.8[a] (−1.3 to −2.6)
mid	9.5 (6.2 to 13.3)	−15.9 (−10.0 to −21.0)	−4.6 (−3.2 to −7.1)	3.3[a] (2.1 to 5.0)	−1.6[b] (−1.1 to −2.3)
apical	8.7 (5.0 to 12.4)	−10.7 (−6.5 to −15.3)	−3.9[†] (−1.9 to −5.8)	2.8[†b] (1.7 to 4.5)	−1.2[a] (−0.8 to −1.8)

De/Da and De/S ratios were calculated. Different letters indicate significant difference between positions. For each wall and each ratio, the overall significance level is 5%.

[†]Number of subjects = 140.

From Kapusta et al. [39] with permission.

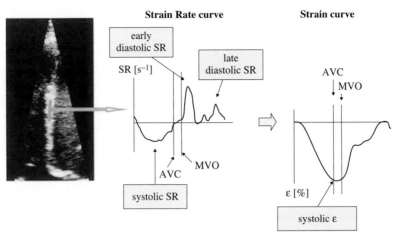

Figure 7.14 Illustration demonstrating derivation of the strain rate and strain curves using Doppler tissue imaging in the longitudinal plane. From Weidemann *et al.* [35] with permission.

echocardiography. Longitudinal strain can be assessed by imaging the heart in the four chamber apical view and interrogating a segment of myocardium as it shortens or lengthens toward or away from the transducer, respectively. Radial strain can be assessed in the parasternal short axis view as the posterior wall of the ventricle, or the ventricular septum, thickens or thins relative to the center point of the ventricle. A strain rate curve can be generated for the complete cardiac cycle, which is similar to the myocardial tissue velocity curve pattern described previously (Fig. 7.14). The first derivative of the strain rate curve is the *strain*, defined as the amount of local deformation caused by an applied force. Hence the strain rate, expressed as strains per second, is the *rate* of deformation of a segment of myocardium. As instantaneous strain values are obtained, the strain is expressed as a percentage of initial value at time zero.

In the radial dimension, myocardial thinning (diastole) is characterized by a negative strain rate and strain value percentage, while thickening (systole) is characterized by a positive strain rate or strain value percentage. In the longitudinal dimension, shortening is characterized by a negative strain rate and strain value percentage, while lengthening is characterized by a positive strain rate or strain value percentage. Both radial and longitudinal strain rates and strain values have been defined for various regions of the myocardium in normal healthy children, as well as for a variety of disorders including ischemic heart disease and cardiomyopa-

thy [44,45]. The beauty of strain analysis lies in its potential to allow for regional characterization of regional segmental myocardial pathophysiology—a methodology hitherto unavailable. Echocardiographic myocardial strain imaging provides for a unique and more elegant understanding of disease processes within the heart.

Summary

Echocardiography allows for a variety of techniques that can be used to assess myocardial blood flow and ventricular function. Doppler assessment of blood flow provides for hemodynamic information via blood flow velocities, while the study of various patterns of flow provides insight into various physiological states. Myocardial function can be evaluated by a change in dimensions via the methods of shortening fraction, ejection fraction, or automated border detection. Velocity of circumferential fiber shortening to wall stress relationship incorporates afterload into the assessment of myocardial function. The myocardial performance index utilizes geometry-independent measures of time intervals for the assessment of global function. Doppler tissue imaging is a new and exciting technique that allows for direct assessment of myocardial dynamics with the ability to derive sophisticated indices of regional myocardial function via strain and strain rate analysis. Further advancements in ultrasound technology will continue to enhance and expand the tools available to the clinician and investigator interested in blood flow and myocardial function in children with heart disease.

References

1. Tworetzky W, McElhinney DB, Brook MM, *et al.* Echocardiographic diagnosis alone for the complete repair of major congenital heart defects. J Am Coll Cardiol 1999; 33:228–233.
2. Goldberg SJ, Allen HD, Marx GR, *et al.* Doppler Echocardiography, 2nd edn. Lea & Febiger, Philadelphia, PA, 1988.
3. Chin AJ, Fogel MA. Noninvasive Imaging of Congenital Heart Disease: Before and After Surgical Reconstruction. Futura Publishing Co, Mt Kisco, NY, 1994.
4. Stevenson JG, Sorenson GK, Garman DM, *et al.* Transesophageal echocardiography during repair of congenital cardiac defects: Identification of residual problems necessitating reoperation. J Am Soc Echocardiogr 1993; 6:356–365.
5. Rosenfeld HM, Gentles TL, Wernovsky G, *et al.* Utility of intraoperative transesophageal echocardiography in the assessment of residual cardiac defects. Pediatr Cardiol 1998; 19:346–351.
6. Ungerleider RM, Kisslo JA, Greeley WJ, *et al.* Intraoperative echocardiography during congenital heart operations: Experience from 1,000 cases. Ann Thorac Surg 1995; 60:S539–S542.
7. Rhodes JF, Qureshi AM, Preminger TJ, *et al.* Intracardiac echocardiography during transcatheter interventions for congenital heart disease. Am J Cardiol 2003; 92:1482–1484.
8. Colan SD, Borow KM, Neumann A. Left ventricular end-systolic wall stress – velocity of fiber shortening relation: A load – independent index of myocardial contractility. J Am Coll Cardiol 1984; 4:715–724.
9. Banerjee A, Brook MM, Klautz RJ, *et al.* Nonlinearity of the left ventricular end-systolic wall stress velocity of fiber shortening relation in young pigs: A potential pitfall in its use as a single – beat index of contractility. J Am Coll Cardiol 1994; 23:514–524.
10. Rowland DG, Gutgesell HP. Noninvasive assessment of myocardial conotractility, preload, and afterload in healthy newborn infants. Am J Cardiol 1995; 75:818–821.
11. Rowland DG, Gutgesell HP. Use of mean arterial pressure for non-invasive determination of left ventricular end-systolic wall stress in infants and children. Am J Cardiol 1994; 74:98–99.
12. Silber JH, Cnaan A, Clark BJ, *et al.* Enalapril to prevent cardiac function decline in long-term survivors of pediatric cancer exposed to anthracyclines. J Clin Oncol 2004; 22:820–828.
13. Donofrio MT, Jacobs ML, Spray TL, *et al.* Acute changes in preload, afterload, and systolic function after superior cavopulmonary connection. Ann Thorac Surg 1998; 65:503–508.
14. Snider AR, Serwer GA. Echocardiography in Pediatric Heart Disease, Year Book Medical Publishers, Chicago, IL, 1990.
15. Rein AJ, Tracey M, Colan SD, *et al.* Automated left ventricular endocardial border detection using acoustic quantification in children. Echocardiography 1998; 15:111–120.
16. Helbing WA, Bosch HG, Maliepaard C, *et al.* On-line automated border detection for echocardiographic quantification of right ventricular size and function in children. Pediatr Cardiol 1997; 18:261–269.
17. Mahle WT, Coon PD, Wernovsky G, *et al.* Quantitative echocardiographic assessment of the performance of the functionally single right ventricle after the Fontan operation. Cardiol Young 2001; 11:399–406.
18. Senzaki H, Chen CH, Masutani S, *et al.* Assessment of cardiovascular dynamics by pressure–area relations in pediatric patients with congenital heart disease. J Thorac Cardiovasc Surg 2001; 122:535–547.
19. Riggs TW, Rodriguez R, Snider AR, *et al.* Doppler echocardiographic evaluation of right and left ventriculardiastolic function in normal neonates. J Am Coll Cardiol 1989; 13:700–705.
20. Schmitz L, Koch H, Bein G, *et al.* Left ventricular diastolic function in infants, children, and adolescents. Reference values and analysis of morphologic and physiologic determinants of echocardiographic Doppler flow signals during growth and maturation. J Am Coll Cardiol 1998; 32:1441–1448.
21. Abdurrahman L, Hoit BD, Banerjee A, *et al.* Pulmonary venous flow Doppler velocities in children. J Am Soc Echocardiogr 1998; 11:132–137.
22. Oh JK, Appleton CP, Hatle LK, *et al.* The noninvasive assessment of left ventricular diastolic function with two-dimensional and Doppler echocardiography. J Am Soc Echocardiogr 1997; 10:246–270.
23. Ito T, Harad K, Takada G. Changes in pulmonary venous flow patterns in patients with ventricular septal defect. Pediatr Cardiol 2002; 23:491–495.
24. Rychik J, Fogel MA, Donofrio MT, *et al.* Comparison of patterns of pulmonary venous blood flow in the functional single ventricle heart after operative aortopulmonary shunt versus superior cavopulmonary connection. Am J Cardiol 1997; 80:922–926.
25. Penny DJ, Rigby ML, Redington AN. Abnormal patterns of intraventricular flow and diastolic filling after the Fontan operation: Evidence for incoordinate ventricular wall motion. Br Heart J 1991; 66:375–378.
26. Olivier M, O'Leary PW, Pankratz S, *et al.* Serial Doppler assessment of diastolic function before and after the

Fontan operation. J Am Soc Echocardiogr 2003; 16:1136–1143.

27. Tei C. New non-invasive index for combined systolic and diastolic ventricular function. J Cardiol 1995; 26:135–136.

28. Eidem BW, Tei C, O'Leary PW, et al. Nongeometric quantitative assessment of right and left ventricular function: Myocardial performance index in normal children and patients with Ebstein anomaly. J Am Soc Echocardiogr 1998; 11:849–856.

29. Tei C, Nishimura RA, Seward JB, et al. Noninvasive Doppler derived myocardial performance index: Correlation with simultaneous measurements of cardiac catheterization measurements. J Am Soc Echocardiogr 1997; 10:169–178.

30. LaCorte JC, Cabreriza SE, Rabkin DG, et al. Correlation of the Tei index with invasive measurements of ventricular function in a porcine model. J Am Soc Echocardiogr 2003; 16:442–447.

31. Burgess MI, Bright-Thomas RJ, Yonan N, et al. Can the index of myocardial performance be used to detect acute cellular rejection after heart transplantation? Am J Cardiol 2003; 92:308–311.

32. Eidem BW, O'Leary PW, Tei C, et al. Usefulness of the myocardial performance index for assessing right ventricular function in congenital heart disease. Am J Cardiol 2000; 86:654–658.

33. Moller JE, Poulsen SH, Egstrup K. Effect of preload alternations on a new Doppler echocardiographic index of combined systolic and diastolic performance. J Am Soc Echocardiogr 1999; 12:1065–1072.

34. Rychik J, Tian ZY. Quantitative assessment of myocardial tissue velocities in normal children with Doppler tissue imaging. Am J Cardiol 1996; 77:1254–1257.

35. Weidemann F, Eyskens B, Sutherland GR. New ultrasound methods to quantify regional myocardial function in children with heart disease. Pediatr Cardiol 2002; 23:292–306.

36. Harada K, Tamura M, Yasuoka K, et al. A comparison of tissue Doppler imaging and velocities of transmitral flow in children with elevated left ventricular preload. Cardiol Young 2001; 11:261–268.

37. Frommelt PC, Ballweg JA, Whitstone BN, et al. Usefulness of Doppler tissue imaging analysis of tricuspid annular motion for determination of right ventricular function in normal infants and children. Am J Cardiol 2002; 89:611–613.

38. Watanabe M, Ono S, Tomomasa T, et al. Measurement of tricuspid annular diastolic velocities by Doppler tissue imaging to assess right ventricular function in patients with congenital heart disease. Pediatr Cardiol 2003; 24:463–467.

39. Kapusta L, Thijssen JM, Cuypers MH, et al. Assessment of myocardial velocities in healthy children using tissue Doppler imaging. Ultrasound Med Biol 2000; 26:229–237.

40. Swaminathan S, Ferrer PL, Wolff GS, et al. Usefulness of tissue Doppler echocardiography for evaluating ventricular function in children without disease. Am J Cardiol 2003; 91:570–574.

41. Fyfe DA, Mahle WT, Kanter KR, et al. Reduction of tricuspid annular Doppler tissue velocities in pediatric heart transplant patients. J Heart Lung Transplant 2003; 22:553–559.

42. Kapusta L, Thijssen JM, Groot-Loonen J, et al. Discriminative ability of conventional echocardiography and tissue Doppler imaging techniques for the detection of subclinical cardiotoxic effects of treatment with anthracyclines. Ultrasound Med Biol 2002; 27:1605–1614.

43. Rein AJ, O'Donnell C, Geva T, et al. Use of tissue velocity imaging in the diagnosis of fetal cardiac arrhythmias. Circulation 2002; 106:1827–1833.

44. Kapusta L, Thijssen JM, Groot-Loonen J, et al. Tissue Doppler imaging in detection of myocardial dysfunction in survivors of childhood cancer treated with anthracyclines. Ultrasound Med Biol 2000; 26:1099–1108.

45. Weidemann F, Eyskens B, Jamal F, et al. Quantification of regional left and right ventricular radial and longitudinal function in healthy children using ultrasound-based strain rate and strain imaging. J Am Soc Echocardiogr 2003; 15:20–28.

CHAPTER 8

Magnetic Resonance Imaging

Mark A. Fogel, MD, FACC, FAAP

Introduction

Cardiac magnetic resonance imaging (CMRI) is becoming the premier imaging modality to assess ventricular function and blood flow in congenital heart disease. The capabilities of CMRI overlap the capabilities of other imaging modalities and procedures such as echocardiography (e.g., average velocity in a vessel), cardiac catheterization (e.g. cardiac output), and angiography (e.g., anatomic visualization and qualitative ventricular functional analysis). However, CMRI has some very special features that other modalities cannot duplicate such as, calculating the velocity in a 1-mm voxel anywhere in three-dimensional space in the vessel or noninvasive myocardial tagging [1,2]. Indeed, investigators using CMRI have obtained unique insights into ventricular function (e.g. *in vivo* regional ventricular strain and wall motion [3–6]) and fluid mechanics (e.g. *in vivo* visualizing velocity profiles [7,8]). CMRI has also demonstrated that it can add greater accuracy to readily accepted standard measures of ventricular function and blood flow (e.g. cardiac output, ventricular volumes and mass [9]), enabling pharmaceutical firms, for example, to markedly decrease the amount of patients needed in clinical drug trials with ventricular function or fluid mechanics as endpoints [10]. Because of the rapid advance of technology, it is clear that many more unique insights will be found in the near future. In addition, many CMRI techniques are at present still in development clinically, and should come into mainstream use soon. Since many of the present experimental techniques will, without a doubt, come into clinical practice one day, the reader should be aware of these as well.

A general overview of CMRI techniques useful in assessing ventricular function and fluid mechanics in congenital heart disease is presented in this chapter with a few examples of how CMRI images lead us to a better understanding of these subjects. The physics of CMRI as it relates to ventricular function and blood flow can encompass a whole textbook, so it will only be touched on in this chapter since a limited understanding of each technique is important. The reader is referred to other textbooks with a more comprehensive treatment of this subject.

The challenges of CMRI in children

In the world of CMRI, many trade-offs are made in the technical part of the imaging to make it quicker and simpler. For example, spatial resolution can be increased at the cost of temporal resolution and vice versa. These trade-offs are of particular importance in children since the pediatric patients require increased spatial resolution because of their size as well as increased temporal resolution because of their relative high heart rates. These trade-offs, which can be taken full advantage of in adults, can only partially be availed of in children. In addition, some of these trade-offs take advantage of the ability of the subject to hold their breath. Since children under 7–9 years of age cannot usually cooperate and therefore need sedation, the specialized sequences designed for breath-holding are useless. Since this is the mainstay of adult CMRI, "work-arounds" have been created and continue to be developed. It is therefore clear that CMRI in children is a specialized field in itself for just the technical part, not to mentioned knowledge of the physiology, function, and anatomy of congenital heart disease. Many modifications or new approaches have been needed to successfully image children. Any person working with these scans needs a fundamental understanding of all this.

There are a few limitations to CMRI in general. The technique requires the subject to hold still, which can be a difficult, even in adults. Young patients usually require sedation and is always a consideration as mentioned above. Even if the patient can hold still, cooperation in a child may be problematic; breath-holding is a good example. Most intravascular coils (e.g., those that are used to close a patent ductus arteriosus), wires used to close the sternum and clips may all cause artifact problems if they are near the structure of interest. Different cardiac MRI techniques are variably affected, with gradient echo sequences, for example, affected more than T_1 spin echo sequences. Claustrophobia may be a problem for some individuals, although lying in different positions (e.g., on stomach with the patient's feet in the scanner first) and some mild sedation can help in addition to the new "short bore" and "open" magnets.

CMRI is not as good at echocardiography just yet in imaging rapidly moving leaflets of valves and chordae, although with faster sequences such as true-FISP (fast imaging with steady state precession) [11] and "slice tracking" technologies, this is becoming less of an issue. Echocardiography is still advantageous if portability to the bedside is necessary, since a critically ill patient would need to be moved to the CMRI scanner to be imaged. This is more a convenience than anything else, as even patients from the intensive care unit are generally imaged by CMRI safely and successfully. Finally, congenital heart disease surgery or Wolf–Parkinson–White syndrome, for example, may cause arrhythmias which might interfere with proper data acquisition; other patients may have bizarre T waves or bundle branch blocks, which may not allow the scanner to trigger properly. This is also becoming less of a concern with the advent of "single shot" CMRI (whole image reconstructed in one heart beat) "real time" CMRI (images continually being reconstructed without regard to ECG triggering) [12] and sequences with arrhythmia rejection. Pacemakers still present a problem and patients who have them inserted usually do not undergo CMRI [13].

CMRI techniques

CMRI is an extremely broad-based tool with multiple types of techniques available for use in evaluating ventricular function and blood flow. There are also many variations on each theme. For example, cine CMRI can construct images with one phase-encoded line of information for each radiofrequency pulse or it can obtain, for example, nine lines of information for each radiofrequency pulse, asking the patient to hold his or her breath (segmented K space). In another example, the CMRI physician can use gradient-echo sequences or true-FISP [12] to image the moving heart. Each technique and its variations have their advantages, disadvantages, and indications.

Techniques used to assess ventricular function

There are five general types of CMRI that are in common use today in varying degrees to assess ventricular function:

1 General cine CMRI [14]
2 Myocardial tissue tagging (e.g., SPAMM, i.e., spatial modulation of magnetization) [1–6]
3 Phase-encoded velocity mapping techniques
  ○ Blood [15–17]
  ○ Myocardial velocimetry [18]
4 Stress CMRI [19] and coronary flow reserve [20]
5 Perfusion [21] and viability [22]
Each one of these is discussed below.

General cine CMRI

This technique can be divided into two categories: (A) gradient echo/FLASH [14] and (B) true-FISP [12] (Fig. 8.1). These are the "workhorses" of ventricular function; blood appears with high signal intensity and other tissue appear with a lower amplitude signal. In true-FISP, this contrast between blood and tissue is markedly enhanced, and relies on this for its superb image quality. Images can be obtained extremely quickly (true-FISP quicker than the gradient echo sequences) and consist of multiple, time-resolved images that are acquired at different phases of the cardiac cycle. Different forms of cine CMRI are available which can acquire up to eight slice levels in a single scan. In addition, there are real-time cine CMRI sequences that do not need triggering to the ECG and in development—a "self-gated" technique

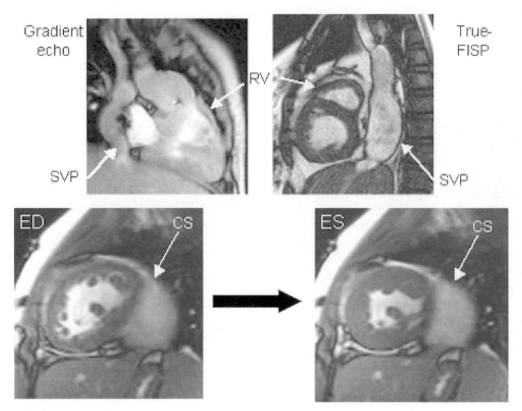

Figure 8.1 Gradient echo and True-FISP cardiac cine MRI. (Top left) Gradient echo CMRI of a patient with hypoplastic left heart syndrome after Fontan reconstruction is shown. This long axis view demonstrates the neo-aorta as well as the systemic venous pathway (left in image). (Top right) True-FISP CMRI of a patient with supero-inferior ventricles and crisscross atrioventricular relations after Fontan reconstruction is shown. The reason why it is called supero-inferior ventricles is demonstrated nicely in this off-axis sagittal image, with the systemic venous pathway seen on the right of the image. (Bottom) True-FISP cine MRI of the short axis view of a patient with single ventricle and a markedly dilated coronary sinus is shown at both end-diastole (ED) and end-systole (ES). CS = coronary sinus, RV = right ventricle, and SVP = systemic venous pathway.

where the movement of the heart itself is used to re-construct the image without an ECG. Temporal resolution with cine CMRI can be as high as 10 msec. These techniques can be done with a breath-hold by (obtaining multiple lines in k-space at once for speed of imaging) or without a breath-hold using multiple signal averages (a necessity for young children) and true-FISP can be performed as "single shot" or "segmented." In addition, there are "shared echo" sequences that speed up cine image acquisition greatly for patients who cannot hold their breath very long.

Although there is a move to image the heart faster and faster, there are advantages to taking time. CMRI is unique in that many of the ways used to create images are performed over hundreds of heartbeats, "averaging out" the ventricular performance in the process. This stands in contrast to images obtained using, for example, echocardiography and angiography, where each image represents the ventricular performance at that instant in time. The physician reading the echocardiographic study or the angiographic images must then view the many heartbeats and "average out" the ventricular performance in his or her mind. In CMRI, this "averaging out" can be documented in the image itself.

Another very important concept used in this technique involves the presence of turbulent blood flow. If present, cine CMRI will display a signal void in the region of turbulence [23] (Figs. 8.2–8.4). This is mentioned here simply because this property is taken advantage of to detect valvular stenosis and insufficiency, which is necessary to assess when evaluating ventricular function. Caution must be used, however, when using this signal void to grade the

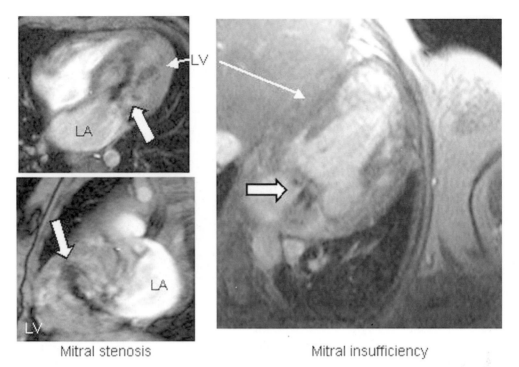

Mitral stenosis

Mitral insufficiency

Figure 8.2 Cine MRI used to assess atrioventricular valve insufficiency or stenosis. The images on the left are from a patient with Shone's complex with a parachute mitral valve. The four-chamber (top left) and two-chamber (bottom left) views demonstrate the loss of signal due to turbulent flow in diastole across this valve. The image on the right is from a patient with congenital mitral insufficiency. In all the images, arrows point to the region of signal void due to flow disturbances. LA = left atrium and LV = left ventricle.

ED   AS – mid systole   AR – mid diastole

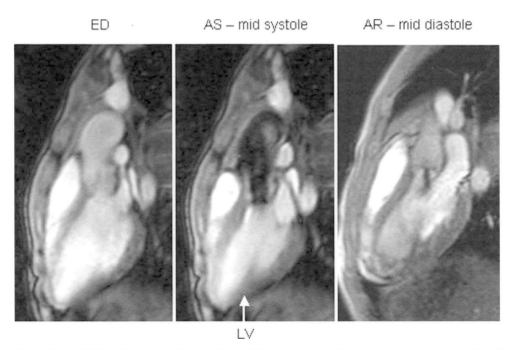

LV

Figure 8.3 Cine MRI used to assess semilunar valve insufficiency or stenosis. The images are from a patient with a bicuspid aortic valve after unsuccessful balloon dilation. The equivalent of a parasternal long axis view by echo is shown here. The image on the left is taken at end-diastole (ED). In mid-systole (middle image), the signal void is seen in the aorta indicating turbulent flow and aortic stenosis (AS). In mid-diastole (image on the right), the signal void is seen in the left ventricle (LV) indicating turbulent flow and aortic regurgitation (AR).

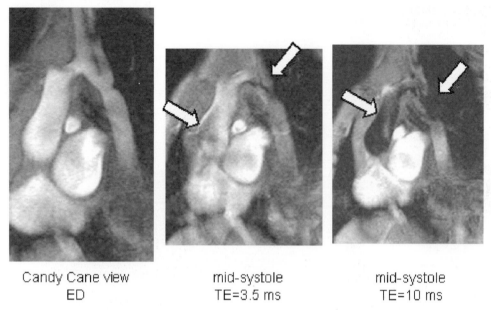

Candy Cane view
ED

mid-systole
TE=3.5 ms

mid-systole
TE=10 ms

Figure 8.4 The effect of echo time (T_E) on the signal void of cine MRI. The candy-cane views are from a patient with a bicuspid aortic valve, aortic stenosis, and coarctation. The image on the left is taken at end-diastole (ED). In mid-systole with a $T_E = 3.5$ msec (middle image), small signal void is seen in the aorta and at the coarctation site is visualized indicating turbulent flow. In mid-systole with a $T_E = 10$ msec (rightmost image), the signal void is much more prominent than with the middle image, "blacking out" almost the entire ascending and proximal descending aorta. Arrows point to the signal voids.

amount of regurgitation or stenosis. The flow void must be viewed in light of the physics of CMRI, just as the interpretation of echocardiographic images must be interpreted only with a thorough understanding of the technology (e.g., frame rate, angle of incidence, etc.). The size of the flow void is a function of a number of factors including the echo time (T_E), where longer echo times increase the size of the signal void and shorter times decrease it (Fig. 8.4). The rough parallel in echocardiography would be adjusting the Nyquist limit or the gain on color Doppler interrogation of the valve. In addition, the size of the flow void is also a function of the direction of the regurgitant jet relative to the orientation of the image voxel. Finally, true-FISP imaging may underestimate the flow void seen on FLASH sequences and it is always best, if a flow void is present on true-FISP imaging, to confirm its size on FLASH sequences.

As in echocardiography, single or multiple short-axis views of the ventricle can be obtained to both qualitatively and quantitatively assess myocardial shortening [9]. Of course, views orthogonal to this plane (four-chamber view and the ventricular long-axis view) can be used to complement the short-axis data. Myocardial thickening and regional wall

motion can be grossly visualized in this manner. However, the major strength of CMRI is the accurate assessment of ventricular mass, volume, stroke volume, ejection fraction, and cardiac index [9,10, 24–27]. Since CMRI can acquire contiguous, parallel, tomographic slices, all major assumptions of ventricular shape, which are needed for calculations of volumes in other imaging modalities, are avoided (Fig. 8.5). This is particularly poignant in congenital heart disease, with the highly variable ventricular shapes found in many lesions. In addition, it is usually when the ventricular shape changes to a form where geometric formulas do not apply is where the clinician is most interested in assessing ventricular volume and mass. CMRI has been validated and used to evaluate right and left ventricular geometry and performance in multiple studies including congenital heart disease [9,10,24–27].

Assessment of wall motion
As with echocardiography, global and regional wall motion, wall thickening (systole) and thinning (diastole) may be assessed using cine CMRI. Multiple views, as mentioned above, should be obtained to fully assess ventricular wall motion from

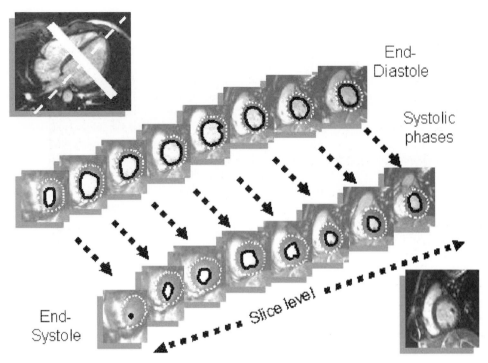

Figure 8.5 Steps to assessment of ventricular mass/volume and ejection phase parameters: A true four-chamber view is obtained (upper left) and images perpendicular to this and the long axis (an imaginary line drawn through the mitral valve and left ventricular apex, dashed line) is the short axis (solid line). A typical short axis is shown in the bottom right image. Contiguous short axis slices are obtained from atrioventricular valve to apex with phases throughout the cardiac cycle (middle images). The endocardial (black lines) and epicardial borders (dashed white lines) are then traced and the areas measured. See text for calculations of ventricular mass, volume, and ejection phase parameters.

a qualitative standpoint (Fig. 8.1). Myocardial tissue tagging (see below), however, allows for more quantifiable results and greater regional specificity than does cine CMRI alone. In addition, with more advanced hardware and software, the endocardial and epicardial surfaces throughout the cardiac cycle can be contoured to produce a three-dimensional beating heart by using finite element analysis. This results in a mathematical description of the positions of the epicardium and endocardium at all phases of the cycle. Therefore, a three-dimensional qualitative assessment of wall motion as well as calculation of global and regional indices of ventricular performance such as ejection fraction, wall thickening, etc., can be obtained.

Assessment of ventricular volumes, ejection phase parameters, and mass
To obtain ventricular volumes and mass (with subsequent cardiac index and ejection fraction calculations), multiple contiguous sets of cine CMRI runs are performed through the entire ventricle at the same temporal resolution (Fig. 8.5). The following protocol is used:

1 Localizers are performed to locate the heart in the chest.

2 *Anatomical survey:* A full set of contiguous axial images is obtained as a general survey of anatomy in order to interpret the functional information in the context of the anatomy. These images are also used as localizers to set up for the short-axis views needed to obtain ventricular volumes. Two types of sequences are generally used: (a) T_1 spin echo (turbo can be used) or (b) steady-state free precession.

3 *Multiplanar reconstruction (MPR) for localization of the ventricular short axis:* MPR is a software package that can stack the axial images atop each other and can then "reslice" it in any plane needed to obtain orientations and slice positions. To obtain the short axis of the ventricle, the following method is used:

○ A short-axis plane of the atrioventricular valves is obtained (viewing these structures en-face).

○ From the short-axis plane of the atrioventricular valves, a plane going through the center of both valves is created (from inferior/anterior right atrioventricular groove to superior/posterior left atrioventricular groove). From this newly created plane, another plane perpendicular to this (a long-axis view of the ventricle) is used to find the apex of the heart.

◦ From this long-axis view, a plane bisecting the atrioventricular valve and apex will yield a "true four-chamber view."
◦ From the four-chamber view, short-axis slices are simply the plane parallel to the atrioventricular valve and perpendicular to the long axis of the ventricle.

4 Using FLASH or steady state free precession techniques, short-axis slices extending from atrioventricular valve to apex are used to obtain ventricular volumes. Usually 8–12 short-axis levels are obtained at a temporal resolution of 20 msec.

This entire part of the exam can be as short as 10 min. The data is then sorted by time [9] and the results are multiple full volume datasets. By tracing the endocardial borders on all images at the phase or at the phases of interest (usually end-diastole, which is defined at the first phase after the R wave on the ECG trace and end-systole, which is usually defined as the phase with the smallest cavity area), ventricular volumes are obtained. This is the product of the measured areas and the slice thickness, with the results summed across all slice levels (use Simpson's rule) [9]. Ejection phase indices are then calculated in the usual fashion:

• Stroke volume is the difference in the cavity volumes at end-diastole and end-systole.
• Ejection fraction is stroke volume divided by the end-diastolic volume.
• Cardiac index is the product of stroke volume and the average heart rate during image acquisition divided by body surface area.

By tracing the epicardial borders and performing the same exercise outlined above with the endocardial borders, total ventricluar volume is obtained. When ventricular cavity volume is subtracted from this total ventricular volume at end-diastole, ventricular mass is obtained [9].

Assessment of valvar stenosis and insufficiency
Visualization of the flow void indicating the turbulent flow that accompanies valvular insufficiency can be graded similar to color Doppler echocardiography. Multiple views need to be obtained for both the flow void of valvar insufficiency as well as stenosis to optimize the ability to visualize this flow void; once the insufficiency or stenosis is visualized, slices in orthogonal directions are mandatory to fully evaluate the jet. This is similar to the sweeps an echocardiographer would use. Volumetric assessment of the regurgitant flow as well as the maximum velocity of the insufficiency and stenosis jet should be calculated using phase-encoded velocity techniques (see below). Phase-encoded velocity mapping can also be used in combination with cine CMRI techniques for the volumetric information (see section Phase-Encoded Velocity Mapping Techniques below). Of course, gradients may be calculated utilizing peak velocities as in echocardiography.

Myocardial tissue tagging

One of the unique capabilities of CMRI is to magnetically tag tissue [1–6,28–32]. This is usually accomplished using a modified cine CMRI technique on most machines (lately spin echo is used), which, prior to imaging, destroys all the spins in a given plane which in turn results in a signal void in the form of a line on the image. For example, in spatial modulation of magnetization (SPAMM), there are:

• multiple radiofrequency pulses of $130°$ separated in time and
• a series of gradient radiofrequency pulses

that produce saturated spins (the hydrogen atoms become incapable of producing a signal during the subsequent radiofrequency pulse) in two sets of parallel stripes perpendicular to each other. A standard cine CMRI sequence then follows, which divides the wall into "cubes of magnetization" as it has been termed [4–6]. The translation, rotation, and deformation of the cubes can then be tracked and assessment of wall strain, motion, and regional wall thickening can then be obtained (Fig. 8.6) in both two and three dimensions. As a side benefit, since the sequence is a spoiled gradient echo one, atrioventricular and semilunar valve insufficiency and stenosis may also be observed. This tagging can be performed during systole or diastole (Fig. 8.6) and images can be obtained with a high temporal resolution if necessary (e.g. 20 msec). The trade-off for the high temporal resolution is that the stripes tend to degrade and blur progressively as the number of acquired images increases, "smearing" the "cubes of magnetization" in the later images. This can be compensated for by

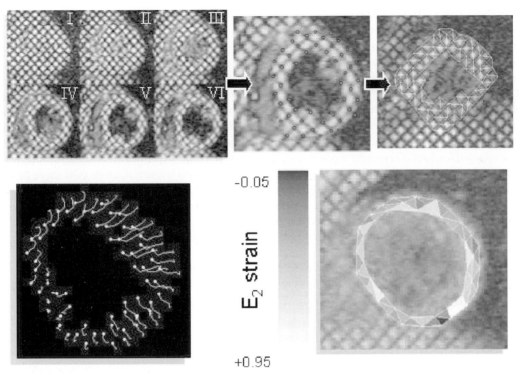

Figure 8.6 Myocardial tissue tagging in systole. These images are from an infant. These left ventricular SPAMM images are created by multiple radiofrequency pulses, dividing the wall into "cubes of magnetization." The top-left set of images are a series of six diastolic phases (roman numerals). On each imaged phase, the intersection points are identified (top, middle) and Delaunay triangulation is used to create nonoverlapping triangles. Tracking this movement and distortion of the "cubes of magnetization" allows for assessment of wall motion (lower left) and deformation (strain, lower right image). Both strain components are then derived from this deformation and coded into a grayscale map (lower right). This grayscale is then mapped onto the anatomic image (lower right). Wall motion is also imaged from the movement and visualized graphically (lower left). Dots represent the starting position at end-diastole and the tails represent the subsequent motion in systole.

performing a number of separate runs at a given slice level (which increases the acquisition time) and combining the images and sorting them temporally. In practice, however, this is rarely necessary as 6–7 images in systole or diastole are sufficient to track the motion and deformation with little tag degradation.

The initial step in analyzing SPAMM images is to track the magnetically tagged grid intersections on the image throughout the phase of interest, which can be done manually or semiautomatically. A triangular grid is created for each image utilizing Delaunay triangulation [33], which ensures uniform, nonoverlapping triangles, and the following analysis can then be performed:

• *Strain analysis (Fig. 8.6)*: Myocardial regional deformations can be characterized using finite strain analysis on the deforming triangles [34], the

methodology of which has been validated in a phantom [35]. This validation demonstrated that strain analysis produced unbiased estimates of the principal strains, principal angles, and orientations of the principal axes. The mathematics of strain analysis is beyond the scope of this chapter and is outlined in the literature [4]. Briefly, for the two-dimensional model (as mentioned earlier, three-dimensional models can also be used), the complex myocardial deformation patterns utilizing continuum mechanics [34] for analysis has been used *in vivo* in the literature. In one approach, the Lagrangian (Green's) strain tensor, $\mathbf{E}$, is computed for each triangle, and the strain tensors are diagonalized to be independent of any coordinate system. The local deformations can be described by two principal strains, E_i, and the orientation of the principal axes relative to the original coordinate system. The first principal strain E_1 is defined as the most negative strain (solution of the eigenvalues of the diagonalized matrix) and the second principal strain E_2, which is orthogonal to E_1, is defined as the most positive strain. In diastole, for example, E_1 can be thought of as "radial thinning" strain, whereas E_2 can be thought of as "circumferential lengthening" strain. The strains can then be mapped onto a grayscale (Fig. 8.6) or color coded and superimposed onto the anatomic image.

• *Wall motion calculation*: The centroid of each triangle can be used to calculate regional wall motion (linear as well as rotational movements) in relation to any point in space, which is usually the center of mass of the ventricular cavity. Some investigators prefer the center of mass of the total ventricle (enclosed by the epicardial surface) and some prefer to use a "moving" center of mass (recalculation of the center of mass for each phase imaged). The

mechanics of wall motion can be characterized by parameters such as wall twist (using angles), radial wall motion (indexed to, for example, end-diastolic volume to account for size differences), or wall thickening or thinning, which can be measured by the distance between "cubes of magnetization" as tracked through the phase of interest. Similar to strain data, wall motion data can be displayed graphically as well as quantitatively (Fig. 8.6). In one type of graphical representation of diastolic wall motion shown in the figure, "dots" represent the triangular centroid location at end systole and the "tails" represent the subsequent diastolic motion. For the analysis, the myocardial wall is typically divided into anatomic regions (e.g., septal, inferior, lateral, and anterior walls in the ventricular short axis and short-axis level along the ventricular long axis).

Tagging can also be performed in the so-called "one dimension" as well, where just one set of parallel

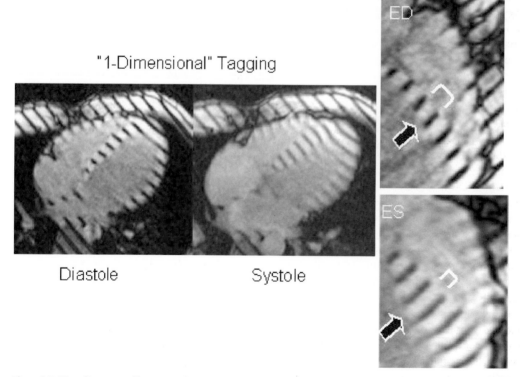

Figure 8.7 "One-dimensional" tagging. The images on the left and in the middle are four chamber views of a patient who was scanned to assess for right ventricular dysplasia in diastole (left) and systole (middle). The one-dimensional tag is laid down as a set of parallel lines perpendicular to the direction of travel of the myocardium. The distance between the tags can be seen to become smaller (ventricular shortening) and the myocardium thickening. The two images on the right are zoomed images of the right ventricle at end-diastole and end-systole and demonstrate how the distance between the tags can be measured (arrows). Regional shortening fractions can then be obtained.

lines are laid down on the myocardium (Fig. 8.7). Some investigators have utilized this type of tagging for strain measurements and have obtained excellent results, similar to the SPAMM technique. This type of tagging has also found great utility in labeling relatively thin structures, such as the right ventricular myocardium with subsequent analysis of regional myocardial shortening both qualitatively as well as quantitatively [36]. To be performed correctly for this purpose, the tags are laid down perpendicular to the direction of myocardial motion (e.g., in the four-chamber view, tags are laid down perpendicular to the long axis of the ventricle). For quantification, the distance between the signal poor areas of the tag are measured at end-diastole and end-systole, and a regional shortening fraction is obtained.

Phase-encoded velocity mapping techniques

Both blood phase encoded velocity mapping [15–17] and myocardial velocimetry [18] fall under this rubric and utilize the same principles to obtain functional data. Blood phase encoded velocity mapping will also be discussed in section Techniques Used to Assess Blood Flow later in the chapter. (It is mentioned in this section because of the ability of the technique to obtain stroke volume, cardiac index and regurgitant fraction which are obvious parameters used to assess ventricular function.) Myocardial velocimetry, however, is detailed in this section.

How it works

The underlying principles of both types of imaging are the same and a simplified approach will be delineated in this chapter. The interested reader is referred to major MRI textbooks for greater detail. Key to the discussion is understanding what "phase" means. When a radiofrequency pulse excites tissue, the subsequent energy release sends out a signal (for example, a sine wave) that can be described by its frequency (how many cycles per second or hertz), its amplitude (the strength of the signal), and its phase (where in the sine wave cycle the signal is at a given period of time). For example, in Fig. 8.8, two sine waves are drawn (A and B). If the Y-axis is signal strength and the X-axis is time in seconds, both waves have a frequency of one cycle per second or hertz and a signal strength of one unit. Therefore, they are identical except they appear to be shifted relative to one another; their phases are not the same as they are in different parts of their cycle at a given

time (e.g., in the figure, during the peak of sine wave A, sine wave B is still on the upswing). Another way to think about this is that the same part of each cycle occurs at a different period of time (e.g., the peak of sine wave A occurs prior to the peak of sine wave B).

The principle underlying phase-encoded (also called phase shift or phase contrast) MRI is simply that moving tissue within a magnetic field changes phase after a radiofrequency pulse imparts energy to it. More correctly, whenever anything moves along the axis of an applied gradient, the phase of the spinning vectors in that object becomes altered relative to the stationary object. This method, therefore, can selectively "label" moving tissue and utilizes what is called a "bipolar" gradient—a gradient that goes from positive to negative and then from negative to positive (e.g., composed of two lobes with opposite signs). This is done with two sequences back to back. When the first lobe is applied both stationary and moving tissue accumulate phase; when the second lobe is applied immediately afterwards, stationary tissue loose their phase and accumulate a net phase of zero. Moving tissue in this time period experiences unequal positive and negative gradients and accumulates a phase shift. Therefore, this will yield a zero phase change for stationary objects in both sequences, a positive phase change for moving tissue in one sequence, and a negative phase change for moving tissue in the other. By subtracting, pixel by pixel, the phases of one sequence from the other, background phase changes of stationary objects are cancelled out and the phase shift of the moving tissue is amplified. Then, usually, the "phase difference" method is used to map the phase shift angles into signal intensities. Velocity is calculated by

$$\Delta \text{ phase} = g v T A_{\text{g}}$$

where g is the gyromagnetic ratio, v the velocity, T the duration of the gradient pulse, and A_{g} is the area of each lobe of the gradient pulse.

A VENC (velocity encoding) is used to tailor the strength of the gradient to the anticipated velocities to be measured (similar to the Nyquist limit in echocardiography). Using the VENC and the signal intensity, the velocity of moving tissue in each pixel can then be encoded. This can occur with either blood (hence blood phase encoded velocity mapping) or with myocardial tissue (hence myocardial velocimetry).

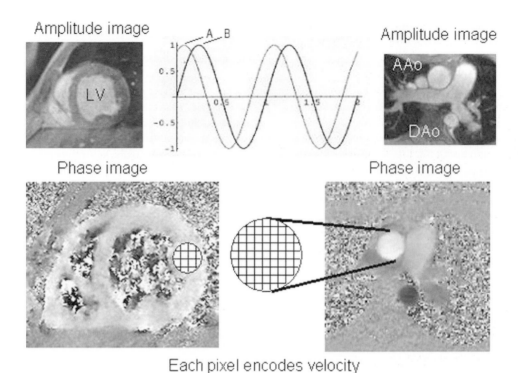

Figure 8.8 *Phase-encoded velocity mapping.* The left images are amplitude (top) and through plane phase (bottom) images of the short axis of the left ventricle (LV) when performing myocardial velocimetry. The VENC is 10 cm/sec. The right images are amplitude (top) and through plane phase (bottom) transverse images from a patient with a ventricular septal defect at the level of the ascending (AAo) and descending aorta (DAo). The image is optimized to map the velocity in the descending aorta (DAo) as it is exactly perpendicular to the flow, but ascending aortic (AAo) can also be visualized. The velocities are mapped to a grayscale and superimposed onto the anatomic image. Flow toward the apex of the heart (left lower image) and foot (AAo flow, right lower image) has a high intensity signal and flow toward the base of the heart (left lower image) and head (DAo flow, right lower image) has a low intensity signal. The top middle image is an example of two identical sine waves that have the same amplitude and frequency but not the same phase. The lower middle image demonstrates that each pixel encodes velocity.

Types of velocity mapping

There are also two basic ways to encode velocity in the image: spatially as well as temporally. In the "spatial" category, in "through-plane" phase encoded velocity mapping (Figs. 8.8–8.10), each pixel encodes velocity into and out of the plane of the image. In-plane phase encoded velocity mapping (Fig. 8.9), as the name implies, is similar to Doppler echocardiography in that velocities are recorded within the plane of the image; however, unlike Doppler, the velocities are recorded in either the *Y*- or the *X*-direction of the image. This is advantageous in that each pixel can encode velocity in three orthogonal planes. In both types, motion in one direction is mapped onto the anatomic image as bright with signal intensity, and motion in the other direction appears dark and signal poor and stationary tissue appears gray (Fig. 8.8–8.10).

In the "temporal" category, images can be constructed with "prospective" or "retrospective" triggering to the ECG. This will be discussed in greater detail in section Techniques Used to Assess Blood Flow.

Myocardial velocimetry

Myocardial velocimetry (Fig. 8.7) [18] is the MRI equivalent to Doppler tissue imaging in echocardiography; velocities of the myocardial tissue can be recorded. Myocardial velocimetry, however, can give a much more comprehensive measurement of myocardial velocities in that, as mentioned above, each pixel can encode velocities in three orthogonal planes hence creating a three-dimensional velocity map of the myocardium. In addition, myocardial velocimetry can determine velocities in any part of the myocardium as opposed to Doppler tissue imaging where only the myocardium traveling in

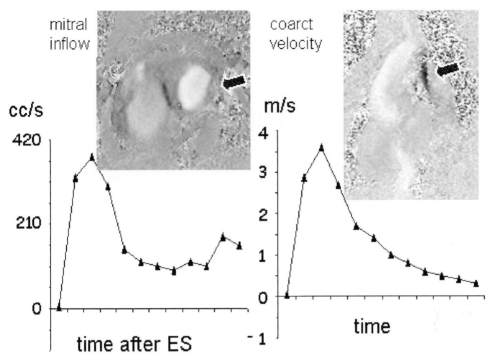

Figure 8.9 In-plane versus through-plane phase encoded velocity mapping. The left image is through-plane phase encoded velocity mapping of the mitral valve (en face) in a patient with transposition of the great arteries after arterial switch procedure. The image is optimized for flow through the mitral valve (arrow), although tricuspid valve inflow can be seen. Flow toward the apex is signal intense. The graph is a "flow" versus time graph through the valve (VENC is 100 cm/ses). The right image is in-plane phase encoded velocity mapping of the aorta (candy cane view) in a patient with coarctation (coarct). The image is optimized for flow through the coarct site (VENC is 3.5 m/sec), encoding velocity of the high signal jet (arrow) in the supero-inferior dimension (flow toward the head is signal intense and flow toward the feet is signal poor). The graph is a "velocity" versus time graph through the coarct site. Note the difference in the ordinate axis units of "flow" in the "through-plane" case (velocity can also be measured in through plane at that level) and "velocity" in the "in-plane" case. ES = end systole.

the direction of the Doppler beam can be accurately recorded; any deviation in direction incurs an error on the order of the cosine of the angle. Both myocardial velocimetry in MRI and Doppler tissue imaging in echo suffer from the same drawback: They do not in reality measure the velocity of a specific piece of myocardium but rather a point in three space is identified and the velocity of myocardium moving into and out of that point is being measured. Only MRI myocardial tagging truly measures this noninvasively. An excellent review comparing the merits of myocardial velocimetry to myocardial tagging was published in 1996 [37].

Stress CMRI/coronary flow reserve

This will not be discussed extensively because of space limitation; however, the reader should be familiar with these techniques.

Stress CMRI

This [19] is similar to other imaging techniques that utilize either physiologic (via exercise) or pharmacological methods to stress the patient. It is indicated when the resting state may not accurately reflect the clinical state of the patient. Any of the above three MRI techniques (cine MRI, myocardial tissue tagging, or phase-encoded velocity mapping methods) can be used in conjunction with stress, depending upon the desired parameter to be measured. Typically, baseline imaging is obtained prior to the application of the stress and subsequently, imaging is performed again in the same views at or immediately following peak stress. Modifications of the MRI parameters need to be performed to accommodate for the increased heart rate and motion of the patient (if exercise). A comparison is then performed between the unstressed and maximally stressed state to

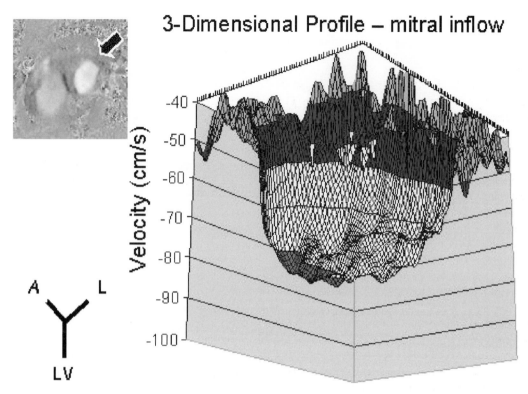

Figure 8.10 The three-dimensional nature of through-plane phase encoded velocity mapping. The left image is through-plane phase encoded velocity mapping of the mitral valve (arrow) of the same patient as in Fig. 8.9 with transposition of the great arteries after arterial switch procedure. The graph on the right is the three-dimensional velocity profile of the inflow of the mitral valve at maximum flow in diastole, derived from the through plane map. A = anterior, L = left, and LV = left ventricle.

determine the effect of the stress on ventricular function. Regional wall motion abnormalities and changes in cardiac index, for example, may be assessed using this method. In the MRI scanner, exercise can be performed utilizing a nonferromagnetic bicycle and less preferably utilizing handgrips. For pharmacological manipulation, dobutamine is most commonly used and has been reported as early as 1992 [38].

There are limitations to the technique, which include the usual CMRI contraindications including claustrophobia, pacemakers, etc. However, the efficacy of stress CMRI in patients with arrhythmias and left ventricular hypertrophy is still to be proven. In addition, it has been pointed out that studies with dobutamine stress MRI have had a relatively high pretest probability of having coronary artery disease and that other patients without such a high pretest probability have not been studied. A good review of

stress MRI was published by Rerkpattanapipat *et al.* [39].

Coronary flow reserve
The ability of the coronary artery system to increase the blood supply to the myocardium proportionate to the metabolic demands of the body is an important functional parameter. Obviously, if a mismatch occurs, ventricular function may suffer. Administration of adenosine, which is a coronary vasodilator, can be used to increase coronary blood flow. The difference between coronary blood flow with and without adenosine is one indicator of the ability of the heart to increase its blood supply. CMRI, utilizing phase-encoded velocity mapping of the blood (see below), can be used to measure coronary blood flow in the native state as well as with adenosine administration. Some studies have used phase-encoded velocity mapping of the coronary artery directly [40,41] and

others have measured coronary venous flow via the coronary sinus [20].

Perfusion/viability

This will not be discussed extensively because of space limitation; however, the reader should be familiar with these techniques.

Perfusion

Regional myocardial perfusion is another parameter important in ventricular function [21]. Regional wall motion abnormalities, for example, may be caused by a lack of blood supply to a certain region of the myocardium. CMRI, utilizing gadolinium enhancement, has the ability to assess regional wall perfusion by using a "first pass" injection technique. Typically, short-axis views of the ventricle as described in the cine MRI section are obtained and the sequence set up is such that the heart is imaged relatively motionless. Gadolinium is injected intravenously while the scanner continuously images the ventricle (up to 4–5 short-axis slices may be imaged at once) and the gadolinium bolus is followed from right ventricular cavity to left ventricular cavity to ventricular myocardium. Defects in perfusion show up as dark portions of the myocardium while the rest of the ventricle is signal intense. This is performed with and without adenosine because of technical considerations and because perfusion defects are more likely to be revealed with adenosine infusion.

Viability

Infarcted myocardium is less of an issue in congenital heart disease than it is in adults. Nevertheless, native lesions such an anomalous left coronary artery from the pulmonary artery or operations that scar the myocardium (e.g. most repaired tetralogy of Fallot) may manifest myocardial infarction and scarring. Gadolinium is avidly taken up by scarred myocardium and can remain in the scarred tissue for an extended period of time while it is subsequently "washed" out by coronary blood flow in perfused myocardium. This is to say that the signal intensity–time curves separate, with the infarcted myocardium gadolinium curve remaining highly signal intense after 5 min, whereas normal myocardium becomes much less so. CMRI pulse sequences, first described in the literature in the mid-1980s [42], have taken advantage of this property to be able to image infarcted myocardium. With the recent development of segmented inversion recovery fast gradient echo sequences and other techniques such as steady-state free precession, signal intensity differences between normal and infarcted myocardium of up to 500% have been achieved [22]. The technique has been shown to accurately delineate the presence, extent, and location of acute and chronic myocardial infarction.

After preliminary scout images and cine sequences are obtained, 0.1–0.2 mmol/kg of intravenous gadolinium is injected. CMRI sequences to visualize infarcted myocardium are used approximatelys 5–20 min after this injection and make use of a nonselective 180° inversion pulse, which spoils all the spins in the myocardium (black on the image). This has the effect of causing the magnetization of tissue to go from +1 to −1. Perfused myocardium and scar tissue begin to recover their spins; however, scar tissue recovers much quicker than normal myocardium because of the gadolinium embedded in the scar tissue. A time delay is placed after the 180° inversion pulse (TI) to image the ventricle at just the point where the normal myocardium is about to regain signal again (and because the scar tissue recovers spins much quicker, it can give off signal). This allows for maximizing the difference in signal intensity between scared and normal myocardium and the ventricle is imaged in mid-diastole.

As can be surmised, choosing the correct TI is a critical component to this whole procedure and is chosen to optimally "null" the myocardium (i.e., the time at which normal myocardium crosses the "zero" point of signal intensity), where the difference between signal intensity in normal and infarcted tissue is maximized. If the TI time is too short, normal myocardium will be below the zero point and the difference between signal intensities of the two types of tissues will not be maximized. Indeed, since the image intensity is a function of the magnitude of the magnetization vector, normal myocardium may become hyperenhanced and scar tissue may become nulled if the TI is shortened enough. At the other extreme, if the TI is too long, the myocardium will be a shade of gray and although the scar tissue will have a higher signal, relative contrast will be reduced. Another factor that affects the choice of TI is the time after gadolinium administration the patient is imaged. Since the gadolinium tends to wash out from the myocardium over time, the TI will have to be adjusted upward the longer the time after injection.

To make the choice of TI more foolproof, some investigators have developed "TI scouts," which obtain multiple images at various increments of TI and the MRI physician can choose the TI on the image that looks best. Other investigators have developed sequences that allow for phase sensitive reconstruction of the inversion recovery data, which will provide consistent contrast between normal and scarred tissue over a wide range of TIs.

There are a few pitfalls in this type of imaging. In patients with arrhythmias as well as in patients who cannot breath-hold, image quality may be degraded. These drawbacks, however, may be overcome by using "single shot" techniques and navigator sequences (for patients who cannot hold their breath). Ghosting artifacts can occur from tissue that have long T1 values, such as pericardial effusion.

Techniques used to assess blood flow

There are three general types of CMRI that are in common use today in varying degrees to assess blood flow (Figs. 8.8–8.12):

1 Phase-encoded velocity mapping of blood [15–17]
   ○ through plane (Figs. 8.8–8.10)
   ○ in-plane (Fig. 8.8)
2 Bolus tagging [7,8,43] (Figs. 8.11–8.13)
3 cine MRI [14] (Figs. 8.1–8.4)

Each one of these is discussed below.

Phase-encoded velocity mapping of blood

The concepts behind phase-encoded velocity mapping were delineated in the previous section with reference to myocardial velocimetry. These may be applied to blood flow as well except that it is blood, not myocardial tissue, which is in motion and is labeled by phase. This technique may be used to measure flow and velocity in any blood vessel; for example, relative flows to both lungs may be obtained by placing through-plane velocity maps across the cross section of the right and left pulmonary arteries. An internal check to these measurements would be placing a through-plane velocity map across the cross section of the main pulmonary artery and ensuring that the blood flow to the right and left pulmonary arteries equals the blood flow in the main pulmonary artery.

Applications

Phase-encoded velocity mapping of blood has many applications in congenital heart disease:

a Shunt flow may be calculated simply by placing velocity maps across both vessels in question and measuring flow; for example, relative flows to both the pulmonary and systemic circulations (Q_p/Q_s) in a patient with an atrial septal defect is as simple as placing velocity maps over both the ascending aorta (Fig. 8.8) and main pulmonary artery and measuring flow [44].

b Regurgitant volumes and regurgitant fraction are important parameters in the assessment of ventricular function and blood flow in patients pre- and postoperatively in congenital heart disease (e.g., regurgitant volume of a patient with Ebstein's anomaly of the triscupid valve or postoperative pulmonary regurgitant fraction in a patient with tetralogy of Fallot with a transannular patch [45]). With CMRI, the regurgitant fraction of a semilunar valve is easily obtained by utilizing through-plane phase encoded velocity mapping just above the semilunar valve and measuring the forward and reverse area under the flow–time curve generated. The regurgitant fraction is simply the area under the reverse flow (regurgitant volume) divided by the area under the forward flow (forward volume) multiplied by 100. Also, one can use a combination of cine MRI techniques (measure ventricular volume at end-diastole and end-systole to obtain the total amount of blood ejected by the ventricle) and phase-encoded velocity mapping (the amount of forward flow from the ventricle) to determine atrioventricular value insufficiency.

c As with echocardiography, gradients across stenotic vessels or valves or ventricular pressure estimates may be assessed by placing a velocity map across the area of vessel narrowing (either using in-plane or through-plane techniques, Fig. 8.8–8.10) or atrioventricular valve regurgitation and utilizing the Bernoulli equation [46].

From an investigational standpoint, CMRI utilizing phase-encoded velocity mapping is unparalleled as a noninvasive tool for measuring flow and velocity-related phenomenon. With the ability to encode velocity in each pixel in both through- and in-plane velocity techniques (Figs. 8.8–8.10), blood flow mechanics can be mapped in any part of the three dimensions of the vessel (see, e.g. Figs. 8.9 and 8.10, blood flow in anterior vs. posterior segments of the aorta) [17,47]. Similarly, since blood flow can be encoded in three orthogonal planes, the three-dimensional direction and velocity of blood may also be obtained [47]. This is useful when investigating both the primary and secondary flow patterns of the vessel, which in the aorta, for example, has been found to be helical [47]. In addition, velocity-mapping data has been used as input information in creating a computational fluid dynamic model of blood flow, such as in the systemic venous pathway of the Fontan reconstruction [48].

How to analyze the images

To determine the flow volume utilizing through-plane phase encoded velocity mapping, the images perpendicular to flow (i.e., a cross-sectional area of the vessel) are used [17]. In general, software allows the identification of the region of interest on the "magnitude" images, which are then simultaneously traced via the software onto the "phase" image, which can sometimes be difficult to read (although one can manually trace the region of interest on the "phase" image as well). The average velocity in the region of interest (in this case, the cross-sectional area of the vessel) is multiplied by the cross-sectional area to obtain the flow volume measurement at that phase of the cardiac cycle. This is equivalent to the sum of the product of the velocity in each pixel by the area of each pixel. If the flow volume of all phases of the cardiac cycle are calculated and plotted on a time–flow graph, the integrated area under the curve will yield the flow during one heartbeat. Multiplying this result by the heart rate will yield cardiac output.

Through-plane phase encoded velocity mapping can also be used to assess the maximum velocity through a blood vessel or valve. If the proper cross-sectional area is obtained (i.e., the images perpendicular to flow in the region where the maximum velocity is occurring), the highest velocity in any pixel in the region of interest at any phase in the cardiac cycle is used in the simplified Bernoulli equation. Care should be taken, of course, to make sure that it is indeed the proper cross-sectional area; angled views not perpendicular to flow or views at a level not where the maximum flow will underestimate the maximum velocity. This is similar to Doppler echocardiography where Doppler interrogation angled obliquely to the jet of interest or the two-dimensional sector not in the area of maximum velocity will underestimate the maximum velocity.

Encoding velocity parallel to flow (Fig. 8.9), similar to Doppler techniques (in-plane velocity encod-

ing), is predominantly used to measure peak flow velocities such as in obstructed pulmonary veins [49], and its reliability is a function of a few factors such as slice thickness ("partial volume" effects may induce inaccuracies in velocity calculations) and the angle of the jet (the jet needs to be aligned perpendicular to the direction of phase encoding and therefore, parallel to the read encoding direction, similar, in some sense, to Doppler flow measurements). It has an advantage over the through-plane technique in measuring maximum velocities in that velocities can be measured all along a jet of interest in the direction the jet is pointing. Newer advances allow the jet to be aligned by rotating the entire field of view to make one side exactly parallel to the jet. The peak flow velocities can then be translated into pressure gradients via the simplified Bernoulli equation ($\Delta P = 4v^2$, where ΔP is the pressure gradient in mm of mercury and v is the peak velocity in m/sec). The phase maps on present day scanners can give a temporal resolution of about 15 msec.

Temporal imaging

As mentioned earlier in this chapter, images can be obtained "temporally" by either "prospective" or "retrospective" triggering to the ECG. In the prospective case, the CMRI scanner is programmed to monitor the ECG and once a QRS is sensed, it begins to acquire data for image reconstruction. There is also typically a "dead time" after the data is acquired before the scanner can begin to acquire the next set of data in the next cardiac cycle. With this method, if the time to acquire the data runs over onto the next QRS or if the next QRS occurs during the "dead time," the scanner would need to wait until the following QRS before more data could be acquired, which could double the time for imaging. In the retrospective case, the CMRI scanner is programmed to acquire data to reconstruct the images continuously and records the ECG during this time period. After all the data is collected, the software "retrospectively" goes back and reconstructs the images based on where the data was collected in relation to the ECG. In this case, the drawback in the prospective case is averted. This is especially important in flow phenomenon since the drawback of the prospective case either does not allow for detection of flow across the entire cardiac cycle or can double the time for image acquisition.

Limitations

These phase-encoded velocity mapping techniques have a few limitations. If the VENC is not chosen properly, erroneous results may occur. For example, if the VENC chosen (maximum velocity detectable) is too low, aliasing similar but not identical to exceeding the Nyquist limit in Doppler echocardiography will occur. If the VENC chosen is too high for the velocity measurement, sensitivity will be lost and a less accurate measurement will be obtained. This is similar to Doppler interrogation of venous flow where the spectral scale is set to a maximum velocity of 5 m/sec. Another way to think of this kind of inaccuracy is the difference when measuring a 402 cup of fluid in an 8 oz measuring cup (appropriate setting of the VENC or Nyquist limit) versus a gallon measuring cup (inappropriate setting of the VENC or Nyquist limit)

For through plane measurements, the imaging plane needs to be as perpendicular to flow as possible. The more angled the imaging plane is to the direction of travel of the blood, the greater the error (similar to not aligning the Doppler beam directly with the blood flow). Similarly, as mentioned above, in-plane measurements need to be parallel to the direction of flow; again, the more angled the imaging plane is to the direction of travel of the blood, the greater the error. This needs to be corrected by the cosine of the angle between the direction of the measured flow and the true flow. Besides not measuring flow in the correct direction, another contributing reason for the error would be "partial volume" effects, where stationary tissue is "averaged in" with moving tissue in the same pixel. This, in effect, dilutes out the phase change effect and will underestimate the velocity and therefore the flow. For example, with "in-plane" velocity mapping of a coarctation of the aorta (Fig. 8.9) to assess for a maximum velocity to calculate a gradient, if the narrowing is 3 mm and the slice thickness is 6 mm, 3 mm of stationary tissue surrounding the narrowing will be averaged in with the high-velocity jet. Since the stationary tissue has zero velocity, this tissue will dilute out the phase information from the blood and underestimate the velocity.

There are other limitations. With calculation of a gradient, as mentioned, care should be taken to ensure that the region of interest contains the area where maximum flow will occur; if this does not occur, an underestimation will result. In addition, very small vessels are poorly assessed by phase-encoded velocity mapping; the general rule of thumb is that the blood vessel must be at least 4 pixels across to get accurate data. Further, flow-related signal loss and loss of phase coherence within a voxel may occur. Shorter echo times (TE), longer TR, and decreasing voxel size may alleviate some of these factors.

Blood (bolus) tagging

As noted in the previous section on myocardial tissue tagging, CMRI is unique in its ability to tag tissue noninvasively. The same way myocardial tissue is tagged allows for blood to be tagged as well. This type of tagging has been called "bolus" or blood tagging and is a gradient echo sequence similar to myocardial tissue tagging [7,8,43]. Instead of a "grid" being laid down on the myocardium or a series of parallel lines (one-dimensional tagging), it utilizes a radiofrequency pulse to produce saturated spins along a single line designated by the user (a black stripe on the image) across a blood vessel. Unlike myocardial tissue tagging, however, a saturation pulse precedes each phase of the cardiac cycle imaged; with myocardial tissue tagging, the saturation pulse is only applied immediately preceding the first phase. The tag from the previous phase typically fades away prior to the next imaged phase if the temporal resolution of the sequence is set correctly. Blood flow displaces this band of saturation, whereas stationary structures (e.g. chest wall and spine) maintain the saturation band's original position (Figs. 8.11 and 8.12). Each image represents blood displacement between tagging and image acquisition.

Velocity can be calculated at any point along the band by measuring the movement of the saturation band placed on the blood relative to the stationary structures (Fig. 8.12) [7,8]; the time between the saturation band being placed and image creation is known and it is a simple calculation to divide the distance of tag displacement by the time. Flow can be calculated using a number of assumptions (circular blood vessel, similarity of velocity profile across the cross-section of the vessel) by measuring the area between the saturation band displaced by the blood and the line made between the saturation band on the chest wall and spine. Converting this area to a volume using the assumptions above and dividing by the time between tagging and image acquisition yields flow during that particular phase of the cardiac cycle. The summation of the flows in all images across the

Bolus tagging – tricuspid inflow - HLHS

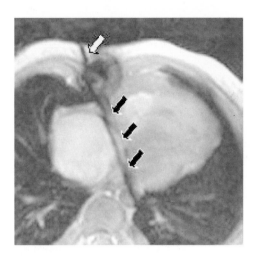 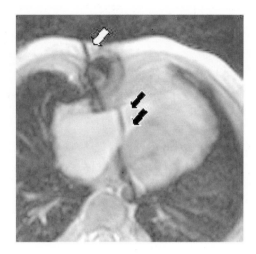

Systole   Diastole

Figure 8.11 Blood (bolus) tagging of atrioventricular valve inflow. The images are from a patient with hypoplastic left heart syndrome (HLHS) that had an aortic to pulmonary artery anastomosis. This gradient echo sequence utilizes radiofrequency pulses to produce saturated spins along a single line and in this particular instance, the line (also called the tag) is placed across the tricuspid valve (black arrows) and chest wall (white arrows), perpendicular to the direction of flow. The left image is near end-systole and the right image is in mid diastole. Note how the tag (black arrows) has moved relative to its original position in systole and stationary structures (e.g., chest wall, white arrow). This essentially visualizes the velocity profile in this plane.

cardiac cycle will be the stroke volume and multiplying by the heart rate yields cardiac output.

Essentially, bolus tagging enables direct visualization of velocity profiles in a blood vessel *in vivo* (Figs. 8.11 and 8.12). Similar to phase-encoded velocity mapping of the blood, individual regions of the blood vessel may be studied to evaluate flow dynamics. These flow dynamics are not limited to the primary flow patterns (e.g. the forward or reverse flow); even secondary flow patterns (blood flow perpendicular to the primary flow) have been visualized by investigators by this technique (Fig. 8.13) [50]. Essentially, the saturation band is placed on the blood vessel in long axis, parallel to the direction of blood flow, and then the blood vessel is imaged perpendicular to the blood flow (e.g., across the cross-sectional area of the vessel). The resultant cine demonstrates blood flow "twisting" (as in the aorta) or lack thereof in the axial plane, representing the secondary flow pattern. The rotation of the blood can be quantified by measuring the angle between bands on successive images.

Akin to the bolus tagging technique, a novel application of presaturation tagging of blood allows for selective labeling of flow from more than one input source to determine how much flow from each input goes to each output [51]. For example, in the Fontan reconstruction for single ventricle physiology, the inferior and superior vena cavae (two inputs) are connected to the confluent right and left pulmonary arteries (two outputs). Presaturation tagging of blood was used to determine how much blood from each cavae went to each pulmonary artery [51]. The way this was done was by performing gradient-echo cine MRI in the bifurcation view of the pulmonary arteries (off-axis axial) and measuring the signal intensity in both branch pulmonary arteries just distal to the superior vena cava-to-pulmonary artery anastomosis. By placing a saturation pulse (essentially a wide tissue tag) on blood just inferior to the imaging plane and performing the exact same cine sequence, a decrease in signal intensity will occur in the pulmonary arteries proportional to the amount of blood entering each pulmonary artery from the inferior

Selected systolic phases

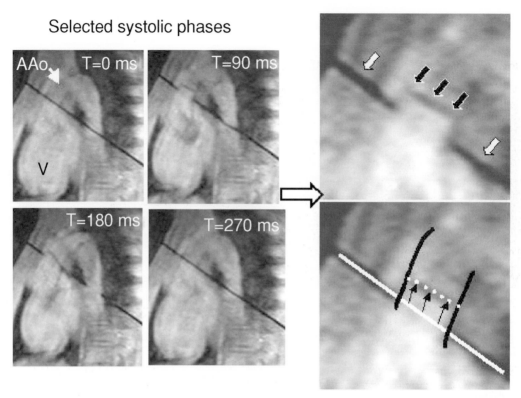

Figure 8.12 Quantification of bolus tagging image information. The image is a candy cane view of a native aorta (i.e., did not have an aortic to pulmonary anastamosis) of a patient with single ventricle after Fontan reconstruction. Four selected images on the left are of bolus tagging across the ascending aorta (AAo) with the time (T) after the R wave in milliseconds. (See Fig. 8.11 and text for more on how this technique creates the tag.) The tag is seen to move at $T = 90$ and 180 msec but not at $T = 0$ msec(end-diastole) and $T = 270$ msec (early diastole). The top right image is a zoom of the ascending aorta at $T = 90$ msec with the white arrows pointing to the tag laid down in its original position; the thick black arrows demonstrate the tag being moved by aortic outflow. The lower-right image demonstrates how to measure velocity from the image in the right-upper panel. The original tag position (white line), the anterior and posterior walls of the aorta (black curves) and the displaced tag (velocity profile, dotted white curve) are traced. The distance the tag has been displaced at any point along the diameter of the aorta can be measured (thin black arrows) and since the time between tagging and image acquisition is known, velocity can be easily calculated.

vena cava. The same concept applies when the saturation tag is applied to blood from the superior vena cava.

In the study by Fogel *et al.* [51], 10 Fontan patients underwent the three cines of the pulmonary arteries mentioned: (I) no presaturation pulse, (II) a presaturation pulse labeling inferior vena cava blood with decreased signal, and (III) a presaturation pulse labeling superior vena cava blood with decreased signal. The relative signal decrease is proportional to the amount of blood originating from the labeled cava. This method was validated in a phantom. While $60 \pm 6\%$ of superior vena cava blood flowed into the right pulmonary

artery, $67 \pm 12\%$ of inferior vena cava blood flowed toward left pulmonary artery. Of blood in the left pulmonary artery and right pulmonary artery, $48 \pm 14\%$ and $31 \pm 17\%$, respectively, came from the inferior vena cava blood. Inferior vena cava blood blood contributed $40 \pm 16\%$ to total systemic venous return. The distribution of blood to each lung was nearly equal (right pulmonary artery/left pulmonary artery blood flow $= 0.94 \pm 11$).

Cine MRI

The previous section on ventricular function delineates the role of cine MRIs use to detect valvar

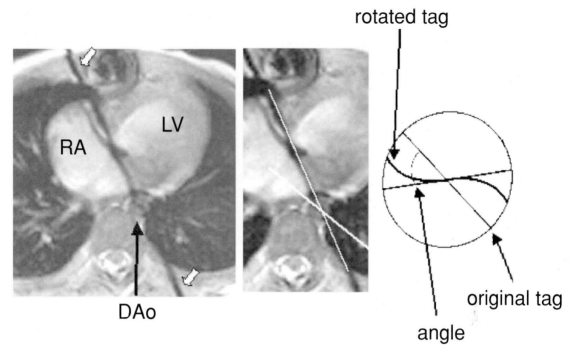

Figure 8.13 Secondary flow patterns visualized by bolus tagging. The images are from a patient with tricuspid atresia and normally related great arteries with a normal aorta. The tag is laid down in the "candy cane view" of the aorta and imaged perpendicular to the direction of flow at the level of the atria (left image). The left image is a still frame in systole (note the tag has not been displaced at the tricuspid valve level) and the tag has not moved from the chest wall and back (white arrows). However, over the descending aorta, the tag has "twisted" counterclockwise on this image. The middle image is a zoom, demonstrating how the original position of the tag and the displacement of the tag are traced (white lines). The measurement of the twisting angle is shown in the diagram on the right. DAo = descending aorta, LV = left ventricle, and RA = right atrium.

stenosis and insufficiency as well as vessel stenosis. See the previous section for further details.

Examples of the techniques mentioned in cardiac MRI

Cardiac MRI has been used to help understand physiology and function in a number of different disease states in congenital heart disease. An example each from ventricular function and blood flow is brought. See Chapter 17 "Considerations in the Single Ventricle" for further CMRI examples.

Ventricular function

The deconditioned left ventricle: The left ventricle can adapt to many loading conditions and although much is known about adaptation from a hemodynamic standpoint, very little is known about the biomechanics of this. A study [3] published in 1996

compared the strain and wall motion of the left ventricles (in short axis) of 11 patients who had transposition of the great arteries after atrial inversion procedures (Senning or Mustard operations) (S/P TGA) with 7 controls using myocardial tissue tagging (SPAMM). This study demonstrated that S/P TGA patients had the greatest strain (regional myocardial deformation: -0.20 ± 0.02 at the atrioventricular valve septal wall), and in 6/8 regions was significantly greater than controls. In addition, the distribution of strain between S/P TGA and controls as well as within the S/P TGA group were markedly different. The septal wall, followed by the lateral wall, appeared affected the most. In terms of LV rotation, S/P TGA patients (10 of 11) twisted clockwise in the lateral or inferior walls and counterclockwise in other walls, creating a region of no twist, whereas control LVs twisted uniformly counterclockwise. S/P TGA patients had no paradoxical wall motion and the lateral wall demonstrated the greatest radial inward motion.

The conclusion was that marked increased regional strain occurs in S/P TGA patients along with abnormalities in the distribution of strain. Abnormal clockwise twist and increased lateral wall motion was also observed in S/P TGA patients. It may be that marked chronic afterload reduction may alter fiber angle orientation to cause the abnormal twisting observed.

Blood flow

Asymmetry of blood flow in the right aortic arch: Right aortic arches can be a cause of a vascular ring or be associated with such congenital heart diseases such as truncus arteriosus, double outlet right ventricle, or tetralogy of Fallot. Flow dynamics in the right aortic arch, as in the left aortic arch, is important for organ perfusion, cardiac energetics, and Doppler flow calculations. A study published in early 2003 used through-plane phase encoded velocity mapping to define flow dynamics in this type of rare aortic arch in 14 children [52]. Although there are complex secondary flow patterns, bulk axial flow makes up the majority of energy utilization and hence, the use of through-plane velocity mapping. Through-plane phase encoded velocity mapping was performed in the ascending and descending aorta to determine flow volume symmetry and velocity. The aortic cross section was divided into four quadrants aligned along the long axis of the aorta. This study demonstrated in the ascending aorta that the posterior right quadrant demonstrated significantly greater blood flow than the other quadrants across the entire cardiac cycle (28% vs. 23–25% of the flow) and at the point of maximum flow (29% vs. 22–25% of the flow). There was also flow asymmetry in the descending aorta; significantly more flow was demonstrated in the posterior quadrants than the anterior quadrants in total flow across the cardiac cycle (28% vs. 21–23% of the flow) as well as at the point of maximum flow (27–28% vs. 20–24% of the flow). The time to maximum flow was significantly shorter in the ascending than the descending aorta (18 vs. 24% of the cardiac cycle). In 10 out of 14 patients, maximum velocity occurred in the right half of both the ascending and descending aorta. Flow reversal at end-systole was haphazard, occurring in all quadrants.

Conclusion

CMRI has come a long way since its beginnings and has evolved into an extremely useful tool to evaluation of ventricular function and blood flow in many types of congenital heart disease, both in the preoperative and postoperative setting. CMRI will play an important role in finding the answers to the many questions that remain, both on a research basis and in clinical application. This chapter has only touched on some of the abilities of MRI to answer these important questions. Promising advances such as oxygen sensitive MRI (detection of the oxygen content of tissues), T_2^* for the detection of myocardial iron stores, spectroscopy, "self gating" sequences, and others will certainly add even further understanding in the future into the physiology and function in congenital heart disease.

References

1. Axel L, Dougherty L. Heart wall motion: Improved method of spatial modulation of magnetization for MR imaging. Radiology 1989; 172:349–350.
2. Axel L, Dougherty L. MR imaging of motion with spatial modulation of magnetization. Radiology 1989; 171:841–845.
3. Fogel MA, Gupta K, Baxter MS, et al. Biomechanics of the deconditioned left ventricle. Am J Physiol Heart Circ Physiol 1996; 40:H1193–H1206.
4. Fogel MA, Gupta KB, Weinberg PW, et al. Regional wall motion and strain analysis across stages of Fontan reconstruction by magnetic resonance tagging. Am J Physiol Heart Circ Physiol 1995; 38:H1132–H1152.
5. Fogel MA, Weinberg PM, Fellows KE, et al. A study in ventricular–ventricular interaction: Single right ventricles compared with systemic right ventricles in a dual chambered circulation. Circulation 1995; 92:219–230.
6. Fogel MA, Weinberg PM, Gupta KB, et al. Mechanics of the single left ventricle: A study in ventricular–ventricular Interaction II. Circulation 1998; 98:330–338.
7. Fogel MA, Weinberg PM, Hoydu A, et al. Effect of surgical reconstruction on flow profiles in the aorta using magnetic resonance blood tagging. Ann Thorac Surg 1997; 63:1691–1700.
8. Fogel MA, Weinberg PM, Hoydu A, et al. The nature of flow in the systemic venous pathway in Fontan patients utilizing magnetic resonance blood tagging. J Thorac Cardiovasc Surg 1997; 114:1032–1041.
9. Fogel MA, Weinberg PM, Chin AJ, et al. Late ventricular geometry and performance changes of functional

single ventricle throughout staged Fontan reconstruction assessed by magnetic resonance imaging. J Am Coll Cardiol 1996; 28:212–221.

10. Bellenger NG, Davies LC, Francis JM, *et al.* Reduction in sample size of studies of remodeling in heart failure by the use of cardiovascular magnetic resonance. J Cardiovasc Mag Reson 2000; 2:271–278.

11. Carr JC, Simonetti O, Bundy J, *et al.* Cine MR angiography of the heart with segmented true fast imaging with steady state precession. Radiology 2001; 219:828–834.

12. Lee VS, Resnick D, Bundy JM, *et al.* MR evaluation in one breath hold with real-time true fast imaging with steady-state precession. Radiology 2002; 222:835–842.

13. Shellock FG, Tkach JA, Ruggieri PM, *et al.* Cardiac pacemakers, ICDs, and loop recorder: Evaluation of translational attraction using conventional ("long bore") and "short bore" 1.5- and 3.0 Tesla MR systems. J Cardiovasc Mag Reson 2003; 5:387–397.

14. Chung KJ, Simpson IA, Newman R, *et al.* Cine magnetic resonance imaging for evaluation of congenital heart disease: Role in pediatric cardiology compared with echocardiography and angiography. J Pediatr 1988; 113:1028–1035.

15. Meier D, Meier S, Boseger P. Quantitative flow measurements on phantoms and on blood vessels with MR. Magn Reson Med 1988; 8:25–34.

16. Rebergen SA, Niezen RA, Helbing WA, *et al.* Cine gradient-echo MR imaging and MR velocity mapping in the evaluation of congenital heart disease. Radiographics 1996; 16:467–481.

17. Fogel MA, Weinberg PM, Haselgrove J. Non-uniform flow dynamics in the aorta of normal children: A simplified approach to measurement using magnetic resonance velocity mapping. J Mag Reson Imaging 2002; 15:672–678.

18. Wedeen VJ. Magnetic resonance imaging of myocardial kinematics. Technique to detect, localize and quantify strain rates of the active human myocardium. Magn Reson Med 1992; 27:52–67.

19. Hundley WG, Hamilton CA, Thomas MS, *et al.* Utility of fast cine magnetic resonance imaging and display for the detection of myocardial ischemia in patients not well suited for second harmonic stress echocardiography. Circulation 1999; 100:1697–1702.

20. Schwitter J, Demarco T, Kneifel S, *et al.* Magnetic resonance-based assessment of global coronary flow and flow reserve and its relation to left ventricular function: A comparison with positron emission tomography. Circulation 2000; 101:2696–2702.

21. Wilke NM, Jerosch-Herold M, Zenovich A, *et al.* Magnetic resonance first-pass myocardial perfusion imaging: Clinical validation and future applications. J Magn Reson Imaging 1999; 10:676–685.

22. Simonetti OP, Kim RJ, Fieno DS, *et al.* An improved MRI technique for the visualization of myocardial injury. Radiology 2001; 218:215–223.

23. Sechtem U, Pflugfelder PW, White RD, *et al.* Cine MRI: Potential for the evaluation of cardiovascular function. AJR 1987; 148:239–246.

24. Boxt LM, Katz J. Magnetic resonance imaging for quantification of right ventricular volume in patients with pulmonary hypertension. J Thorac Imaging 1993; 8:92–97.

25. Culham JA, Vince DJ. Cardiac output by MR imaging: An experimental study comparing right ventricle and left ventricle with thermodilution. Can Assoc Radiol J 1988; 39:247–249.

26. Dell'Italia LJ, Blackwell GG, Pearce DJ, *et al.* Assessment of ventricular volumes using cine magnetic resonance imaging in the intact dog. A comparison of measurement methods. Invest Radiol 1994; 29:162–167.

27. Katz J, Milliken MC, Stray-Gundersen J, *et al.* Estimation of human myocardial mass with MR imaging. Radiology 1988; 169:495–498.

28. Buchhalter MB, Weiss JL, Rogers WJ, *et al.* Noninvasive quantification of left ventricular rotational deformation in normal humans using magnetic resonance imaging myocardial tagging. Circulation 1990; 81:1236–1244.

29. Donofrio MT, Clark BJ, Ramaciotti C, *et al.* Regional strain and wall motion of the transplanted left ventricle in pediatric patients using magnetic resonance tagging. Am J Physiol Regul Integr Comp Physiol 1999; 277(46):R1481–R1487.

30. Rademakers FE, Rogers WJ, Guier WH, *et al.* Relation of regional cross-fiber shortening to wall thickening in the intact human heart: Three-dimensional strain analysis by NMR tagging. Circulation 1994; 89:1174–1182.

31. Maier SE, Fischer SE, McKinnon GC, *et al.* Evaluation of left ventricular segmental wall motion in hypertrophic cardiomyopathy with myocardial tagging. Circulation 1992; 86:1919–1928.

32. Oxenham HC, Young AA, Cowan BR, *et al.* Age-related changes in myocardial relaxation using three-dimensional tagged magnetic resonance imaging. J Cardiovasc Mag Reson 2003; 5:421–430.

33. Lee DT, Schachter BJ. Two algorithms for constructing a Delaunay triangulation. Int J Comput Infor Sci 1980; 9:219–242.

34. Waldman LK, Fung YC, Covell JW. Transmural myocardial deformation in the canine left ventricle. Circ Res 1985; 57:152–163.

35. Young AA, Axel L, Dougherty L, *et al.* Validation of tagging with MR imaging to estimate material deformation. Radiology 1993; 188:101–108.

36. Menteer JD, Weinberg PM, Fogel MA. Quantifying right ventricular regional systolic function: Tetralogy of fallot versus normals using MRI 1-D myocardial tagging. J Am Coll Cardiol. 2003; 41:496A (Abstract 891-2).

37. McVeigh ER. MRI of myocardial function: Motion tracking techniques. Mag Reson Imaging 196; 14:137–150.

38. Pennell DJ, Underwood SR, Manzara CC, *et al.* Magnetic resonance imaging during dobutamine stress in coronary artery disease. Am J Cardiol 1992; 70: 34–40.

39. Rerkpattanapipat P, Link KM, Hamilton CA, *et al.* Detecting left ventricular myocardial ischemia during intravenous dobutamine with cardiovascular magnetic resonance imaging (MRI). J Cardiovas Mag Reson 2001; 3:21–25.

40. Edelman RR, Manning WJ, Gervino E, *et al.* Flow velocity quantification in human coronary arteries with fast breath-hold MR angiography. J Mag Reson Imaging 1993; 3:699–703.

41. Keegan J, Firmin D, Gatehouse P, *et al.* The application of breath-hold phase velocity mapping techniques to the measurement of coronary artery blood flow velocity: Phantom data and initial invivo results. Magn Reson Med 1994; 31:526–536.

42. McNamara MT, Tscholakoff D, Revel D, *et al.* Differentiation of reversible and irreversible myocardial injury by MR imaging with and without gadolinium-DTPA. Radiology 1986; 158:765–769.

43. Edelman RR, Mattle HP, Kleefield J, *et al.* Quantification of blood flow with dynamic MR imaging and pre-saturation bolus tracking. Radiology 1989; 171:551–556.

44. Beerbaum P, Korperich H, Barth P, *et al.* Noninvasive quantification of left-to-right shunt in pediatric patients. Phase-contrast cine magnetic resonance imaging compared with invasive oxymetry. Circulation 2001; 103:2476–2482.

45. Rebergen SA, Chin JGL, Ottenkamp J, *et al.* Pulmonary regurgitation in the late post-operative follow-up of tetralogy of Fallot: Volumetric quantification by nuclear magnetic resonance velocity mapping. Circulation 1993; 88:2257.

46. Martinez JE, Mohiaddin RH, Kilner PJ, *et al.* Obstruction in extracardiac ventriculopulmonary conduits: Value of nuclear magnetic resonance imaging with velocity mapping and Doppler echocardiography. J Am Coll Cardiol 1992; 20:338.

47. Kilner PJ, Yang GZ, Mohiaddin RH, *et al.* Helical and retrograde secondary flow patterns in the aortic arch studied by three-directional magnetic resonance velocity mapping. Circulation 1993; 88:2235–2247.

48. Migliavacca F, Kilner PJ, Pennati G, *et al.* Computational fluid dynamic and magnetic resonance analyses of flow distribution between the lungs after total cavopulmonary connection. IEEE Trans Biomed Eng 1999; 46:393–399.

49. Videlefsky N, Parks WJ, Oshinski J, *et al.* Magnetic resonance phase-shift velocity mapping in pediatric patients with pulmonary venous obstruction. J Am Coll Cardiol 2001; 38:262–267.

50. Hoydu AK, Bergey PD, Haselgrove JC. A MRI bolus tagging method for observing helical flow in the descending aorta. MRM 1994; 32:794–800.

51. Fogel MA, Weinberg PM, Rychik J, *et al.* Caval contribution to flow in the branch pulmonary arteries of Fontan patients using a novel application of magnetic resonance presaturation pulse. Circulation 1999; 99:1215–1221.

52. Fogel MA, Weinberg PM, Haselgrove J. Flow volume asymmetry in the right aortic arch in children utilizing magnetic resonance phase encoded velocity mapping. Am Heart J 2003; 145:154–161.

CHAPTER 9

Nuclear Cardiology and Positron Emission Tomography

Bruce Y. Lee, MD & Martin Charron, MD

Introduction

Nuclear cardiology has been a mainstay in the evaluation of heart disease in adults. However, its use in children, especially for the diagnosis and management of congenital heart disease, has been limited by the poor anatomic detail it provides, making it difficult to delineate structural abnormalities as accurately as echocardiograms, magnetic resonance imaging, and cardiac catheterization. Nonetheless, with the proper equipment and techniques, nuclear cardiology can be a useful complement to anatomic studies, by offering important physiologic information and quantification of function and volume. Additionally, in those occasions where adequate anatomic studies cannot be obtained, nuclear cardiology studies are relatively safe and noninvasive means of revealing sufficient anatomic detail to aid clinical management.

In nuclear medicine, understanding the techniques used is as important as being able to read the images generated. Motion artifact, the quality of the radiopharmaceutical, improper positioning of the patient, poor injection technique, inadequate gating (in gated studies), and inadequate hardware and software can each have significant impact on the quality and interpretability of the study. Therefore, this chapter will first discuss the general technology and techniques behind cardiac scintigraphy. This will be followed by reviewing four studies that have been used in pediatric patients with congenital heart disease: (1) Technetium-99m labeled macroaggregated albumin (MAA), (2) first pass radionuclide radioangiography, (3) gated blood pool angiocardiography (radionuclide ventriculography), and (4)

myocardial perfusion scintigraphy. Next, the current and potential future use of positron emission tomography (PET), a growing, powerful technology, in such patients will be addressed. Finally, the advantages of cardiac scintigraphy and PET will be summarized.

Basic technology and techniques

General principles

After a radioisotope is injected intravenously into the patient, it either stays in the blood circulation or enters specific tissue (e.g., myocardium) depending on the isotope. Once the isotope has traveled to its target, the patient is imaged using a gamma camera system consisting of detector(s), a frame supporting the detector(s), hardware, and software.

From inside the patient, the radiopharmaceutical emits a γ-ray that travels through the patient's body and hits the detector either directly or passes through a collimator placed between the detector and the patient before hitting the detector (which is composed of numerous scintillation crystals). The collimator, usually composed of lead, is either a single hole or series of holes that acts as a filter, excluding unwanted γ-ray photons. The collimator allows only those γ-rays traveling in certain directions and from a given area to hit the scintillation crystals. The four most common types of collimators are (1) pinhole, which is a single hole and functions like a pinhole camera, (2) parallel hole, which only allows parallel rays through, (3) converging, which magnifies images, and (4) diverging, which shrinks images. Of these, the parallel hole collimator is most frequently used in cardiology studies.

Planar imaging versus single photon emission tomography (SPECT)

In nuclear cardiology, there are two general ways of acquiring images: (1) Planar imaging and (2) SPECT. The differences between these two techniques are similar to those between plain X-ray films and computerized tomography (CT). In planar imaging, the camera is fixed relative to the patient, just as the film is fixed in plain X-rays. Each image then represents one "view" of the patient from a single vantage point. Radiation coming from above and below a given organ is superimposed on radiation coming directly from the organ, reducing the amount of contrast. In other words, it may be difficult to distinguish the heart from structures that lie above and below the heart [1]. The most common planar projections used in myocardial imaging are the ones that get the camera closest to the heart: anterior, 45° left anterior oblique (LAO), and left lateral view.

SPECT cameras have one to three camera heads. The more the heads, the better the resolution, because extra heads mean more data can be acquired from different angles simultaneously. The gamma camera detector(s) rotates around the patient, just as the radiation detector does in CT. The camera takes a picture every several degrees until multiple pictures are taken through at least a 180° loop. These pictures are then reconstructed to form two-dimensional images and generate cross-sectional images (i.e., slices through the body).

The detector(s) can rotate anywhere from 180° to 360° around the patient. However, 180° (from 45° RAO to LPO) rotation has thus far been used most commonly. This is because many believe that images acquired over the rest of the circle are too far away from the heart and therefore subject to too much tissue attenuation (radiation is absorbed or deflected by the patient's body before it reaches the detector) and scatter (when γ-rays bounce off atoms and are redirected in new directions) [2]. However, as the systems become faster and able to acquire more data, the use of 360 degrees collection continues to increase [3].

The detectors can rotate in either a circle or a patient-contoured orbit (the camera stays at a constant distance from the patient's body). A patient-contoured orbit theoretically improves resolution because the camera is closer to the heart, but may result in more artifact because the orbit is not held constant from patient to patient [4]. There is still no clear consensus on which technique is better.

Reconstruction, processing, and analysis

The acquired data is reconstructed into images. During reconstruction the data is often filtered, that is, certain frequencies of radiation are eliminated to enhance the resolution of the picture. During processing, the reconstructed images are repositioned and resliced to account for patient-to-patient variability in body habitus and location of body structures. A comprehensive discussion on image reconstruction is beyond the scope of this chapter. Nonetheless, it is important to point out that various image reconstruction techniques are used in nuclear cardiology, and the most popular one is back-projection. Algebraic reconstruction is used less frequently. Software programs can correct for tissue attenuation, motion artifact, scatter, and the loss of resolution that occurs with body structures located deep from the body surface.

Prepared images can be analyzed in many different ways. In general, they can be viewed either as a motion picture (cinematic or cine view) or as static images. Regions of interest (ROI) can be drawn around selected parts of the images. A computer measures the number of counts inside each ROI. Time–activity curves (TAC), a graph of the number of counts (y-axis) as a function of time (x-axis), can be generated for any ROI.

Gating

Gating can be performed where data is collected over many cardiac cycles, and the images generated are actually averages over a long time period of time. In nongated studies, averaged images can be adversely affected by cardiac motion (contraction, relaxation, and movement of the entire heart). For example, at certain times during a study, an infarcted portion of myocardium (no radiotracer uptake) may occupy a given group of pixels a fixed distance from the detector. At other times normal myocardium (normal radiotracer uptake) may move into that same group of pixels. Then, the average images will show radiotracer uptake and no defect in that area. Also, when myocardium contracts it gets brighter, which throws off the average images. Knowing when during a cardiac cycle each piece of data is acquired will prevent, for example, end-systole data from being mixed with mid-diastole data.

In gated studies, scintigraphic data acquisition is linked to a marker of cardiac contraction such as an electrocardiogram (EKG), pulse wave tracing, or

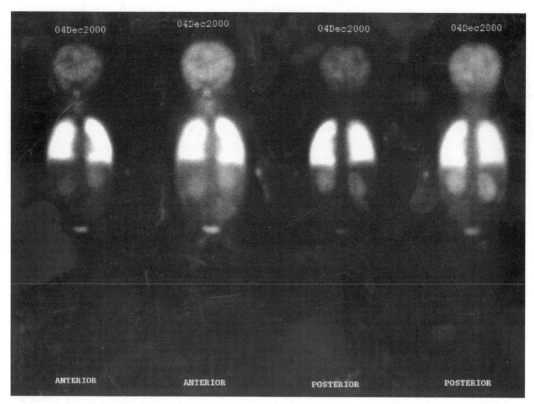

Figure 9.1 Technetium-99m labeled macroagrregated albumin (MAA) for right-to-left shunt detection. In patients without right-to-left shunts, only the lungs should be visualized as the Tc-99m-MAA becomes lodged in the pulmonary circulation and does not reach the systemic circulation. However, in this patient with a right-to-left shunt, the brain and the kidneys are seen, particularly in the later anterior and posterior images.

heart sounds. In other words, the gating tells the computer what set of image data corresponds to what part of the cardiac cycle. To adequately perform gating, the following conditions must be met: regular heart rate and rhythm, limited beat-to-beat variability in cardiac function during the study, minimal patient motion, minimal diaphragmatic motion, large intravascular location of the tracer, and sufficient count density. Computer software can correct some of these inadequacies, if they are minor.

Technetium-99m labeled macroaggregated albumin for detection and quantitation of right-to-left shunts

General principles

Macroaggregated albumin (MAA) is commonly used in lung perfusion scans. Albumin particles are too large to travel through capillaries and get lodged in the first capillary bed they encounter. Therefore, in normal patients after intravenous administration, the agent will pass through the right side of the heart and become trapped in pulmonary capillaries, generating activity only in the lungs. However, in patients with right-to-left shunts, a portion of the radiotracer will travel through the shunt and enter the systemic circulation (Fig. 9.1). Therefore, the more the radiotracer present in the systemic circulation, the larger the right-to-left shunt.

Radiopharmaceutical

Both the size and number of particles administered must be carefully determined. Particles too large can cause clinically significant occlusion of blood vessels. Particles too small may pass through the capillary beds. Too many particles may lead to clinically significant embolism. Too few particles may result in inadequate radiotracer activity. Particle sizes ranging from 10 to 50 μm and an injection of 30 000–150 000 particles is recommended [5].

Imaging technique

Sequential whole body planar imaging follows injection. Ideally, both anterior and posterior images are obtained and the geometric mean of these images used. However, in practice, imaging is done in either the anterior projection or posterior projection. Patient crying or Valsalva during the procedure increases pulmonary resistance and spuriously increases shunting. Activity in the bladder indicates free Tc-99m (not attached to MAA), which traveled through the pulmonary circulation to the systemic circulation and falsely increases total body counts and invalidates the study [5].

Analysis and applications

Quantification of left-to-right shunts

The percentage of right-to-left shunt is calculated by the following formula: (Total body counts − Total lung counts)/(Total body counts). This technique correlates well with the Fick oximetry method conducted during cardiac catheterization ($r = 0.82$) in quantifying right-to-left shunts [6].

While the MAA technique accurately quantifies known left-to-right shunts, it is not accurate in diagnosing shunts. False negatives occur in total anomalous pulmonary venous return, since the high pulmonary to systemic flow ratio results in most of particles accumulating in the lungs, despite the presence of a right-to-left shunt. False positives occur in patients with pulmonary hypertension, a patent foramen ovale, and no structural congenital heart disease (e.g., patients with persistent fetal circulation) [5].

Evaluating the adequacy of surgical systemic-to-pulmonary shunts

The MAA technique also evaluates the adequacy of surgical systemic-to-pulmonary shunts. Blood that flows from the right side of the heart into the lungs has a high concentration of MAA. Blood that flows through a surgical systemic-to-pulmonary shunt into the lungs has a relatively low concentration of MAA, since it is diluted by MAA-poor blood from the left side of the heart. A properly functioning shunt increases MAA lung uptake, but the increase is less than the total increase in blood flow. However in practice, many factors, such as the type of surgical anastomosis and the resistance in the right and left pulmonary arteries, affect this distribution and confound results [3].

First pass radionuclide angiocardiography

General principles

First pass radionuclide angiocardiography (FRPA) involves the intravenous administration of a radiopharmaceutical that immediately returns to the heart via the venous system and then passes through the cardiac chambers and the pulmonary circulation and enters the systemic circulation. Thus, the radionuclide serves as a "contrast" agent that demonstrates the path that blood takes through the cardiopulmonary circuit. This study's two primary applications in assessing congenital heart disease are (1) quantifying ventricular function (cardiac output and ejection fraction) and (2) diagnosing and evaluating a multitude of abnormal shunts and cardiac chamber wall defects.

Radiopharmaceutical

An ideal radiopharmaceutical for FRPA stays predominantly in the blood pool during imaging and then quickly clears from the body, so that the study may be repeated frequently to serially monitor the effects of any medical intervention (e.g., drugs, exercise, and devices) on ventricular function. Radiopharmaceuticals with long half-lives linger in the body after the first study, generating significant background counts that interfere with subsequent studies. As with every nuclear medicine study, there is a fine balance between resolution and safety. Higher doses generate more counts and better images, but pose greater risks to the patient. Therefore, smaller children require smaller doses, resulting in poorer resolution. Radiopharmaceuticals with shorter half-lives clear faster from the body, result in less radiation exposure, and allow for higher doses and better resolution.

Tc-99m (pertechnetate) is the most commonly used radiopharmaceutical for FRPA. Its relatively long half-life (6 h) limits study repetition. Tc-99m-MAG3 and T_c-99m-DTPA clear from the blood faster than Tc-99m and may be more effective for repeated studies [7].

Another complication of using pertechnetate is its significant uptake by the thyroid gland, which results in unnecessary radiation exposure to the thyroid and background interference. Giving intravenous sodium perchlorate or oral potassium perchlorate, prior to administering the pertechnetate can prevent this from happening. The thyroid gland does not take up Tc-99m that is bound to molecules such as MDP or DTPA. Therefore, no perchlorate is necessary when Tc-99m-DTPA or T_c-99m-MAG2 are used.

Imaging technique

In shunt evaluations, the patient is positioned supine and the gamma camera (with a parallel hole high sensitivity collimator) is placed across the anterior chest from the suprasternal notch to just below the xiphoid to cover both lung fields.

In ventricular function evaluations, the patient may be supine, sitting, or standing. The gamma camera with a 30° slanted parallel hole collimator is positioned horizontally across the anterior chest. When the heart is in an abnormal position, the collimator is moved to include the entire heart. For example, in patients with levocardia, the collimator is positioned in a left anterior oblique position. Incorrect positioning often results in inadequate or improperly interpreted studies.

After the patient is properly positioned, the radiopharmaceutical is administered intravenously, usually through an antecubital vein. It is essential to deliver the radiopharmaceutical in a single, rapid bolus. Doses that are fragmented or delivered too slowly result in activity in multiple places in the cardiopulmonary circuit at a given time, making it difficult to ascertain the true path of the radiopharmaceutical and adversely affecting measurements of ventricular function. Moreover, crying or Valsalva maneuvers during the injection cause rapid variations in intrathoracic pressure that delays venous return to the heart and fragment the dose. Therefore, great care must be taken to keep the patient calm and use a proper injection technique, which includes minimizing extravasation, injecting with a rapid continuous motion, and using a saline flush either simultaneously or immediately after the injection.

Imaging begins concurrently with radiotracer injection, and in most cases, lasts for a total of 25 sec. Images are acquired more frequently for ventricular function quantification (at least 25 frames/sec) than for shunt evaluation (2–4 frames/sec) [7].

Analysis and applications

Ventricular function analysis

Reviewing the images in cinematic mode gives a global view of ventricular wall motion and function and an assessment of the technical adequacy of the study (i.e., whether there is excessive background activity, sufficient contrast, and proper positioning of the patient). Next, TACs, calculated from the ROIs drawn around each ventricle, identify the end systolic and diastolic images. The images with the maximum activity (i.e., the most blood) in the ventricles represent end-diastole, and the images with the minimum activity (i.e., the least blood) represent end-systole. The end-diastolic images over several cardiac cycles are summed, as are the end-systolic images. The composite end-systolic image is then subtracted from the composite end-diastolic image, resulting in a stroke volume image used to identify the atrioventricular plane. ROIs are then drawn around each ventricle in the composite end-diastolic and end-systolic images. The ejection fraction for each ventricle is calculated by the following formula: $EF = (EDC - ESC)/(EDC)$, where EF is ejection fraction, EDC is the end-diastolic counts, and ESC is the end-systolic counts. If the ROIs are drawn carefully, this can be an extremely accurate means of measuring ejection fraction [8].

Cardiac output can be determined using the following formula: Cardiac output = (blood volume × equilibrium heart count rate)/(area) under the first transit TAC. To calculate the denominator for this formula, an ROI is drawn around the heart and is used to generate a TAC that measures activity during the radionuclide's first passage through the heart. A mathematical method (called the gamma variate method) can substract that part of the TAC that represents blood returning to the heart for a second time after going through the systemic circulation. The area under the resulting curve becomes the denominator for the equation. The same ROI can be used to measure the equilibrium cardiac count rate, which is in the numerator. Finally, total body blood volume can be estimated. While this method may overestimate cardiac output, it compares favorably to the Fick method [3].

Left-to-right shunt detection

Viewing the images in cinematic mode helps identify gross abnormalities and assess the quality of the study. To determine the quality of the injection, a TAC is calculated from an ROI drawn over the superior vena cava. Acceptable injections have a single peak of less than 3 sec wide. Several peaks indicate dose fragmentation. A peak wider than 3 sec suggests that the bolus was delivered over too long a period of time. Following an inadequate injection,

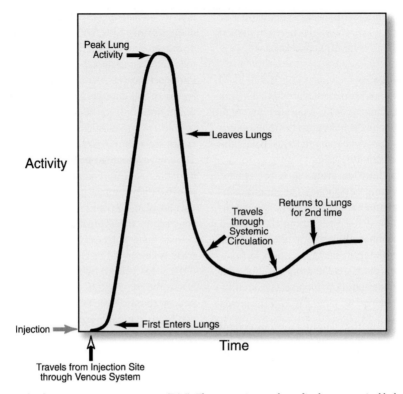

Figure 9.2 Normal pulmonary time–activity curve (TAC). The curve rises as the radiopharmaceutical bolus enters the pulmonary circulation, falls when it leaves the lungs, and then rises slightly again after the radiopharmaceutical has traveled through the systemic circulation and returns to the pulmonary circulation.

the study may be repeated with twice the dose after 20 min. Should this repeated study also be inadequate, the study must be performed at a later date, since too much background activity remains from the two initial studies.

The order in which different structures appear mirrors the flow of blood. ROIs should be drawn over both lung fields (while carefully excluding other structures), and a TAC should be plotted. A normal TAC is shown in Fig. 9.2. Note that the curve begins flat as the radiotracer travels through the superior vena cava and right side of the heart. A single peak occurs when the bolus enters the lungs. The peak drops almost completely back to the baseline once the bolus has passed into the left side of the heart. After this "valley," a second smaller peak occurs when the radiotracer has gone through the systemic circulation and returns for a second time through the right side of the heart back into the lungs. The second peak is much shorter than the first one because the bolus has since become diluted.

In left-to-right shunts, the radiotracer initially passes through the lungs, enters the left side of the heart, returns to the right side of the heart and then back into the lungs, before all of the initial bolus of radiotracer has cleared from the lungs. Therefore, the initial peak on the pulmonary TAC is much broader and the pulmonary activity does not return completely to the baseline (Fig. 9.3). In fact a second peak occurs while the initial peak is sloping down, representing the bolus reentering the lungs after traveling through the left-to-right shunt. Moreover, since much of the tracer returns quickly to the right side of the heart, the left side of the heart and the aorta are often poorly visualized. The order that different structures appear directly corresponds to the flow of blood as seen in the following conditions:

• Tetrology of Fallot: Here the blood (and hence the radiopharmaceutical) flows through the right side of the heart (the right atrium and right ventricle are visualized first) and then into the aorta with some going into the pulmonary circulation (the lungs and systemic vasculature are visualized simultaneously). From the pulmonary circulation, the blood returns to the left side of the heart (the left ventricle is visualized later). The greater the severity of the

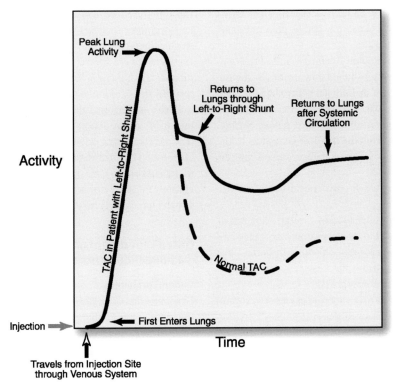

Figure 9.3 Time–activity curve (TAC) in a patient with a right-to-left shunt. After leaving the lungs for the first time, a portion of the radiopharmaceutical crosses through the septal defect, patent ductus arteriosus, or other right-to-left communication and returns to the pulmonary circulation early, creating a "hump" on the downslope of the TAC.

pulmonary stenosis, the less blood flow to the lungs and the less activity is seen in the lungs and left ventricle [8].

• Transposition of the great vessels with intact ventricular septum: The blood initially flows through the right side of the heart (the right atrium and right ventricle are visualized first) and then into the aorta and systemic circulation (systemic activity is seen right after right atrium and right ventricle). Since much of the blood is bypassing the pulmonary circulation, pulmonary activity appears late and is usually reduced. Imaging the patient from a left lateral position may demonstrate the anterior aorta or the absence of the pulmonary artery in pulmonary atresia [8].

• Conditions usually associated with an atrial septal defect (ASD) such as Ebstein's anomaly, persistent fetal circulation, and tricuspid atresia: In these conditions, blood flows directly from the right atrium to the left atrium (appearance of activity in the left atrium right after the right atrium) [8].

• Persistent cardinal vein: In this condition, blood goes directly from the left superior vena cava to the

left atrium. Therefore, injecting the radiotracer into a left upper extremity vein or the left internal jugular vein demonstrates activity through the left superior vena cava and followed by the left atrium [9].

• Total anomalous pulmonary venous return above the diaphragm: In this condition, blood returns from the pulmonary circulation through the pulmonary veins and back into the right side of the heart. This left-to-right shunt results in marked persistent activity in the lungs [10].

• Total anomalous pulmonary venous return below the diaphragm: In this condition, blood goes from the pulmonary circulation to the inferior vena cava, and activity occurs in the abdomen immediately after pulmonary activity is seen and before left-sided cardiac activity appears [10].

• Complete obstruction of a pulmonary artery results in the ipsilateral absence of lung flow unless bronchial arterial flow is present.

FPRA also can help assess the success and complications of surgical repair of congenital heart problems. In the immediate postoperative period after a right-to-left shunt is closed to repair a cyanotic lesion, left-to-right shunt representing persistent bronchial arterial blood may still be present in part or all of both lungs.

• Successful Senning or Mustard repair of transposition of great vessels: Blood flow occurs in the following order: right atrium, left ventricle, lungs, left atrium, right ventricle, and systemic circulation.

• Baffle obstruction after Mustard repair: Normal rapid blood flow from the superior vena cava to the atrium is disrupted, and collateral vessels may be seen.

• Baffle leak: There is an early appearance of activity in the right heart.

• Fontan procedure: Blood flow through the conduit from the right atrium to the pulmonary artery can be seen easily and residual shunting from the right atrium to the left atrium may be seen in some patients with persistent cyanosis [11].

• Surgically placed aorticopulmonary shunts (Blalock–Taussig and Waterston shunts): In this case, increased blood flow to the lung on the side of the shunt is seen. Stenosis or kinking at the anastomosis site may lead to predominant flow to the contralateral side.

• Glenn shunts (SVC to RPA): Following upper extremity vein injections, the superior vena cava is first seen, followed by the right lung, left ventricle, and then the aorta. After lower extremity injections, the right atrium, right ventricle, and left lung are seen sequentially [12].

Left-to-right shunt quantification
FPRA is also useful for quantifying left-to-right shunts. The shunt fraction is Q_p/Q_s, where Q_p is the blood flow through the shunt and Q_s is the blood flow though the systemic circulation. When bi-directional shunting occurs, FRPA can only quantify the left-to-right component. Shunts can be quantified by determining proportion of radiotracer that travels through the shunt. This can be accomplished by the gamma variate method, which uses curve fitting. The basic principle behind curve fitting is that a pulmonary TAC is actually a composite of several events after the injection of radiotracer. The first event is the initial passage of radiotracer through the pulmonary circulation. The second event occurs only if a shunt is present, that is, radiotracer returning to the lungs after passing through the left-to-right shunt. The third event occurs in all patients: radiotracer returning to the lungs after it has passed

through the entire systemic circulation. Mathematical formulas can be used to generate curves that resemble the TACs for the first and third events. When these curves are subtracted from the patient's pulmonary TAC, a curve estimating the second event results [3].

FPRA outperforms the Fick method in identifying atrial septal defects (ASD) because in ASD a true MVO_2 cannot be obtained. The gamma variate method is sensitive enough to identify shunting in patients with Q_p/Q_s ratios as low as 1.2 and accurately measure ratios up to about 3.0–3.5, above which increasing errors occur [13].

Gated blood pool angiocardiography (radionuclide ventriculography)

General principles
Gated blood pool angiography is similar to FPRA in that after the radiopharmaceutical is injected intravenously, it remains in the blood and passes through the cardiac chambers, permitting the evaluation of ventricular function and detection of valvular regurgitation. The primary difference between FPRA and gated blood pool angiocardiography is that the latter observes the heart over many cardiac cycles and the data acquired are averages over these cardiac cycles.

As the name implies, gated blood pool angiography is gated, and the images are acquired over 20–30 min. Since recording takes place over such a long period of time, the patient may need to be sedated. By contrast, FPRA is not gated and takes less than 30 sec to perform, making image acquisition significantly easier.

There are several advantages of gated blood pool angiography over FPRA. Injection technique is not as important in gated blood pool angiography as in FRPA, since the radiopharmaceutical makes many loops and eventually equilibrates in the circulation. Also, global and regional ventricular function as well as valve function can be better evaluated.

Disadvantages of gated blood pool angiography include its long study time (20–30 min vs. <30 sec for FRPA), sometimes requiring sedation of the patient. There is also much higher background activity (60–80% vs. <20% for FRPA) since over time the radiopharmaceutical will leave the vascular space. Moreover, gated blood pool angiography is inadequate for shunt evaluation since averaging images over a long period of time makes it difficult to ascertain the path the radiopharmaceutical takes and the time it takes to travel [7].

Radiopharmaceutical

The agent of choice is technetium labeled red blood cells (RBCs). Tc-99m labeled human serum albumin (which was the first radiotracer used for gated blood pool angiocardiography) has become obsolete in nuclear cardiology, as labeled RBCs are a cheaper alternative.

Imaging technique

Patients can be imaged in any position: supine, sitting, or upright. EKG leads are placed on both shoulders and the left costal margin. The gamma camera along with a 30° slanted parallel hole collimator is placed on the chest LAO and tilted posteriorly to separate the left ventricle from the right ventricle. The LAO view offers information about the free wall of the right ventricle, the relative size of the right ventricle, and the right ventricular ejection fraction. Anterior and left anterior oblique views are routinely obtained. When information on the posterior wall is needed, a left lateral decubitus view is helpful. Images are taken at 32 frames per heartbeat on either a 64×64 pixel matrix or 128×128 pixel matrix for a total of 5–10 million counts. The data recording speed is 40 msec/frame, but may be adjusted depending on the heart rate. Software can correct for mild arrhythmias up to an R–R interval of 100 msec or 10% aberrancy.

Analysis can be manual or automated and consists of general visual inspection of either a series of images or a cinematic film (Fig. 9.4). ROIs are drawn over the ventricles. Since the count rate is directly proportional to the blood volume, ventricular function and volumes (chamber sizes, wall motion abnormalities, global cardiac function, global ejection fraction, ejection rate, and filling rate) can all be measured.

Analysis and applications

When aortic or mitral regurgitation is present, gated blood pool angiography can quantify the amount of regurgitation and assess the need for repair or the adequacy of repair. The regurgitant volume index (also known as the stroke volume ratio or stroke count ratio) is the standard measure used and is calculated by the following formula: Stroke volume ratio = Change in count rates in left ventricle between end-diastole and end-systole/Change in count rates in right ventricle between end-diastole and end-systole.

This ratio is 1.0 in normal patients. The normal range for children is 0.70–1.5 [14,15]. The ratio is elevated with aortic or mitral regurgitation. A ratio of 2.0–3.0 is consistent with moderate-to-severe regurgitation. Greater than 3.0 suggests severe regurgitation. This test cannot detect mild regurgitation and is unreliable at low left ventricular ejection fractions.

Other volume and ventricular function indices can be calculated by measuring counts in end-diastolic images (end-diastolic volume) and changes in counts between end-systole and end-diastole (cardiac output, stroke volume, and ejection fractions). Finally, focal wall motion abnormalities can be seen, and while these are rare in children, they do occur is some congenital diseases, such as anomalous left coronary artery departing from the pulmonary artery [7].

Myocardial perfusion scintigraphy

General principles

Myocardial perfusion imaging is commonly used in adults, especially for the diagnosis and assessment of coronary artery disease (CAD), but is used much less frequently in children because CAD is rare among children (except for those with Kawasaki's disease). However, myocardial perfusion scintigraphy can play a significant role in the evaluation or treatment of congenital heart disease.

The general principle behind myocardial perfusion imaging is that injected radiotracer will accumulate more in areas with greater blood flow and myocardial mass, but less in areas with decreased blood flow or myocardial mass. In myocardial perfusion studies, imaging at rest and at stress (either the patient exercises or is injected with a pharmaceutical that simulates exercise) is obtained, although sometimes only stress or rest images are acquired. Adenosine (which stimulates vasodilatation), dipyrimadole (which increases concentrations of adenosine in the body by inhibiting its degeneration and uptake by the vascular endothelium), or dobutamine (an inotropic agent) is used for pharmaceutical stress. Studies may be gated.

In normal left ventricles radiotracer accumulation should be relatively homogenous, both at stress and at rest. (Normal right ventricles usually are barely

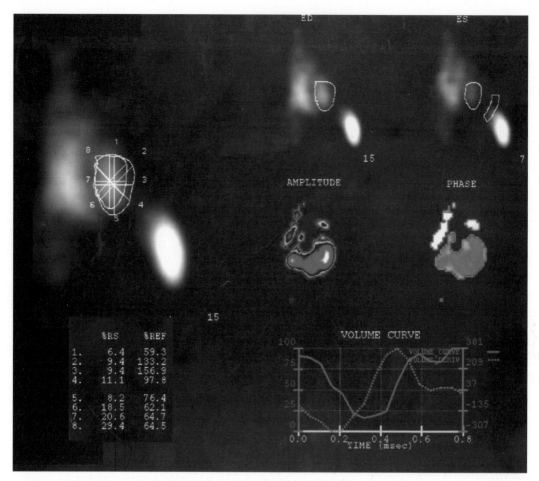

Figure 9.4 Gated radionuclide ventriculography with Tc-99m labeled RBCs in a patient with an ejection fraction of 84%. As shown, a region of interest (ROI) is drawn around the left ventricle (thick arrow) and a second ROI (thin arrow) is drawn to subtract the counts due to the body background. The background ROI should not be drawn around any major vascular structures.

visualized at rest, secondary to the small amount of myocardial mass relative to the left ventricle. However, during stress, the blood flow to the right ventricle increases and visualization improves.) Decreased blood flow, abnormally decreased myocardial mass, and scarring all result in "perfusion defects," which are manifested by decreased or zero tracer uptake (Fig. 9.5).

Radiopharmaceutical

The two commonly used radiotracers in myocardial perfusion scintigraphy are technetium-99m sestamibi and thallium-201.

Technetium-99m sestamibi

The average injected dose of technetium is 0.25 mCi (9.25 MBq)/kg, ranging from 4 mCi (148 MBq) to 10 mCi (370 MBq). Following intravenous administration, most of the technetium remains free in the circulating blood (less than 1% is bound to proteins in plasma). It clears rapidly from the blood ($t_{1/2} = 4.3$ min and after 5 min less than 8% remains in blood) and then accumulates in the thyroid gland, myocardium, kidneys, and striated muscle. At rest, 1.5% of the injected radiotracer is taken up by the myocardium, where it remains fixed and does not redistribute. Since it does not redistribute, separate injections are required for rest and stress images. Its biological half-life in the myocardium is 6 h with an effective half-life of 3 h (taking into account the 6-h physical half-life of the radiotracer).

The major route of radiotracer elimination is the hepatobiliary system, and radiotracer will appear in the intestine within an hour. Significant radiotracer

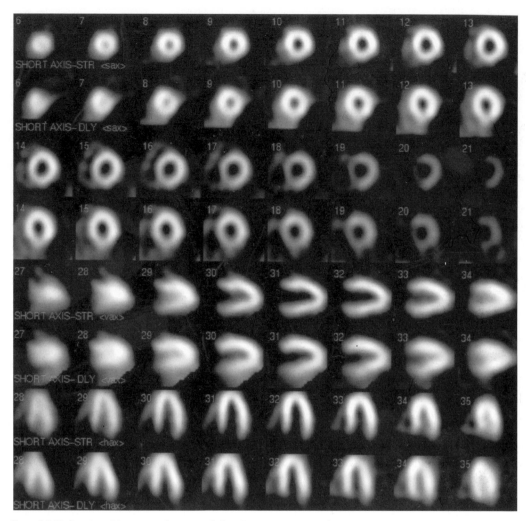

Figure 9.5 Technetium-99m-sestamibi myocardial perfusion images. A1: Short-axis stress images; A2: short-axis rest images; B1: vertical long-axis stress images; B2: vertical long-axis rest images; C1: horizontal long-axis stress images; C2: horizontal long-axis rest images.

activity in the liver and bowel interferes with proper visualization of the left ventricular inferior wall. (Giving the patient a fatty meal to promote gallbladder contraction and accelerate hepatobiliary excretion does not improve image quality.) The biological half-life in the liver is 30 min with an effective half-life of 28 min. After 48 h, 27% of the injected dose is present in the urine and 33% in the feces.

If the rest and stress imaging are done on separate days, the same dose can be used [0.25 mCi (9.25 MBq)/kg with a range of 4.0 mCi/kg (92.5 MBq) to 10 mCi/kg (370 MBq)]. However, if they are done on the same day, the stress injection should be increased to 0.75 mCi/kg (27.7 MBq) [range 10 mCi/kg (185 MBq) to 30 mCi/kg (1110 MBq)] to overcome

background activity remaining from the rest injection (the rest dose remains of 0.25 mCi/kg) [7].

Thallium-201

Thallium-201, which is produced in cyclotron, has a physical half-life of 73 h and decays by electron capture, producing mercury K X-rays of 69–83 keV (10% abundance). The doses range from 0.150 to 2.0 mCi. Thallium is a potassium analogue that penetrates the myocardial cell membranes through the Na^+K^+ ATPase. Like Tc-99m, it clears rapidly from the blood (half-life < 1 min). The myocardium takes up 3–4% of the injected tracer with maximum uptake after 10 min. Unlike Tc-99m, it is not fixed in the myocardium and redistributes with time, exercise, drugs, and ischemia. Therefore, only a single injection of thallium-201 is required for rest and stress portions of the study [7].

The main advantage of Tc-99m over thallium is that since the former is given in a higher dose, the images typically have higher count density and less low energy scatter. However, as mentioned above, Tc-99m can suffer more from subdiaphragmatic activity.

Imaging technique

For the rest portion of the study, the patient is injected with radiopharmaceutical, followed by a 45–60 min wait before being imaged supine. This provides ample time for proper radiotracer uptake and (in the case of Tc-99m) sufficient transit through the hepatobiliary system. Either planar or SPECT images can be obtained, usually using an ultra-high-resolution collimator. (The imaging protocol is often tailored to each individual SPECT system.) In a stop-and-shoot or pseudocontinuous mode, the detectors usually make 40 stops (each stop lasting for 30 sec), for a total of 20-min imaging time. Images are reconstructed and reoriented along the long axis of the left ventricle.

To allow adequate clearance of the radiotracer, there should be at least a 2–4-h wait after the rest imaging is completed before the stress portion of the exam is commenced. If gating is used, the patient should be fitted with the proper gating device, usually an ECG machine. For pharmacological stress, imaging is performed either 5 min (for thallium) or 60 min (for Tc-99m sestamibi) after the dipyrimadole, adenosine, or dobumtamine is delivered. For physical stress, injection is given during peak exercise, and the patient continues exercising for 30–60 sec after the injection to allow for adequate radiotracer uptake. Imaging is performed 15 min after exercise is completed [7].

Analysis and applications

Myocardial perfusion imaging is useful in evaluating the presence and degree of CAD in patients with Kawasaki's disease and the degree of perfusion in transplanted hearts. Additionally, it can be employed to evaluate severe types of congenital heart defects and myocardial ischemia from surgical procedures to correct them:

• Arterial switch operation (ASO): The long-term success of the ASO depends on continued patency and adequate functioning of the coronary arteries. Myocardial perfusion defects following ASO are very common. These perfusion defects often do not have corresponding wall motion abnormalities and therefore are difficult to detect by echocardiogram. Many of these defects are consequences of intraoperative aortic cross clamping [16].

• Pulmonary atresia with intact ventricular septum: In many of these patients, the coronary sinusoids (instead of the coronary ostia) perfuse large portions of the myocardium (so-called "right ventricular coronary dependence"). During surgical repair of pulmonary atresia, the right ventricle is decompressed, often causing significant myocardial ischemia, which can be detected with perfusion imaging postrepair [17].

• Anomalous left coronary artery: Diagnosis of this condition is usually made through history, physical, EKG, and echocardiogram with color Doppler. So while scintigraphy does not play a pivotal role in diagnosis, it can assess the severity of myocardial hypoperfusion in patients with anomalous left coronary artery and, following repair, serially evaluate recovery of function and perfusion [18].

• Right ventricular hypertrophy and hypertension: As mentioned previously, a visible right ventricle on myocardial perfusion scintigraphy suggests right ventricular hypertrophy. This can occur in tetrology of Fallot (pre- and postoperatively), transposition of the great arteries (following Senning or Mustard repair when the right ventricle is at systemic pressure or after an ASO with residual supravalvular pulmonary stenosis and secondary RVH) [19].

• Asymmetric septal hypertrophy: This is manifested by abnormal distribution of left ventricular myocardial mass. Thalium-201 imaging may detect and determine the size of the ventricular septum in children with a possible single ventricle.

Positron emission tomography

General principles

Positron emission tomography (PET) has only recently moved from the research arena to the clinical arena in the study of the heart. New applications continue to emerge. PET was first applied to the heart in the early 1970s by researchers at Washington University in St. Louis, MO, who used two different isotopes, F-18 deoxyglucose and C-11 palmitate, to study myocardial metabolism [20].

In PET, compounds similar to those normally used by the heart are labeled with isotopes of oxygen, carbon, nitrogen, or fluorine and employed to evaluate myocardial perfusion and metabolically important biochemical reactions. When administered intravenously, these labeled compounds behave the same as or similarly to their naturally occurring analogous compounds. For example, intravenously injected glucose labeled with C-11 will be used by myocardial tissue that actively metabolizes glucose.

PET has some decided advantages over conventional scintigraphy (which uses compounds taken up by relevant structures but are not used in any regular metabolic pathways) and provides more information about the biochemical activity of a structure or tissue of interest. Compared to the isotopes used in conventional scintigraphy, those used in PET have relatively short half-lives, minimizing radiation exposure to the patient, allowing studies to be repeated more frequently, and offering the opportunity to dynamically follow effects of an intervention. The short half-lives also allow higher administered dosages and in turn higher count rates and better temporal and spatial resolution (as low as 3 mm for PET vs. 5–8 mm for SPECT). Moreover attenuation correction for PET, which typically is performed by obtaining a transmission scan utilizing Ga-68, further improves resolution. Finally, PET can quantify function more accurately than other techniques. PET does have its limitations. Detector "dead time" (to be described later) and mispositioning of counts, especially at high-count rates, can be troublesome. Scatter effects are usually small as long as myocardial activity is high and lung activity is low [20].

Radiopharmaceutical

Some radiotracers are produced by generators, whereas others are produced in a cyclotron. In the latter, a stable element is bombarded with protons, deuterons, or helium nuclei, which results in a very unstable isotope with excessive protons that decay by positron emission. The isotope emits a positron that travels only 4–5 mm before it interacts with an electron, yielding two 511 keV photons that travel in directions 180° opposite from each another (the so-called *annihilation reaction*). The occurrence and location of this event can be detected by two detectors on opposite ends of the body through a process called *coincidence counting*. When one detector detects a photon coming from a location in the body

and the opposite detector detects another photon coming from an adjacent location shortly thereafter (within 5–20 ns of the first photon), the machine registers an event occurrence at that part of the body. In other words, if each detector detects a photon at nearly the same time, it is assumed that the two photons come from the same annihilation reaction (Fig. 9.6). The radiotracers used will be discussed in detail in section Analysis and Applications.

Imaging technique

Most PET machines consist of three or more rings around the patient. These rings contain detectors with numerous scintillation crystals, which are made of bismuth germinate oxide (BGO), lutetium oxyorthosilicate (LSO), or thallium-doped sodium iodide (NaI(Tl)). Each photon hits a detector scintillation crystal, producing a flash of light that is sensed by a photomultiplier tube (PMT) located behind the crystal. Once a crystal is activated, there is a period of time during which it discharges its energy to the PMT and cannot be activated again ("dead time"). Once this dead time has elapsed, the crystal may be reactivated. Like SPECT, the PMT generates electrical currents that are converted into data that subsequently are reconstructed into images. A number of reconstruction algorithms have been used including back-projection, confidence weighting, and time of flight [21]. Tracer activity in different tissues can be quantified as well, providing more accurate measurements than images alone.

PET resolution is limited by the fact that positrons travel only a short distance before undergoing the annihilation reaction (so the exact origin of the positron often cannot be determined). Moreover, the two photons generated by the same reaction do not always travel exactly 180° (it can vary by ±0.5° otherwise known as the full-width half-maximum (FWHM)) from each other. Although moving the opposite detectors closer to each other (i.e., reducing the diameter of the ring) improves resolution, it increases scatter, since more randomly traveling photons are more likely to hit the detectors. Increasing the number of crystals improves spatial resolution.

The large blood chambers of the right and left ventricles allow simultaneous measurements of radioactivity in blood and tissue. Measuring the change in radiotracer activity in the blood and myocardium over time can quantify the rates of tracer uptake and clearance from tissue. In turn, depending on the

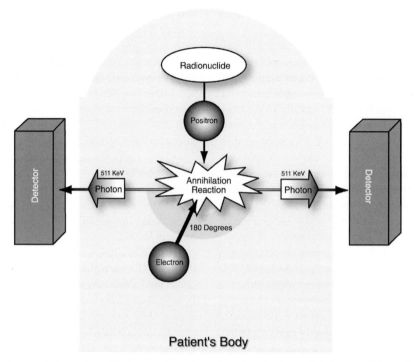

Figure 9.6 Positron emission and annihilation reaction. The positron is emitted, travels 4–5 mm, collides with an electron, undergoes an annihilation reaction, and emits two photons. The photons then travel approximately 180° from each other and hit the detectors.

tracer used, myocardial blood flow, metabolic rate, and tissue tracer retention can be estimated.

Analysis and applications

PET is considered the gold standard in evaluating myocardial viability. Unlike other imaging modalities that furnish indirect measures of viability such as wall motion or blood flow, PET delivers the most direct measure of viability, myocardial metabolism.

Myocardial perfusion

PET can provide absolute quantification of regional myocardial blood flow. This is particularly useful in congenital heart disease where myocardial perfusion abnormalities may be diffused and thus are not restricted to sharply delineated areas detectable in SPECT studies. Three types of radiotracers have been used for myocardial perfusion studies: (1) microspheres (9–10 μm in diameter particles labeled with Ga-68 or C-11 that are not used in routine clinical situations), (2) tracers that are extracted and retained by the heart, and (3) diffusible tracers.

Tracers that are extracted and retained by heart include N-13 ammonia, rubidium-82 chloride, and copper-62-pyruvaldehyde-bis-(N^4-methylthiosemi-carbazone) (PTSM). The primary assumption is that these tracers are taken up and released by myocardial cells in a uniform manner directly proportional to the amount of coronary blood flow and that local variations in metabolism do not affect tracer distribution.

• N-13 ammonia, NH4+ is converted to glutamine via the glutamine synthetase pathway in the myocardium. It boasts a high extraction fraction (70–80% at physiologic flow rates) and prolonged retention in the heart (with a biological half-life of 80–400 min). Typically PET scans are obtained at rest and after dipyrimadole injection. Unfortunately, anything that affects the glutamine synthetase pathway affects uptake. There is also minimal breakdown of N-13 ammonia into urea and amino acids. Pulmonary disease and smoking can increase lung radiotracer uptake. Since net uptake plateaus at blood flows of 2.0–2.5 mL/(g min), beyond this level of blood flow the scan becomes less sensitive. Wall thinning and wall motion abnormalities can cause artifacts [22,23].

• Rb-82 chloride is generator-produced and has a very short physical half-life (76 sec), making it an ideal agent for sequential studies, which can be performed up to every 8 min. Net uptake plateaus at flows greater than 2.5–3 mL/(g min) [24].

• PTSM is limited by extensive uptake by the liver (which causes inferior wall defect artifacts) and diminished uptake with dipyrimadole.

Diffusible tracers were developed because extraction and retention of tracers is not linearly related to the rate of blood flow. O-15 has a short physical half-life (2.1 min) and can be produced rapidly. Most studies have used H_2O-15, since infarcted regions (scar) of myocardium cannot rapidly exchange H_2O. Scans should be performed in rapid succession (every 2–5 sec) over 1–5 min. Since a fair amount of the tracer does not diffuse into the myocardium and instead remains in the vascular space, a separate scan using inhaled O-15 labeled carbon monoxide must be performed. The O-15 CO labels RBCs (and hence delineates the vascular pool), which can be subtracted from the H_2O images. Analysis of images involves drawing an ROI over the left atrium or left ventricle and generating TACs for arterial blood and myocardium (which can be used to calculate the perfusable tissue index (PTI)) to distinguish viable from nonviable myocardium [25,26].

Assessment of myocardial metabolism

Abnormal cardiac contractility results from abnormal myocardial metabolism, which may be a consequence of either abnormal perfusion or primary metabolic abnormalities. During ischemia, the heart moves from relying predominantly on oxidation of free fatty acids (which supply 40–60% of the myocardial fuel vs. 20–40% for glucose) to relying mainly on glycolysis (or aerobic metabolism of glucose to lactate) for energy. Therefore, measuring myocardial metabolism may be a more accurate way of determining myocardial viability. To study cardiac metabolism with PET, two general approaches have been used. One is to use radionuclides to label normal metabolic substrates. The other is to use labeled compounds similar to metabolic substrates, but those that are not completely metabolized. In this latter approach, standard correction factors called *lumped constants* must be applied to results in order to ac-

count for the fact that substrate analogs may accumulate more or less than normal metabolic substrates. Of course, the lump constant will vary depending on the isotopes used [27].

Carbon-11 palmitate has been one of the two compounds most commonly used in PET studies. Palmitate normally comprises of 25–30% of circulating fatty acids and 50% of the myocardial energy originated from the oxidation of fatty acids. Once in the heart, it clears in three phases: vascular washout of nonextracted or back-diffused tracer, beta-oxidation (biological half-life of 20 min), and incorporation of tracer into triglyceride and phospholipid pools (biological half-life of several hours). A TAC around the heart can be drawn. With ischemia, the TAC is altered, since back-diffusion of unmetabolized palmitate increases and there are fewer viable myocardial cells to covert palmitate into forms that can be cleared via the last two phases [28].

The most extensively studied tracer in PET is fluorine-18-2-flouro-2-deoxyglucose (FDG). C-11 labeled glucose was initially used in studies, but was found to be broken down into too many useless labeled intermediates. FDG is transported across the sarcolemma of the myocardial cell. A portion of it back-diffuses out of the cell and the remainder is phosphorylated and retained intracellularly. FDG is not converted to glycogen or pyruvate, but remains intact in the cell for hours, slowly diffusing back into the blood. FDG uptake is affected by the patient's nutritional state. During fasting, fatty acid content in the arteries is elevated, which provides the heart with sufficient fuel and limits FDG uptake. After a meal, FDG uptake increases. Catecholamines, glucose levels, oxygen, and insulin can also affect FDG uptake. FDG uptake can occur in areas of myocardial infarction, but not necessarily in quantities that will significantly alter the study's sensitivity and specificity [29].

FDG studies of the myocardium are interpreted by comparing myocardial function with perfusion and FDG uptake (Fig. 9.7). Dysfunctional areas with diminished perfusion and FDG uptake is likely scar that does not recover with revascularization. On the other hand, dysfunctional areas with diminished perfusion but preserved FDG uptake may be viable. Early in the course of infarction, the changing patterns of metabolism can confound the interpretability of this study. Anaerobic glycolysis may occur in areas

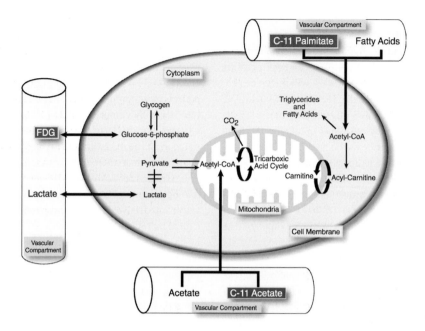

Figure 9.7 Myocardial metabolism and positron emission tomography (PET) radiopharmaceuticals.

of dying myocardium that cannot be rescued, and FDG uptake cannot distinguish between aerobic and anaerobic respiration.

A number of other compounds (e.g., C-11 labeled lactate, pyruvate, and amino acids) have been proposed as PET radiotracers. An alternative approach is using compounds called hypoxic sensitizers (e.g., fluorine-18 fluoromisonidazole) that readily diffuse into the myocardium. When oxygen levels are normal, these compounds are metabolized in a cycle back into the parent compound, which subsequently can diffuse out of the cell. During hypoxic conditions, these compounds are reduced and incorporated into insoluble protein constituents. Using these compounds, which measure low oxygen content, is a more direct measure of ischemia than techniques that measure only blood flow. There is no accumulation of hypoxic sensitizers in infarcted myocardium, which lacks the appropriate reducing enzymes [3].

Advantages and future directions

Nuclear cardiology spans the continuum of established techniques and developing techniques, particularly in PET. Even though they have been available for years, nuclear cardiology studies are still underused by some clinicians who do not recognize the advantages of these techniques. Some of these are listed below:

• Extensive validation: Nuclear cardiology studies have stood the test of time. Years of experiments and clinical use have provided a plethora of supporting data. Moreover, since nuclear studies have long been entrenched in the clinical decision algorithms, pediatric cardiologists and surgeons are very familiar with the implications of scan results.

• Good contrast: Few imaging studies even approach the signal-to-noise ratio of nuclear studies.

• Well-established safety profile: Years of study and use have confirmed the safety of nuclear medicine studies. They are minimally invasive and result in minimal radiation exposure.

• Few contraindications: Pacemakers, appliances, and surgical clips do not affect and are not affected by the studies. Dye allergies are also not an issue. The open design of gamma cameras allows close monitoring of critically ill patient and intrastudy interventions.

• Sedation usually not required: Since the gamma camera does not significantly enclose the patient, claustrophobia is rarely a problem. Most nuclear image acquisition protocols are relatively quick to perform, so usually sedation or anesthesia is not necessary.

• Accurate volumetric measurements: Nuclear studies are excellent at quantifying volumes and consequently, stroke volume and right and left ventricular ejection fractions. Since volume is directly proportional to radiotracer accumulation, volume measurements do not depend on the shape of the heart or the positioning of cross-sectional slices. In anatomic cross-sectional imaging, where the slices are made can lead to under- or overestimation of volume.

• True physiologic imaging: While anatomic imaging detects the anatomic sequelae of physiologic disturbances, they do not directly demonstrate physiologic processes, as do conventional scintigraphy and PET, which provides unrivaled physiologic information. Current studies evaluating the use of PET to assess for the presence, number, and distribution of myocardial receptors for various drugs, chemicals, and compounds may provide even more comprehensive methods of evaluating ventricular function and metabolism

• Availability: Nuclear cardiology techniques are readily available in nearly every hospital.

• Serial monitoring: Since nuclear cardiology studies are less expensive, faster, and easier to perform than are magnetic resonance studies, they are better suited to serially follow the results of surgical repair of congenital heart problems.

• Ability to exercise the patient and use electrocardiograms: Neither the cameras nor the radioisotope interfere with electrocardiogram recording or the patient's ability to exercise during the study.

The anatomic detail of conventional nuclear medicine and PET studies also continues to improve, ensuring their future role in the evaluation of congenital heart disease and potentially offering new possibilities.

References

1. Thrall JH, Ziessman HA. Nuclear medicine: The requisites. In: Thrall JH, ed., The Requisites. Mosby, Philadelphia, p. 371, 1995.
2. Maublant J, Peycelon P, Kwiatkowski F, et al. Comparison between 180 degrees and 360 degrees data collection in technetium-99m MIBI SPECT of the myocardium. J Nucl Med 1989; 30:295–300.
3. Gerson MC. Cardiac Nuclear Medicine. McGraw-Hill, New York, p. 830, 1997.
4. Maniawski P, Morgan H, Wackers F. Orbit-related variation in spatial resolution as a source of artifactual defects in thallium-201 SPECT. J Nucl Med 1991; 32:871–875.
5. Gates G. Radionuclide Scanning in Cyanotic Heart Disease. Thomas, Springfield, IL, 1974.
6. Gates G, Orme H, Dore E. Cardiac shunt assessment in children with macroaggregated albumin technetium-99m. Radiology 1974; 112:649–653.
7. Treves ST. Pediatric Nuclear Medicine. Springer-Verlag, New York, 1995.
8. Kurtz D, Ahnberg DS, Freed M, et al. Quantitative radionuclide angiocardiography. Determination of left ventricular ejection fraction in children. Br Heart J 1976; 38:966–973.
9. Park HM, Smith ET, Silberstein EB. Isolated right superior vena cava draining into left atrium diagnosed by radionuclide angiocardiography. J Nucl Med 1973; 14:240–242.
10. Hagan AD, Friedman WF, Ashburn WL, et al. Further applications of scintillation scanning technics to the diagnosis and management of infants and children with congenital heart disease. Circulation 1972; 45:858–868.
11. Janos GG, Gelfand MJ, Schwartz DC, et al. Postoperative evaluation of the Fontan procedure by radionuclide angiography. Am Heart J 1982; 104:785–793.
12. Miller JH, Gelfand MJ. Pediatric Nuclear Imaging. W.B. Saunders, Philadelphia, PA, 1994.
13. Askenazi J, Ahnberg DS, Korngold E, et al. Quantitative radionuclide angiocardiography: Detection and quantitation of left to right shunts. Am J Cardiol 1976; 37:382–387.
14. Parrish MD, Graham TP Jr, Born ML, et al. Radionuclide stroke count ratios for assessment of right and left ventricular volume overload in children. Am J Cardiol 1983; 51:261–264.
15. Hurwitz RA, Treves S, Freed M, et al. Quantitation of aortic and mitral regurgitation in the pediatric population: Evaluation by radionuclide angiocardiography. Am J Cardiol 1983; 51:252–255.
16. Mayer JE Jr, Jonas RA, Castaneda AR. Arterial switch operation for transposition of the great arteries with intact ventricular septum. J Card Surg 1986; 1:97–104.
17. Gentles TL, Colan SD, Giglia TM, et al. Right ventricular decompression and left ventricular function in pulmonary atresia with intact ventricular septum. The influence of less extensive coronary anomalies. Circulation 1993; 88:II183–II188.
18. Hurwitz RA, Caldwell RL, Girod DA, et al. Clinical and hemodynamic course of infants and children with anomalous left coronary artery. Am Heart J 1989; 118:1176–1181.
19. Rabinovitch M, Fischer KC, Treves S. Quantitative thallium-201 myocardial imaging in assessing right

ventricular pressure in patients with congenital heart defects. Br Heart J 1981; 45:198–205.

20. Sandler MP, Coleman RE, Wackers FJT, *et al.* Diagnostic Nuclear Medicine, Vol. 1. Williams and Wilkins, Philadelphia, PA, 1988.

21. Budinger TF. Time-of-flight positron emission tomography: Status relative to conventional PET. J Nucl Med 1983; 24:73–78.

22. Beanlands RS, Muzik O, Hutchins GD, *et al.* Heterogeneity of regional nitrogen 13-labeled ammonia tracer distribution in the normal human heart: comparison with rubidium 82 and copper 62-labeled PTSM. J Nucl Cardiol 1994; 1:225–235.

23. Schelbert HR, Phelps ME, Huang SC, *et al.* N-13 ammonia as an indicator of myocardial blood flow. Circulation 1981; 63:1259–1272.

24. Selwyn AP, Allan RM, L'Abbate A, *et al.* Relation between regional myocardial uptake of rubidium-82 and perfusion: Absolute reduction of cation uptake in ischemia. Am J Cardiol 1982; 50:112–121.

25. Bergmann SR, Herrero P, Markham J, *et al.* Noninvasive quantitation of myocardial blood flow in human subjects with oxygen-15-labeled water and positron emission tomography. J Am Coll Cardiol 1989; 14:639–652.

26. Iida H, Rhodes CG, de Silva R, *et al.* Myocardial tissue fraction—correction for partial volume effects and measure of tissue viability. J Nucl Med 1991; 32:2169–2175.

27. Camici P, Ferrannini E, Opie L. Myocardial metabolism in ischemic heart disease: Basic principles and application to imaging by positron emission tomography. Prog Cardiovasc Dis 1989; 32:217–238.

28. Fox KA, Abendschein DR, Ambos HD, *et al.* Efflux of metabolized and nonmetabolized fatty acid from canine myocardium. Implications for quantifying myocardial metabolism tomographically. Circ Res 1985; 57:232–243.

29. Buxton DB, Schelbert HR. Measurement of regional glucose metabolic rates in reperfused myocardium. Am J Physiol 1991; 261:H2058–H2068.

CHAPTER 10

Exercise Testing

Stephen Paridon, MD

Introduction

Current methods for the assessment of ventricular function and myocardial blood flow generally share one common characteristic: they all measure these functions in the resting state. Exercise evaluation of ventricular performance and myocardial blood flow is the exception to this rule. Since children are seldom completely sedentary during their waking hours, it is obviously important to have some method of assessing cardiac performance during conditions that will be encountered in daily living. Exercise testing uniquely fills this role.

Perhaps the major advantage of exercise testing over other testing modalities is its usefulness in assessing myocardial performance under a variety of physiologic states. Preload, afterload, and inotropy are all altered significantly by exercise from their resting states. Abnormalities of myocardial performance that are not apparent in the resting state maybe identified under these circumstances. In addition, abnormalities of the interaction of the heart with other organ systems, such as the pulmonary system, that are not obvious at rest may become apparent during an exercise test.

Exercise testing has a more limited utility in the assessment of myocardial blood flow in congenital heart disease and little is known about myocardial blood flow patterns either at rest or exercise in most of the complex congenital heart lesions. The reasons for this are several: There are no good animal models for most of these lesions that could be used to invasively measure patterns of regional myocardial blood flow. There is great heterogenecity in these lesions, which prevents generalization of findings from one group of lesions to another. Noninvasive measurements of regional myocardial blood flow and coronary flow reserve have been done only in select types of lesions and in relatively small numbers. The lack of age- and sex-specific normative data remains a major obstacle to their widespread use.

In this chapter basic exercise physiology as it relates to cardiovascular performance will be reviewed. Particular focus will be on those measurements that directly or indirectly serve as indicators of cardiac performance. The normal response of the cardiovascular system and its interactions with the exercising muscles and other support organs will be reviewed. This will include the changes in myocardial blood flow associated with the increased cardiac output of exercise. In the second part of this chapter, techniques for the measurement of cardiovascular performance during exercise will be discussed. These will include both invasive and noninvasive techniques. Special attention will focus on the information needed to perform a metabolic exercise test to noninvasively evaluate cardiovascular function in the current era.

Basic cardiovascular exercise physiology

Exercise performance requires a continuous meshing of multiple organ systems all functioning correctly [1,2]. This can be seen in Fig. 10.1 in which the various organ systems involved in exercise are represented by a series of meshing gears. The overarching role of this system is the production of chemical energy, its conversion to mechanical energy, and the elimination of the byproducts of this activity all while maintaining the body's chemical and thermal homeostasis within a relatively narrow range.

As can be seen (from left to right) in Fig. 10.1, adenosine triphosphate (ATP) is produced by the

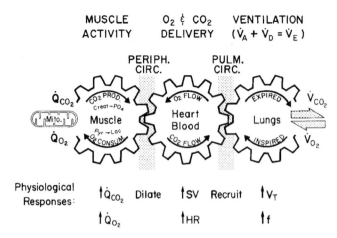

Figure 10.1 An illustration of the functional interdependence of multiple organ systems during exercise. The meshing gears represent the musculoskeletal and the cardiopulmonary systems interacting to assure adequate oxygen delivery and byproduct removal from the exercising muscles. The smooth continuous interaction of these multiple physiologic systems are essential for proper muscle function during exercise. (See the text for detailed discussion.) From Wasserman *et al.* [1] with permission.

exercising muscle in small amounts in the cytosol by anaerobic metabolism and in large amounts in the mitochondria by aerobic metabolism. ATP is then used to drive the excitation contraction coupling in the exercising muscle resulting in the conversion of chemical energy into mechanical energy, heat, and motion. The aerobic metabolism requires oxygen to serve as the terminal electron receptor in the mitochondrial electron transport chain with the net production of carbon dioxide (CO_2) and water. Anaerobic metabolism results in the production of pyruvate, which is subsequently converted to lactate for the same purpose. For this process to continue oxygen must be continuously delivered and the byproducts of this metabolism, CO_2, lactate, organic, and inorganic phosphates, and hydrogen ions must all be removed [1–3].

The circulatory and pulmonary systems act as service organs providing the exercising muscle with the substrate needed for exercise metabolism and the removal of the byproducts of that metabolism.

Effects of exercise on the cardiovascular system
Cardiac output
In order to fulfill its role as a service organ, the cardiovascular system must be able to increase the blood supply to the exercising muscles commiserate with their metabolic demands. In a well-conditioned adult this will result in a four- to fivefold increase in cardiac output over the resting levels. Cardiac output is the product of stroke volume and heart rate [3,4]. Both of these increase during exercise but their relative contributions to cardiac output

are different (Fig. 10.2). At rest, stroke volume is approximately 60% of its maximal value. At the onset of exercise a combination of increased venous return and sympathetic tone will cause stroke volume to increase. This occurs as a consequence of two mechanisms. The increased preload augments the stretch on the myocardium resulting in changes in the Starling forces. The increase in sympathetic tone results in an increased inotropic state of the myocardium. This increased inotropic state improves the active tension developed for any given preload thus further augmenting stroke volume.

As can be seen from Fig. 10.2, the changes in stroke volume do not occur evenly throughout increasing levels of exercise. Almost all the augmentation of stroke volume occurs at levels at or below 30–40% of an individual's maximum oxygen consumption (VO_2). The net effect of these changes is that increased stroke volume results in a relatively small contribution to the overall increase in cardiac output at higher workloads.

Increased chronotropy is the primary mechanism for the increased cardiac output, especially at higher work rates. This is reflected in the essentially linear relationship between heart rate and VO_2 as work rates increase (Fig. 10.2). Therefore, the ability to increase heart rate in a normal fashion with exercise is essential to achieving a normal aerobic workload. Conditions that impair chronotropic response, such as those that commonly occur in many types of congenital cardiac conditions, usually result in impaired exercise performance [6–8].

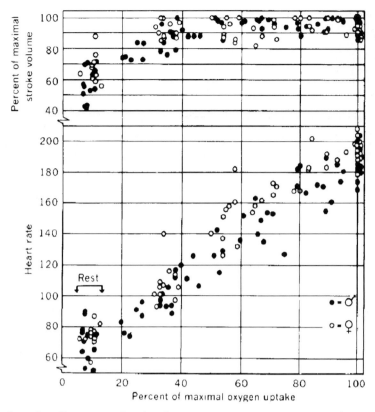

Figure 10.2 The relationship of heart rate and stroke volume to increasing oxygen consumption during cycle ergometry in 23 male and female subjects. Note that stroke volume reaches its maximal value at approximately 30–40% of the maximal oxygen uptake. Heart rate continues to rise in a linear fashion throughout exercise. From Astrand and Rodahl [5] with permission.

Distribution of cardiac output

In order to maintain the exercising muscles' efficiency, the increased cardiac output with exercise must be preferentially distributed to these muscles. Under normal circumstance (as shown in Fig. 10.3) this is in fact the case. At peak exercise the blood flow to the exercising muscle may be 80% or more of the total maximal cardiac output. This distribution of blood flow is achieved by a combination of autonomic and metabolic vasoregulatory mechanisms [5].

Exercise is essentially a state of increased sympathetic nervous system tone, which is regionally overridden by metabolic vasodilation. The increase in sympathetic tone associated with exercise results in a generalized constriction of the precapillary resistance arterioles. At the same time, the sympathetic tone increases heart rate and inotropy resulting in increased cardiac output [5,9].

At the level of the exercising muscle, vasodilation occurs as a result of local metabolic changes. Aerobic and anaerobic metabolism, excitation–contraction coupling, and breakdown of adenosine triphosphate all result in the release of potent vasodilators into the interstitial spaces. These dilators include free potassium and hydrogen ions, carbon dioxide, lactate, adenosine dyphosphate, and inorganic phosphate. The result is a profound vasodilatation of the vascular bed in the exercising muscles.

The net effect of these two states is the preferential shunting of blood to the exercising muscles. The vasoconstriction of the splanchnic vascular bed results in either no change or a decrease in gut and renal blood flow. The effect on the overall peripheral vascular resistance depends on the size of the exercising muscle groups. In exercise that is dynamic and uses a large amount of the skeletal muscles, such as running, the net result is a significant drop in

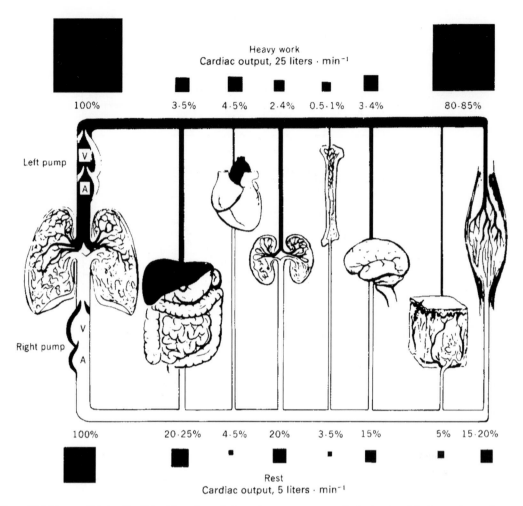

Figure 10.3 The parallel circuits of blood flow through the various organ systems both at rest and during peak exercise. Note that the cardiac output increases by approximately fivefold from rest to strenuous exercise. However, the relative distribution of blood flow to the various organ systems is significantly different from rest to peak exercise. In both states, the black squares are proportional to the percentage of cardiac output received by the organ system. Note that the blood flow to the muscle increases from approximately 15–20% of cardiac output at rest to 80–85% of the cardiac output at peak exercise. Astrand and Rodahl [5] with permission.

systemic vascular resistance despite an overall increase in sympathetic tone.

Oxygen consumption as a surrogate of cardiac output

Measurement of cardiac output during exercise is often impractical. Direct measurement of cardiac output requires invasive instrumentation. As will be discussed in subsequent sections, this usually requires the patient to undergo exercise in the cardiac catheterization laboratory. Noninvasive methods of measuring cardiac output are either technically difficult to perform during actual exercise or require a physiologic state that is not found in many congenital heart conditions or both.

For these reasons, oxygen consumption has become a surrogate of cardiac output in many clinical and research settings [2,5,10]. The utility of using VO_2 as a surrogate of cardiac output can be seen in Fig. 10.4. Over a broad range of VO_2 there is a nearly linear relationship between VO_2 and cardiac output. There is a tendency for the linearity to decrease with a flatting of the rise in cardiac output at near maximal levels of VO_2 (Fig. 10.4).

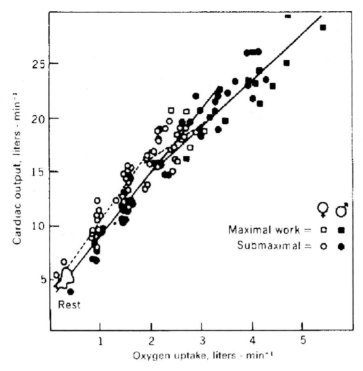

Figure 10.4 The relationship of cardiac output to oxygen consumption measured in 23 male and female subjects during sitting cycle ergometry. These data are from the same subjects shown in Fig. 10.2. (See text for discussion.) Astrand and Rodahl [5] with permission.

The reasons for this change in the VO_2–cardiac output relationship at high work rates and high VO_2 are several, but all result from a widening of the arterial–venous oxygen difference (AVO_2 difference) at high levels of exercise. VO_2 is determined by the amount of delivered oxygen in the blood, which is extracted by the metabolically active tissues. During exercise this extraction is determined by the myoglobin content of the exercising muscle and the isoenzyme characteristics of the muscle, as well as the physiological milieu in which the muscle is working [2,5]. The physiologic state will have a great impact on the oxygen–hemoglobin dissociation curve. As stated early, there are multiple byproducts of muscle metabolism released into the intercellular space during exercise. These include hydrogen ions and carbon dioxide both of which shift the oxygen hemoglobin dissociation curve to the right [2]. The local increase in muscle temperature during exercise has the same effect. The net result is an increase in oxygen unloading to the exercising muscle especially at higher levels of work. This causes the

AVO_2 difference to widen and VO_2 to rise even in the presence of a flattening or plateauing of the rise in cardiac output near peak exercise [2,5,9].

As can also be seen in Fig. 10.4, there is a tendency for females to have a somewhat higher cardiac output for any given VO_2 and to have a lower maximal VO_2 [5]. The reasons for these findings have to do with the hemoglobin contact of the blood. The presence of the anemia will diminish the O_2 content and will require a higher cardiac output to deliver an equivalent VO_2. The presence of a lower hemoglobin content in adolescent and adult females will be reflected in this slightly higher cardiac output. This effect is more pronounced in states of pathologic anemia. The ability to use VO_2 as a surrogate of cardiac output will be significantly impaired when these conditions exist.

Oxygen pulse

In a clinical setting, the practitioner is frequently interested in assessing the intrinsic inotropic state of the myocardium during exercise. As was stated earlier, this state is primarily reflected by the stroke volume of the heart. A noninvasive measurement of stroke volume is a useful tool to assess myocardial function. This has given rise to the use of the oxygen pulse (O_2 pulse) during exercise testing [11]. The O_2 pulse is simply the VO_2 (usually expressed as mL/min) divided by the heart rate at any given point during the exercise test. Like VO_2, over a wide range, the rise in O_2 pulse is a reflection of the stroke volume of the heart.

The O_2 pulse is perhaps most useful in assessing changes in myocardial performance over time or following therapeutic interventions in an individual patient. Assuming no change in the hemoglobin content or large weight changes, the VO_2 required to perform a given amount of work for an individual patient is constant. Therefore, any increase in the O_2 pulse measured at a given work rate would reflect a lower heart rate needed to achieve the VO_2 and as a consequence a higher stroke volume. The converse would be true for a falling O_2 pulse. This does presume the hemoglobin content of the blood has not changed and that the chronotropic state of the heart is also unchanged. A significant change in either of these will limit the usefulness of the O_2 pulse to act as a marker of stroke volume during exercise.

Work rate as a surrogate of VO_2 and cardiac output

Over a broad range of ages and body size, the amount of oxygen required to perform a given amount of work is surprisingly constant. This amount is generally in the range of $10–11$ mL of O_2/min/W when measured on a cycle ergometer [2]. This has allowed work rate during exercise to be used as a surrogate of VO_2, and by reflection, of cardiac output. The utility of using this measurement is its simplicity. Accurately measuring work rate requires only a well-calibrated ergometer. This equipment is relatively cheap especially when compared with the metabolic carts needed to measure expired gases for VO_2 and noninvasive cardiac output. It also allows measurement during exercise in locations were a large amount of equipment maybe cumbersome. Special nonferrous ergometers are available to permit measurement of work during MRI imaging where other equipment would not be permitted.

There are several pitfalls in using work rate as an estimate of VO_2 or cardiac output. One of the most common is that ergometers measure only "external" work performed by the patient. In the presence of significant obesity the additional "internal" work needed to move the adipose tissue through the cycling process would not be reflected in the work registered by the ergometer. In such a state the actual VO_2 of the subject would be underestimated at any given workload [11]. There are also occasional musculoskeletal or neurological conditions such as hemiparesis that could result in a particular patient having a significant low mechanical efficiency. Under these circumstances VO_2 would again be underestimated for any given work rate. A much less common occurrence is the opposite state such as seen in certain elite athletes. These individuals may have an extremely efficient cycling or running cadence. Under these circumstances work rate may significantly overestimate the VO_2.

Invasive measurements during exercise

Invasive measurements of cardiac function during exercise have become primarily of historic interest. The development of newer technologies over the last 20 years has resulted in much less of the need to perform these procedures. Nonetheless, direct measurement of cardiac performance during exercise occasionally may be extremely useful in an individual clinical setting.

The vast majority of invasive exercise testing in pediatric patients occurs in the cardiac catheterization laboratory [12–15]. These studies are usually combined with additional diagnostic or interventional procedures. They are restricted to older children because of the need for significant patient participation and cooperation during the study. In most cases, some degree of sedation is still usually required. This will limit the ability of the patients to exercise and therefore almost all studies are submaximal.

Catheter placement requires that the patients are generally supine. The frequent use of femoral vein and artery access usually requires that the patient must remain supine even during the exercise testing. The ergometers used for these studies are usually hand cranks that are designed to attach to the catheterization table allowing the patient to perform arm exercise while in a recumbent position. Rarely, a leg ergometer that attaches to the base of the table maybe used in older patients where arm and neck access is utilized for catheter placement.

The type and placement of catheters used during exercise would depend upon the nature of the cardiac lesion and the information being sought during the study. Cardiac output can be measured by thermodilution techniques in those patients without significant intracardiac shunts. Direct Fick measurements can be used in many other subjects. This will require the measurement of oxygen consumption during exercise. This is readily available in most laboratories using commercially available metabolic carts designed for this precoedure [13].

The biggest advantage of invasive exercise testing is the ability to measure those hemodynamic values not readily assessed using current noninvasive technology. These include primarily oximetry and pressure measurements. Of these two, the pressure measurements are frequently the most useful. Changes in diastolic pressures and gradients across valves and vessels can be useful in assessing the severity of lesions. They can also be useful in monitoring the response of the heart to surgical and medical intervention.

Figure 10.5 shows how this type of testing was used in a classic study by Moller of children with valvular pulmonary stenosis. The effects of the severity of the valve stenosis on the end diastolic pressure during exercise are shown in Fig. 10.5a. The subsequent improvement in both stroke volume and right ventricular end diastolic pressure following surgical relief of the obstruction is shown in Fig. 10.5b [12].

Figure 10.6 shows a recent study by Derrick et al. [14] that demonstrates the use of both invasive and noninvasive assessment of cardiac performance in a group of patients who had undergone the Mustard operation for repair of D-transposition of the great arteries. In this case, dobutamine was used as a pharmacologic replacement for exercise during the cardiac catheterization. Pharmacologic stress has the advantage of not requiring the patient to actively cooperate in the performance of the study. This is particularly useful in younger patients where performing a cardiac catheterization in a nonsedated or lightly sedated state may not be practical. In addition, there is not a problem with motion artifact that can distort catheter pressure racings during ergometry. The disadvantage of pharmacologic stress is that it is not identical to exercise in its effects on the myocardium and especially in its effects on the peripheral vasculature. It maybe difficult to generalize

the findings from pharmacologic stress to exercise for these reasons. Nonetheless, as can be seen from Fig. 10.6, the findings with the two modalities are often quite similar. Pharmacologic stress will be discussed in more detail later in this chapter as it relates to the evaluation of regional myocardial blood flow where it probably has its greatest utility.

Noninvasive exercise testing

Exercise laboratory, environment, and safety precautions

It is essential that any exercise laboratory have sufficient space and environmental controls to assure successful exercise testing. These requirements assure that the patient is comfortable and calm throughout the exercise test. The space should be adequate to accommodate various ergometers as well as additional equipment used in the exercise physiology laboratory. As a rule, a minimum of at least 250 ft^2 is required for a single station exercise laboratory. This is usually the minimum space required. If multiple ergometers are to be employed frequently a minimum of 500 ft^2 per exercise station may be required [15,16].

Climate control is also an important consideration. The area should be properly thermal regulated during the exercise test. The room should be well ventilated. This is particularly a concern in smaller spaces. Ideally, the temperature should be maintained between 20 and 23°C. This range will permit the child to exercise comfortably but still allow adequate heat dissipation. Humidity should also be controlled to approximately 50% to ensure free perspiration during exercise [15].

Although exercise testing can generally be performed at extremely low risk in the pediatric population, even in the presence of complex cardiovascular disease, proper safety precautions for a rare significant complication are essential in any exercise physiology laboratory [17,19]. The personnel staffing of the exercise laboratory should include at least one physician who is well trained in pediatric exercise testing. All exercise technicians staffing the exercise laboratory should be familiar with pediatric exercise testing and at least one of these technicians should be trained in advanced pediatric life support. A well-stocked crash cart and a defibrillator should be present at the time of exercise testing. In addition, a system for delivering oxygen and a system for

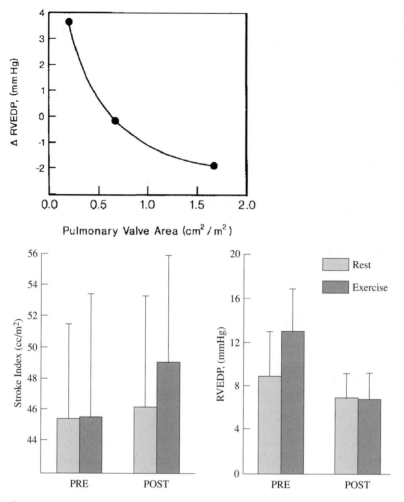

Figure 10.5 Data from exercise testing during cardiac catheterization in 64 children with pulmonary valve stenosis. (a) The change in right ventricular end diastolic pressure from rest to exercise based on the pulmonary valve area. Note that right ventricular end diastolic pressure tends to rise abnormally in those subjects with significantly reduced valve area. (b) The change from rest to exercise during cardiac catheterization of both the stroke volume index and the right ventricular end diastolic pressure in 20 children before and after undergoing surgical pulmonary valvulotomy. Note the rise in the stroke volume index and fall in the right ventricular end diastolic pressure following successful surgical valvulotomy in these subjects. From Moller [13] with permission.

negative pressure to be used for suction should also be readily available in the exercise laboratory [19].

Much of patient safety is dependant on proper education and preparation prior to the exercise testing. All patients and families should be thoroughly instructed in the techniques that will be required of the child during the exercise testing. Prior to arrival in the laboratory the patient should be instructed to fast for approximately 2 h [16,19]. They should also be instructed to wear appropriate clothing that is loose fitting such as shorts and tee shirts. In addition, they should wear comfortable athletic shoes to allow them to safely utilize the exercise lab ergometers.

Skin preparation with an abrasive to remove the superficial layer of epidermis and to improve electrical pick-up is essential [19,20]. This will allow an accurate artifact-free monitoring of the patient's electrocardiogram throughout the exercise test. The patient should be instructed on special procedures that may be necessary for the exercise test prior to beginning the study. This may include

Exercise

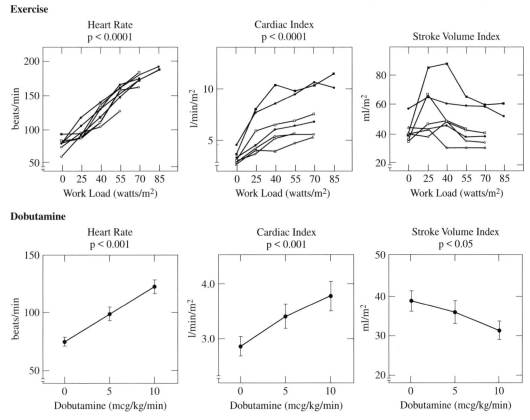

Figure 10.6 Comparison of the response of subjects who have undergone the Mustard operation for D-transposition of the great arteries to exercise and dobutamine stress testing. Note the overall similar response of heart rate, cardiac index, and stroke volume index to both modalities of testing. From Derrick *et al.* [14] with permission.

such maneuvers as resting spirometry as well as the collection of expired gases using a metabolic cart. The presence of a mouthpiece for this type of testing will prevent talking during the testing. It is therefore essential for the patient to be instructed in nonverbal communications using simple hand signals to indicate any distress or symptoms. The use of a perceived exertion scale such as the BORG scale can be particularly helpful with this type of nonverbal communication [19,21].

Depending on the type of exercise testing performed, a physician may or may not be actually present during the exercise test. In such cases that a physician is not required to be present, there should be immediate access to a physician should the need arise. Table 10.1 includes a list of exercise testing indications for which the American Heart Association has indicated that a physician's presence may

not be required [22]. It should, however, be remembered that these are guidelines and individual assessment of the risk for any given patient is essential.

Equipment

Ergometers

The two most commonly used ergometers in a pediatric exercise laboratory are the treadmill and the upright cycle ergometer. There are advantages and disadvantages to both types of ergometers. In addition, there are certain types of testing that can only be performed on one or the other type of ergometer. For this reason, it is generally best that both types of ergometers are available for use in a pediatric exercise laboratory. Table 10.2 lists the relative merits of the treadmill versus the cycle ergometer in exercise testing [19,23].

Table 10.1 Indications for Exercise Testing That May Not Require a Physician's Presence.

1	Assessment of working capacity in healthy children for research.
2	Evaluations of chest pain of noncardiac origin
3	Postoperative follow-up of patients with good hemodynamics to assess working capacity or rehabilitation screen.
4	Evaluation of isolated PAC's or PVC's in a healthy child with a normal QTc.
5	Routine follow-up of known arrhythmias or pacemakers.
6	Kawasaki disease or other coronary abnormalities without a known history of ischemia.
7	Asymptomatic mild aortic stenosis.
8	Evaluation of asymptomatic mild congenital or acquired cardiac malformations.

Adapted from Guidelines for Pediatric Exercise Testing, Circulation 1994; 90:2166–2179. From Paridon [9] with permission.

Table 10.2 Treadmill versus Cycle Ergometer.

Features	Treadmill	Cycle
Patient familiarity	+	
Higher work rates and VO$_2$	+	
Greater pediatric experience		+
Quantification of work performed		+
EKG and blood pressure artifact		+
Safety		+
Expense		+
Noise		+

From Paridon [9] with permission.

Treadmill The greatest advantage of the treadmill over the cycle ergometer is the familiarity to the patients of the walking or running required in the use of this type of ergometer [24]. Most children even at a young age can quickly adapt the gate necessary to performing an exercise test on a treadmill. There is also no lower limit for height, which can often limit the ability to use a cycle ergometer in young children. More muscle groups are exercised using a treadmill ergometer than a cycle ergometer. For this reason, the maximum VO$_2$ and the maximum O$_2$ pulse tend to be approximately 10% greater on a treadmill when compared to a cycle ergometer for the same subject [23,24].

There are significant disadvantages to the treadmill [19]. The motor is noisy and may frighten young children. In addition, it may sometimes make communication among the laboratory staff difficult. Most importantly, the increased upper body motion associated with walking or running often results in much greater distortion of the electrocardiographic signal. In addition, it may often make auscultation of blood pressure significantly more difficult. The safety concerns are greater with a treadmill than with a cycle ergometer. The patient must be closely monitored to quickly detect any problems with gate that may place the patient a risk for falling. It is also essential that the patient be instructed about the importance of not attempting to either suddenly get off the moving treadmill or stop abruptly during the testing. External physical work cannot be accurately measured on a treadmill. This makes treadmill ergometry unacceptable in a clinical situation where accurate measurement of physical working capacity is an essential piece of information needed by the clinicians.

Cycle ergometers The cycle ergometer offers several advantages compared to the treadmill. Because of decreased movement in the upper portion of the body, there is significantly less artifact when measuring electrocardiographic and blood pressure data. This may be particularly important in patients where electrocardiographic evaluation of changes in ST segments or arrhythmias are of paramount importance. Blood pressure is often easier to measure in a cycle ergometer since there is significantly less motion of the upper extremities [19].

The cycle ergometer can measure externally performed work rate accurately. This does require that the workload on the ergometer be relative independent of pedal rate and that the ergometer is regularly calibrated for accuracy. Neither of these issues are usually a problem in the currently available modern electronically braked cycle ergometer that is typically employed in the exercise physiology laboratory [19,23,24].

The disadvantages of cycle ergometry are, as stated above, that the oxygen consumption is generally 10% lower than that achieved with a treadmill test. Children are less familiar with proper cycling techniques and often require more coaching and instruction to obtain an adequate exercise test. Seating arrangement and crank arm size can frequently be a problem with smaller children. Most cycle ergometers even when modified with pediatric use are not suitable for exercise testing in children under approximately 130 cm in height [19].

Electrocardiographic recorders
There are many high-quality commercial electrocardiographic recording systems designed for exercise testing. These are primarily geared toward the evaluation for left ventricular myocardial ischemia in adult patients. None of these are specifically designed for pediatric use. Fortunately, most of these systems are acceptable for pediatric use without any modification. Requirements for these systems should include the ability to continuously monitor multiple ECG leads as well as obtain a 12 lead ECG at appropriate time intervals [19,20]. Automated arrhythmia detection algorithms signal averaging capabilities to eliminate baseline drift, and background artifact are features usually found on most modern systems. These features are particularly valuable for interpreting QRS and ST-segment changes [19].

Blood pressure monitors
There are a number of commercially available blood pressure measuring devices specifically designed for exercise testing. Most of these systems rely on a microphone placed over the brachial artery to directly auscultate the blood pressure. Although cumbersome, a mercury monometer and stethoscope are still frequently used in many laboratories. Because of the significant problems with noise in the exercise lab and arm motion especially during treadmill testing a system that relies on direct auscultation either through a microphone or a stethoscope is preferable over automated methods for the determination of blood pressure [19,22].

Respiratory gas exchange analyzers
Measurement of expired gas has become routine in pediatric exercise testing. There are several commercially available metabolic carts for the measurement of VO_2 and VCO_2 that are suitable for pediatric use. Most of the systems provide additional pulmonary function data such as minute ventilation, tidal volume, and respiratory rate. Most of these systems are able to analyze data on a continuous basis. This allows data to be analyzed on either a breath-by-breath basis or to be analyzed following averaging by various algorithms using either time or respiratory rate [10,19].

Noninvasive measurements of cardiac output
There are several methods that have been employed in an attempt to measure cardiac output during exercise testing. No method is without a significant source of possible error. Most systems are cumbersome. This has lead to much less frequent use of these measurements compared to the measurements of oxygen consumption obtained from the metabolic carts. As was stated earlier in this chapter, the inability to easily measure cardiac output with exercise has lead to the widespread use of oxygen consumption as its surrogate during exercise.

The most common systems used to noninvasively estimate cardiac output with exercise have been those that measure effective pulmonary blood flow. In the absence of a significant intrapulmonary or intracardiac shunt, effective pulmonary blood flow should be equal to cardiac output. Unfortunately, in the pediatric population, residual intracardiac communications and residual pulmonary abnormalities are frequently encountered. Therefore, this system is restricted in its utility to those cardiac lesions without these residual problems.

Inert gas rebreathing is most commonly used in these types of cardiac output systems. During the measurement of pulmonary blood flow, the patient breathes through a closed system containing a known volume of gas. A nondiffusible gas such as helium is used to measure lung volume. A diffusible gas such as acetylene is then absorbed into the blood stream in proportion to total pulmonary blood flow. The decay of the acetylene concentration in the expired gases is used to calculate the effective pulmonary blood flow. An example of a cardiac

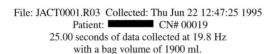

File: JACT0001.R03 Collected: Thu Jun 22 12:47:25 1995
Patient: ██████████ CN# 00019
25.00 seconds of data collected at 19.8 Hz
with a bag volume of 1900 ml.

←,→,+,− – Move Cursor, SPACE BAR – Select Point, < , > – move start
(,) – move end, ENTER – Calculate Q, ↑↓ – Axis Scale, ESC – Exit

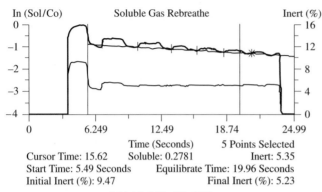

Cursor Time: 15.62   Soluble: 0.2781   Inert: 5.35
Start Time: 5.49 Seconds   Equilibrate Time: 19.96 Seconds
Initial Inert (%): 9.47   Final Inert (%): 5.23

Initial Soluble (%): 0.76
Q: 11.26 1/minute VT: 1211 ml   VS: 2930 ml   Qstd: 9.48 1/minute
M: −0.0275   B: −0.7060   Intcpt: 0.7686   Kb: 0.8515

Figure 10.7 A noninvasive cardiac output measurement by the diffusible gas technique. Time is on the x-axis, and the natural log of the concentration of the diffusible gas (acetylene) is on the y-axis. The lower curve shows the helium concentration that equilibrates between the lungs and the rebreathing bag after several breaths. This allows calculation of the lung volume. The slope of the decay of the acetylene is calculated for the top curve and is used to measure pulmonary blood flow that should equal systemic cardiac output (in this case 11.26 L/min) in the absence of pulmonary disease or intracardiac shunting. From Paridon [9] with permission.

output calculation using this method is shown in Fig. 10.7 [19,25,26].

The other type of system for estimating effective pulmonary blood flow uses carbon dioxide rebreathing. This system employs an indirect Fick mechanism to estimate cardiac output. Unfortunately, there are a number of assumptions that are necessary in order to estimate arterial PCO_2, which is needed for calculations in this method. The presence of intrapulmonary or cardiac shunting will again result in significant inaccuracies in patients with residual congenital defects. The maneuvers required by the patient to use these systems are usually more complex than the inert gas rebreathing system. As such they are less suitable for use during exercise and in smaller children with higher respiratory rates [19].

Other less commonly used measurements of cardiac output include Doppler echocardiography to measure aortic blood flow. Movement and noise artifact make this technique quite difficult to perform during exercise. This has lead to this technique being used primarily at rest and then immediately following the cessation of exercise rather than during active exercise testing [25,26]. There have been attempts to use bioimpedience to measure cardiac output. This has the advantage of requiring no significant patient cooperation. Motion artifact remains a big problem with this type of system. Studies that have compared bioimpedience to the various types of diffusible gas methods have shown poor correlation between the two systems [26].

Exercise protocols
There is no one exercise testing protocol that is clearly superior to any of the others. The choice of which exercise protocol to use in a particular individual is often dictated by the type of data required from the exercise test.

Treadmill protocols The Bruce treadmill protocol and its modifications are still the most commonly used protocols in both adult and pediatric exercise physiology laboratories [24]. The protocol consists of 3-min stages that increase in both treadmill speed and grade at each stage. The incremental increase in the workload for the Bruce protocol between each stage is quite large, making this protocol difficult to use in younger children. The relatively long duration of each stage (3 min) makes interpretation of metabolic data more difficult. The duration of exercise with the Bruce protocol is often 15–18 min in children. This can result in younger children becoming distracted with a decrease in their compliance to the testing procedures [19].

More recently developed treadmill protocols have generally used shorter stages (1 min or less) and smaller incremental work increases [23]. The most popular of these protocols generally consist of the subject walking at a fixed speed throughout the protocol. The grade of the treadmill is then increased in an incremental fashion until the patient achieves exhaustion. This type of protocol is more suitable to the measurement of expired gases and collection of metabolic data. Examples of treadmill protocols are shown in Fig. 10.8.

Cycle protocols Cycle protocols have been more commonly used in the pediatric population than in the adult population. There are several reasons for the more common use of cycle protocols. Cycling is generally a more common activity in the pediatric population than in adult population and as such children are often more comfortable than adults in performing cycle ergometry. The importance of a stable platform for metabolic measurements and the measurement of an accurate work rate are also often more important to pediatric exercise testing than to adult exercise testing. Both of these would favor the use of cycle ergometry over treadmill [19].

The James cycle protocol has been in the past the most commonly used pediatric protocol [27]. It consisted of 10 stages, each lasting 3 min. The incremental work increase and work rate between the stages was chosen based on the body surface area of the child undergoing exercise testing (Fig. 10.9). The long work stages (3 min) of the James protocol raises the same problems for measurement of metabolic data that are encountered with the Bruce protocol.

In the last 10–15 years the use of ramp cycle ergometry has become increasingly common in pediatric exercise testing. In this type of protocol there is a smooth continuous rise in work rate throughout the exercise test. This has several advantages for the pediatric exercise test [23,24]. There is a smooth rise in work rate, which allows easy measurements of metabolic data. With current technology, the slopes of the ramps can be modified over a wide range allowing the protocol to accommodate patients with a wide range of ages, sizes, and physical conditioning. An example of various ramp protocols is shown in Fig. 10.9.

Evaluation of myocardial blood flow and coronary flow reserve during exercise

The evaluation of myocardial blood flow in congenital heart disease both at rest and exercise remains a challenge. This is true for both global as well as regional myocardial blood flow. The reasons for these difficulties are several.

There is no way to currently, noninvasively, quantitatively assess global myocardial blood flow with exercise. The recent developments of intracoronary Doppler echocardiography has allowed estimates of both right and left coronary artery flow [28]. This technique can also be used to assess coronary flow reserve following pharmacologic vasodilation. This procedure is obviously invasive and requires the patient to undergo the study in the cardiac catheterization laboratory. All the problems associated with exercise with invasive monitoring listed previously apply to this situation. This technique measures the flow only in the large areas of the myocardium and does not allow assessment of regional flows or regional flow reserves.

Noninvasive assessment of myocardial blood flow during exercise usually consists of either indirect measurement of myocardial ischemia or qualitative measurement of regional myocardial blood flow using radiopharmaceuticals as measures of myocardial blood flow. Both modalities have been utilized in most congenital heart lesions. Despite this, the data for any of these techniques is sparse when compared to the large number of studies in adult patients. This is due to the small numbers of congenital patients with any one type of defect when compared to the vast numbers of adult subjects with coronary artery disease. The heterogenecity of patients within certain types of defects such as single ventricles makes the comparison even with these small groups problematic. Nonetheless, these studies are being performed with increasing frequency despite these limitations.

Assessment of myocardial ischemia
ST segment depression has been used for decades to assess myocardial ischemia in congenital heart defects. Neither the sensitivity nor the specificity of ST segment changes are known when compared with different measures of myocardial perfusion, such as nuclear imaging, or when compared to coronary angiography [19,20].

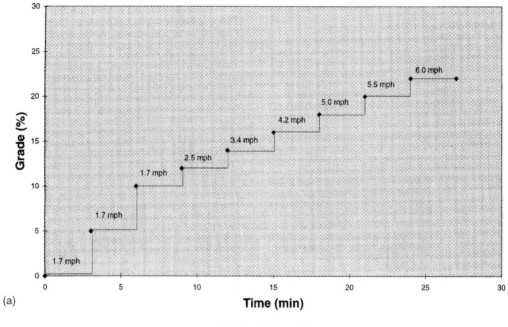

(a)

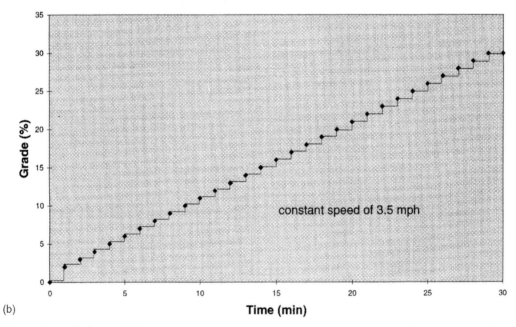

(b)

Figure 10.8 Treadmill protocols. (a) Bruce protocol consists of 3-min stages with an increase in both speed and grade. The first two stages are often omitted in healthy adult testing. (b) Balke protocol: The grade is increased from 0 to 2% after the first minute and increased 1% in each subsequent minute. The treadmill speed is held constant at 3.5 MPH. From Paridon [9] with permission.

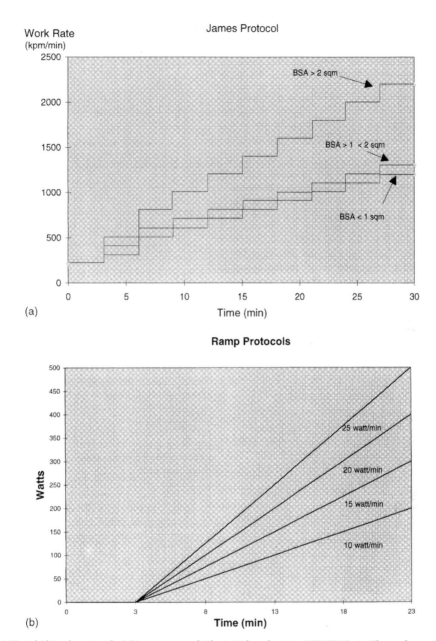

Figure 10.9 Upright bicycle protocols. (a) James protocol: The initial work rate is 200 KPM/min. The work rate is increased every 3 min by different amounts depending on the patients body surface area (BSA). (b) Ramp protocol: The patient initially pedals for 3 min with unloaded cycling to establish a baseline metabolic state. Work rate is then increased continuously at a chosen level based on the patient's physical condition, age, and size. From Paridon [9] with permission.

Studies of congenital heart defects that report ST segment changes are primarily those that involve the coronary arteries such as anomalous origins or courses of the coronary arteries. The other large groups are those defects that require coronary movement and reimplantation as part of their surgical corrections. These include ᴅ-transposition of the great arteries and certain types of aortic valve surgery such as the Ross procedure [29–32].

Stress echocardiography has been used over the last decade in an attempt to improve on ST segment change alone in the assessment of exercise-induced myocardial ischemia in certain congenital lesions [33]. This technique has been useful in such lesions as D-transposition of the great arteries after the arterial switch operation. In this situation, the cardiovascular anatomy has been essentially restored to normal. This allows assessment of regional left ventricular wall motion both at rest and during exercise using the same criteria utilized in adult patients with coronary artery disease. The same is true for primary lesions of the coronary arteries such as anomals origin of the left coronary artery from the pulmonary artery. There are no large series of patients with any congenital heart defect that have reliably reported sensitivity and specificity of stress echocardiography compared to angiography or nuclear myocardial imaging. In more complex defects this technique is less useful. Unusual ventricular anatomy such as a systemic right ventricle and the presence of artificial material such as patches and baffles makes assessment of wall motion changes much more difficult. Also many of these hearts have various degrees of electrocardiographic conduction abnormalities, which can make wall motion difficult to interpret both at rest and during exercise.

In patients with congenital lesions, measurement of wall motion immediately after exercise by echocardiography can often be difficult. This may be due to poor echo windows as a result of complex anatomy or previous surgery. These patients are often younger children who have a high respiratory rate at peak exercise compared to adults. This high respiratory rate can often impair imaging. Cooperation in very young patients is also an issue.

These problems have lead to the use of pharmacologic stress testing in certain subgroups of patients when performing stress echocardiography. The stressing agents are usually either an intravenous inotropic medication, most frequently dobutamine, or a coronary vasodilator such as adenosine or dipyridamole [33,34]. The choice of agent to use is based on the type of defect being studied and the reason for the evaluation. Inotropic agents will increase cardiac output and myocardial oxygen consumption. These are more commonly used in stress echocardiography. Coronary vasodilators are usually chosen when a stenotic coronary lesion is suspected and are more commonly employed with nuclear perfusion imaging.

In the typical dobutamine stress test, the resting images are obtained for a baseline comparison.

The dobutamine is then infused usually at a starting dose of 5 mcg/(kg min). The dose is then escalated at a fixed time interval (often 3 min) to either a predetermined maximal level or the development of rate-related symptoms. Assessment of wall motion changes are usually made at the completion of each dosing increment.

Nuclear perfusion imaging

Measurement of regional myocardial blood flow in congenital heart disease using nuclear imaging has become increasingly common over the last decade. This is occurring despite the lack of data on the sensitivity and specificity of these types of studies in children or various types of congenital defects. The most commonly employed method is single photon emission computer tomography (SPECT). Positron emission tomography (PET) is being used with increasing frequency in certain centers and has some advantages and disadvantages when compared to SPECT imaging in the study of congenital defects.

Single photon emission computer tomography
In SPECT imaging, a nuclear-labeled radiopharmaceutical is injected into the blood stream. In the current era, this is usually labeled with technetium-99 (Tc-99). The Tc-99 is taken up by the myocardium in proportion to the regional myocardial blood flow. A gamma camera is used to measure the isotope's uptake. Images are routinely reconstructed using computer tomography into multiple slices in a horizontal long axis, a vertical long axis, and a short axis plane. Qualitative differences in regional myocardial blood flow are assessed in these multiple planes [30, 35–37].

The typical SPECT imaging protocol utilizes rest and stress imaging studies. These are typically done on the same day with adequate time between the two imaging sessions to allow washout of the radioisotope. Comparison between the resting and stress imaging allows qualitative assessment of relative decreased perfusion in regions of the myocardium.

Exercise testing using the standard protocol discussed earlier in this chapter is usually the mode of stress for SPECT studies in patients who are old enough and can cooperate with exercise testing. Pharmacologic stress is frequently utilized in younger children when exercise testing is not feasible.

Electrocardiography is routinely used during the exercise or pharmacologic stress test. This permits a comparison of ST segment changes during exercise that may suggest myocardial ischemia with the findings of the stress-induced SPECT imaging. With increasing frequency, stress echocardiograph is also employed in combination with SPECT imaging as yet a third way to simultaneously assess regional myocardial blood flow and ischemia [33,36].

Recent advances in SPECT technology have made possible the study of complex cardiac defects. This includes the ability to accurately image systemic morphologic right ventricles [37]. Although the various structures of a complex heart defect can be accurately identified, the implications of differences in regional myocardial blood flow are questionable. Even more so than in simple defects, there are no data regarding the sensitivity and specificity of regional perfusion in these complex lesions.

Positron emission tomography
Positron emission tomography (PET) utilizes extremely short-lived positron-emitting radioisotopes in the assessment of regional myocardial blood flow. Like SPECT imaging, these isotopes are taken up by the myocardium in proportion to the regional myocardial blood flow. Ammonia labeled with N-13 is the most commonly used isotope for this type of study.

Because of the extremely short half-life of the positron-emitting isotopes, exercise testing is usually not practical. This has resulted in pharmacologic stress testing being the modality of choice for PET studies. The studies are usually performed with the subject in the PET scanner in order to allow immediate acquisition of images following completion of the intravenous drug infusion protocol. This short half-life obviously limits the utility of PET imaging in circumstances where additional data regarding exercise performance such as maximal VO_2 or working capacity are desired. The short half-life also requires that the isotope be generated on site. This requires a nuclear lab with a cyclotron and particle accelerator adjacent to the PET scanner. These facilities greatly increase the cost of the PET scan when compared to SPECT imaging.

Despite these limitations, PET does have some significant advantages over SPECT. The radiation dose with positron emitting isotopes is extremely low when compared to SPECT. These doses are low enough to allow their use in research studies on healthy adults. In addition, PET data acquisition technology allows quantification of regional myocardial blood flow. This results in rest and stress absolute flows for all the regions of interest of the myocardium and permits calculation of coronary flow reserve (CFR) for regions of interests in the myocardium. Coronary flow reserve is defined as the difference between the maximal coronary flow and the resting coronary flow for each region of interest. The ability to measure regional CFR permits quantitative measurements of regional differences in myocardial flow rather than qualitative differences seen with more conventional SPECT imaging.

Studies of congenital heart defects utilizing PET technology have been in those lesions involving the manipulation of coronary arteries as part of their repair. These have included D-TGA and aortic vale disease [32,38,39]. There are also studies in pediatric subjects with acquired coronary artery disease, typically from Kawasaki disease [40]. All of these studies compare regional coronary blood flow to data from young healthy adults. Even with the extremely low radiation dose, it has not been feasible to ethically collect data on regional myocardial blood flow in healthy children and adolescents using PET technology. The assumption in current PET studies is that myocardial response to pharmacologic vasodilatation and coronary flow reserve are similar in children and young adults. Since there are no data regarding this assumption, this remains a significant concern in the interpretation of the findings of current PET studies in the pediatric population.

References

1. Wasserman K, Hansen JE, Sue DY, *et al.* Exercise testing and interpretation: An overview. In: Principles of Exercise Testing and Interpretation, 2nd edn. Lea & Febiger, Philadelphia, Ch. 1, pp. 1–8, 1994.
2. Wasserman K, Hansen JE, Sue DY, *et al.* Physiology of exercise. In: Principles of Exercise Testing and Interpretation, 2nd edn. Lea & Febiger, Philadelphia, Ch. 2, pp. 9–51, 1994.
3. Astrand P, Rodahl K. The muscle and its contraction. In: Textbook of Work Physiology, Physiological Bases of Exercise, 3rd edn. McGraw-Hill, New York, Ch. 2, pp. 12–53, 1986.
4. Rowland TW. Response to endurance exercise: Cardiovascular system. In: Developmental Exercise Physiology. Human Kinetics, Champaign, IL, Ch. 8, pp. 117–140, 1996.

5. Astrand P, Rodahl K. Body fluids, blood and circulation. In: Textbook of Work Physiology, Physiological Bases of Exercise, 3rd edn. McGraw-Hill, New York, Ch. 4, pp. 127–208, 1986.

6. Mulla N, Simpson P, Sullivan NM, et al. Determinants of aerobic capacity during exercise following complete repair of tetralogy of fallot with transannular patch. Pediatr Cardiol 1997; 18(5):350–356.

7. Mulla N, Paridon SM, Pinsky WW. Cardiopulmonary performance during exercise in patients with repaired tetralogy of fallot with absent pulmonary valve. Pediatr Cardiol 1995; 16(3): 120–126.

8. Paridon SM, Humes RA, Pinsky WW. The role of chronotropic impairment during exercise after the mustard operation. J Am Coll Cardiol 1991; 17(3): 729–732.

9. Paridon, SM. Exercise physiology and capacity. In: Rychik J., Wernovsky G., eds., Hypoplastic Left Heart Syndrome. Kluwer, Boston, Ch. 18, pp. 329–346, 2003.

10. Freedson PS, Goodman TL. Measurement of oxygen consumption. In: Rowland TW., ed., Pediatric Laboratory Exercise Testing: Clinical Guidelines. Human Kinetics, Champaign, IL, pp. 91–113, 1993.

11. Wasserman K, Hansen JE, Sue DY, et al. Measurements during integrative cardiopulmonary exercise testing. In: Principles of Exercise Testing and Interpretation, 2nd edn. Lea & Febiger, Philadelphia, Ch. 3, pp. 52–79, 1994.

12. Stone FM, Bessinger FB Jr, Lucas RV Jr, et al. Pre- and postoperative rest and exercise hemodynamics in children with pulmonary stenosis. Circulation 1974; 49:1102–1106.

13. Moller JH. Exercise responses in pulmonary stenosis. Prog Pediatr Cardiol 1993; 2(3):8–13.

14. Derrick GP, Narang I, White PA, et al. Failure of stroke volume augmentation during exercise and dobutamine stress is unrelated to load-independent indexes of right ventricular performance after the mustard operation. Circulation 2000; 102(suppl III):154–159.

15. Barber G. Pediatric exercise testing—Methodology, equipment, and normal values. Prog Ped Cardiol 1993; 2(2):4–10.

16. Tomassoni TL. Conducting the pediatric exercise test. In: Rowland TW., ed., Pediatric Laboratory Exercise Testing: Clinical Guidelines. Human Kinetics, Champaign, IL, pp. 1–17, 1993.

17. Alpert BS, Verrill DE, Flood NL, et al. Complications of ergometer exercise in children. Pediatr Cardiol 1983; 4:91–96.

18. Freed M. Exercise testing in children: A survey of techniques and safety. Circulation 1981; 64(suppl IV):IV–278 (abstract).

19. Paridon, SM. Exercise testing. In: Garson A, Bricker JT, Fisher DJ, Neish SR, eds., The Science and Practice of Pediatric Cardiology, Vol. 1, 2nd edn. Lippincott, Philadelphia, PA, Ch. 40, pp. 875–888, 1998.

20. Bricker JT. Pediatric exercise electrocardiography. In: Rowland TW., ed., Pediatric Laboratory Exercise Testing: Clinical Guidelines. Human Kinetics, Champaign, IL, pp. 43–65, 1993.

21. Borg G. Psychophysical bases of perceived exertion. Med Sci Sport Exerc 1982; 14:377–381.

22. Washington RL, Bricker JT, Alpert BS, et al. Guidelines for exercise testing in the pediatric age group. Circulation 1994; 90(4):2166–2179.

23. Wasserman K, Hansen JE, Sue DY, et al. Protocols for exercise testing. In: Principles of Exercise Testing and Interpretation. Lea & Febiger, Philadelphia, pp. 96–111, 1994.

24. Rowland TW. Aerobic exercise testing protocols. In: Rowland TW., ed., Pediatric Laboratory Exercise Testing: Clinical Guidelines. Human Kinetics, Champaign, IL, pp. 19–41, 1993.

25. Driscott DJ, Staats BA, Beck KC. Measurements of cardiac output in children during exercise: A review. Pediatr Exerc Sci 1989; 1:102–115.

26. Washington RL. Measurement of cardiac output. In: Rowland TW., ed., Pediatric Laboratory Exercise Testing: Clinical Guidelines. Human Kinetics, Champaign, IL, pp. 131–140, 1993.

27. James FW, Kaplan S, Glueck CJ, et al. Responses of normal children and young adults to controlled bicycle exercise. Circulation 1980; 61:902–912.

28. Oskarsson G, Pesonen E, Munkhammar P, et al. Normal coronary flow reserve after arterial switch operation for transposition of the great arteries. An intracoronary Doppler guidewire study. Circulation 2002; 106:1696–1702.

29. Mahle WT, McBride MG, Paridon SM. Exercise performance following the arterial switch operation for D–transposition of the great arteries. Am J Cardiol 2001; 87:753–758.

30. Paridon SM, Farooki ZQ, Kuhns LR, et al. Exercise performance after repair of anomalous origin of the left coronary artery from the pulmonary artery. Circulation 1990; 81(4):1287–1292.

31. James FW. Exercise responses in aortic stenosis. Prog Pediatr Cardiol 1993; 2(3):1–7.

32. Singh TP, DiCarli MF, Sullivan NM, et al. Myocardial flow reserve in long-term survivors of repair of anomalous left coronary artery from pulmonary artery. JACC 1998; 31(2):437–443.

33. Kimball TR. Pediatric stress echocardiography. Pediatr Cardiol 2002; 23:347–357.

34. Dodge-Khatami A, Tulevski II, Bennink GBWE, et al. Comparable systemic ventricular function in

healthy adults and patients with unoperated congenitally corrected transposition using MRI dobutamine stress testing. Ann Thorac Surg 2002; 73:1759–1764.

35. Paridon SM, Galioto FM, Vincent JA, *et al.* Exercise capacity and incidence of myocardial perfusion defects after Kawasaki disease in children and adolescents. J Am Coll Cardiol 1995; 25(6):1420–1424.

36. Weindling SN, Wernovsky G, Colan SD, *et al.* Myocardial perfusion, function and exercise tolerance after the arterial switch operation. J Am Coll Cardiol 1994; 23:424–433.

37. Lubiszewska B, Gosiewska E, Hoffman P, *et al.* Myocardial perfusion and function of the systemic right ventricle in patients after atrial switch procedure for complete transposition: Long–term follow-up. J Am Coll Cardiol 2000; 36:1365–1370.

38. Bengel FM, Hauser M, Duvernoy CS, *et al.* Myocardial blood flow and coronary flow reserve late after anatomical correction of transposition of the great arteries. J Am Coll Cardiol 1998; 32:1955–1961.

39. Hauser M, Bengel FM, Kuhn A, *et al.* Myocardial blood flow and flow reserve after coronary reimplantation in patients after arterial switch and ross operation. Circulation 2001; 103:1875–1880.

40. Muzik O, Paridon SM, Singh TP, *et al.* quantification of myocardial blood flow and flow reserve in children with a history of Kawasaki disease and normal coronary arteries using positron emission tomography. J Am Coll Cardiol 1996; 28(3):757–762.

PART III
Ventricular Function in Specific Categories

CHAPTER 11

Ventricular Function in Pressure Overload Lesions

Steven D. Colan, MD

Cardiac pressure overload lesions in children can be encountered in both congenital and acquired forms of heart disease (see Table 11.1). The range of primary lesions leading to pressure overload is considerably less complex than is the case for volume overload lesions, but this list is deceptive in its simplicity. One of the most challenging aspects of congenital heart disease is the frequency with which cardiac anomalies appear in combination. Aortic stenosis can be seen in isolation, but is often associated with one or more other left-heart lesions including mitral stenosis and regurgitation, aortic regurgitation, subaortic stenosis, and coarctation. Coarctation of the aorta is often associated with ventricular septal defect, left ventricular inflow, and outflow tract obstruction, and can occasionally be encountered in virtually all forms of complex congenital heart disease. Pulmonary stenosis is one of the more common forms of congenital heart disease, both as an isolated lesion and in conjunction with atrial septal defect, ventricular septal defect, and most other forms of congenital heart disease. Understanding the impact of pressure overload on the myocardium is significantly more difficult when compounded by other factors that can impact myocardial function, including volume overload and cyanosis. Most investigations into myocardial mechanics, both in humans and in animals, have therefore focused on these lesions in isolation. There are surprisingly few available data examining the impact of combined pressure and volume overload, but the work that has been done indicates that there is by no means a simple additive effect. However, given this paucity of data, the current discussion will focus primarily on the myocardial response to isolated pressure overload lesions.

Pathophysiology of myocardial response to pressure overload

The fate of the myocardium when faced with an increased pressure load is primarily determined by a complex interplay between load, hypertrophy, and function. Experimental studies in surgically instrumented animals with acute supravalvar aortic stenosis have helped to clarify the cardiac adaptations to pressure overload. The pattern which is observed after acute imposition of a pressure load is quite similar to that observed in severe congenital aortic stenosis, and consists of dilation with wall thinning, elevation in wall stress, and fall in ventricular function. Over the ensuing weeks, the process of compensation manifests as normalization of ventricular volume and function concurrent with a rise in myocardial mass. This compensatory hypertrophy appears to be essential to this process. If obstruction is progressively increased in excess of the rate of acquisition of mass, experimentally forcing a persistent elevation of systolic wall stress, ventricular dysfunction does not resolve and over a period of weeks depressed myocardial contractility supervenes [1]. Similar to animal models, acute surgical obstruction of left ventricular outflow in infants leads to ventricular dilation and severely depressed function [2]. Myocardial hypertrophy, which is initiated within a period of hours and is sufficiently rapid to result in a doubling of ventricular mass in less than 1 week, is associated with recovery of systolic function. The dynamic equilibrium between hypertrophy and systolic performance is a dominant theme at all stages of the clinical course of pressure overload hypertrophy.

Table 11.1 Common Forms of Heart Disease in Children Associated with Pressure Overload.

Left-sided pressure overload	Right-sided pressure overload
Aortic stenosis (subvalvar, valvar, and supravalvar)	Pulmonic stenosis (subvalvar, valvar, and supravalvar)
Aortic coarctation	Pulmonary artery stenosis
Systemic hypertension	Pulmonary hypertension

As discussed in Chapter 12, control of the cardiac hypertrophic response is generally believed to function as a servomechanism, with stress and strain as the controlling feedback variables. Strain is the change in length from the initial or resting length. Stress is the total force per unit cross-sectional area, and for a thin-walled cylindrical chamber *wall stress* can be approximated by the Laplace relation: $(pr)/2h$, where p is the transmural left ventricular pressure, r the left ventricular radius, and h the wall thickness. Since the mechanical load of systolic contraction is mediated by the myofibers, we are primarily interested in the forces exerted on and by these fibers, known as *fiberstress*. Although often discussed as if they are synonymous, ventricular wall stress and myocardial fiberstress are not equivalent [3]. This divergence arises because the myocardium is composed of ordered, circumferentially oriented fibers, resulting in mechanical attributes that have different values in the radial and circumferential directions (anisotropism) [4], and that respond differentially to longitudinal and transverse strain [5]. With regard to control of hypertrophy, when there is a sustained alteration in cardiac workload, the altered systolic force or tension generated by the myocardial fibers elicits myocardial hypertrophy or atrophy until the load per fiber is again returned to the normal range. Systolic stress, similar to blood pressure, is a time-varying process, with peak stress achieved early in systole, falling almost linearly to the lower end-systolic values (Fig. 11.1). Peak systolic stress appears to be the major mechanical determinant of concentric hypertrophy, whereas end-systolic stress is the primary determinant of the extent of the systolic shortening (Fig. 11.2) [6]. Although these forms of "afterload," end-systolic, and peak-systolic stress are generally closely correlated, and therefore changes in mass and function are closely related, there are circumstances such as aortic stenosis that disrupt this process. The im-

portance of this phenomenon is discussed below in relationship to aortic stenosis. The trophic response to elevated stress is an intrinsic property of myocardium that can occur even without neural or hormonal mediation, although these other modulating influences play an important role *in vivo*, as discussed in Chapter 12.

Impact of concentric hypertrophy on systolic function

Teleologically, compensatory hypertrophy serves its primary purpose insofar as it successfully normalizes systolic function and cardiac output. Although the early hypertrophic response is characterized by normal or even enhanced myocardial contractility [7,8], chronic pressure overload myocardial hypertrophy is known to lead to depressed myocardial function in animals and adult humans [9]. The pathophysiology of the transition from compensated myocardial hypertrophy to contractile dysfunction remains incompletely understood. It is clear that once the myocardium fails, abnormalities of nearly every cellular component and system are present. Interventions at the later stages of the disease seem less likely to be effective in reversing the process, leading most investigators to focus on the early events in this transition. The assumption is that identification of a premiere cause of the onset of myocyte contractile dysfunction would enable targeted interventions to prevent or delay this transition. Relevant to this effort is the hypothesis that has been put forward by a number of observers that hypertrophy is inherently maladaptive [10]. The essence of this argument is the theory that the cellular modifications of compensatory hypertrophy are intrinsically harmful to the cell, perhaps most succinctly summarized as the notion that cell hypertrophy is the first stage of cell death. If true, unless the maladaptive and compensatory aspects of cell hypertrophy can be uncoupled or the

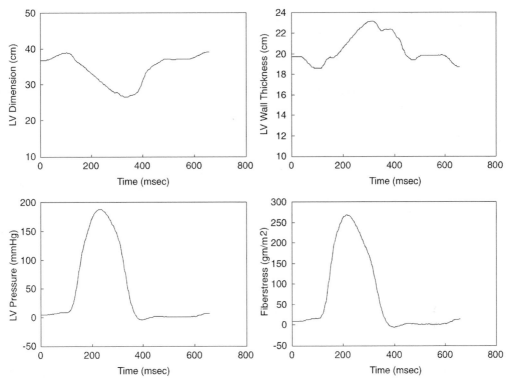

Figure 11.1 The time course of stress over the course of the cardiac cycle is determined by the temporal variance in wall thickness, cavity dimension, and cavity pressure. These data are for a single cardiac cycle recorded in an experimental animal with implanted ultrasound crystals and a high-fidelity left ventricular pressure catheter. Peak stress is an early systolic event, following which stress falls almost linearly to end-systole. Early diastolic stress decay is exponential, interrupted by a gradual rise in passive stress due to ventricular filling.

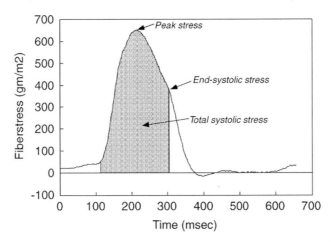

Figure 11.2 The several indices measurable from the stress–time curve have particular importance for ventricular mechanics. Peak stress is the primary determinant of hypertrophy, end-systolic stress is the primary determinant of the extent of systolic shortening, and total systolic stress is a primary determinant of myocardial oxygen consumption. Under normal circumstances, there is a tight association between these three indices of afterload. However, under certain hemodynamic circumstances such as aortic stenosis and coarctation of the aorta, the time course of arterial pressure over the course of systole is sufficiently altered so that the normal relationship among these three indices is disturbed.

maladaptive changes are reversible, only prevention of cell hypertrophy can avoid cell injury. It is therefore of some importance to summarize the evidence that adverse changes are intrinsically linked to the process of hypertrophy.

Myocyte hypertrophy is associated with depressed peak contraction rate and slowed relaxation, related to alteration in the Ca^{2+} transient [11]. However, it is also clear that this change is not intrinsic to the change in cell size, because contractile function remains normal during the most rapid and marked phase of cellular expansion [12]. In pathologic hypertrophy, the increase in cell size is not closely associated with impaired myocyte function. Physiologic hypertrophy secondary to intense athletic participation is perhaps the most extreme example of dissociation between hypertrophy and contractile dysfunction [13].

Based on observations in small mammals, it has been hypothesized that altered expression of myosin isoforms is one mechanism whereby myocardial performance could be affected in response to pressure overload hypertrophy. A transition in expression of myosin isoforms from V1 to V3 has been documented in small mammals in response to myocardial infarction and hemodynamic stress, a shift that results in increased myocardial efficiency, but has been hypothesized to contribute to the onset of contractile failure. In humans, down-regulation of α-myosin heavy chain mRNA has been reported in failing compared with normal myocardium, which results in a transition from the normally small but significant V1 isoform content to failing myocardium that is 100% V3. However, this transition does not appear to contribute to the onset of contractile dysfunction, since there is no difference between the failing and nonfailing ventricular myosin with regard to isometric force, unloaded shortening, half-maximal calcium activation, velocity of shortening, or average force [14].

Myocardial hypertrophy could potentially involve both myocyte hypertrophy and hyperplasia. One of the more contentious issues in cardiology is the long-held belief that mature cardiac myocytes are terminally differentiated and are incapable of reentering the cell cycle. The current status of this issue has been recently reviewed in detail [15]. The primary basis for the belief that adult myocytes are incapable of replication is the observed inability of cardiac myocytes to regenerate and replace myocardium damaged by infarction. Nonetheless, proliferation of neonatal myocytes in a number of species has been demonstrated, where a large proportion of cells synthesize DNA and undergo mitotic division. More recently, DNA replication, nuclear mitotic division, and myocyte proliferation have been described in myocardial infarction models with overt cardiac failure [16,17]. Thus, it is clear that similar to most other tissues, the myocardium retains the full panoply of remodeling potentialities, including myocyte hypertrophy and proliferation, in conjunction with apoptotic and necrotic myocyte death. However, it is germane to the present discussion to note that elevated diastolic wall stress appears to be a consistent factor in the initiation of myocyte division [18], whereas systolic overload has not been an effective model in eliciting this type of cellular growth [19]. Therefore, with regard to understanding the progression from pressure overload hypertrophy to myocardial dysfunction, myocyte proliferation appears to play a role only after myocardial failure ensues.

Inadequate neovascularization has long been speculated to contribute to the myocardial deterioration associated with pressure overload hypertrophy. New formation of intracellular contractile material accounts for the expansion of myocytes. This hyperplasia of myofibrillar units results in an increase in oxygen utilization and requires a proportional growth of mitochondria responsible for oxygen consumption and energy supply. Early investigations suggested a reduction of the mitochondria to myofibrillar volume ratio in pressure overload hypertrophy, but subsequent work indicated that mitochondrial content increases in proportion to adaptive cellular growth [20]. Limitations in coronary vascular reserve have been observed in adult animal and human models of pressure overload hypertrophy, with magnitude of vascular dysfunction correlating with severity of hypertrophy [21]. This can be attributed to a disproportionate increase in ventricular mass compared to the microvascular growth, a rarefaction of the arteriolar bed, abnormal coronary vascular resistance, and/or extravascular compression by the ventricular mass. There is a fundamental age-related difference in this regard, with maintenance of normal neovascularization in immature but not adult animals with a supracoronary aortic stenosis pressure overload model [22–24]. In humans as well young age appears protective against the capillary rarefaction that accompanies pressure overload hypertrophy [25]. This may well contribute to the extreme infrequency with which myocardial dysfunction supervenes in congenital compared with acquired aortic stenosis.

Cell loss has been identified as an important component in the transition from compensated hypertrophy to myocardial failure. In mouse knockout models myocyte apoptosis has been identified as a critical element in the transition from compensated cardiac hypertrophy and heart failure during acute pressure overload [26]. The two main cellular events that have been identified as having the capacity to induce apoptosis are hypoxia and mechanical loading [27], both of which could be important in pressure overload hypertrophy. However, even though progressive cell loss was found in association with myocardial decompensation in humans with aortic stenosis, apoptosis did not contribute substantially [19]. Instead, these patients have myocyte degeneration and death with replacement fibrosis in proportion to the severity of systolic dysfunction.

Importance of hypertrophy to maintenance of systolic function

The dynamic tension between hypertrophy as a mechanism to normalize fiberstress and maintain normal function versus cell growth as the mediator of myocyte dysfunction raises the important issue as to whether and how much hypertrophy is required. Sustained elevation of myocardial stress in animal models quickly leads to myocardial failure [1]. In humans, hypertrophy is a critical factor in the recovery of ventricular function after imposition of acute pressure overload [28]. Inadequate hypertrophy, with sustained elevation of afterload, is believed to be a primary factor in the chronic myocardial injury associated with volume overload hypertrophy. Nonetheless, there are now several models where hypertrophy has been blocked despite sustained pressure overload with apparently improved outcome. In rats with pressure overload hypertrophy due to banding of the ascending aorta, administration of an angiotensin converting enzyme inhibitor (fosinopril) attenuated the hypertrophic response, resulting in sustained elevation of wall stress, but treatment nonetheless inhibited or prevented the progressive impairment of systolic and diastolic function [29]. In pressure-overload model in mice, calcineurin

inhibition with cyclosporine completely inhibited hypertrophy without adverse impact on ventricular function or mortality, whereas untreated mice had significant hypertrophy though they did not progress to cardiac failure [30]. Inhibition of the GTP pathway in hypertensive rats inhibited hypertrophy and improved contractility without dropping blood pressure, but there was no decrease in interstitial fibrosis [31]. Transgenic mice with blunted ventricular hypertrophy in response to pressure overload manifest higher end-systolic stress, but better preservation of systolic function compared to wild-type mice [32]. These observations suggest that hypertrophy and normalization of wall stress in response to pressure overload may not be necessary to maintain cardiac function.

It is clear that many evolved compensatory mechanisms solve a short-term problem at the expense of long-term adverse effects. Conforming to this perspective, myocardial hypertrophy has been described both as savior and villain, and simultaneously adaptive and maladaptive. Nevertheless, it is at best counterintuitive that, as suggested by the foregoing reports, the complex hypertrophic response to pressure overload is unnecessary. That is, the concept that the carefully regulated process of normalization of stress is superfluous to maintenance of systolic function, as has been suggested [33], is difficult to accept from an evolutionary point of view. With reference to this, it is worth noting that for each of the above reports, contradictory data also exist. Meguro *et al.* demonstrated in a mouse model that attenuation of myocardial hypertrophy in response to calcineurin inhibition with cyclosporine A increased heart failure-related mortality [34]. Ding *et al.* found that cyclosporine A did not prevent hypertrophy in mice with aortic stenosis even though calcineurin activity was severely depressed [35]. Mukawa *et al.* found that in rats inhibition of ACE activity alone without lowering blood pressure did not prevent cardiac hypertrophy [36]. Thus, although primary blockade of hypertrophy may appear to represent an attractive therapeutic target, at present it appears premature to reach the conclusion that hypertrophy is superfluous [37].

Impact of concentric hypertrophy on diastolic function

Increased diastolic filling pressure has long been known to accompany concentric hypertrophy

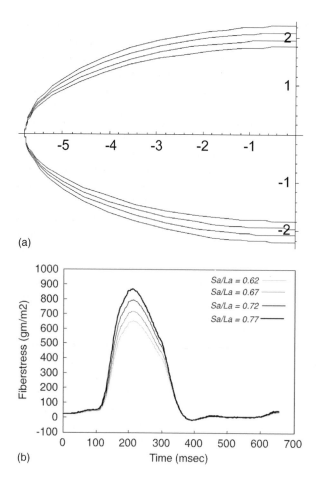

(a)

(b)

Figure 11.3 Illustration of the variation in stress as a function of ventricular sphericalization. (a) The left ventricle is modeled as a prolate ellipsoid with a constant long axis dimension but variable short axis dimension.. (b) Ventricular mass was assumed to be constant and fiberstress was calculated at each of these short axis (Sa) to long axis (La) dimension ratios. As shown, global stress rises in proportion to the deviation toward a more spherical shape.

secondary to pressure overload such as aortic stenosis and coarctation. There are both myocardial and ventricular factors that contribute to this. The change in geometry of the left ventricle is important in two respects. Because of the inverse relationship of stress to wall thickness, the process of concentric hypertrophy reduces wall stress by increasing the mass-to-volume ratio. Although this is advantageous for handling the elevated pressure load during systole, this increased wall thickness also means that during diastole a higher pressure is required to achieve a normal level of wall stress. If myocardial compliance is normal, that is, there is a normal relationship between stress and strain, a normal diastolic stress must be achieved in order to stretch the myocardium to a normal length. This implies that the elevation in wall thickness relative to diameter necessitates a rise in diastolic pressure to achieve a normal filling volume, even if myocardial

properties are normal. The second geometric factor is the altered ventricular shape to a more prolate spheroid, with a fall in the short axis to long axis ratio. For a given left ventricular mass, global stress falls in proportion to the magnitude of deviation from a spherical shape (Fig. 11.3). Again, this is an example of how ventricular remodeling in response to pressure overload improves the force generating capacity at the expense of diastolic function. The contrast to adaptation to volume overload is worth noting. Optimization of diastolic volume capacity occurs when the ventricle becomes more spherical and mass-to-volume ratio is normal or low. Optimization for systolic force generation occurs when the ventricle becomes less spherical and the mass-to-volume ratio rises. In terms of changes in ventricular geometry, the contrast between remodeling in response to pressure overload and volume overload illustrates the direct opposure between changes that improve systolic function and those that improve diastolic passive properties.

Myocardial material properties can also be altered by the hypertrophic response to pressure overload. The myocardial extracellular matrix surrounds the cardiac myocytes and myocardial microcirculation and interlinks cardiac myocytes and myofibrils. Adjacent cardiomyocytes are connected by collagen fibers referred to as struts, which play an important role in force transmission, and are surrounded by a collagen mesh that serves to maintain muscle fiber and cardiac myocyte alignment and to determine the size and shape of the cardiac chambers [38]. The importance of the fibrillar collagen matrix to the transmission of force generated by myocytes has been demonstrated by recent work using plasmin treatment to cause matrix metalloproteinase activation and collagen degradation. In this model, acute disruption of the fibrillar collagen network caused a decrease in myocardial systolic performance but had no impact on cardiomyocyte contractility [39]. Since fibrillar collagen facilitates transduction of cardiomyocyte contraction into myocardial force development and helps to maintain normal myocardial systolic performance, it is not surprising that interstitial myocardial collagen content increases by 40–150% in pressure overload hypertrophy [40]. The increase in collagen content has been observed in both right and left ventricular pressure overload in neonates as well as in older children [41]. Collagen is a rather inelastic material and elevated concentrations are associated with less compliant myocardium. Pressure overload hypertrophy also invariably involves myocyte hypertrophy, and it is therefore reasonable to inquire whether hypertrophy *per se* is an important contributor to abnormal diastolic myocardial properties. There are animal data to indicate that alterations in the constituitive properties of myocytes contribute to the increased myocardial stiffness seen in pressure overload hypertrophy [42], independent of changes in the extracellular matrix. Nevertheless, trained athletes manifest significant myocardial hypertrophy but have normal or even enhanced myocardial diastolic function [13], indicating that reduced myocardial compliance is not intrinsic to the hypertrophic process. In contrast, animal models have identified a direct correlation between myocardial collagen content and myocardial stiffness in rats and nonhuman primates with hypertension [43]. Fibrillar collagen therefore appears to be the primary contributor to the increased myocardial stiffness associated with pressure overload hypertrophy [44].

It is important to note that collagen deposition does not always result in increased myocardial stiffness. Although volume overload, pressure overload, heart failure, myocardial infarction, and physiological hypertrophy are each associated with increased left ventricular mass, the resulting impact on passive myocardial properties is profoundly different between these models. A significant reduction in collagen volume content accompanies volume overload hypertrophy and myocardial compliance improves [45]. The ventricle also becomes more compliant in conjunction with the remodeling stimulated by experimental myocardial infarction, but in this case marked fibrosis is present [46]. In contrast, the rise in myofibrillar collagen content appears to be the primary cause of the diminished myocardial compliance that accompanies pressure overload hypertrophy [38]. There is now considerable data indicating that the extent of collagen cross-linking is a primary determinant of the diverse relation that exists between myocardial fibrosis and changes in myocardial stiffness [47]. These observations point out the importance of considering both the quantity and quality of newly synthesized collagen when attempting to understand the impact on passive myocardial properties.

Aortic stenosis

Aortic valve disease represents perhaps the purest form of isolated left ventricular pressure and/or volume overload since no other chambers of the heart are directly affected by the hemodynamic abnormality. Because of this as, well as the clinical importance of aortic valve disease, there is a substantial body of experimental and clinical data that has accumulated concerning the effects on the myocardium. It is clear that the consequences for the myocardium depend on the age of onset, the duration of the hemodynamic load, the relative severity of pressure versus volume overload, the adequacy of the adaptive response, and the nature and success of therapeutic interventions. Although for any particular individual a mixture of valve stenosis and regurgitation is quite common, one or the other generally predominates. For this reason, most investigative work has addressed the two lesions separately.

In children, valvar stenosis is seen in two clinically distinct patterns, depending the time of onset and severity of stenosis. Many children who have mild or absent left ventricular outflow tract obstruction at birth have progressive aortic stenosis over time. The clinical picture in these patients has notable differences from adults with aortic stenosis: They have greater hypertrophy relative to the severity of pressure overload, systolic function is invariably normal to hyperdynamic, and they are at negligible risk for development of ventricular or myocardial dysfunction. The second and far more rare syndrome of aortic stenosis is seen in infants with severe stenosis who present early in life with a syndrome of low cardiac output, variable degrees of left ventricular hypoplasia, severe ventricular dysfunction, and congestive heart failure. Intervention to relieve the outflow obstruction can result in clinical recovery and normalization of ventricular function, but restenosis is nearly universal. The presentation in infancy is associated with afterload mismatch related to muscle mass that is inadequate to overcome the outflow impedance. If managed medically, some patients develop sufficient hypertrophy to recover a normal output and to normalize ventricular function, indicating that deterioration of function primarily relates to the fact that there is insufficient cardiac muscle to carry the load. Deficient hypertrophy at birth implies that the left ventricle has been relatively protected from the hemodynamic overload prior to delivery. Prenatal flow redistribution across the atrial septal defect can reduce the volume flow through the left side, thereby protecting the left ventricle from excess pressure load (Fig. 11.4). Under these circumstances, the afterload mismatch and secondary ventricular dysfunction arise with the obligatory rise in left ventricular load at the time of postnatal ductal closure and increase in pulmonary blood flow. In the most extreme form of this syndrome, flow through the left ventricle is so severely reduced that marked left ventricular hypoplasia results, and a two-ventricle heart is not achievable. If the left ventricular structures are adequate in size and the afterload mismatch is relieved in the postnatal period by compensatory hypertrophy, with or without relief of left ventricular outflow obstruction, the subsequent physiology is similar to that in other patients with aortic stenosis.

Effects of aortic stenosis on systolic myocardial mechanics

Cardiac function in congenital aortic stenosis has represented somewhat of an enigma. The inverse relation between myocardial shortening and the force resisting shortening would seem to predict that ejection performance should be depressed by the elevated outflow impedance. However, ejection fraction is usually above normal and in fact rises in proportion to the pressure gradient. This apparent paradox can be explained in part by considering the nature of myocardial afterload. As discussed previously, the normal response to the mechanical stimulus of pressure overload is compensatory hypertrophy, which persists until the increase in wall thickness is sufficient to normalize fiberstress. Conceptually, new fibers are added until the load per fiber is normalized and systolic function is restored. However, this mechanism would predict that systolic function should be normal rather than enhanced. The simplest explanation for the observed elevation in function is that pressure overload hypertrophy leads to enhanced contractility. Although this possibility has not been excluded, there are at least three alternative explanations that have been put forward to explain the observed enhanced function in congenital aortic stenosis.

First, there is evidence that elevated systolic function relates to alterations in the time course of wall stress during systole [48]. Although peak systolic pressure is elevated in aortic stenosis, end-systolic pressure is normal since at the time of aortic valve closure left ventricular pressure must fall below aortic pressure (Fig. 11.5). As shown by a number of investigators, peak systolic stress is the major determinant of hypertrophy. That is, it is the peak load per fiber that serves as the feedback mechanism for formation of new fibers. In aortic stenosis it is the normal end-systolic pressure despite an elevated peak pressure that results in a proportionally lower end-systolic stress. Functionally, the marked hypertrophy that is required to normalize the elevated peak pressure results in "excess" muscle relative to the normal end-systolic pressure, and consequently end-systolic stress is lower than normal. In contrast to the control of hypertrophy, the force limiting the extent of shortening is end-systolic wall stress. Thus, normalization of peak stress leads to subnormal end-systolic stress with the consequent enhanced

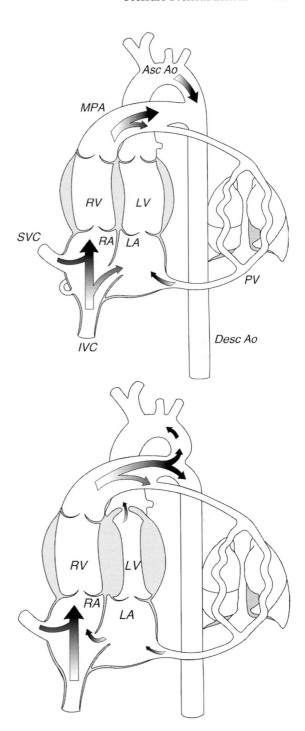

Figure 11.4 Pattern of prenatal flow redistribution in fetuses with aortic stenosis. (a) The normal flow pattern and (b) the changes that occur with aortic stenosis. Flow reversal across the atrial septal defect from the left atrium (LA) to the right atrium (RA) reduces the volume flow through the left ventricle (LV) and antegrade into the ascending aorta. The increased flow through the right ventricle (RV) and flow reversal in the distal arch supplies blood to the head and neck vessels, compensating for the diminution of antegrade aortic flow.

systolic performance. Since end-systolic stress represents the afterload that is relevant to systolic shortening, one is faced with the rather counter-intuitive observation that myocardial afterload is reduced in aortic stenosis. Supranormal function is isolated to the affected ventricle, consistent with the hypothesis that local loading is responsible. Further support for this concept derives from the observation that

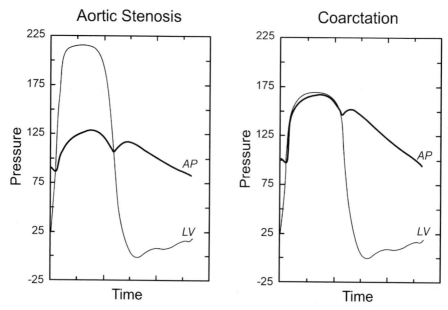

Figure 11.5 Time course of left ventricular (LV) and arterial pressure (AP) in aortic stenosis and coarctation. Although peak systolic pressure is elevated in aortic stenosis, end-systolic pressure is normal since at the time of aortic valve closure left ventricular pressure must fall below aortic pressure. In contrast, both peak and end-systolic pressure are elevated in coarctation, and the percent elevation in end-systolic pressure often exceeds the relative elevation in peak pressure.

relief of stenosis is followed by a rise in end-systolic stress toward normal with consequent reduction in function [49].

The second factor that contributes to the observed elevation in systolic function in patients with aortic stenosis is the use of endocardial function indices to evaluate function. For geometric reasons discussed in detail below under the discussion of aortic coarctation, endocardial indices overestimate global systolic fiber shortening [50]. At the myocardial level, fiber shortening is determined by fiberstress, contractility, and preload. Overestimation of the magnitude of fiber shortening secondary to reliance on endocardial indices leads to an artifactual perception of elevated contractility. This issue has been explored in some detail in patients with hypertension and with coarctation, but has not been investigated in congenital aortic stenosis. Therefore, the importance of this artifactual misrepresentation of the magnitude of fiber shortening relative to the other factors is unknown.

The third observation that has been proposed to explain the elevation in systolic performance is an alteration in intrinsic myocardial trophic properties. This explanation is also based on the concept that ex-

cess hypertrophy leads to low afterload, but in this case the excess hypertrophy is thought to be a consequence of the age of onset of the pressure load. According to this hypothesis, pressure load early in life elicits a proportionally greater myocardial hypertrophic response, a property that persists if the aortic stenosis is not fully relieved. This phenomenon may represent a persistence of the increased trophic response seen in normal infants [51], which is elicited by the presence of aortic stenosis from birth. Total (integrated) systolic wall stress is the primary hemodynamic determinant of myocardial oxygen consumption [52]. Therefore, reduced total systolic stress also predicts that per gram myocardial oxygen consumption should be reduced—a finding which has also been confirmed [53]. This pattern of supra-normal function with low end-systolic stress is far less often seen in patients who develop stenosis later in life, although it appears to be more common in women than in men [54].

Timing of intervention in aortic stenosis

Systolic dysfunction is rarely encountered beyond the neonatal period in children with congenital aortic stenosis. In contrast to aortic regurgitation, where clinical management and timing of intervention are largely based on evidence of systolic myocardial dysfunction, management of aortic stenosis has been primarily based on the magnitude of pressure overload and symptomatic limitations. Symptoms and signs of congestive heart failure are considered ominous findings in adults with aortic valve stenosis, and half or more of patients with congestive heart failure due to valvar aortic stenosis have normal systolic function [55]. Diastolic dysfunction, related to either intrinsic alteration of the hypertrophied myocardium or as a consequence of ischemia, is observed even in patients without systolic dysfunction, and appears to precede the onset of systolic dysfunction. Although impaired diastolic function has been documented in congenital aortic stenosis, the natural history of the process and the contribution this may make to onset of symptoms or exercise limitations is not known.

Although there is a general agreement that onset of symptoms warrants intervention, indications for intervention for asymptomatic children with congenital aortic stenosis remain uncertain. Transcatheter or surgical valvotomy incurs the risk of valvar insufficiency and the potential need for valve replacement. Valve replacement, either to eliminate the outflow obstruction or because of the aortic regurgitation, carries both the risk of surgery and the long-term hazards associated with a prosthetic valve. Virtually all studies of outcome after aortic valve replacement have found an annual mortality of at least 1%, with morbidity rates that are even higher. Although the potential for sudden death is occasionally suggested as a justification for intervention, the risk of sudden death is in fact orders of magnitude higher after valve replacement [56] and cannot be used to justify valve replacement or a procedure that increases the risk of valve replacement. Reduction in risk of sudden death after intervention for aortic stenosis has not been demonstrated and indeed the risk has been reported to be higher than in nonintervention groups [57]. Systolic dysfunction and symptoms are reversible in adults with aortic stenosis, leading to the recommendation that early intervention is not indicated to prevent irreversible myocardial damage in patients with isolated aortic stenosis. Chronic pressure overload is far better tolerated in children than in adults with remodeling resulting in hyperdynamic function and inevitably normal cardiac function after correction. Despite the risks associated with intervention, it is a common practice in pediatric cardiology to intervene at an arbitrary pressure gradient rather than wait for symptoms or evidence of ventricular dysfunction. Prevention of progressive and irreversible myocardial dysfunction is the usual justification for this practice, which almost certainly results in most patients having intervention before it is needed. Unfortunately, stenosis tends to be recurrent and intervention often results in compounding pressure with volume load due to new or increased valve insufficiency. All of these factors as well as the risk of sudden death need to be considered when recommending timing for intervention in aortic stenosis. Considerable data in children are accumulating concerning the success and recurrence rates for balloon dilation of congenital aortic stenosis and the incidence and severity of iatrogenic valve insufficiency, but fewer data concerning myocardial outcome in children have been reported.

Aortic coarctation

Coarctation of the aorta can be seen as an isolated lesion but is often associated with other forms of congenital heart disease. Because of the complexity of differentiating between the effects of aortic arch obstruction and those of coexistent hemodynamically significant defects, virtually all investigations of myocardial mechanics in these patients have been conducted in the isolated form. Similar to aortic stenosis, coarctation of the aorta can be seen in the neonatal period with either acute and at times even catastrophic onset or as a chronic condition. The neonatal presentation with congestive heart failure secondary to afterload excess parallels the presentation of critical aortic stenosis in infancy, and similarly resolves with elimination of the elevated wall stress, either through surgical treatment of the arch obstruction or through compensatory hypertrophy. However, beyond the neonatal period the natural histories of coarctation and aortic stenosis are quite distinct. Although rarely observed today, patients with untreated coarctation are at high risk for congestive heart failure and myocardial dysfunction in their third and fourth decade. In contrast, patients with congenital aortic stenosis are at extremely low risk of myocardial failure, even though the absolute level of pressure overload is frequently far higher in aortic stenosis. Although the pathophysiology of this difference is not entirely understood, there are several pertinent observations.

Effects of coarctation on systolic myocardial mechanics

In contrast to the enhanced systolic function that is typical of aortic stenosis, with coarctation systolic function is normal or depressed, even when contractility is normal. Both observations are related to the differences in ventriculoarterial interactions in the two diseases. As shown in Fig. 11.5, coarctation is associated with elevated end-systolic pressure, and indeed the pressure at end-systole is often more elevated than pressure earlier in systole. The hypertrophic response, driven by peak stress, is sufficient to normalize peak stress, which occurs in early systole, but is inadequate to normalize end-systolic stress. As a result of the elevated end-systolic stress, myocardial shortening is depressed. The chronic elevation of wall stress has been observed in other circumstances to lead to myocardial injury and failure, possibly because it is associated with elevated per-fiber myocardial oxygen consumption.

In contrast to the risk for excess afterload, depressed function, and impaired contractility associated with unrepaired coarctation, increased systolic function and enhanced load-independent indices of contractility have been reported in patients following successful repair of coarctation of the aorta during childhood [50]. The etiology of these persistent changes of myocardial mechanics remains unclear. Persistent elevation of myocardial contractility in these patients is difficult to explain, particularly as chronic ventricular hypertrophy is known to be associated with contractile dysfunction in older patients and in animal models. As discussed above with regard to aortic stenosis, these observations may in fact at least in part be secondary to misrepresentation of fiber shortening through reliance on endocardial-based indices of ventricular function. In the reports of enhanced function in patients after coarctation repair, left ventricular performance has been assessed using indices based on the phasic variation in chamber size, such as ejection fraction and fractional shortening. Endocardial-derived indices correctly quantify chamber properties of the left ventricle since they indicate the change in chamber volume that occurs over the course of the cardiac cycle. As such they are appropriate for assessing the pump function of the heart as reflected by stroke volume and cardiac output. However, muscle function of the heart is most correctly measured as myocardial fiber shortening. Depending on ventricular configuration, chamber volume reduction during systole may not correlate closely with fiber shortening. Under such circumstances, endocardial indices do not accurately reflect myocardial function. The issue can be conceptualized by modeling the left ventricle as a series of concentric shells (Fig. 11.6). Myocardial contraction is accompanied by wall thickening with greater inward movement of the endocardial and subendocardial myocardium than the subepicardial myocardium (Fig. 11.7). In fact, there is a progressive, nonlinear rise in fiber shortening from the subepicardial to the subendocardial fibers. Estimates of fiber shortening based on endocardial excursion therefore overestimate average transmural fiber shortening—an effect that is directly related to the thickness-to-dimension ratio [50]. This implies that fiber shortening is most severely overestimated by endocardial indices in the presence of hypertrophy [58]. Hence, transmural mean myocardial fiber shortening may be depressed despite normal endocardial excursion; less intramural shortening is required for the same total systolic wall thickening and endocardial displacement in ventricles with concentric hypertrophy. This misrepresentation of fiber mechanics has been found to be clinically important in subjects with left ventricular hypertrophy secondary to systemic hypertension, where it can lead to a failure to recognize depressed fiber shortening [9].

In studies of midwall and endocardial left ventricular mechanics in normal children and young adults compared with a group of patients who had varying degrees of residual arch obstruction after coarctation repair, indices derived from endocardial dimensions were found to overestimate myocardial function and contractility in the postcoarctation patients [50]. Based on the analysis of midwall mechanics, this misrepresentation was found to relate to the known failure of endocardial indices to reflect the magnitude of transmural variation in fiber shortening. As predicted by theory, the extent of this misrepresentation was proportional to the end-systolic thickness-to-dimension ratio and was therefore most significant in patients with concentric hypertrophy. Although the magnitude of elevation of

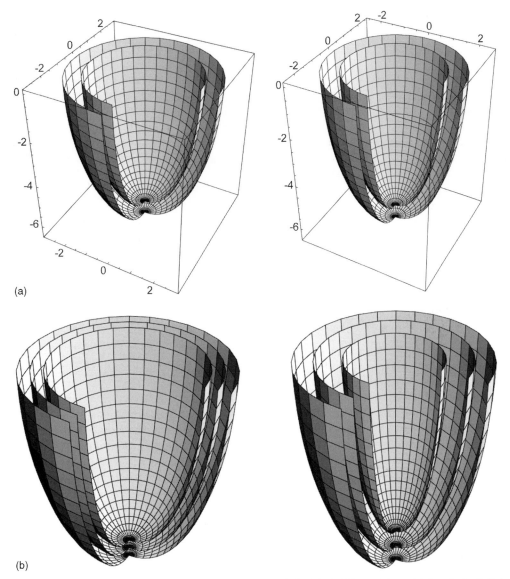

Figure 11.6 The ventricle can be modeled as a series of concentric shells. (a) The left ventricle modeled as single-shelled prolate ellipsoid with the endocardial and epicardial surfaces shown at end-diastole (left figure) and end-systole (right figure). (b) The endocardial, midwall, and epicardial shells are shown at end-diastole (left figure) and end-systole (right figure), dividing the myocardium into an inner shell between the endocardial and midwall surfaces and an outer shell between the midwall and epicardial surfaces. The greater thickening of the inner shell is evident (a phenomenon that is presented quantitatively in Fig. 11.7 for this model).

contractility in patients after coarctation repair was less marked when midwall indices were used, it was still significant, indicating that this effect may not be purely artifactual. There is at present no clear explanation for the finding of persistently elevated myocardial contractility in these postcoarctation repair patients. In animal models with experimentally in-

duced pressure overload, and in adult humans with hypertension, left ventricular hypertrophy is commonly associated with a gradual deterioration in left ventricular function and contractility. Similar evaluation of myocardial mechanics using indices based on midwall indices has not been reported in children with aortic stenosis, who, as described above, have

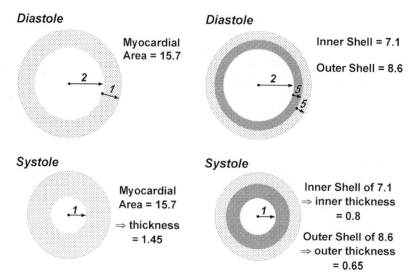

Figure 11.7 Myocardial contraction is accompanied by wall thickening with greater inward movement of the endocardial and subendocardial myocardium than the subepicardial myocytes secondary to geometric factors. Standard endocardial indices for the short axis plane are shown in the left diagrams with a percent wall thickening of 45%. The difference in thickening for inner and outer shells for the same magnitude of shortening calculated using midwall shortening is illustrated in the right diagrams. The percent wall thickening is greater for the inner shell (60%) than for the outer shell (30%).

also been reported to manifest enhanced contractility based on endocardial-derived indices. Thus, at present we are left with the interesting but unexplained possibility that pressure overload hypertrophy in children is indeed associated with an enhanced contractile state.

Right ventricular pressure overload

Chronic right ventricular pressure overload is encountered in many forms of congenital heart disease. Compared with the left ventricle, there have been far fewer clinical studies evaluating the impact on the right ventricular myocardium, but there are several relevant clinical observations. Although exercise capacity is impaired, the long-term natural history of isolated pulmonary stenosis is surprisingly benign, with a normal life expectancy free from onset of irreversible right ventricular failure, suggesting that chronic isolated pressure overload is well tolerated by the right ventricle. In contrast, many patients with previously palliated congenital heart disease have chronic right ventricular dysfunction and right-sided failure in association with right ventricular pressure overload. For example, conduits implanted between the right ventricle and the

pulmonary artery in children for treatment of pulmonary atresia nearly always develop obstruction over time, with right ventricular pressure often rising to suprasystemic levels in association with right ventricular dysfunction, leading to the clinical syndrome of congestive heart failure. The situation for these patients is obviously complex. The right ventricle has been subject to one or more surgical procedures including a right ventriculotomy. The conduits are also invariably associated with significant regurgitation and secondary right ventricular volume overload. Differentiating which of volume overload, right ventricular scar, and pressure overload in these patients is responsible for the myocardial injury is generally not possible.

In animals, contractility of the right ventricle, based on load-independent indices of contractility derived from pressure–volume relations, rises above normal acutely after pulmonary artery banding [59] and after sustained right ventricular pressure overload of 8 weeks' duration [60]. Despite this, cardiac output and right ventricular ejection fraction fall. Whether a similar situation exists in humans with chronic pressure overload is unclear due to the paucity of studies using load-independent indices of contractility in the right ventricle. An important implication of these observations is that myocardial injury cannot be presumed simply because right ventricular systolic performance is impaired. Impaired ejection fraction despite enhanced contractility implies that afterload (fiberstress) is elevated, preload is reduced, or both. There have been few clinical investigations of right ventricular wall stress in children, primarily because the complex anatomy and irregular shape of the right ventricle prevents utilization of standard geometric-based formulas. Nevertheless, there is no evidence that the control mechanisms for ventricular hypertrophy are substantially different for the right compared with the left ventricular myocardium, indicating that hypertrophy with normalization of stress is the anticipated compensatory response. In contrast, there is reason to expect that pressure overload hypertrophy would diminish preload reserve. The impact of right ventricular hypertrophy in response to pressure or volume overload on right ventricular diastolic properties parallels that of the left ventricle with diminished right ventricular compliance in pressure overload hypertrophy and increased right ventricular compliance in right ventricular volume overload [61]. Similarly, right ventricular pressure overload results in impaired right ventricular relaxation, whereas volume overload has little or no effect on relaxation [62]. Elevated systemic venous pressure is more poorly tolerated than similar elevations in pulmonary venous pressure and has a far more profound impact on venous return. Abnormal right ventricular diastolic function consequent to pressure overload would therefore be predicted to impair right ventricular preload, ejection fraction, and cardiac output, even if contractility is normal.

Chronic right ventricular pressure overload also affects left ventricular size and function. There is generally a significant reduction in left ventricular diastolic volume, related to two apparent mechanisms. First, the diminished right ventricular output results in reduced pulmonary venous return and left ventricular filling. This is the series aspect of ventricular interdependence. Second, elevation in right ventricular pressure abolishes the normal transseptal pressure gradient, displacing the interventricular septum leftward to a neutral or even reversed position, changing the shape and reducing the diastolic capacitance of the left ventricle. This represents the parallel aspect of ventricular interaction. The phenomenon of diastolic and systolic ventricular interdependence is a well-documented phenomenon, as recently reviewed by Santamore and Dell'Italia [63]. Right ventricular pressure overload leads to reduced left ventricular diastolic and end-systolic volume, stroke volume, and ejection fraction. These changes are primarily related to perturbations in left ventricular geometry and are immediately reversible upon elimination of right ventricular hypertension.

References

1. Aoyagi T, Fujii AM, Flanagan MF, *et al.* Transition from compensated hypertrophy to intrinsic myocardial dysfunction during development of left ventricular pressure-overload hypertrophy in conscious sheep. Systolic dysfunction precedes diastolic dysfunction. Circulation 1993; 88:2415–2425.
2. Boutin C, Wernovsky G, Sanders SP, *et al.* Rapid two-stage arterial switch operation: Evaluation of left ventricular systolic mechanics after an acute pressure overload stimulus in infancy. Circulation 1994; 90:1294–1303.
3. Gentles TL, Colan SD. Wall stress misrepresents afterload in children and young adults with abnormal left ventricular geometry. J Appl Physiol 2002; 92:1053–1057.
4. Vendelin M, Bovendeerd PHM, Engelbrecht J, *et al.* Optimizing ventricular fibers: Uniform strain or stress, but not ATP consumption, leads to high efficiency. Am J Physiol Heart Circ Physiol 2002; 283:H1072–H1081.
5. Gopalan SM, Flaim C, Bhatia SN, *et al.* Anisotropic stretch-induced hypertrophy in neonatal ventricular myocytes micropatterned on deformable elastomers. Biotechnol Bioeng 2003; 81:578–587.
6. Colan SD. Noninvasive assessment of myocardial mechanics—A review of analysis of stess-shortening and stress-velocity. Cardiol Young 1992; 2:1–13.
7. Takaoka T, Esposito G, Mao L, *et al.* Heart size-independent analysis of myocardial function in murine pressure overload hypertrophyh. Am J Physiol Heart Circ Physiol 2002; 282:H2190–H2197.
8. Cingolani OH, Yang XP, Cavasin MA, *et al.* Increased systolic performance with diastolic dysfunction in adult spontaneously hypertensive rats. Hypertension 2003; 41:249–254.
9. De Simone G, Devereux RB, Celentano A, *et al.* Left ventricular chamber and wall mechanics in the presence of concentric geometry. J Hypertens 1999; 17:1001–1006.
10. Katz AM. Maladaptive growth in the failing heart: The cardiomyopathy of overload. Cardiovasc Drugs Ther 2002; 16:245–249.

11. Kiss E, Ball NA, Kranias EG, *et al.* Differential changes in cardiac phospholamban and sarcoplasmic reticular Ca^{2+}-ATPase protein levels—Effects on Ca^{2+} transport and mechanics in compensated pressure-overload hypertrophy and congestive heart failure. Circ Res 1995; 77:759–764.

12. Naqvi RU, Del Monte F, O'Gara P, *et al.* Characteristics of myocytes isolated from hearts of renovascular hypertensive guinea pigs. Am J Physiol Heart Circ Physiol 1994; 266:H1886–H1895.

13. Colan SD. Mechanics of left ventricular systolic and diastolic function in physiologic hypertrophy of the athlete heart. Cardiol Clin 1997; 15:355–372.

14. Noguchi T, Camp P Jr, Alix SL, *et al.* Myosin from failing and non-failing human ventricles exhibit similar contractile properties. J Mol Cell Cardiol 2003; 35:91–97.

15. Anversa P, Olivetti G. Cellular basis of physiologic and pathologic myocardial growth. In: Page E, Fozzard HA, Solaro RJ, eds., Handbook of Physiology, Section 2: The Cardiovascular System, The Heart, Vol I. Oxford University Press, Oxford, pp 75–144, 2001.

16. Beltrami AP, Urbanek K, Kajstura J, *et al.* Evidence that human cardiac myocytes divide after infarction. N Engl J Med 2001; 334:1750–1757.

17. Kajstura J, Leri A, Finato N, *et al.* Myocyte proliferation in end-stage cardiac failure in humans. Proc Natl Acad Sci USA 1998; 95:8801–8805.

18. Capasso JM, Bruno S, Cheng W, *et al.* Ventricular loading is coupled with DNA synthesis in adult cardiac myocytes after acute and chronic myocardial infarction in rats. Circ Res 1992; 71:1379–1389.

19. Hein S, Arnon E, Kostin S, *et al.* Progression from compensated hypertrophy to failure in the pressure-overloaded human heart—Structural deterioration and compensatory mechanisms. Circulation 2003; 107:984–991.

20. Nishio ML, Ornatsky OI, Craig EE, *et al.* Mitochondrial biogenesis during pressure overload induced cardiac hypertrophy in adult rats. Can J Physiol Pharmacol 1995; 73:630–637.

21. Kozàkovà M, De Simone G, Morizzo C, *et al.* Coronary vasodilator capacity and hypertension-induced increase in left ventricular mass. Hypertension 2003; 41:224–229.

22. Kolar F, Papousek F, Pelouch V, *et al.* Pressure overload induced in newborn rats: Effects on left ventricular growth, morphology, and function. Pediatr Res 1998; 43:521–526.

23. Flanagan MF, Aoyagi T, Currier JJ, *et al.* Effect of young age on coronary adaptations to left ventricular pressure overload hypertrophy in sheep. J Am Coll Cardiol 1994; 24:1786–1796.

24. Flanagan MF, Fujii AM, Colan SD, *et al.* Myocardial angiogenesis and coronary perfusion in left ventricular pressure-overload hypertrophy in the young lamb: Evidence for inhibition with chronic protamine administration. Circ Res 1991; 68:1458–1470.

25. Rakusan K, Flanagan MF, Geva T, *et al.* Morphometry of human coronary capillaries during normal growth and the effect of age in left ventricular pressure-overload hypertrophy. Circulation 1992; 86:38–46.

26. Hirota H, Chen J, Betz UA, *et al.* Loss of a gp130 cardiac muscle cell survival pathway is a critical event in the onset of heart failure during biomechanical stress. Cell 1999; 97:189–198.

27. Wernig F, Xu QB. Mechanical stress-induced apoptosis in the cardiovascular system. Prog Biophys Mol Biol 2002; 78:105–137.

28. Boutin C, Jonas RA, Sanders SP, *et al.* Rapid two-stage arterial switch operation: Acquisition of left ventricular mass after pulmonary artery banding in infants with transposition of the great arteries. Circulation 1994; 90:1304–1309.

29. Litwin SE, Katz SE, Weinberg EO, *et al.* Serial echocardiographic-Doppler assessment of left ventricular geometry and function in rats with pressure-overload hypertrophy: Chronic angiotensin-converting enzyme inhibition attenuates the transition to heart failure. Circulation 1995; 91:2642–2654.

30. Hill JA, Karimi M, Kutschke W, *et al.* Cardiac hypertrophy is not a required compensatory response to short-term pressure overload. Circulation 2000; 101:2863–2869.

31. Satoh S, Ueda Y, Koyanagi M, *et al.* Chronic inhibition of Rho kinase blunts the process of left ventricular hypertrophy leading to cardiac contractile dysfunction in hypertension-induced heart failure. J Mol Cell Cardiol 2003; 35:59–70.

32. Esposito G, Rapacciuolo A, Prasad SVN, *et al.* Genetic alterations that inhibit in vivo pressure-overload hypertrophy prevent cardiac dysfunction despite increased wall stress. Circulation 2002; 105:85–92.

33. Sano M, Schneider MD. Still stressed out but doing fine—Normalization of wall stress is superfluous to maintaining cardiac function in chronic pressure overload. Circulation 2002; 105:8–10.

34. Meguro T, Hong C, Asai K, *et al.* Cyclosporine attenuates pressure-overload hypertrophy in mice while enhancing susceptibility to decompensation and heart failure. Circ Res 1999; 84:735–740.

35. Ding B, Price RL, Borg TK, *et al.* Pressure overload induces severe hypertrophy in mice treated with cyclosporine, an inhibitor of calcineurin. Circ Res 1999; 84:729–734.

36. Mukawa H, Toki Y, Shimauchi A, *et al.* Pressure overload per se rather than cardiac angiotensin converting enzyme activity may be important in the development of rat cardiac hypertrophy. J Hypertens 1997; 15:1027–1032.

37. Morisco C, Sadoshima J, Trimarco B, *et al.* Is treating cardiac hypertrophy salutary or detrimental: The two faces of Janus. Am J Physiol Heart Circ Physiol 2003; 284:H1043–H1047.

38. Janicki JS, Brower GL. The role of myocardial fibrillar collagen in ventricular remodeling and function. J Card Fail 2002; 8:S319–S325.

39. Baicu CF, Stroud JD, Livesay VA, *et al.* Changes in extracellular collagen matrix alter myocardial systolic performance. Am J Physiol Heart Circ Physiol 2003; 284:H122–H132.

40. Janicki JS, Matsubara BB. Myocardial collagen and left ventricular diastolic dysfunction. In: Gaasch WH, LeWinter MM, eds., Left Ventricular Diastolic Function. Lea & Febiger, Philadelphia, pp 125–140, 1993.

41. Schwartz SM, Gordon D, Mosca RS, *et al.* Collagen content in normal, pressure, and pressure-volume overloaded developing human hearts. Am J Cardiol 1996; 77:734–738.

42. Harris TS, Baicu CF, Conrad CH, *et al.* Constitutive properties of hypertrophied myocardium: Cellular contribution to changes in myocardial stiffness. Am J Physiol Heart Circ Physiol 2002; 282:H2173–H2182.

43. Yamamoto K, Masuyama T, Sakata Y, *et al.* Myocardial stiffness is determined by ventricular fibrosis, but not by compensatory or excessive hypertrophy in hypertensive heart. Cardiovasc Res 2002; 55:76–82.

44. Stroud JD, Baicu CF, Barnes MA, *et al.* Viscoelastic properties of pressure overload hypertrophied myocardium: Effect of serine protease treatment. Am J Physiol Heart Circ Physiol 2002; 282:H2324–H2335.

45. Brower GL, Janicki JS. Contribution of ventricular remodeling to pathogenesis of heart failure in rats. Am J Physiol 2001; 280:H674–H683.

46. Jugdutt BI, Joljart MJ, Khan MI. Rate of collagen deposition during healing and ventricular remodeling after myocardial infarction in rat and dog models. Circulation 1996; 94:94–101.

47. Badenhorst D, Maseko M, Tsotetsi OJ, *et al.* Cross-linking influences the impact of quantitative changes in myocardial collagen on cardiac stiffness and remodelling in hypertension in rats. Cardiovasc Res 2003; 57:632–641.

48. Borow KM, Colan SD, Neumann A. Altered left ventricular mechanics in patients with valvular aortic stenosis and coarctation of the aorta: Effects on systolic performance and late outcome. Circulation 1985; 72:515–522.

49. Dorn GW II, Donner R, Assey ME, *et al.* Alterations in left ventricular geometry, wall stress, and ejection performance after correction of congenital aortic stenosis. Circulation 1988; 78:1358–1364.

50. Gentles TL, Sanders SP, Colan SD. Misrepresentation of left ventricular contractile function by endocardial indexes: Clinical implications after coarctation repair. Am Heart J 2000; 140:585–595.

51. Colan SD, Parness IA, Spevak PJ, *et al.* Developmental modulation of myocardial mechanics: Age- and growth-related alterations in afterload and contractility. J Am Coll Cardiol 1992; 19:619–629.

52. Akinboboye OO, Reichek N, Bergmann SR, *et al.* Correlates of myocardial oxygen demand measured by positron emission tomography in the hypertrophied left ventricle. Am J Hypertens 2003; 16:240–243.

53. Schwitter J, Eberli FR, Ritter M, *et al.* Myocardial oxygen consumption in aortic valve disease with and without left ventricular dysfunction. Br Heart J 1992; 67:161–169.

54. Carroll JD, Carroll EP, Feldman T, *et al.* Sex-associated differences in left ventricular function in aortic stenosis of the elderly. Circulation 1992; 86:1099–1107.

55. Hess OM, Villari B, Krayenbuehl HP. Diastolic dysfunction in aortic stenosis. Circulation 1993; 87(suppl 4):IV73–IV76.

56. Colan SD. The adult athlete with congenital heart disease. In: Williams RA, ed., The Athlete and Heart Disease: Diagnosis, Evaluation, and Management. Lippincott Williams & Wilkins, Philadelphia, 1998, pp 79–107.

57. Keane JF, Driscoll DJ, Gersony WM, *et al.* Second natural history study of congenital heart defects: Results of treatment of patients with aortic valvar stenosis. Circulation 1993; 87(suppl):I16–I27.

58. Aoyagi T, Mirsky I, Flanagan MF, *et al.* Myocardial function in immature and mature sheep with pressure-overload hypertrophy. Am J Physiol 1992; 262:H1036–48.

59. Hon JK, Steendijk P, Khan H, *et al.* Acute effects of pulmonary artery banding in sheep on right ventricle pressure-volume relations: Relevance to the arterial switch operation. Acta Physiol Scand 2001; 172:97–106.

60. Leeuwenburgh BPJ, Helbing WA, Steendijk P, *et al.* Biventricular systolic function in young lambs subject to chronic systemic right ventricular pressure overload. Am J Physiol Heart Circ Physiol 2001; 281:H2697–H2704.

61. Pasipoularides A, Shu M, Shah A, *et al.* Right ventricular diastolic function in canine models of pressure overload, volume overload, and ischemia. Am J Physiol Heart Circ Physiol 2002; 283:H2140–H2150.

62. Pasipoularides AD, Shu M, Shah A, *et al.* Right ventricular diastolic relaxation in conscious dog models of pressure overload, volume overload, and ischemia. J Thorac Cardiovasc Surg 2002; 124:964–972.

63. Santamore WP, Dell'Italia LJ. Ventricular interdependence: Significant left ventricular contributions to right ventricular systolic function. Prog Cardiovasc Dis 1998; 40:289–308.

CHAPTER 12

Ventricular Function in Volume Overload Lesions

Steven D. Colan, MD

Exposure of one or more chambers of the heart to an increased output characterizes most forms of congenital heart disease. Some of these lesions, particularly those involving valvar insufficiency, can also be encountered in acquired forms of heart disease, where the physiology is quite similar despite differences in anatomic substrate. Despite apparent similarities, the myocardial response to the excess workload varies depending on the particular lesion involved. Thus, although it is both possible and useful to develop a paradigm for the impact on the myocardium of excess volume work, it is also necessary to account for the fact that volume overload of similar magnitude may have markedly different impact depending on the underlying cause. This approach will be taken in this presentation, utilizing aortic regurgitation as a model of the myocardial response to volume overload, recognizing this as a prototype of "pure" left ventricular volume overload, and certainly the lesion for which there is the largest body of relevant data. Subsequently, the other forms of volume overload (Table 12.1) will be examined with respect to their impact on myocardial function and the potential reasons for observed differences from aortic regurgitation will be explored.

Pathophysiology of myocardial response to volume overload

The primary albeit not the only mechanism for the secondary cardiac structural alterations in response to chronic volume overload is believed to be direct load-induced hypertrophy. It has been shown that mechanical load is a sufficient and perhaps a primary factor responsible for growth regulation in adult mammalian myocardium [1]. Mechanotransduction is the biochemical cellular response to mechanical stimuli, and is an important although incompletely understood factor in cardiac pathophysiology [2]. Load induction of growth appears to be mediated by regulation of gene expression in response to the direct physical effects of cellular stress and strain mediated through a large number of cytosolic signaling pathways (reviewed by Molkentin and Dorn [2]). The structural changes in the myocardium that occur in response to these stimuli have been labeled myocardial *remodeling*, which can be defined as the molecular, cellular, and interstitial changes within the myocardium that result in changes in ventricular size and function. The term *reverse remodeling* is commonly used to refer to reversal of these changes, although it is worth noting that the latter term is to a large degree redundant since direction of change is not necessarily implied in the term *remodeling*. To add to the confusion, some authors use the term *remodeling* in a much more restrictive sense to refer exclusively to the progressive dilation that accompanies myocardial failure [3]. The term is more generally used in the broader sense as defined above, and this convention is used here.

The description of the heart in terms of its mechanical behavior has been a productive endeavor that has elucidated many aspects of cardiac growth and function. However, the terminology used in discussions of cardiac mechanics is sometimes unfamiliar to students of medicine, who are usually more familiar with biochemical and biologic processes than with engineering terms for the mechanical

Table 12.1 Common Forms of Heart Disease in Children with Volume Overload.

Left-sided volume overload	Right-sided volume overload	Biventricular volume overload
Aortic regurgitation	Pulmonic regurgitation	Ventricular septal defect
Mitral regurgitation	Tricuspid regurgitation	Chronic anemia
Patent ductus arteriosus	Atrial septal defect	Complete heart block
Aortopulmonary shunts	Anomalous pulmonary veins	Single ventricle

properties of materials. The potential for confusion has been compounded by the fact that many terms that have a precise meaning in the engineering world have other more general use that leads to an intuitive but often incorrect understanding. Certain of these terms are used pervasively in the discussions that follow, and it is therefore worthwhile to provide explicit definitions. From a mechanical point of view, *stress* is the intensity of force and is expressed as the force per unit cross-sectional area. For the ventricle, wall stress refers to total force in the ventricular wall. Calculation of wall stress is derived from the Laplace relationship, which states that wall stress is proportional to (pressure)(radius of curvature)/(wall thickness). The implications of this equation are that higher pressure, larger cavity size, or thinner walls will increase wall stress (see Fig. 11.1 in Chapter 11). *Fiberstress* refers to the stress exerted on individual myofibers, taking into consideration the absence of radially oriented fibers and the impact of the transmural hydrostatic pressure gradient on the individual fibers [4]. The term *strain* refers to the deformation produced by the application of a force, a dimensionless quantity that is the fractional or percent change relative to an initial or unstressed state. For example, when a myofiber lengthens in response to diastolic fiberstress, the percent lengthening relative to the unstressed length is the *strain* and the speed at which the fiber lengthens is the *strain rate*. The mechanical characterization of materials is based on the experimentally determined relationship between stress and strain for that material, relationships that are called the *constitutive equations*.

The pattern of myocardial growth in response to increased ventricular workload (Fig. 12.1 and 12.2) can be conceptually divided into addition of myofibrils in series (increase in chamber volume) and in parallel (increase in wall thickness) [5]. The increase in diastolic wall stress that results from an increased volume of diastolic filling causes elongation of the individual myofibers. The myocardial response to this

(a)

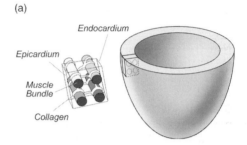

(b) Concentric Hypertrophy

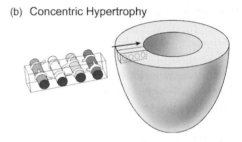

(c) Eccentric Hypertrophy and
Dilated Cardiopathy

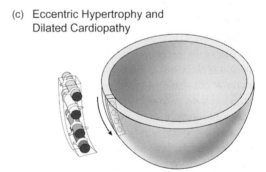

Figure 12.1 Hypertrophy can be divided conceptually into concentric hypertrophy, where fibers are added in parallel, increasing wall thickness without a change in cavity volume, and eccentric hypertrophy, where fibers are added in series, resulting in an increase in volume with little change in wall thickness.

increased preload (diastolic fiber length) is the formation of new fibers in series. The addition of additional of fibers in series increases the diastolic capacitance of the ventricle, thereby reducing diastolic

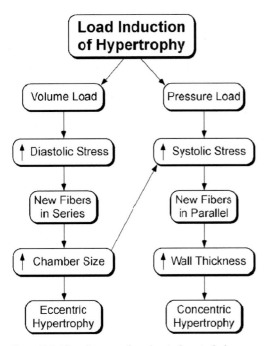

Figure 12.2 Flow diagram of mechanical control of hypertrophy. See text for description.

wall stress. This process of eccentric hypertrophy, defined as a proportional rise in ventricular mass and volume, continues until diastolic wall stress is normalized, thereby turning off the stimulus to hypertrophy [6]. A similar servomechanism controls concentric hypertrophy (rise in ventricular mass without an equivalent increase in volume), although in this case the stimulus for addition of fibers in parallel is peak systolic wall stress. Hemodynamic circumstances that lead to an elevation of peak wall stress stimulate the addition of parallel fibers—a process that continues until the rise in the ratio of wall thickness to cavity dimension is sufficient to reduce peak systolic wall stress to the equilibrium point. It is important to note that because of the dependence of wall stress on the ratio between thickness and dimension, in eccentric hypertrophy the increase in cavity volume that results from the addition of fibers in series would result in a rise in systolic wall stress were there no increase in wall thickness. In fact, the cardiac adaptation to volume overload involves the addition of sufficient new fibers in series to normalize diastolic wall stress and the addition of sufficient fibers in parallel to normalize the thickness-to-dimension ratio. These two servomechanisms operate independently to maintain diastolic and systolic fiber loads

in the normal range in spite of higher operant volume. The ventricular structural modifications parallel adaptations at the cellular level where myocardial structural changes in response to pressure overload manifest as an increase in myocyte cross-sectional area, whereas increased volume load due to physiologic growth or aortocaval fistula leads to proportional growth of myocyte length and diameter (the increase in cross-sectional area accounts for about two thirds of the increase in myocyte volume and increase in length accounts for the other third) [7]. This concept has acquired further support from observations in an isolated myocyte preparation that permitted observation of the hypertrophic response to stretching forces applied during different periods of the cell cycle. When a stretching force was applied during diastole (analogous to increased diastolic stress), cell elongation was noted, whereas application of systolic force caused the cells to become thicker [8].

Although mechanical factors represent the underlying stimulus to hypertrophy in hemodynamic overload lesions, age, sex, genetic, and neurohumoral influences play important modulating roles. Clinically, it has long been appreciated that widely divergent magnitudes of hypertrophy can be encountered in patients with seemingly similar severity of hemodynamic overload. Age modulation of the hypertrophic response has been identified in normal children [9]. Similarly, athletes engaged in similar training programs manifest a broad range of physiologic hypertrophy [10]. The contribution of genetic variation to the hypertrophic response has been verified in an animal model of aortic stenosis [11], where an identical degree of pressure overload for an identical period of time in animals of the same size and sex resulted in hypertrophy that varied from inadequate to exuberant. Interestingly, in this animal model the wall thickness prior to creation of aortic stenosis was highly predictive of the hypertrophic response.

The role of the neurohumoral systems in the hypertrophic response has been the subject of intense investigation, in particular with regard to the potential for pharmacologic interventions. Initially, investigations in the infarct model indicated that mechanical load was not the sole determinant of hypertrophy. There followed a series of experimental and clinical intervention studies supporting the hypothesis that hormonal systems contribute substantially to the remodeling process [12]. These observations laid the foundation for the broad spectrum of physiologic, cellular, and molecular studies that now characterize the study of myocardial remodeling. Manipulation of the neurohumoral systems will impact the remodeling process in a predictable fashion through heart rate and blood pressure changes. More controversial and less well understood are the potential direct effects on the myocardium, independent of altered hemodynamics [13]. For example, in pressure overload and congestive heart failure models, there is evidence that the renin–angiotensin system may be a critical component in the mechanotransduction of hemodynamic stress to cardiac hypertrophy. Pharmacologic inhibition of angiotensin converting enzyme (ACE) can slow or prevent remodeling in both of these circumstances. The influence of this system on the volume overload appears to be significantly different. For example, although cardiac angiotensin-II is upregulated in animal models of volume overload, in an ACE knockout model in mice, ACE underexpression did not prevent volume overload cardiac hypertrophy or left ventricular dysfunction [14]. In a canine model of acute mitral regurgitation, administration of ACE receptor blockers not only failed to attenuate the remodeling process, there was in fact greater elongation of cardiomyocytes in the treated animals, despite decreased systemic vascular resistance and reduced local expression of the renin–angiotensin system [15]. Similarly, ramipril therapy in dogs with chronic mitral regurgitation suppressed angiotensin II to normal levels but had no effect on ventricular dilation or hypertrophy [16]. In contrast to pressure overload hypertrophy, volume-overload-induced hypertrophy appears related to a decreased rate of protein degradation without a substantial increase in the rate of protein synthesis [17]. In addition to the obvious implications concerning the potential nonutility of ACE inhibitor therapy in mitral regurgitation, these observations illustrate the potential pitfalls in assuming that observations in one model of ventricular hypertrophy will be applicable in another.

Aortic regurgitation

Aortic regurgitation in children is occasionally a primary but more commonly a secondary lesion. As a primary disorder, it is typically a slowly progressive lesion with adequate time for ventricular compensation. Sudden onset can be encountered as a consequence of aortic valvotomy for valve stenosis, surgical valve injury, or due to endocarditis, with the potential to overwhelm the capacity for ventricular adaptive mechanisms. Valvar aortic regurgitation is not the most common cause of ventricular volume overload in congenital heart disease, but it represents a relatively "pure" form of increased diastolic load without the complicating issues of left-to-right shunts, pulmonary hypertension, and biventricular overload. It, therefore, serves as a reasonable model to consider the impact of volume overload on the myocardium.

Effects of aortic regurgitation on systolic myocardial mechanics

Numerous studies have permitted the natural history of myocardial mechanics in aortic regurgitation to be described in some detail. The sequence of events in chronic aortic regurgitation can be divided into four stages of variable duration (Fig. 12.3). During the first and the most prolonged period, ventricular dilation is accompanied by proportional compensatory hypertrophy. Because of the appropriate matching between the increase in volume and mass, the mass-to-volume ratio, fiberstress, and ventricular performance all remain within the normal range. The second phase is characterized by the first manifestations of the failure of the compensatory mechanisms. Ventricular volume continues to rise, but hypertrophy fails to keep pace, resulting in a state of inadequate hypertrophy as manifested by a fall in the mass-to-volume ratio and persistent elevation of peak systolic stress. The elevated afterload (end-systolic stress) results in a fall in the rate and magnitude of systolic fiber shortening, clinically detectable as reduced shortening fraction and velocity of fiber shortening. At least for some period of time after the appearance of inadequate hypertrophy, contractility remains normal. Adequate hypertrophy is also a critical factor for maintenance of normal left ventricular geometry, since the initially normal configuration of the ventricle becomes more spherical as mass-to-volume ratio falls. In the third phase, afterload mismatch increases with a further rise in wall stress and fall in function, but at this stage the ventricular dysfunction is exacerbated by reduced myocardial contractility. Over the short term, the impaired contractility may be fully reversible, and valve replacement results in complete recovery of function and contractility. After a variable period of time, the

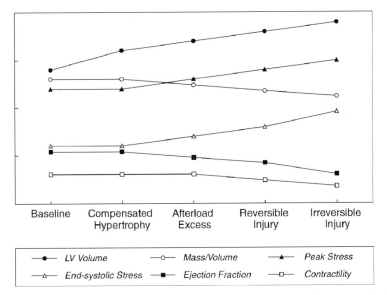

Figure 12.3 Stages in the natural history of aortic regurgitation. The timing and relative changes in each of the variables are illustrated. See text for more details.

stage of irreversible myocardial injury is reached. At this stage in the disease, valve replacement may still be tolerated and is likely to be beneficial but does not restore myocardial mechanics to normal.

The sequence of events in acute aortic regurgitation depends on the severity of regurgitation, but may include the rapid onset of congestive heart failure. The pace of the ventricular response to severe acute aortic regurgitation is entirely distinct from chronic aortic regurgitation, but the pathophysiology is quite similar. Because of the absence of a period of compensatory hypertrophy, the patient is thrown immediately into the second stage of the sequence described above, with inadequate hypertrophy, afterload mismatch, and impaired function. At this stage, a rapid increase in mass can lead to normalization of afterload and function. However, it is frequently the case that adequate hypertrophy is not achieved, and the patient rapidly passes into the stage of reversible followed by irreversible contractile dysfunction.

Effects of aortic regurgitation on diastolic ventricular mechanics

Ventricular remodeling in response to volume overload is teleologically a process designed to increase ventricular capacitance. The ventricular adaptation to chronic volume overload and to the elimination of volume overload has been studied in a number of human and animal models. Chronic volume overload in

both humans and animals is associated with a rightward shift of the diastolic pressure–volume relationship (Fig. 12.4). Because of the adaptation to chronic volume overload, for any given filling volume the end-diastolic pressure will be lower than would be found in a normal heart at the same volume. In addition to the aforementioned mechanism of cellular elongation and addition of fibers in series, there is considerable evidence that alterations in collagen content and structure contribute to this change in ventricular compliance. For example, creation of

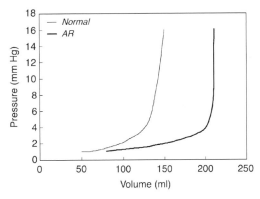

Figure 12.4 Change in the left ventricular diastolic pressure–volume relation in response to left ventricular volume overload. The diastolic pressure–volume curve is shifted to the right, with a lower slope value in the operant range, consistent with improved compliance.

an aortocaval fistula is associated with activation of myocardial matrix metalloproteinases within 12 h, and after 1 week there is nearly a 50% reduction in myocardial collagen content with shift of the end-diastolic pressure–volume curve to the right [18]. Collagen is not the only protein that has been associated with altered ventricular compliance. Titin, the largest known protein, constitutes 10% of the myofibrillar protein mass of the myocardium and is the main source of passive resistance to stretch in the cardiac myocyte. Variable expression of titin isoforms is an effective method of modulating passive muscle stiffness. Changes in titin and collagen are currently believed to explain most of the variation in passive properties of cardiac muscle [19]. In contrast, there is little evidence that "myocyte slippage" contributes to chamber dilation in volume overload [20].

The reduction in collagen content and increase in myocardial compliance early in the disease stands in contrast to the later phases where myocardial fibrosis and impaired myocardial compliance are typical and appear to play an important role in the transition to ventricular dysfunction [21]. In animal models, severe fibrosis of aortic regurgitation is associated with normal collagen content and in fact accumulation of noncollagen elements within the extracellular matrix, specifically fibronectin, accounts for the fibrosis and appears to be a primary response to the augmentation of cyclic strain [21].

In addition to the direct effects of altered extracellular matrix composition on myocardial compliance, the extracellular matrix also appears to play an important role in maintenance of ventricular shape. Progressive ventricular dilation is associated with a transition to a more spherical configuration. From a geometric perspective, this change in shape maximizes diastolic ventricular capacitance. For any given surface area, the sphere is the geometric shape with the maximum contained volume. Therefore, the transition to a spherical ventricular shape can be seen as an adaptation that optimizes the ventricle for diastolic capacitance. For any given ventricular mass, a larger ventricular volume can be accommodated by the transition from a prolate spheroid to a sphere. Thus, if indeed the limits to hypertrophy have been reached, the only means by which the ventricle can increase its diastolic volume is to become more spherical. Unfortunately, this change in configuration comes at a cost with respect to systolic workload and function since the fall in mass-to-volume ratio associated with the transition to a spherical configuration results in a higher global average fiber-stress. The rise in ventricular afterload that is associated with ventricular ensphering causes a fall in systolic function and may well play a role in the progressive deterioration in contractility that generally follows.

Mechanism of decompensation

Because of the potential therapeutic implications, the sequence of events involved in the transition from compensated to inadequate hypertrophy and from reversible to irreversibly impaired contractility has been a particular focus of investigation. The onset of inadequate hypertrophy is the first of these two events and in fact appears to create the circumstances that lead to the onset of contractile dysfunction [22]. For example, we have shown that sustained elevation of wall stress in animals results in the rapid appearance of impaired contractility [23]. Wall stress is a major determinant of myocardial oxygen consumption, myocardial blood flow is impeded by elevated wall stress (particularly in diastole), and myocardial neovascularization is generally reduced in hypertrophy, all of which could contribute to a chronic substrate deficit. Afterload reduction has been shown to slow the rate of progression of myocardial dysfunction, supporting the concept that inadequate hypertrophy with secondary elevation in wall stress plays an important primary role. The factors that control hypertrophy and may determine this transition from compensated to inadequate hypertrophy are therefore of primary importance to understanding the pathophysiology of this disease.

It is uncertain why the normal feedback control mechanism for hypertrophy fails, but abnormalities of diastolic function provide a potential mechanism. The mechanical coupling between load and induction of hypertrophy is stretch-induced distortion of the cell membrane. Therefore, if changes in diastolic properties of the ventricle disrupt the transmission of the signal and the increase in load does not result in the expected distortion of the cell membrane, the normal compensatory hypertrophy mechanism fails. This is the mechanism for myocardial atrophy in patients with constrictive pericarditis. Although the process of ventricular remodeling in response to volume overload improves *ventricular* compliance, patients with severe aortic regurgitation manifest depressed *myocardial* compliance in the more advanced stages of the disease. Furthermore, the presence of severe fibrosis and the onset of impaired myocardial compliance precedes the onset of inadequate hypertrophy and depressed myocardial contractility in patients with aortic regurgitation [21].

The fact that despite enhanced ventricular capacitance severe aortic regurgitation is associated with impaired myocardial compliance demonstrates the fallacy in certain commonly held beliefs about aortic regurgitation. Aortic regurgitation has been described as a preload-enhanced condition in which augmented preload may mask the effects of contractile dysfunction. This misunderstanding is in part related to ambiguity in the use of the term "preload." Although clinically end-diastolic pressure and stress are often used as indices of preload, in terms of myocardial function preload refers to the Frank–Starling mechanism, wherein increased end-diastolic myocardial length results in greater systolic shortening. The conclusion that preload is elevated in aortic regurgitation is based on the observation that end-diastolic stress and pressure are often elevated in patients with severe aortic regurgitation. Inasmuch as the preload effect is determined by end-diastolic fiber length, elevated diastolic stress will result in elevated end-diastolic fiber length only if the myocardium has a normal stress–strain relationship. However, elevation of filling pressures and diastolic stress secondary to aortic regurgitation is seen only in patients who have depressed myocardial compliance. By definition, the noncompliant myocardium experiences less than normal fiber stretch for any given diastolic stress. Therefore, filling pressure and diastolic stress are not valid indices of myocardial preload in patients with severe aortic regurgitation. Preload conditions are normal during the compensated stages of the disease, since the process of compensatory dilation and hypertrophy described above leads to normalization of diastolic stress and pressure with preserved myocardial compliance. As the disease progresses, decreased compliance develops before the onset of inadequate hypertrophy and depressed myocardial contractility. There is, in fact, an inverse relation between myocardial compliance and ejection fraction [24], indicating that the poorly compliant ventricle results in a *reduced* preload state in spite of elevated diastolic stress and pressure. Thus, augmented preload probably exists only in the acute phase of the disease, before compensatory hypertrophy and dilation ensue, whereas chronic aortic regurgitation is characterized by normal or reduced preload.

Cardiac mechanics in children with aortic regurgitation

There are surprisingly few data on cardiac mechanics in infants and children. There have been considerable relevant data gathered in adults, but there are obstacles to their direct application in young patients, as will be discussed. Nevertheless, it is clear that the natural history of aortic regurgitation in all age groups is characterized by a prolonged period of compensated hypertrophy that insidiously gives way to myocardial decompensation. Intervention for symptoms or exercise limitation alone is rarely necessary because these are rarely encountered without ventricular dysfunction, thereby allowing aortic valve replacement to be delayed until the risk of irreversible myocardial injury exceeds surgical risk. Aortic valve replacement may not reverse abnormalities in contractility even though loading conditions and function may improve. It is also well documented that the incidence of sudden death in aortic regurgitation is vanishingly rare [25]. The decision as to when to intervene for chronic aortic regurgitation therefore depends primarily on the potential for normalization of ventricular and myocardial mechanics after valve repair or replacement. Although there are many published studies in adults examining risk factors for poor outcome after aortic valve replacement, there are no published data in children. The best that can be done at this time is to review the experience in adults [25] and attempt to extrapolate this to children.

Timing of intervention in aortic regurgitation

The severity of aortic regurgitation is an important factor in the decision to intervene. Moderate aortic regurgitation (regurgitant fraction <40%) is extremely well tolerated and benefit from intervention at this stage of the disease is unlikely. There are a number of methods of assessing severity of regurgitation. Regurgitant *volume*, the volume of blood that reenters the left ventricle through the aortic valve during diastole, is determined by the regurgitant orifice area, arterial impedance and capacitance, diastolic properties of the left ventricle, and the length of diastole. Regurgitant *fraction*, the percent of ventricular stroke volume that the regurgitant volume represents, is additionally dependent on forward stroke volume, which is determined by the interplay of ventricular and vascular properties. Regurgitant fraction is the best measure of the relative magnitude of the additional volume load imposed on the left ventricle and can be determined by a variety of noninvasive methods, the most accurate of which is magnetic resonance imaging [26]. Myocardial contractility is only one of the many factors that determine regurgitant fraction, making it a poor predictor of outcome after aortic valve replacement. Although many pediatric cardiologists recommend intervention for aortic regurgitation based on severity alone, this approach cannot be recommended. Regurgitant index reflects the severity of regurgitation and therefore the severity of the hemodynamic burden, but gives little indication of the adequacy of compensatory mechanisms or of temporal location in the long natural history of this disorder.

Ventricular dilation is one of the primary compensatory mechanisms in volume overload lesions, a process that has been described in some detail above. During the compensated stage of the disease, myocardial function is preserved and the magnitude of dilation is proportional to the severity of regurgitation. After the transition to inadequate hypertrophy with or without contractile dysfunction, normalization of end-diastolic pressure and stress fails, and additional dilation may ensue. However, as discussed above, the myocardium is relatively noncompliant at this stage of the disease, limiting ventricular dilation despite the onset of contractile failure. Since contractile state is at most an indirect determinant of end-diastolic pressure and volume, the numerous other factors upon which they depend reduce their utility in detecting the onset of myocardial contractile failure. Consequently, absolute left ventricular end-diastolic volume or short axis dimension have been found to be weak predictive of outcome after surgery in some series in adults, but an equal number of series have found that even very marked dilation was not predictive [27].

Systolic function, assessed as ejection fraction or shortening fraction, represents the end result of the interaction of intrinsic myocardial properties (contractility, compliance, hypertrophic response) and extrinsic factors (severity of regurgitation, vascular properties, autonomic tone). Even though systolic function is an unreliable measure of contractility in these patients, postoperative survival and ventricular function correlate with preoperative ejection

fraction [28]. The load dependence of ejection fraction and all ejection phase indices limits their capacity to distinguish abnormal contractility from altered loading conditions. Each of the adverse changes that are characteristic of the natural history of myocardial mechanics would be expected to reduce ejection fraction: onset of diminished myocardial compliance with secondary fall in preload effect, afterload excess secondary to inadequate hypertrophy, and myocardial contractile deficit. Systolic dysfunction is therefore a sensitive though not specific indicator of myocardial dysfunction, but is generally accepted as an indication for intervention on the regurgitant aortic valve. However, due to the lack of specificity of this index, if systolic dysfunction is used to select patients for intervention then many patients will undergo surgery prematurely.

Ejection fraction response to exercise has been suggested as a measure of functional reserve that improves on the specificity of the resting ejection fraction, but prospective trials found that this index was not prognostically significant in patients with aortic regurgitation. Exercise elicits a complex interplay of vascular and autonomic reflexes, abnormalities of which could either mask or mimic myocardial dysfunction. The loading changes that occur in response to exercise are therefore unlikely to be similar in patients with and without heart disease. As an example of this, exercise-induced tachycardia disproportionately reduces diastolic time, reducing absolute and relative regurgitant volume. In patients with aortic regurgitation, regurgitant fraction falls during exercise secondary to the tachycardia-induced fall in net diastolic time. Therefore, in contrast to normals, exercise results in preload reduction in patients with aortic regurgitation, inducing a fall in ejection fraction even if contractility is normal. This explains why the major correlates of the change in ejection fraction during exercise are severity of regurgitation and peripheral vascular response with a very weak relationship to myocardial contractility.

End-systolic fiber length is determined only by afterload and contractility. This preload independence makes this a potentially attractive index, particularly in patients with volume overload lesions such as aortic regurgitation. Virtually all studies that have evaluated end-systolic ventricular size have found outcome to be related to absolute end systolic volume or dimension. However, the magnitude of systolic dilation that represents an incremental risk has varied enormously among studies (end-systolic volume index 90–200 mL/m^2, end-systolic diameter 48–60 mm). Although associated with outcome, absolute end-systolic ventricular size has not been found to be highly predictive of outcome. This limitation is predictable from the afterload dependence of end-systolic volume, since afterload excess often precedes depressed contractility in this disease.

Several investigators have reported the evaluation of myocardial contractility in severe aortic regurgitation using indices based on pressure–volume analysis. The slope of the end-systolic pressure–volume relation (E_{max}) is a load-independent index of contractility. When determined from end-systolic pressure and volume points obtained during changes in afterload induced by methoxamine or nitroprusside infusions during atrial pacing, E_{max} correlated with normalization of systolic function after aortic valve replacement [29]. Although these data confirm the observation that contractility is a major determinate of outcome, E_{max} is extremely cumbersome to use for routine clinical use and there are many technical issues associated with its use. For example, E_{max} is dependent on absolute ventricular size and the correct method for adjusting for ventricular size has not been determined—a limitation that is particularly problematic in growing children with aortic regurgitation.

An alternative method of separating the contribution of impaired contractility from excess afterload is to adjust ejection-phase indices for afterload (end-systolic stress) [30]. In a long term and comprehensive study comparing many of the indices that have been reported to be useful in predicting outcome after aortic valve replacement, the change in stress-adjusted ejection fraction from rest to exercise was found to be the single best predictor of all cardiac end-points [31]. The practical obstacles to the methodology used in this study are considerable, particularly in children. An additional important observation in this report was that stress-adjusted fractional shortening at rest was not significantly predictive of outcome. The limitations to the ability of this index to detect impaired contractility are primarily related to its dependence on preload, as has been shown in other clinical situations [32]. In contrast to ejection phase indices that reflect only percent fiber shortening (fractional shortening and ejection fraction), indices based on rate of fiber shortening such as the velocity of circumferential fiber shortening

are independent of preload and overcome the limitations of stress-adjusted shortening indices [33]. The stress-adjusted velocity of shortening index has not been evaluated in adult patients with aortic regurgitation. In our own experience in children, this load-independent index of contractility has been highly predictive of the onset of symptoms and ventricular dysfunction, but the number of patients who have undergone aortic valve replacement or repair has been too small to provide a meaningful evaluation of the utility of this index in assessing the risk for postoperative ventricular dysfunction.

There are no published recommendations for timing of intervention in children with aortic regurgitation. The guidelines for the management of patients with valvular heart disease published by the joint task force of the American College of Cardiology and the American Heart Association [25] include recommendations for adolescents and young adults. In the absence of meaningful data in this age group, these recommendations were based on extrapolation from the adult series. The recommended indications for intervention include onset of symptoms, ventricular dysfunction (ejection fraction <50%), and diastolic ventricular dimension more than 4 standard deviations (SD) beyond the body surface area adjusted normal value.

The controversial aspect of these recommendations relates to criteria for intervention in asymptomatic patients and how to manage younger children. In comparison to adult risk factors, the criteria that were selected are biased toward early intervention. The magnitude of ventricular dysfunction, assessed as ejection fraction, that has been identified as a risk factor in 10 published series in adults has ranged from 30 to 45% with a median value of 45%. The most recent series to have evaluated end-diastolic dimension as a risk factor found that even a value of 5.6 SD above the normal mean was not predictive [34]. Our personal experience in children has been similar to that described in the series by Klodas et al. [34], with many children who have extreme ventricular dilation experiencing no evidence of deterioration for many years. Figure 12.5 illustrates this phenomenon in one patient who would have been operated at a body surface area considerably below his adult stature had he undergone surgery when his end-diastolic dimension was 4 SD above the mean. As illustrated, his ventricular recovery after aortic valvuloplasty was rapid and dramatic, with

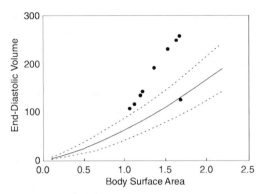

Figure 12.5 Example of the natural history of left ventricular volume in a growing child with severe aortic regurgitation and the response to aortic valvuloplasty. The solid and interrupted lines are the normal mean and 95% confidence intervals, respectively, for end-diastolic volume (mL) versus body surface area (m^2). The solid dots show the progressive rise in end-diastolic volume out of proportion to the rise in body surface area, with the last point representing the dramatic and rapid normalization of end-diastolic volume following successful surgical aortic valvuloplasty.

an end-diastolic dimension at the mean for body surface area within 2 weeks of surgery. End-systolic dimension more than 4.5 SD above normal has been consistently identified as a risk factor in adult series, but is not included in the criteria for young adults. Until better data are available concerning outcome in children and adolescents, intervention for asymptomatic patients with normal ventricular function will remain highly controversial.

Mitral regurgitation

Mitral regurgitation is also encountered as both a congenital and acquired lesion in children. The vast majority of children with mitral regurgitation have an underlying congenital anomaly of the mitral valve, regardless of whether regurgitation is present early in life. Although it is difficult to find population statistics, at Boston Children's Hospital the most common cause of moderate to severe mitral insufficiency is atrioventricular canal defects (also known as atrioventricular septal defects) of one form or another. Although the valve in this defect may be insufficient from the time of birth, often the severity of regurgitation increases following closure of the ventricular septal defect. The natural history of this

disease is complicated by the coexistence of atrial and ventricular defects and the need for surgical repair of the associated defects. Mitral regurgitation can also be encountered in association with many other forms of congenital and acquired heart disease. However, at least in the United States, the occurrence of chronic moderate to severe mitral regurgitation in children who have no other cardiac abnormalities is actually quite rare. Defining the natural history of the disease in children is therefore far more complex because of the confounding effects of the coexistent cardiac lesions.

Physiology of mitral regurgitation

The factors that influence the severity of mitral regurgitation, as defined by the Torricelli principle, include the systolic pressure gradient between the left ventricle and the left atrium, the duration of systole, and the effective regurgitant orifice area, as

$$V_{MR} = ROA \, C \, T_s (P_{LV} - P_{LA})^{0.5}$$

where V_{MR} is the mitral valve regurgitant volume, ROA the regurgitant orifice area, C the constant, T_s the duration of systole, P_{LV} the left ventricular mean systolic pressure, and P_{LA} is the mean left atrial pressure during ventricular systole. Although changes in ventricular and atrial pressure are theoretically important, the range over which the pressure gradient between the ventricle and atrium varies is small and the importance is further reduced by the square root relationship. For example, in a patient with $V_{MR} = 30$ mL, $P_{LV} = 100$, and $P_{LA} = 5$, dropping the mean systolic pressure to 90 will only reduce the regurgitant volume to 28.4 mL. In general, the regurgitant orifice area makes the largest contribution to changes in severity of mitral regurgitation. Left ventricular size and geometry are important determinants of mitral regurgitant orifice area both chronically in response to progressive ventricular dilatation and acutely in response to inotropic and vasodilator interventions. Reduction in left ventricular end-diastolic diameter results in concomitant reduction in the diameters of the subvalvar area and mitral valve apparatus, improving mitral valve closure. The reduction in the regurgitant orifice area decreases regurgitant volume.

Mitral valve anatomy is a primary determinant of the magnitude of variation in the regurgitant orifice area. For example, a calcified valve with a fixed systolic orifice tends to undergo minimal change in the regurgitant orifice over the course of systole. Intrinsically, dynamic valve abnormalities such as mitral valve prolapse have a variable regurgitant orifice both over the course of the cardiac cycle and also in response to positional changes in ventricular filling. So-called "functional" mitral regurgitation in association with ventricular dysfunction and dilation generally improves in conjunction with improved function and reduced cavity size. The valve anatomy typical of the postoperative atrioventricular septal defect typically manifests significant variability of regurgitant orifice size, with the largest regurgitant orifice in early systole progressively falling over the course of ejection, and progressing chronically in conjunction with annular dilatation.

Effects of mitral regurgitation on systolic myocardial mechanics

There has been considerable debate about ventricular mechanics in mitral regurgitation. Because the regurgitant volume is ejected into the low pressure left atrium [35], mitral regurgitation has been described by some authors as characterized by reduced ventricular afterload, thereby possessing the potential to mask myocardial dysfunction. This notion persists in the literature despite considerable evidence to the contrary. In fact, the "Guidelines for the management of patients with valvular heart disease" sponsored by a joint working group of the American Heart Association and the American College of Cardiology presents this theory in their discussion of chronic mitral regurgitation [25]. According to this hypothesis, the ventricular dysfunction becomes apparent only after valve replacement eliminates the "low impedance leak" into the left atrium. There are two assumptions intrinsic to this hypothesis: (1) mitral regurgitation represents a low impedance leak and (2) the low impedance leak reduces ventricular afterload, with the potential to mask ventricular dysfunction. Although possible under certain acute conditions, both of these assumptions are generally incorrect with regard to chronic mitral regurgitation. The presence of mitral regurgitation creates parallel circuits exiting the left ventricle. As in any flow circuit, the relative impedance in each circuit determines the proportion of flow that goes into each circuit. Clinically, severe mitral regurgitation is characterized by a regurgitant fraction of about 50%; that is, an approximately equal volume is ejected into the aorta and into the left atrium. Equal volumes of flow

exiting in both directions implies that even in severe regurgitation the impedances in both circuits are about equal. Patients with less severe regurgitation have regurgitant fractions less than 50%, physiology that is possible only if impedance to ejection into the left atrium is higher than the aortic impedance. Thus, in patients with chronic mitral regurgitation, the impedance to flow into the left atrium is at a minimum approximately equal to aortic impedance, which does not really qualify as a "low impedance leak."

Nevertheless, the presence of a parallel circuit invariably reduces the *net* impedance to flow out of the ventricle. When the ventricle has an additional outlet, the overall impedance to ejection is less than it would be if only one mode of egress were present. This is the case for ventricular septal defects with left-to-right flow as well. Therefore, although the concept of a "low impedance leak into the left atrium" is incorrect, it is correct that the presence of mitral regurgitation reduces the impedance to ejection compared to what it would be without the mitral regurgitation, assuming aortic impedance does not change. If aortic impedance rises, as is often the case in patients with reduced cardiac output and neurohumoral activation, net impedance to ejection may be elevated despite the presence of mitral regurgitation.

The second assumption in the foregoing hypothesis is the notion that reduced ejection impedance leads to subnormal ventricular afterload. Afterload is a somewhat nonspecific term that has been used in a general sense to refer to the force resisting myocardial shortening and is not synonymous with impedance to ejection. As discussed above, this force is quantifiable as fiberstress. The extent of myocardial systolic shortening is determined by myocardial contractility and end-systolic fiberstress. Therefore, from the point of view of myocardial shortening, end-systolic fiberstress is the appropriate measurement of afterload. Fiberstress is directly related to pressure and volume and inversely related to wall thickness. Ejection impedance contributes to end-systolic fiberstress insofar as it is one of the determinates of ventricular pressure. However, even if ejection pressure were low in mitral regurgitation (which is generally not the case), this is not a sufficient condition to create a state of low fiberstress, that is, reduced afterload. In fact there has now been a great deal of work showing that in *acute* mitral regurgitation, arterial pressure and fiberstress may be low; but in *chronic* compensated mitral regurgitation, fiberstress is normal to elevated; and in *chronic* decompensated mitral regurgitation, fiberstress and wall stress are invariably elevated [15,36–40]. This issue has been reviewed in a recent editorial by Gaash [41].

Effects of mitral regurgitation on diastolic myocardial mechanics

Compared with aortic regurgitation, there is far less information available concerning diastolic function in mitral regurgitation. Chamber stiffness has been reported to be below normal, as would be expected after remodeling in response to chronic volume overload [39]. In contrast, muscle stiffness was normal, emphasizing the dissociation between chamber and muscle properties that frequently accompanies the remodeling process.

Timing of intervention in mitral regurgitation

Similar to the aortic regurgitation, the decision as to when intervention is justified in chronic mitral regurgitation is based on data examining risk factors for poor outcome after mitral valve replacement. The situation in mitral valve disease is more complex than in aortic disease, because left ventricular dysfunction is seen commonly after mitral valve replacement even in patients with normal ventricular function preoperatively. Although, as discussed above, there has been a common misconception that there is a sudden rise in afterload after mitral valve replacement that is secondary to elimination of a "low impedance leak" into the left atrium, there is in fact ample evidence to indicate that end-systolic fiberstress is similar or lower after valve replacement, regardless of whether there has been deterioration in ventricular function [39]. In fact, ejection performance commonly deteriorates even in patients who have a fall in afterload (end-systolic fiberstress), indicating that some other mechanism is responsible. Importantly, the new appearance of ventricular dysfunction is a common observation in valve replacement, but not after valve repair. This argues strongly that this is not a hemodynamic effect.

Based on a number of investigations in animal models and in humans, an understanding has developed that this postoperative deterioration is related in part to the disruption of the internal organization of the left ventricle due to removal of the mitral valve apparatus. In humans undergoing mitral valve replacement, retention of chordae and papillary muscles is associated with better postoperative function. In animal models, chordal detachment is associated with a decline in maximum elastance, and reattachment results in a return to normal. Preservation of the chordae tendineae and papillary muscles during mitral valve replacement is now accepted as a requisite to preserve postoperative regional and global function. Because of the confounding effect of the surgical technique, it is much more difficult to interpret studies reporting risk factors for mitral valve replacement. Most reported adult series have found ventricular dysfunction to be a negative prognostic factor. However, it is not clear whether severe dilation with normal systolic function represents a predictor of poor outcome. In adults, elevated end-systolic dimension (>45 mm) has been found to be a risk factor for death and persistent ventricular dilation, but is rarely present in patients with normal ventricular function. In one series in children, ventricular end-diastolic dimension, end-systolic dimension, and shortening fraction were not related to postoperative outcome [42]. There was a marked fall in ventricular end-diastolic dimension in the immediate postoperative period, accompanied by a significant reduction in fractional shortening. This is the anticipated response to valve replacement or successful valve repair, with radical reduction in filling volume leading to acute preload reduction. Importantly, ventricular size and function returned to normal at late follow-up, even in the subjects with preoperative reduced ventricular function. Again, similar to the circumstances for aortic insufficiency, in children the relevance of risk factors derived in adults with mitral regurgitation is questionable. The utility of load-independent indices in predicting outcome after mitral valve repair has not been explored.

Ventricular septal defect

The natural history of ventricular septal defects is strikingly different from aortic or mitral regurgitation. In contrast to the generally chronic and slowly progressive hemodynamic load of valve regurgitation, the relative volume overload from ventricular septal defects tends to increase rapidly within the first few months of life and diminish thereafter. A large left-to-right shunt secondary to a ventricular septal defect will generally prompt intervention early in life because of congestive heart failure and concerns about pulmonary vascular injury. The acute impact on ventricular mechanics and the potential for recovery after surgical closure have been studied, but there are no data about the long-term ventricular response to these large volume loads. At the other end of the spectrum, small ventricular defects are not associated with significant left ventricular volume overload. The intermediate sized defects that do not result in elevated pulmonary pressure but are associated with a significant left ventricular volume overload do prompt concerns about the potential long-term impact on left ventricular function. Although this concern figures prominently in patient management, there is surprisingly little information about how large the shunt must be to create a risk and how great this risk is. In one study of 9 patients aged 12–24 years (median = 21 years) with a left-to-right shunt of 1.4–2.1 (median = 1.7), the left ventricle was noted to be dilated and hypertrophied but no abnormalities of ventricular function were present [43]. In aortic or mitral regurgitation, a regurgitant fraction of >40% is considered severe and represents a risk for long-term myocardial deterioration. In the presence of a moderate ventricular septal defect, although diastolic left-to-right flow is often present, the modest size of the defect restricts this to the point that most of the volume overload burden is borne by the left ventricle. Since there is twice the normal volume of flow entering the left ventricle, a 2-to-1 pulmonary-to-systemic flow ratio is therefore the equivalent volume overload to that of a 50% regurgitant fraction in aortic or mitral regurgitation. Therefore, extrapolating from the experience in adults with left ventricular volume overload secondary to mitral or aortic regurgitation leads to the conclusion that a ventricular septal defect with a 2-to-1 or greater left-to-right shunt entails the risk of myocardial deterioration over the long term.

The factors that influence the severity of left-to-right shunting in ventricular septal defects include those discussed above concerning mitral regurgitation with several additional complicating features. The volume of flow that traverses the defect during systole relates to the size of the defect, the transseptal pressure difference as determined by systemic and pulmonary arterial impedance and capacitance, and the length of systole. The volume of diastolic flow is also related to the size of the defect and the length of diastole, but in this case the pressure difference across the septum is determined by the diastolic properties of the left and right ventricles. This

is a complex situation because of ventricular interdependence wherein increased diastolic filling of the right ventricle actually diminishes left ventricular capacitance. Except for very large ventricular septal defects, the volume of flow through the defect during diastole is usually a small percentage of the total flow. Also similar to the situation for mitral regurgitation, the presence of the ventricular septal defect reduces the overall impedance to ejection but for the same reasons as discussed in relationship to mitral regurgitation, myocardial afterload assessed as end-systolic fiberstress is normal, not reduced.

During the acute phase, congestive heart failure can be seen and is sometimes though not always associated with depressed contractility [44]. Outcome after closure of ventricular septal defect appears to depend on the age at which surgery is performed. Patients repaired early in life (<2 years) were found to have normal ventricular size, function, wall stress, and contractility at a mean follow-up of 5 years. In contrast, patients who were more than 2 years old at the time of surgery were found to have persistent left ventricular dilation and hypertrophy with a ventricular shape that was persistently more spherical than normal at a mean follow-up of 7 years, despite the fact that their magnitude of volume overload was less than that in the younger cohort. This experience is similar to that in single ventricle patients, who are at risk of irreversible remodeling if volume-unloading surgery is delayed beyond 2 years [45].

Right ventricular volume overload (atrial septal defect and pulmonary regurgitation)

Right ventricular volume overload when the right ventricle is in the subpulmonary position is important both for its potential impact on the right ventricular myocardium and also for the known adverse impact it has on left ventricular function. In many forms of right ventricular volume overload, such as totally anomalous pulmonary venous connection and atrial septal defect, the time of surgical repair is dictated by factors other than the onset of ventricular dysfunction. However, pulmonary regurgitation is a problem of escalating importance in congenital heart disease, as many patients are now experiencing right ventricular failure as a consequence of 20–30 years of hemodynamically significant right ventricular volume overload. In many congenital cardiac anomalies, but particularly in tetralogy of Fallot, successful relief of right ventricular outflow tract obstruction results in an incompetent pulmonary valve. The severity of regurgitation in terms of regurgitant volume is generally modest early after repair but tends to progress for a number of reasons. As discussed with reference to mitral regurgitation, for both the mitral and aortic valve, regurgitant orifice size is the primary determinant of severity of regurgitation. The pressure gradient between the originating and recipient chamber is relatively unimportant for the valves in the systemic circulation inasmuch as the range of variation in the pressure gradient is by necessity quite small. The circumstances are quite different on the pulmonary side, where the regurgitant orifice is generally quite large and severity of regurgitation is determined by other factors. The right ventricle has marked hypertrophy at the time of repair of pulmonary stenosis, thereby reducing its compliance. Because the diastolic pressure difference between the right ventricular and pulmonary artery in the absence of pulmonary artery hypertension is quite low, a moderate rise in diastolic pressure in the right ventricular due to reduced compliance can have a significant impact on regurgitant volume. However, the primary determinant of the severity of pulmonary regurgitation is the capacitance of the central pulmonary arteries. Central pulmonary artery capacitance is generally well below normal in patients with tetralogy of Fallot because of the common association of pulmonary artery hypoplasia. Although both of these circumstances limit pulmonary regurgitation early after surgery, the trend over time toward increased pulmonary artery compliance and right ventricle compliance leads to a progressive rise in regurgitant volume. The clinical experience in these patients has made it clear that the right ventricle, similar to the left, is subject to myocardial injury secondary to the chronic volume overload. Similarly, extrapolating from the experience with the left ventricle with regard to outcome after intervention has resulted in pulmonary valve replacement being undertaken when symptoms appear or if the right ventricle progresses to extreme dilation or manifests moderate to severe dysfunction. At present, there are insufficient data to know whether this is the correct approach.

The secondary effects of right ventricular volume overload on left ventricular function have received considerable attention. Patients with significant right ventricular volume overload are commonly noted to have low normal or mildly depressed left ventricular function, with relatively low left ventricular diastolic volume. The phenomenon has been explained on the basis of adverse diastolic ventricular interaction. Diastolic ventricular interaction is well documented in both the normal and diseased heart. In animal preparations, as left ventricular volume rises the right ventricular pressure–volume curve shifts leftward and becomes steeper. Increased right ventricular volume has the same effect on the diastolic properties of the left ventricle (Fig. 12.6). The decreased chamber compliance of either the left or right ventricle that is observed with independent volume loading of the contralateral ventricle is observed with or without an intact pericardium, although the presence of the pericardium increases the strength of the coupling. The intrinsic nature of the property is related to the anatomic continuity of muscle fibers between the two chambers and the ventricular septum.

Diastolic ventricular interaction is always present, provided there are two separate ventricles, and accounts for a number of physiologic observations [46]. The normal respiratory variation in left ventricular stroke volume relates to a rise in right ventricular filling during inspiration with consequent reduction in left ventricular compliance. The influence of the pericardium on the magnitude of ventricular coupling is readily apparent when the influence of the pericardium rises, as with pericardial constriction or effusion. Under these circumstances, increased diastolic ventricular interaction accounts for the exaggerated effects of respiration on stroke volume characteristic of pericardial tamponade. Less widely appreciated is the fact that this phenomenon is absent when diastolic ventricular interaction is not possible. For example, pulsus paradoxus is never observed in patients with single ventricle physiology, even if tamponade is severe, because ventricular interaction cannot take place. This is an issue of major clinical importance to the postoperative Fontan population, who have a high incidence of pericardial effusion but in whom none of the usual clinical indices of tamponade (pulsus paradoxus, respiratory variation in mitral inflow velocity, diastolic collapse of the right atrium or ventricle) are valid.

The pathophysiology of left ventricular dysfunction in patients with right ventricular volume overload secondary to pulmonary or tricuspid

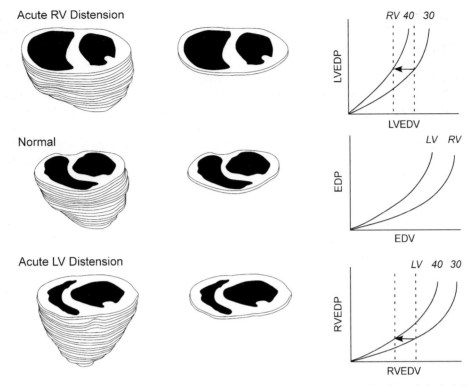

Figure 12.6 Ventricular interaction is bidirectional. Acute elevation of right ventricular (RV) volume shifts the left ventricular (LV) diastolic pressure–volume curve to the left, consistent with decreased compliance. The right ventricle responds in a similar fashion to an acute rise in LV volume.

regurgitation is secondary to increased diastolic ventricular interaction. Although this has been attributed to decreased preload, the situation is in fact more complex than this. Although the increased filling of the right ventricle impairs left ventricular compliance, myocardial compliance remains normal [47]. As discussed above, from the perspective of myocardial function the preload effect relates to end-diastolic fiber length. When the ventricle is noncircular, as is the case with right ventricular volume overload, left ventricular volume is reduced despite the fact that end-diastolic fiber length is normal. Recent work in our laboratory demonstrated the mechanism of the seemingly paradoxical finding that despite reduced ejection fraction, fiber shortening is normal. During early systole fiber shortening results in transformation of the distorted left ventricular shape to a spheroidal configuration with no change in ventricular volume, because a sphere is the geometric shape with the minimum surface area relative to the contained volume. We found that 15–20% of fiber shortening was expended in the process of shape change, prior to the onset of ventricular ejection, resulting in a reduced ejection fraction despite normal fiber shortening (Fig. 12.7).

There are some important differences in ventricular mechanics between the common forms of right ventricular volume overload. The potential for a positive feedback loop exists in pulmonary regurgitation. The rise in left ventricular filling pressure mediated by increased diastolic ventricular interaction can result in more severe pulmonary regurgitation consequent to the transmission of this pressure rise to diastolic pulmonary artery pressure. The absence of this phenomenon in association with tricuspid regurgitation may contribute to the fact that tricuspid regurgitation is less subject to progression compared with pulmonary regurgitation. In contrast to pulmonary regurgitation, a large atrial septal defect is intrinsically associated with equilibration of right and left ventricular diastolic pressure, which means that the elevation in left atrial pressure that would be needed to normalize left ventricular filling in the face of reduced left ventricular compliance is impeded.

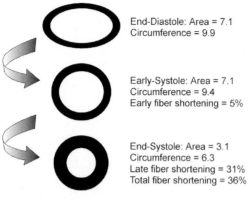

End-Diastole: Area = 7.1
Circumference = 9.9

Early-Systole: Area = 7.1
Circumference = 9.4
Early fiber shortening = 5%

End-Systole: Area = 3.1
Circumference = 6.3
Late fiber shortening = 31%
Total fiber shortening = 36%

Figure 12.7 Illustration of left ventricular shape change during the course of systole in the presence of right ventricular volume overload. The distorted left ventricle expends the initial 5% shortening on conversion of the ventricle to a circular shape, prior to the onset of area change and ventricular ejection. Although the total fiber shortening is 36%, only 31% is actually devoted to ventricular ejection.

The role of diastolic ventricular interaction as the cause of decreased left ventricular function secondary to right ventricular volume overload has important implications with regard to timing of intervention. There is ample evidence that as soon as the volume overload is eliminated, ventricular function normalizes. Perhaps the best model for this is transcatheter device closure of atrial septal defect. Under these circumstances, the change in physiology is virtually instantaneous, without the potentially confounding effects of an open pericardium, thoracotomy, cardiopulmonary bypass, and positive pressure ventilation. Investigations in our laboratory have documented that ventricular function returns to normal immediately, despite persistent right ventricular dilation. It is therefore reasonable to base timing of intervention for pulmonary regurgitation on issues such as symptoms and exercise tolerance and on the potential for right ventricular myocardial injury without concerns about permanent adverse effects on left ventricular function. At present, data concerning right ventricular outcome after pulmonary valve replacement in patients with pulmonary regurgitation are limited. Repair of atrial septal defect in adults is associated with persistent right ventricular dilation [48], whereas closure in children results in complete normalization of right ventricular morphology [49]. Similarly, adults with pulmonary regurgitation secondary to repair of tetralogy of Fallot have incomplete resolution of right ventricular dilation and fail to normalize right ventricular function after pulmonary valve replacement [50,51]. To date, this intervention has generally been undertaken late in the clinical course, since most patients who have undergone pulmonary valve replacement have right ventricular dysfunction at the time of intervention [52,53]. This circumstance is quite similar to the prior experience with aortic regurgitation, where historically intervention was delayed until the onset of symptoms. However, with the availability of sufficient outcome data to indicate that earlier intervention improved the preservation of left ventricular myocardial performance, timing of aortic valve replacement for aortic regurgitation is undertaken when there is evidence of left ventricular dysfunction, even in the absence of symptoms. Progress in determining the optimum timing of pulmonary valve replacement has been impeded by the fact that late survival of postoperative tetralogy of Fallot patients is a relatively recent phenomenon as well as limitations in the methodology for assessing right ventricular function. The more widespread availability of cardiac magnetic resonance imaging, which is unquestionably the most accurate clinically available method of assessing right ventricular function, has already had a considerable impact on the field and promises to drastically impact our management of these patients [50].

Functionally single ventricle hearts

The heart with a single or functionally single ventricle is invariably subject to volume overload early in life in order to sustain a reasonable level of arterial oxygenation. Ventricular function in the univentricular heart is considered separately elsewhere in this volume.

References

1. Ruwhof C, Van der Laarse A. Mechanical stress-induced cardiac hypertrophy: Mechanisms and signal transduction pathways. Cardiovasc Res 2000; 47:23–37.
2. Molkentin JD, Dorn GW. Cytoplasmic signalling pathways that regulate cardiac hypertrophy. Annu Rev Physiol 2001; 63:391–426.

3. Katz AM. Maladaptive growth in the failing heart: The cardiomyopathy of overload. Cardiovasc Drugs Ther 2002; 16:245–249.

4. Gentles TL, Colan SD. Wall stress misrepresents afterload in children and young adults with abnormal left ventricular geometry. J Appl Physiol 2002; 92:1053–1057.

5. Colan SD. The adult athlete with congenital heart disease. In: Williams RA, ed., The Athlete and Heart Disease: Diagnosis, Evaluation, and Management. Lippincott Williams & Wilkins, Philadelphia, pp 79–107, 1998.

6. Yamakawa H, Imamura T, Matsuo T, et al. Diastolic wall stress and ANG II in cardiac hypertrophy and gene expression induced by volume overload. Am J Physiol 2000; 279:H2939–H2946.

7. Gerdes AM, Clark LC, Capasso JM. Regression of cardiac hypertrophy after closing an aortocaval fistula in rats. Am J Physiol 1995; 268:H2345–H2351.

8. Yamamoto K, Dang QN, Maeda Y, et al. Regulation of cardiomyocyte mechanotransduction by the cardiac cycle. Circulation 2001; 103:1459–1464.

9. Colan SD, Parness IA, Spevak PJ, et al. Developmental modulation of myocardial mechanics: Age- and growth-related alterations in afterload and contractility. J Am Coll Cardiol 1992; 19:619–629.

10. Colan SD. Mechanics of left ventricular systolic and diastolic function in physiologic hypertrophy of the athlete heart. Cardiol Clin 1997; 15:355–372.

11. Koide M, Nagatsu M, Zile MR, et al. Premorbid determinants of left ventricular dysfunction in a novel model of gradually induced pressure overload in the adult canine. Circulation 1997; 95:1601–1610.

12. Cohn JN. Structural basis for heart failure: Ventricular remodeling and its pharmacological inhibition. Circulation 1995; 91:2504–2507.

13. Bader M. Role of the local renin-angiotensin system in cardiac damage: A minireview focussing on transgenic animal models. J Mol Cell Cardiol 2002; 34:1455–1462.

14. Perry GJ, Mori T, Wei CC, et al. Genetic variation in angiotensin-converting enzyme does not prevent development of cardiac hypertrophy or upregulation of angiotensin II in response to aortocaval fistula. Circulation 2001; 103:1012–1016.

15. Perry GJ, Wei CC, Hankes GH, et al. Angiotensin II receptor blockade does not improve left ventricular function and remodeling in subacute mitral regurgitation in the dog. J Am Coll Cardiol 2002; 39:1374–1379.

16. Dell'Italia LJ, Balcells E, Meng QC, et al. Volume-overload cardiac hypertrophy is unaffected by ACE inhibitor treatment in dogs. Am J Physiol 1997; 273:H961–H970.

17. Matsuo T, Carabello BA, Nagatomo Y, et al. Mechanisms of cardiac hypertrophy in canine volume overload. Am J Physiol 1998; 275:H65–H74.

18. Janicki JS, Brower GL. The role of myocardial fibrillar collagen in ventricular remodeling and function. J Card Fail 2002; 8:S319–S325.

19. Wu YM, Cazorla O, Labeit D, et al. Changes in titin and collagen underlie diastolic stiffness diversity of cardiac muscle. J Mol Cell Cardiol 2000; 32:2151–2161.

20. Gerdes AM. Cardiac myocyte remodeling in hypertrophy and progression to failure. J Card Fail 2002; 8:S264–S268.

21. Borer JS, Truter S, Herrold EM, et al. Myocardial fibrosis in chronic aortic regurgitation—Molecular and cellular responses to volume overload. Circulation 2002; 105:1837–1842.

22. Brower GL, Janicki JS. Contribution of ventricular remodeling to pathogenesis of heart failure in rats. Am J Physiol 2001; 280:H674–H683.

23. Aoyagi T, Fujii AM, Flanagan MF, et al. Transition from compensated hypertrophy to intrinsic myocardial dysfunction during development of left ventricular pressure-overload hypertrophy in conscious sheep. Systolic dysfunction precedes diastolic dysfunction. Circulation 1993; 88:2415–2425.

24. Villari B, Hess OM, Kaufmann P, et al. Effect of aortic valve stenosis (pressure overload) and regurgitation (volume overload) on left ventricular systolic and diastolic function. Am J Cardiol 1992; 69:927–934.

25. Bonow RO, Carabello B, De Leon AC Jr, et al. ACC/AHA guidelines for the management of patients with valvular heart disease—A report of the American College of Cardiology/American Heart Association Task Force on practice guidelines (Committee on Management of Patients with Valvular Heart Disease). J Am Coll Cardiol 1998; 32:1486–1582.

26. Powell AJ, Geva T. Blood flow measurement by magnetic resonance imaging in congenital heart disease. Pediatr Cardiol 2000; 21:47–58.

27. Tarasoutchi F, Grinberg M, Spina GS, et al. Ten-year clinical laboratory follow-up after application of a symptom-based therapeutic strategy to patients with severe chronic aortic regurgitation of predominant rheumatic etiology. J Am Coll Cardiol 2003; 41:1316–1324.

28. Tornos MP, Olona M, Permanyer-Miralda G, et al. Heart failure after aortic valve replacement for aortic regurgitation: Prospective 20-year study. Am Heart J 1998; 136:618–627.

29. Starling MR, Kirsh MM, Montgomery DG, et al. Mechanisms for left ventricular systolic dysfunction in aortic regurgitation: Importance for predicting the functional response to aortic valve replacement. J Am Coll Cardiol 1991; 17:887–897.

30. Gentles TL, Colan SD, Wilson NJ, *et al.* Left ventricular mechanics during and after acute rheumatic fever: Contractile dysfunction is closely related to valve regurgitation. J Am Coll Cardiol 2001; 37:201–207.

31. Borer JS, Hochreiter C, Herrold EM, *et al.* Prediction of indications for valve replacement among asymptomatic or minimally symptomatic patients with chronic aortic regurgitation and normal left ventricular performance. Circulation 1998; 97:525–534.

32. Colan SD, Sanders SP, Ingelfinger JR, *et al.* Left ventricular mechanics and contractile state in children and young adults with end-stage renal disease: Effect of dialysis and renal transplantation. J Am Coll Cardiol 1987; 10:1085–1094.

33. Colan SD, Borow KM, Neumann A. Left ventricular end-systolic wall stress-velocity of fiber shortening relation: A load-independent index of myocardial contractility. J Am Coll Cardiol 1984; 4:715–724.

34. Klodas E, Enriquez-Sarano M, Tajik AJ, *et al.* Aortic regurgitation complicated by extreme left ventricular dilation: Long-term outcome lifter surgical correction. J Am Coll Cardiol 1996; 27:670–677.

35. Carabello BA. The pathophysiology of mitral regurgitation. J Heart Valve Dis 2000; 5:600–608.

36. Gaasch WH, Zile MR. Left ventricular function after surgical correction of chronic mitral regurgitation. Eur Heart J 1991; 12 Suppl B:48–51.

37. Goldfine H, Aurigemma GP, Zile MR, *et al.* Left ventricular length-force-shortening relations before and after surgical correction of chronic mitral regurgitation. J Am Coll Cardiol 1998; 31:180–185.

38. Zile MR, Gaasch WH, Levine HJ. Left ventricular stress-dimension-shortening relations before and after correction of chronic aortic and mitral regurgitation. Am J Cardiol 1985; 56:99–105.

39. Corin WJ, Sütsch G, Murakami T, *et al.* Left ventricular function in chronic mitral regurgitation: Preoperative and postoperative comparison. J Am Coll Cardiol 1995; 25:113–121.

40. Murakami T, Nakazawa M, Nakanishi T, *et al.* Prediction of postoperative left ventricular pump function in congenital mitral regurgitation. Pediatr Cardiol 1999; 20:418–421.

41. Gaasch WH, Aurigemma GP. Inhibition of the renin-angiotensin system and the left ventricular adaptation to mitral regurgitation. J Am Coll Cardiol 2002; 39:1380–1383.

42. Krishnan US, Gersony WM, Berman-Rosenzweig E, *et al.* Late left ventricular function after surgery for children with chronic symptomatic mitral regurgitation. Circulation 1997; 96:4280–4285.

43. Magee AG, Fenn L, Vellekoop J, *et al.* Left ventricular function in adolescents and adults with restrictive ventricular septal defect and moderate left-to-right shunting. Cardiol Young 2000; 10:126–129.

44. Stewart JM, Hintze TH, Woolf PK, *et al.* Nature of heart failure in patients with ventricular septal defect. Am J Physiol 1995; 269:H1473–H1480.

45. Colan SD. Systolic and diastolic function of the univentricular heart. Prog Ped Cardiol 2002; 16:79–87.

46. Santamore WP, Dell'Italia LJ. Ventricular interdependence: Significant left ventricular contributions to right ventricular systolic function. Prog Cardiovasc Dis 1998; 40:289–308.

47. Satoh A, Katayama K, Hiro T, *et al.* Effect of right ventricular volume overload on left ventricular diastolic function in patients with atrial septal defect. Jpn Circ J 1996; 60:758–766.

48. Jost CHA, Oechslin E, Seifert B, *et al.* Remodelling after surgical repair of atrial septal defects within the oval fossa. Cardiol Young 2002; 12:506–512.

49. Kort HW, Balzer DT, Johnson MC. Resolution of right heart enlargement after closure of secundum atrial septal defect with transcatheter technique. J Am Coll Cardiol 2001; 38:1528–1532.

50. Vliegen HW, Van Straten A, De Roos A, *et al.* Magnetic resonance imaging to assess the hmodynamic effects of pulmonary valve replacement in adults late after repair of tetralogy of Fallot. Circulation 2002; 106:1703–1707.

51. Therrien J, Siu SC, McLaughlin PR, *et al.* Pulmonary valve replacement in adults late after repair of tetralogy of Fallot: Are we operating too late? J Am Coll Cardiol 2000; 36:1670–1675.

52. de Ruijter FT, Weenink I, Hitchcock FJ, *et al.* Right ventricular dysfunction and pulmonary valve replacement after correction of tetralogy of Fallot. Ann Thorac Surg 2002; 73:1794–1800.

53. Discigil B, Dearani JA, Puga FJ, *et al.* Late pulmonary valve replacement after repair of tetralogy of Fallot. J Thorac Cardiovasc Surg 2001; 121:344–351.

CHAPTER 13

The Right Ventricle in a Dual Chambered Circulation

Andrew N. Redington, MD, FRCP(C) (UK)

Introduction

The concept of the right ventricle as "dispensable" [1], or simply an innocent bystander, in a circulation driven by the left ventricle was popularized in the 1970s. Indeed, the evolution of the Fontan circulation—a clear illustration of how a circulation can perform in the absence of a subpulmonary right ventricle—did much to undermine interest and investigation into right ventricular functional performance. To some extent the last 30 years have seen a complete turnaround in our philosophical approach to the right ventricle. Its importance in acquired heart disease is increasingly understood and championed [2], and the realization of the fundamental importance of the right ventricle in the circulation of patients having undergone repair of congenital heart disease has also evolved in a similar way [3].

While it can be argued that philosophical considerations lead, in part, to the relative dearth of information regarding the right ventricle, more pragmatic issues are probably equally important. There is no doubt that the right ventricle is a more difficult structure to analyze, functionally, than is its left ventricular counterpart. There are physiologic, spatial, geometric, and mathematical issues all of which have confounded investigators wanting to learn more. However the last decade, in particular, has seen an explosion of techniques that can equally be applied to right and left ventricular function. Improved echocardiographic techniques, magnetic resonance imaging and angiography, and conductance catheterization have all been applied to the analysis of right ventricular performance. It is outside the scope of this chapter to assess comparative utility of these techniques, rather the chapter will concentrate on describing the information obtained using them.

Right ventricular anatomy

Morphologically, the right ventricle is probably best described as a tripartite structure, consisting of an inlet portion, an apical trabecular portion, and outlet portion. This certainly facilitates the description of disease, but is an artificial separation in terms of analysis of its function. Figure 13.1 shows a painstaking dissection of the deep layers of the myocardial mass. The deeper layers of the normal right ventricular form an entirely separate structure from that of the left ventricle. Its muscle fibers are arranged along a predominately longitudinal axis from the atrioventricular ring to the ventricular apex, and in more radial fashion toward the outlet. This fiber arrangement probably explains why the right ventricle has more rapid long axis acceleration than does the left ventricle during ventricular systole [4,5], as well as the apparent peristaltic motion described between the inlet and outlet portions of the ventricle during contraction [6]. This peristaltic motion is no more than a time delay between the onset of motion of the inlet, which moves toward the apex in early systole, and the subsequent contraction of the outlet portion, in sequential fashion. Consequently, while the left ventricle ejects a significant portion of its stroke volume as a result of torsional shape change [7], right ventricular ejection is much more dependent on myocyte fiber shortening.

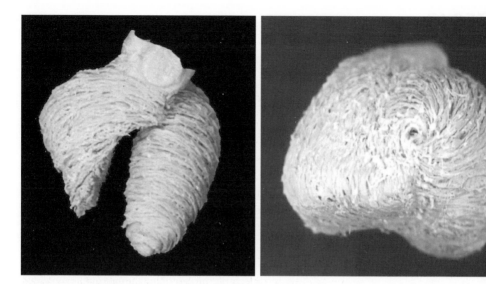

Figure 13.1 Dissection of the deep myofibers of the left and right ventricles (left-hand panel). The left ventricular fibers are oriented circumferentially, while the separate, generally longitudinally orientated right ventricular fibers are clearly seen. The right hand panel shows the superficial fibers. There are common fibers providing myocardium to both right and left ventricles. With permission from Professor R.H. Anderson.

While the deeper myocardial fibers are separate in the normal heart, this pattern is disrupted by congenital abnormalities. In tetralogy of Fallot, for example, there is contiguity of the deep sono-spiral layers of the left and right ventricle [8]. This alone would suggest that there may be marked interdependence between the two ventricles, but more importantly, all hearts have shared myofibers that encircle both right and left ventricles (Fig. 13.1). These superficial fibers run obliquely over the surface of the right ventricle and on to the left ventricle. Again, the orientation and geometry of these fibers varies as the heart is affected by congenital heart disease, but the basic pattern of shared superficial longitudinal fibers is common to all biventricular hearts. This is of crucial importance to the understanding of ventricular crosstalk and right–left heart interactions discussed in detail later.

The variable three-dimensional arrangement of right ventricular muscle fibers underscores its complex spatial geometry in health and disease, and confounds analysis of its function by single plane or orthogonal techniques. This is in contradistinction to the geometrically simpler left ventricle, which can be mathematically modeled on the basis of a prolate ellipsoid [9]. Various geometric models have been proposed to describe the right ventricle (e.g.,

triangular-based pyramids, pyramids with additional cones accounting for the outflow tract [10], etc), but none adequately describe the right ventricle either in health or disease. This is because the inlet of the right ventricle is a complex ellipse, its outlet is approximately circular, and the remainder of the right ventricle, while triangulating at the apex, is variably flattened as it wraps around the left ventricle. Modest degrees of right heart dilatation alter this arrangement significantly. There is therefore no simple way of describing the right ventricle geometrically, and assessment of its size and shape must take account of its three-dimensional complexity. For this reason, most investigative techniques use multiple slice methods to analyze right ventricular form.

Right ventricular physiology

It has proven to be misguided, in virtually every area of physiologic investigation, to apply the concepts and indices developed for the description of left ventricular performance to the right ventricle. There are fundamental differences in both the manifestation of systolic and diastolic performance, an understanding of which allow a robust assessment of circulatory performance. Furthermore, it is only with an understanding of normal physiology that the abnormal

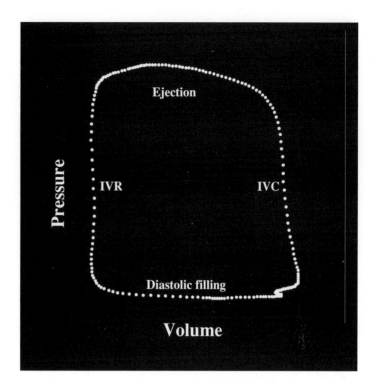

Figure 13.2 Conductance catheter derived left ventricular pressure–volume loop. This is a typical example showing periods of isovolumic contraction (IVC), ejection, isovolumic relaxation (IVR), and diastolic filling.

physiology as imposed by congenital heart lesions and their treatment can be understood.

Right ventricular systolic function

Apart from the geometric considerations, there is much debate as to whether, intrinsically, the right ventricular myofiber behaves differently to that of the left ventricle. It is clearly very difficult to separate out the effects of the very major differences in ventricular load from intrinsic differences at a cellular or metabolic level. Nonetheless, there are some tantalizing data suggesting real differences. In isolated muscle preparations, for example, while peak total tension is identical, the time taken to reach it is much shorter in the right ventricle. These differences persist in the face of varying loading conditions, calcium concentrations, and inotropic agents [11]. The implications of these, albeit subtle, differences remain to be seen, but it is worth emphasizing that there are no data to suggest that the right ventricular myocardium is fundamentally more or less well-adapted to act in either a pulmonary or systemic role. Furthermore, nothing is known about function at a myofiber level that precludes a classical

examination of the relationship between pressure, volume, and flow within the ventricular chamber.

Pressure–volume characteristics

The normal left ventricular pressure–volume curve (Fig. 13.2) demonstrates the features of a square wave pump, with a period of isovolumic contraction, a phase of relatively isotonic ejection, followed by isovolumic relaxation, and diastolic filling. If preload is varied, usually by snaring or balloon occluding the inferior caval vein [12], then a family of pressure–volume loops can be obtained (Fig. 13.3). The linear relationship of pressure–volume points that exist at a defined time point in the cardiac cycle forms the basis of the elastance model to describe contractility [13]. The most commonly analyzed pressure–volume point is the upper left-hand corner of the pressure–volume curve, the so-called "end-systolic point." End-systolic elastance (E_{es}) or maximal elastance (maximum P/V or E_{max}) probably represent the purest description of intrinsic myocardial contractility. This is because their relative linearity excludes preload or afterload dependency, and the slope of their relationship describes changes in contractile

226   Chapter 13

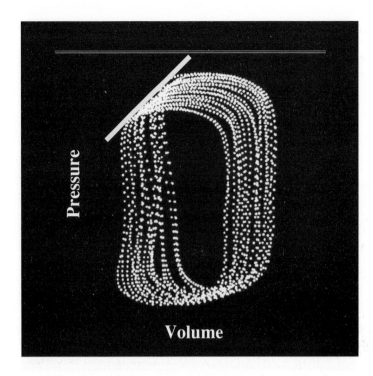

Figure 13.3 A family of left ventricular pressure–volume loops obtained during balloon caval occlusion. Left ventricular pressure and volume full sequentially as preload is reduced. The line describes the endsystolic pressure–volume relationship.

force with changing inotropy. Increased inotropy increases the slope of the end-systolic pressure–volume relationship, while decreased inotropy decreases it.

The right ventricular pressure–volume relationship is substantially different to that of the left ventricle. Figure 13.4 shows a similar family of right ventricular pressure–volume relationships, obtained in the same way as those shown in Fig. 13.3 for the

left ventricle. Unlike the square or rectangular left ventricular pressure–volume curve, the right ventricle has poorly defined periods of isovolumic contraction and relaxation. This is because ejection begins to occur from the ventricle early on during pressure rise and, perhaps more importantly, continues during pressure fall [14]. Consequently, the curve is more triangular or trapezoidal in shape and has

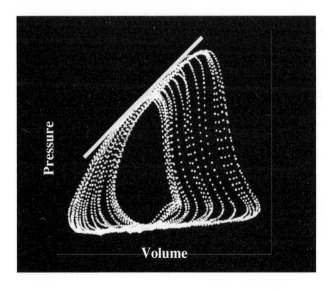

Figure 13.4 Right ventricular pressure–volume loops obtained during caval occlusion. Note how the normal right ventricular pressure–volume relationship is triangular in overall shape, with ejection occurring during pressure rise and during pressure full. There are therefore poorly defined isovolumic periods. The "endystolic" pressure–volume relationship is described by the line and varies with inotropes etc., as in the left ventricle (see text for details).

been shown to be almost entirely a reflection of the different afterload characteristics of the pulmonary vascular bed [15]. The low hydraulic impedance of the pulmonary vascular bed facilitates ejection during right ventricular pressure development and also allows for continued ejection during right ventricular pressure fall. These observations have many implications. Firstly, the energetics of contraction are very different. The area subtended by the pressure–volume curve represents the external mechanical work performed by the ventricle. This is clearly much smaller for the right ventricle, compared with the left ventricle, despite a similar stroke output. While the "square wave pump" of the left ventricle is necessarily required to overcome the systemic vascular resistance, it is energetically wasteful. The stored potential energy in the myocardium at end-systole is not converted into external mechanical work [16]. Conversely, the right ventricle harnesses some of this potential energy and converts it to external work. Consequently, right ventricular ejection has an energy cost approximately one fourth of that of the left ventricle. The disadvantage of this contractile pattern is reflected in the very limited afterload reserve of the right ventricle. The right ventricle is less suited to acute changes in ventricular afterload, with right heart failure much more rapidly for a given percentage change in pulmonary arterial pressure. Indeed, it has been estimated that the right ventricle is 2–3 times more afterload sensitive than is the left ventricle [17]. Secondly, this configuration has implications for the way in which we measure right ventricular function. The lack of a well-defined isovolumic contraction or relaxation period makes interpretation of so-called isovolumic indices of function, much less robust in the right ventricle. Finally, the concept of ventricular elastance is more difficult to understand when there is such a disparity between the point of maximal elastance and end-systolic elastance. Nonetheless, the slope of maximal elastance (maximum P/V) is similarly resistant to changes in loading conditions and varies approximately with inotropic state [18]. While perhaps theoretically flawed the assessment of right ventricular elastance can be used, clinically, to describe right ventricular performance. Another index derived from ventricular pressure–volume relationships is the slope of the end-diastolic volume–stroke work relationship or preload recruitable stroke work. For the left ventricle, this

index is less sensitive to contractile change, but shows less intrinsic variability [12]. Intuitively, it would be a more ideal method of assessing right ventricular systolic function. Indeed, it has been shown to be more linear in response to afterload change, and equally sensitive to changes in contractile state for the right ventricle [19]. However, any technique involving the measurement of pressure–volume relationships must remain essentially experimental. What are the more clinically applicable measurements of right ventricular systolic function?

"Real world" analysis of right ventricular systolic function

The assessment of right ventricular systolic function in the clinical setting has been notoriously difficult. This is because right ventricular ejection fraction and the indices from which it is derived are exquisitely sensitive to loading conditions. Indeed, there is an almost linear inverse relationship between right ventricular ejection fraction and right ventricular afterload. This is adaptive, rather than intrinsic, and therefore changes in right ventricular shortening fraction, ejection fraction, and volumes are difficult to interpret when there are changes in load, and they have failed the test of time when assessing longitudinal change, in response to surgical or pharmacological therapeutic intervention. Thus very few therapeutic algorithms incorporating such measurements (no matter how they are made) have proven robust, and this has severely hampered the development of guidelines regarding timing of treatment in long-term follow-up, etc.

The Holy Grail of a noninvasive, load independent, index of contractility is yet to be fully established. However, recent developments in tissue Doppler echocardiography [20] have improved our ability to separate load-dependant from load-independent changes of right ventricular function. Tissue Doppler echocardiography represents a paradigm shift in our interpretation of color Doppler velocimetry. Previously, software and hardware developments were focused on maximizing the Doppler signal from the blood pool and suppression of the Doppler velocity signals from the myocardium and surrounding tissues. With tissue Doppler echocardiography, the reverse is true. The blood flow signal is suppressed, and the lower velocity signals from the myocardium are displayed. Its temporal resolution continues to

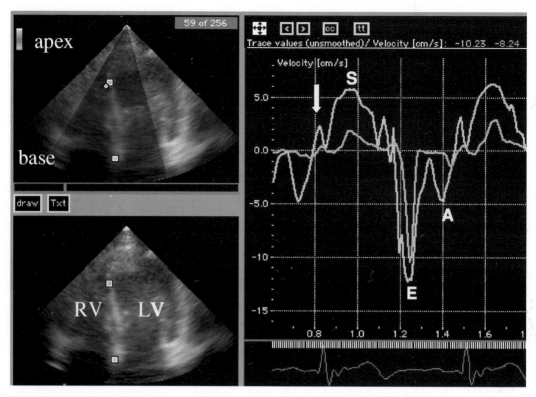

Figure 13.5 Typical tissue Doppler echo recordings from the basal and apical portions of the septum. There is systolic shortening (S), early rapid lengthening (E), and atrial systolic lengthening (A) of the myocardium during the cardiac cycle. The second trace is taken from the apical region and shows reduced amplitudes of systolic shortening in the normal heart. Note also the presystolic spike marked with an arrow (see Fig. 13.6 for details).

improve and this allows a high-fidelity velocity signal to be obtained from almost any area of the myocardium. Figure 13.5 shows a typical example from the right ventricle. As expected, from a four-chamber view, there is a period of systolic shortening with the myocardium moving toward the apex, followed by periods of lengthening during early rapid filling and atrial systole. Unfortunately, both ejection phase shortening indices and diastolic lengthening velocities, derived by tissue Doppler echocardiography, have been shown to be both afterload and preload dependent. Figure 13.5 also highlights a brief, but important, period of acceleration and decceleration occurring during the preejection period. This isovolumic "spike" represents a phase of early ventricular activation both for the right and the left ventricle. Figure 13.6 shows a simultaneous tissue Doppler and right ventricular pressure recording (obtained using a micromonometer). It can be seen that the onset of preejection acceleration occurs

coincidently with the onset of pressure rise. Easily measured by TDE, this isovolumic acceleration has subsequently been shown to be remarkably afterload resistant and preload resistant over a wide physiologic range [4,5]. Furthermore, it tracks changes in right ventricular contractility as influenced by inotropic stimulation with Dobutamine and suppression with esmolol [4]. Interestingly, isovolumic acceleration varies with heart rate. It is thus able to track the force–frequency relationship, or Treppe effect, a fundamental property of myocardial contractile response, so often ignored in the past. While the underlying cellular mechanisms responsible for isovolumic acceleration remain to be determined exactly, it seems likely that it is a reflection of early systolic calcium cycling. As such, it may well provide us with very different insights into myocardial performance in the future, and it has already been used to describe changes in function in the congenitally malformed right ventricle [21] (see below).

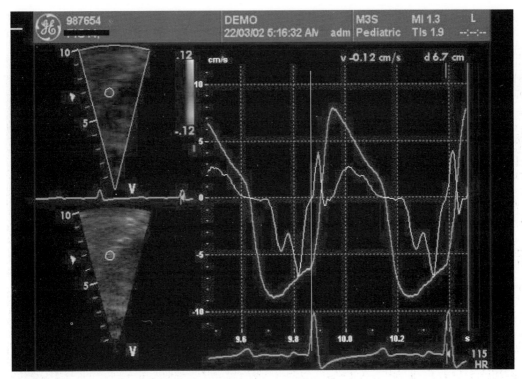

Figure 13.6 Tissue Doppler echo recording obtained with simultaneous micromanometer tipped pressure measurement in the right ventricle and electrocardiogram. The presystolic spike (isovolumic acceleration) starts at the very onset of pressure rise in the ventricle and is completed well before peak pressure development.

Right ventricular diastolic function

The assessment of right ventricular diastolic dysfunction represents an even greater challenge to contemporary analytical techniques than that of systolic function. Again, concepts derived for the left ventricle cannot be transposed to the right ventricle. Left ventricular diastolic function can be described in three phases: relaxation, early rapid filling, and late diastolic filling. Direct measurements of pressure, flow, and volumes, or their surrogates, have long been used to describe the relaxation and compliance characteristics of the left ventricle. These same measurements may be invalid in the right ventricle, however. Again, an understanding of the pressure–volume relationships of the right ventricle helps to understand the potential limitations of some of these measurements in the right ventricle. In the absence of a well-defined isovolumic relaxation period, those measurements requiring isovolumic status for their validity may be flawed. Thus the time constant of right ventricular relaxation and minimum dP/dT may not be measurable as an iso-

volumic event. Early rapid filling is easier to define and indices such as maximal filling rate, and Doppler derived peak E-wave velocity are probably reasonable reflectors of right ventricular restoring forces, albeit varing markedly with respiration, mean airway pressure, etc [22]. In patients with a normal pulmonary vascular resistance, however, end-diastolic indices and the measurement of ventricular compliance are unsound. In order to measure ventricular compliance, the ratio of pressure change (ΔP) per unit volume change (ΔV) is required. This assumes that the ventricular chamber is a closed system, that is, blood flow through the tricuspid valve during atrial systole fills the right ventricular cavity and induces a concomitant pressure rise. Similarly, the end-diastolic pressure–volume relationship should reflect the curvilinear relationship between ΔP and ΔV. Again, this is appropriate only if the ΔP measured truly reflects a predictable change in ventricular volume. This is not always the case for a ventricle in subpulmonary position. As ventricular compliance worsens, the resistance to ventricular filling may exceed the pulmonary vascular resistance. Under these circumstances, right atrial contraction, while still producing transtricuspid flow on a Doppler echocardiogram for example, fails to fill the ventricle and instead leads to ejection into the pulmonary artery during late diastole [23]. Neither the transtricuspid flow characteristics, the ΔV in the right ventricle that occurs as the result of atrial contraction, nor the ΔP can be relied upon as truly reflecting right ventricular dynamics. They will be variably affected by right atrial function, right ventricular compliance, and the pulmonary vascular resistance.

While this fundamental difference in ventricular diastolic physiology obviates the use of many of the indices used to describe left ventricular diastolic function, it also opens up an arena for the, subjective at least, assessment of right ventricular diastolic disease. For example, the presence of antegrade diastolic flow in the pulmonary artery, coincident with atrial systole, represents an excellent surrogate measure for the description for a poor right ventricular diastolic compliance. The understanding of this physiology has lead to the understanding of ventricular responses in the setting of right heart disease, the affects of cardiac surgery, and the long-term effects of right ventricular volume overload for example.

Right–left heart interaction

Implicit to the discussion of right ventricular performance in a biventricular circulation is the influence that one ventricle will have on the other as a result of myocardial cross talk, ventricular–ventricular interdependence, and ventricular–ventricular interference during disease. Many congenital heart diseases are natural models of the potential effects of these interactions. Although, immature, our understanding of right–left heart interactions both in health and congenital heart disease is increasing.

Ventricular cross talk

Given the shared superficial fibers of the right and left ventricle have already been described earlier (Fig. 13.1). It would be extraordinary if there were not ventricular cross talk (the effect of ventricular contraction on one side of the heart significantly affecting contractile properties of the other side of the heart). This is no better demonstrated than in a beautiful physiologic experiment conducted in an animal preparation whereby the ventricles were electrically isolated but mechanically intact [24]. Damiano and colleagues showed that under these circumstances pacing the electrically isolated right ventricle leads to very little left ventricular pressure development (Fig. 13.7). Thus, the contribution of right ventricular contractile force to left ventricular pressure development was shown to be rather limited. Conversely, pacing the left ventricle to induce left ventricular contraction leads to a very marked pressure increment in the electrically isolated right ventricle. This simple experiment therefore demonstrated the marked contribution of the left ventricle to right ventricular

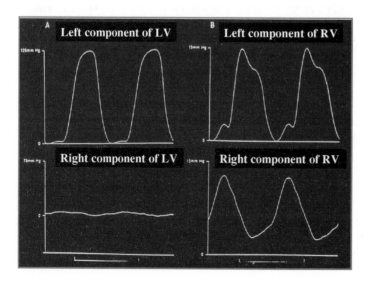

Figure 13.7 Pressure recordings obtained in electrically isolated, but mechanically contiguous right and left ventricles (see text for details). From Damiano *et al.* [24] with permission.

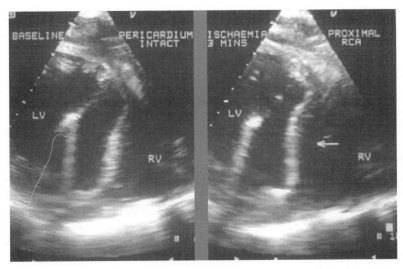

Figure 13.8 The effect of acute right heart dilatation on left ventricular geometry. In this case, the pericardium is intact. As the right ventricle dilates, the septum is moved toward the left ventricle, which is altered in its configuration. This has marked effects on both right and left ventricular function.

force generation. Indeed, it was estimated that approximately 50–60% of right ventricular force was generated as a result of left ventricular contractile activity.

This concept was further elucidated in another elegant surgical model. Hoffman and coworkers replaced the right ventricular free wall myocardium with a noncontractile patch [25]. Despite the lack of right ventricular myocardium, right ventricular pressure development was almost normal, presumably as a result of left ventricular free wall and septal shortening. Interestingly, however, as right ventricular size was increased (by increasing the size of the noncontractile patch) both right and left ventricular pressure development fell. It appeared therefore that not only was right ventricular size predictor of right ventricular pressure development, but it may well be affecting the integrity of left ventricular contraction. However, it was difficult to separate a parallel effect (ventricular interdependence) from a series effect (consequent upon reduced right ventricular output) in this experiment.

Ventricular interference

The notion that dilation of one heart chamber may interfere with the function of other heart chambers is well established. The direct effects of right ventricular dilatation on left ventricular contractile performance were more difficult to show however, because

of the difficulty in separating parallel and series effects described above. Some answers were obtained in a study of isolated right ventricular dilatation, using load-independent indices of left ventricular function [26]. This study, in which right ventricular dilatation was achieved via right coronary artery occlusion, also allowed the description of the influence of importance of pericardial constraint when considering ventricular–ventricular interaction. When the pericardium was intact, there was a reciprocal relationship between right ventricular and left ventricular size. Unsurprisingly, as the right ventricle dilated, there was septal shift with a loss of left ventricular volume (Fig. 13.8). Going along with this, there was a marked reduction in left ventricular intrinsic contractile performance, with a fall in preload recruitable stroke work. This strongly suggests that integrity of both the right and left geometry is required for optimal ventricular performance from either side of the heart. While the effect of right ventricular dilatation on left ventricular contractile performance was somewhat attenuated when the pericardial constraint was released, there was still a significant effect underscoring this point. Although this was an acute study, the effects of ventricular–ventricular interference in the perioperative situation, and more chronically in volume and pressure loaded abnormalities of both the right and left heart, are increasingly understood and are important to consider when assessing global function in specific lesions affecting the right ventricle.

Specific lesions

With the myriad of congenital heart diseases and the very marked interindividual variation of anatomy and physiology, it would be impossible to address all of the issues pertaining to right ventricular dysfunction under all circumstances, in this review. Rather, these issues will be discussed generically, concentrating on the major manifestations of chronic right heart disease so amply illustrated by "naturally" occurring models in operated and unoperated congenital heart disease.

The small right ventricle

There is far more flexibility, in terms of tolerating a reduced ventricular end-diastolic volume, on the right side of the heart. This is largely because of the physiologic redundancy that can be factored into a biventricular repair in the presence of a small right ventricle. Such physiologic redundancy does not exist on the left side. A miscalculation of left ventricular size prior to a proposed biventricular repair can have dire consequences. Even if left ventricular growth could be achieved under those circumstances, the short-term morbidity and mortality precludes success [27]. While there must be a threshold of right ventricular size, beyond which a biventricular repair cannot be sustained, the aim of a biventricular repair, in the presence of a small right ventricle, must be simply to generate sufficient pulmonary blood flow to allow adequate oxygenation and a low right atrial pressure. Importantly, the right ventricular output need not be the same as the systemic output. Superficially, therefore, it should be simple to calculate the right ventricular volume required. If one considers that, for example, a pulmonary blood flow of approximately 1 L/mm^2 is adequate for most infants, then at a heart rate for 100 beats/min and a right ventricular ejection fraction of 50%, it is easy to calculate that an end-diastolic volume of 20 mL/m^2 is required. The situation is more complex than this, however, and must take account of many variables, not only absolute right ventricular size. Right atrial function, the integrity of the atrial septum, the pulmonary vascular resistance, and the possibility of bypassing the right ventricle using a venopulmonary connection are all important in decision-making.

How then, can a small right ventricle be successfully incorporated into a biventricular circulation without right heart failure? In order to understand some of the therapeutic strategies, we must first understand the underlying physiologic problem of the restrictive right ventricle.

Right ventricular restrictive physiology

The concept of restrictive physiology has been discussed earlier. Restrictive physiology can be a manifestation of abnormal ventricular myocardial compliance, in the presence of ventricular disease [23], or simply a manifestation of decreased cavity size, in the absence of myocardial disease [28]. The physiologic and clinical manifestations are similar. As mentioned earlier, the measurement of chamber compliance requires the knowledge of the change in ventricular pressure, imposed by concomitant change in ventricular volume. Intrinsic to this is a closed system in ventricular diastole. Unlike the left ventricle, where the high aortic diastolic pressure maintains aortic valve closure during ventricular filling and left atrial systole, the right ventricle is connected to a low-pressure pulmonary artery. It is therefore relatively easy for the right atrial pressure to exceed the pulmonary artery diastolic pressure during right atrial systole. Under these circumstances, pulmonary blood flow is augmented by right atrial systole, even if right ventricular filling does not occur as the right atrium empties. This is manifested as antegrade diastolic flow in the main pulmonary artery during late diastole, coincident with the P wave on the electrocardiogram (see Fig. 13.9). The phenomenon was first described in congenital heart disease in the setting of pulmonary atresia with intact septum and critical pulmonary stenosis [23]. Under these circumstances, it is probably a manifestation of both a small ventricular cavity and an intrinsically poorly compliant myocardium. Subsequently, it has been described in the patient early after repair of tetralogy of Fallot [29] (where intraoperative myocardial damage appears to be the culprit) as well as other congenital heart disease associated with right ventricular hypoplasia, for example, Ebstein anomaly, unbalanced atrioventricular septal defect, etc. The contribution of antegrade diastolic pulmonary blood flow to the total pulmonary blood flow can be as much as 40% of the total. Add to this, the inhibition of retrograde blood flow (pulmonary regurgitation) and it is easy

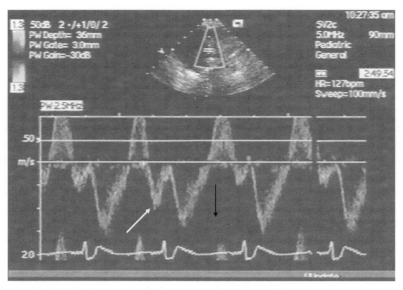

Figure 13.9 Pulsed wave Doppler recording in the main pulmonary artery of a patient after repair of tetralogy of Fallot. The arrow highlights a period of antegrade late diastolic flow after the P wave on the electrocardiogram. The area under the curve accounts for approximately 35% of the total antegrade flow. Antegrade diastolic flow also reduces the duration of pulmonary regurgitation.

to understand that maintenance of this source of cardiac output is fundamental to right heart function, and is particularly important in the perioperative period. Antegrade diastolic pulmonary blood flow occurs as a consequence of a small pressure transient between the right atrium and pulmonary at artery end-diastole. Thus, maintenance of sinus rhythm, maintenance of right atrial preload and pressure, and reduction in right ventricular (right atrial) afterload are all important. In regard to the latter, maintenance of a low mean airway pressure is crucial. In ventilated patients with restrictive physiology the mean airway pressure represents a significant part of the total afterload seen by the right atrium and right ventricle. This is manifested as a waxing and waning of antegrade diastolic flow during positive pressure ventilation. During the inspiratory phase of positive pressure ventilation, antegrade diastolic flow diminishes and hence the cardiac output. Reducing mean airway pressure will conversely increase cardiac output. This can be achieved by minimizing the inspiratory time, avoiding prolonged plateau pressure, and minimizing positive end expiratory pressure. The ultimate goal is to maintain oxygenation and alveolar ventilation at the lowest mean airway pressure until normal spontaneous negative ventilation pressure can be achieved. Taking this a step

further, in physiologic studies in children after cardiac surgery, imposed negative pressure ventilation (using a negative pressure currase device) markedly improved cardiac output after repair of tetralogy of Fallot, for example [30]. Although not in routine clinical use, the use of negative pressure ventilation has been described as salvage therapy prior to extracorporeal support in the sickest of these children [31], but more importantly serves to amplify the potential beneficial effects of modifying adverse "cardiopulmonary" interactions in right heart disease.

While an understanding of the physiology of restrictive right ventricular disease has lead to an improvement in the care and outcome of these patients, there are other ways of avoiding low systemic cardiac output syndrome in these patients. These will be outlined below.

Interatrial communication

In many centers, the use of an atrial septal fenestration, or leaving the patent foramen ovale open, is routine management of the young neonate undergoing biventricular repair, particularly those primarily affecting the right heart. The presence of ventricular hypoplasia, or the super-added influence of restrictive myocardial disease, is obviated by the capacity to shunt from right to left at atrial level, although at the expense of pulmonary blood flow, the right atrium is decompressed and the systemic cardiac output is augmented. Although no formal data have been published, it is likely that despite the resulting hypoxemia oxygen delivery is maintained or enhanced using this strategy. Certainly, there has been a marked improvement in surgical mortality for neonatal repair for tetralogy of Fallot ever since this strategy has been adopted [32,33]. Desaturation, as a manifestation of restrictive physiology, is the norm after surgical or interventional therapy for critical pulmonary stenosis or pulmonary atresia. Indeed, the transition from right-to-left shunting heralds the resolution of restrictive physiology, and ultimately spontaneous closure of the PFO is seen in most. In those patients in whom right-to-left shunting persists, it is possible to contemplate later transcatheter or surgical closure of the atrial septum, but this is of debatable benefit. At the very least, careful testing of the circulation is required, with balloon occlusion of the atrial septum and measurement of cardiac output, before this is performed.

Bidirectional Glenn procedure
In some hearts, either right ventricular cavity size is too small or there are associated anatomic lesions that preclude a "full" biventricular repair. Another method of generating pulmonary blood flow, at the same time as reducing the preload to the right heart, is the incorporation of a bidirectional Glenn anastomosis in the circulation. This can be contemplated only when there is a low pulmonary vascular resistance. This "so called" $1^1/_2$- ventricle repair has been used in the treatment algorithm of patients with critical pulmonary stenosis, pulmonary atresia intact septum, unbalanced atrioventricular septal defect, and Ebstein's anomaly of the tricuspid valve [34]. While the earlier advantages have been amply demonstrated, the long-term issues of a lifetime with a cavopulmonary shunt have yet to be elucidated, although the midterm results remain excellent [35].

The dilated right ventricle

Although some right ventricles have intrinsic limitation to right ventricular dilation, hence their designation as restrictive, progressive dilatation is the normal response to a chronic volume load in normal, "nonrestrictive" ventricles. Thus, chronic left-to-right shunt at atrial level, systemic arteriovenous

fistula, and pulmonary regurgitation all lead to dilatation of the right ventricle usually with a normal or near normal right ventricular systolic pressure. The right ventricular dilatation that occurs as a consequence of atrial shunting, anomalous pulmonary venous return, or arteriovenous fistula is usually treated by surgery or transcatheter interventional occlusion, and is held up as one of the indications for treatment. When performed in early childhood, resolution of ventricular dilatation is the norm and the long-term consequences are minimal. However, postoperative patients with pulmonary regurgitation, usually as a consequence of repair of right ventricular outflow tract obstruction, represent a large group of patients in whom chronic right heart dilatation is a significant issue and in whom decision-making remains uncertain. Before considering these postoperative issues, it is worthwhile to examine the pattern of responses of the normal right ventricle as it is affected by isolated pulmonary regurgitation in the otherwise normal circulation [36]. These patients are asymptomatic for decades, despite marked pulmonary regurgitation and right ventricular dilation. In the fourth, fifth, and sixth decades symptoms begin to occur. These consist of congestive heart failure and reduced exercise tolerance, atrial and ventricular arrhythmias, and even sudden death. It is therefore no coincidence that these same issues are features of the postoperative tetralogy patient, although perhaps with a slightly shorter time of course of evolution. Indeed, pulmonary regurgitation is increasingly recognized as the culprit lesion, at least in part, for all of the major long-term morbidities seen after the repair of tetralogy of Fallot [37]. It is also another illustration of how a "clinical model" of disease allows for unique investigation of adverse hemodynamics that evolve over the course of decades, unobtainable in any experimental preparation.

When one considers the hemodynamic determinants of pulmonary regurgitation, there are three main factors. The first, of course, is the integrity of the pulmonary valve, secondly the nature of the right ventricle and its compliance during diastole, and thirdly, the impedance to pulmonary blood flow, and therefore propensity to reversal, within the pulmonary vascular bed.

While the restriction of pulmonary regurgitation, consequent upon a functionally normal pulmonary valve is intuitive, the converse is not so easy to understand. Some patients without effective pulmonary valve function (after transannular patch repair of tetralogy, for example) have normal or near normal right ventricular size decades after surgery, despite the anatomic substrate for "free" pulmonary incompetence. This again is a manifestation of restrictive right ventricular physiology. The intrinsic myocardial disease in these patients prevents progressive right ventricular dilatation [38]. For some therefore, relative immunity from the morbidity associated with pulmonary regurgitation is conferred by this "abnormality" of diastolic function. While almost certainly there is a spectrum of myocardial compliance, those patients with nonrestrictive physiology can be expected to react in a "normal" way to chronic pulmonary incompetence and its concomitant volume load. That is, in the presence of an incompetent pulmonary valve, progressive right ventricular dilatation is inevitable. Indeed, several studies have shown a linear relationship between the amount of pulmonary regurgitation and right ventricular size and function [39,40]. Accelerated right ventricular dilatation will occur whenever there is increased impedence to pulmonary blood flow. Thus, a raised pulmonary vascular resistance, generalized hypoplasia, or branch pulmonary artery stenosis will all accentuate the propensity to pulmonary regurgitation and right heart dilatation [41]. Aggressive treatment of the latter, by balloon dilation or stenting, can achieve acute reduction in the degree of pulmonary regurgitation [41] and has become an essential part of the management of these patients in early life.

While our understanding of the factors generating right heart dilatation have increased substantially over the last decade or so, our understanding of the issues regarding timing of intervention for right heart dilatation associated with pulmonary remains immature. As with the left heart dilatation associated with chronic mitral or aortic incompetence. The primary aim of intervention is to relieve volume load at a time appropriate for complete reverse remodeling of ventricular size and function to occur. This has been a challenging area even for the easier to measure left ventricle and remains an area of great uncertainty for the right ventricle. The issue of timing is particularly pertinent to childhood and teenage years, where there is a natural tendency to avoid early use of prosthetic valves in a growing child. The currently available data suggests that this strategy of delayed intervention, particularly when

extended into early adult life, does not allow for reverse remodeling of the right ventricle in the setting of chronic pulmonary incompetence after tetralogy repair [42]. The optimal timing of pulmonary valve implantation remains to be determined, although the advent of transcatheter implantable valve devices may improve our ability and further modify our desire to restore pulmonary valve function at an earlier age than previously.

The pressure loaded ventricle

It is now unusual to allow persistent pressure loading of the subpulmonary right ventricle. Transcatheter, or surgical intervention, is performed at an early age and usually relieves significant right ventricular hypertension, albeit frequently, at the expense of pulmonary regurgitation (see above). The best example of chronic right ventricular hypertension, and perhaps the most relevant to contemporary pediatric cardiac practice, is the situation where the right ventricle acts as the systemic ventricle. For both naturally occurring (congenitally corrected transposition CCTGA) and surgically imposed (after atrial redirection procedures), there remains substantial concern regarding the ability of the right ventricle to act as the systemic pumping chamber throughout a normal lifespan.

Despite these significant concerns, there is remarkably little substantive data to support them. Clinical surveys emphasize "abnormalities" of right ventricular function, but have failed to demonstrate temporal decline [43]. Furthermore, as mentioned earlier, there are virtually no data to support any intrinsic biochemical or physiologic difference between the right and left ventricular myofibers. At an anecdotal level CCTGA has been first diagnosed at autopsy in old age. And most patients with systemic right ventricles lead essentially normal lives. It is, however, undoubtedly true, that some patients do not, and most formal studies of maximal exercise performance reveal marked reduced functional capacity [44]. Whether this represents intrinsic right ventricular failure, or reflects the effects of secondary phenomena, remains to be seen. Most of the current available data support the latter however.

Diastolic failure

Much of the justification for transition to the arterial switch as treatment for simple transposition of the great arteries was the improbability of the right ventricle acting as a systemic pump throughout a normal lifespan. This method was abandoned over 20 years ago, and those patients surviving after an atrial switch are a unique and interesting population. Remarkably few have presented in their early adult life with right ventricular failure. Equally, remarkably few patients have a normal exercise tolerance [45] and other issues such as atrial dysrhythmia, overt baffle obstruction, and the tricuspid regurgitation. All this contributes to the decreased functional reserve seen in these patients. Interestingly, despite reduced maximal exercise performance, many of these patients sustain normal submaximal exercise performance [46]. Thus many remain asymptomatic in their daily activities, despite these obvious adverse physiologic sequelae.

Assessment of systemic right ventricular function is particularly difficult. There can be no doubt that right ventricular shortening is reduced when in a subaortic position [47]. Whether this represents intrinsic failure of the myocardium or an adaptive response of the right ventricle to its loading conditions has been notoriously difficult to examine. In a recent study of patients after atrial switch, some of the determinants of decreased functional reserve were examined using load independent indices of right ventricular function [48]. Despite reduced resting ejection fraction, end-systolic elastance appeared to respond appropriately to dobutamine stress, when assessed using a conductance catheter technique (Fig. 13.10). Diastolic responses

to both dobutamine stress and exercise in these patients was highly abnormal, however. There was a failure of augmentation of stroke volume and, in some, a fall in stroke volume with tachycardia. This is highly abnormal and appeared to be related to a fixed ventricular filling rate. Thus the reduced RR interval coincident with induced tachycardia led to reduced stroke volume. This was unlikely to be related to intrinsic myocardial diastolic disease, as time constant of relaxation and minimum dP/dT all behaved appropriately. More likely, diastolic failure under these circumstances was related to abnormal atrioventricular coupling consequent upon the abnormal atrial pathways imposed by the surgery. While clearly not appropriate to all patients after atrial switch, these data emphasized the need to perform detailed investigations, using appropriate indices, when assessing abnormal right heart hemodynamics.

Systolic failure

Clearly, the same abnormalities of atrioventricular coupling cannot explain the reduced exercise performance seen in patients with CCTGA. Once again, right ventricular shortening is demonstrably lower than normal and fails to respond in a normal way to exercise or dobutamine stress [49]. The effect of coexisting anatomic lesions, such as left ventricular outflow tract obstruction, ventricular septal defect, and intrinsic abnormalities of the tricuspid valve, must all be taken into account and contribute to the complex hemodynamic milieau that exemplifies

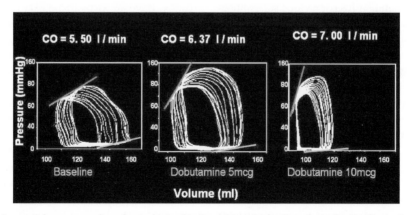

Figure 13.10 Sequential pressure–volume loops obtained in the right ventricle of a patient after the Mustard operation for transposition of the great arteries. Systemic ventricular responses (end-systolic elastance) are appropriate, during increasing doses of Dobutamine. Diastolic function improves. Note, however, how the stroke volume reduces sequentially with increasing tachycardia (see text for details). From Derrick et al. [48] with permission.

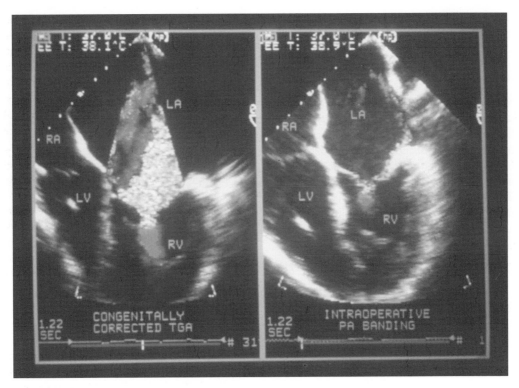

Figure 13.11 Transesophogeal echocardiogram performed during pulmonary artery banding in a patient with congenitally corrected transposition and no associated anatomic lesions, but severe tricuspid valve incompetence. During pulmonary arterial banding the left ventricle enlarges, the septum is moved toward the right ventricle and the septal leaflet is opposed to the other leaflets of the tricuspid valve. Consequently, there is a marked, acute, reduction in tricuspid incompetence and an extraordinary reduction in left atrial size (see text for details).

these patients. However, it is worth reemphasizing that isolated right ventricular myocardial failure is a relative rarity in these patients. More common is progressive right heart dilation and systolic failure in the presence of chronic and worsening tricuspid regurgitation. In this regard, the systemic right ventricle is at a marked disadvantage, compared with its left ventricular counterpart. The anatomic pillar on which the definition of right ventricular and tricuspid valve morphology rests, is the presence or chordal attachments to the interventricular septum. Progressive right heart dilatation, no matter what its cause, leads to septal shift toward the left ventricle. This sets the scene for the development of tricuspid regurgitation, as the septal leaflet is pulled away from the anterosuperior and mural leaflets. Thus a vicious spiral of progressive right heart dilation consequent upon, but leading to worsening, tricuspid regurgitation is established. Understanding this phenomenon allows us to harness, and reverse, these right-left heart interactions. Reversal of the adverse septal shift can be achieved by increasing the pressure in the left ventricle. Banding the pulmonary artery may substantially reduce the degree of tricuspid incompetence [50], without any direct surgery needing to be performed on the tricuspid valve itself. Figure 13.11 shows the acute response of banding of the pulmonary artery of a profoundly regurgitant tricuspid valve in the setting of CCTGA. As the band is tightened, the tricuspid valve regurgitation all but disappears, and the gross left atrial dilatation is reversed almost immediately. Pulmonary artery banding under these circumstances is usually performed as part of a retraining protocol in order to reestablish the left ventricle as the systemic ventricle. This is either as part of a double switch in CCTGA or a Mustard take down and arterial switch after atrial redirection procedures. Such is the improvement in tricuspid regurgitation, and symptoms in many of these patients, that further surgery to complete an "anatomic" repair may not be desired or necessary, at least in the short term.

Summary

In summary, the importance of the right ventricle in the biventricular circulation of patients with both acquired and congenital heart disease is increasingly understood. The past decade has seen a remarkable increase in our understanding of right ventricular physiology, and how it may be modified by naturally occurring models of right heart disease. There is still much to learn, and it is notable that this chapter does not mention pharmacologic therapy for right ventricular dysfunction. Virtually nothing is known in this regard. Nonetheless, with increasing understanding of the basic physiology, a refinement of indications for surgical therapy, and investigation of appropriate pharmaco-therapy, there is a potential for an equally extraordinary change in our understanding of right ventricular performance over the next 10 years.

References

1. Sade RM, Castaneda AR. The dispensable right ventricle. Surgery 1975; 77(5):624–631.
2. La Vecchia L et al. Predictors of right ventricular dysfunction in patients with coronary artery disease and reduced left ventricular ejection fraction. Coron Artery Dis 2002; 13(6):319–322.
3. Redington AN. Right ventricular function. Cardiology Clin 2002; 20(3):341–349.
4. Vogel M, et al. Validation of myocardial acceleration during isovolumic contraction as a novel noninvasive index of right ventricular contractility: Comparison with ventricular pressure-volume relations in an animal model. Circulation 2002; 105(14):1693–1699.
5. Vogel M et al. Noninvasive assessment of left ventricular force-frequency relationships using tissue Doppler-derived isovolumic acceleration: Validation in an animal model. Circulation 2003; 107(12): 1647–1652.
6. Geva T, Powell AJ, Crawford EC, et al. Evaluation of regional differences in right ventricular systolic function by acoustic quantification echocardiography and cine magnetic resonance imaging. Circulation 1998; 98(4):339–345.
7. Gibson DG, Brown DJ. Continuous assessment of left ventricular shape in man. Br Heart J 1975; 37(9): 904–910.

8. Sanchez-Quintana D, Anderson RH, Ho SY. Ventricular myoarchitecture in tetralogy of Fallot. Heart 1996; 76(3):280–286.
9. Kendall SW, Bittner HB, Peterseim DS, et al. Right ventricular function in the donor heart. Eur J Cardiothorac Surg 1997; 11(4):609–615.
10. Ferlinz J. Angiographic assessment of right ventricular volumes and ejection fraction. Cathet Cardiovasc Diagn 1976; 2(1):5–14.
11. Rouleau JL, Paradis P, Shenasa H, et al. Faster time to peak tension and velocity of shortening in right versus left ventricular trabeculae and papillary muscles of dogs. Circ Res 1986; 59(5):556–561.
12. Kass DA et al. Comparative influence of load versus inotropic states on indexes of ventricular contractility: Experimental and theoretical analysis based on pressure-volume relationships. Circulation 1987; 76(6):1422–1436.
13. Sunagawa K. Sagawa K. Models of ventricular contraction based on time-varying elastance. Crit Rev Biomed Eng 1982; 7(3):193–228.
14. Redington AN, Gray HH, Hodson ME, et al. Characterisation of the normal right ventricular pressure-volume relation b biplace angiography and simultaneous micromanometer pressure measurements. Br Heart J 1988; 59(1):3–30.
15. Redington AN, Rigby ML, Shinebourne EA, et al. Changes in the pressure-volume relation of the right ventricle when its loading conditions are modified. Br Heart J 1990; 63(1):45–49.
16. Nozawa T, Cheung CP, Noda T, et al. Relation between left ventricular oxygen consumption and pressure-volume area in conscious dogs. Circulation 1994; 89(2):810–817.
17. Weber KT, Janicki JS, Shroff S, et al. Contractile mechanics and interaction of the right and left ventricles. Am J Cardiol 1981; 47(3):686–695.
18. Dickstein ML, Yano O, Spotnitz HM, et al. Assessment of right ventricular contractile state with the conductance catheter technique in the pig. Cardiovasc Res 1995; 29(6):820–826.
19. Feneley MP et al. Comparison of preload recruitable stroke work, end-systolic pressure-volume and dP/dtmax-end-diastolic volume relations as indexes of left ventricular contractile performance in patients undergoing routine cardiac catheterization. J Am Coll Cardiol 1992; 19(7):1522–1530.
20. McDicken WN, Sutherland GR, Moran CM, et al. Colour Doppler velocity imaging of the myocardium. Ultrasound Med Biol 1992; 18(6–7):651–654.
21. Vogel M, Sponring J, Cullen S, et al. Regional wall motion and abnormalities of electrical depolarization and repolarization in patients after surgical repair of tetraloty of Fallot. Circulation 2001; 103(12):1669–1673.

22. Vermilion RP, Snider AR, Meliones JN, *et al.* Pulsed Doppler evaluation of right ventricular diastolic filling in children with pulmonary valve stenosis before and after balloon valvuloplasty. Am J Cardiol 1990; 66(1):79–84.

23. Redington AN, Penny D, Rigby ML *et al.* Antegrade diasblic pulmonary arterial flow as a marker of right ventricular restriction. Cardiol Young 1992; 2:382–386.

24. Damiano RJ Jr, La Follette P Jr, Cox JL, *et al.* Significant left ventricular contribution to right ventricular systolic function. Am J Physiol 1991; 261(5 Pt 2): H1514–H1524.

25. Hoffman D, Sisto D, Frater RW, *et al.* Left-to-right ventricular interaction with a noncontracting right ventricle. J Thorac Cardiovasc Surg 1994; 107(6): 1496–1502.

26. Brookes C, Ravan H, White P, *et al.* Acute right ventricular dilatation in response to ischemia significantly impairs left ventricular systolic performance. Circulation 1999; 100(7):761–767.

27. Lofland GK *et al.* Critical aortic stenosis in the neonate: A multi-institutional study of management, outcomes, and risk factors. Congenital Heart Surgeons Society. J Thorac Cardiovasc Surg 2001; 12(1):10–27.

28. Cabzuelo-Huerta G, Frontera-Izquierdo P, Vazquez-Perez J. Isolated hypoplasia of the right ventricle with interatrial communication. Study of a case and review of the literature. An Esp Pediatr 1983; 18(1):39–44.

29. Cullen S, Shore D, Redington A. Characterization of right ventricular diastolic performance after complete repair of tetralogy of Fallot. Restrictive physiology predicts slow postoperative recovery. Circulation 1995; 91(6):1782–1789.

30. Shekerdemian LS, Bush A, Shore DF, *et al.* Cardiorespiratory responses to negative pressure ventilation after tetralogy of Fallot repair: A hemodynamic tool for patients with a low-output state. J Am Coll Cardiol 1999; 33(2):549–555.

31. Shekerdemian LS, Schulze-Neick I, Redington AN, *et al.* Negative pressure ventilation as haemodynamic rescue following surgery for congenital heart disease. Intensive Care Med 2000; 26(1):93–96.

32. Di Donato RM, Jonas RA, Mayer JE, *et al.* Neonatal repair of Fallot's tetralogy with and without pulmonary atresia. Nippon Kyobu Geka Gakkai Zasshi 1989; 37(suppl):97.

33. Pigula FA, Khalil PN, Mayer JE, *et al.* Repair of tetralogy of Fallot in neonates and young infants. Circulation 1999; 100(suppl 19):II157–II161.

34. Alvarado O, Sreeram N, McKay R, *et al.* Cavopulmonary connection in repair of atrioventricular septal defect with small right ventricle. Ann Thorac Surg 1993; 55(3):729–736.

35. Van Ardsell GS. One and one half ventricle repairs. Semin Thorac Cardiovasc Surg Pediatr Card Surg Annu 2000; 3:173–178.

36. Shimazaki Y, Blackstone EH, Kirklin JW. The natural history of isolated pulmonary valve incompetence: Surgical implications. Thorac Cardiovasc Surg 1984; 32(4):257–259.

37. Gatzoulis MA *et al.* Risk factors for arrhythmia and sudden cardiac death late after repair of tetralogy of Fallot: A multicentre study. Lancet 2000; 356(9234): 975–981.

38. Gatzoulis MA, Till JA, Somerville J, *et al.* Mechanoelectrical interaction in tetralogy of Fallot. QRS prolongation relates to right ventricular size and predicts malignant ventricular arrhythmias and sudden death. Circulation 1995; 92(2):231–237.

39. Redington AN, Oldershaw PJ, Shinebourne EA, *et al.* A new technique for the assessment of pulmonary regurgitation and its application to the assessment of right ventricular function before and after repair of tetralogy of Fallot. Br Heart J 1988; 60(1):57–65.

40. Rebergen SA, Chin JG, Ottenkamp J, *et al.* Pulmonary regurgitation in the late postoperative follow-up of tetralogy of Fallot. Volumetric quantitation by nuclear magnetic resonance velocity mapping. Circulation 1993; 88(5, pt 1):2257–2266.

41. Chaturvedi RR *et al.* Increased airway pressure and simulated branch pulmonary artery stenosis increase pulmonary regurgitatiion after repair of tetralogy of Fallot. Real-time analysis with a conductance catheter technique. Circulation 1997; 95(3):643–649.

42. Therrien J *et al.* Impact of pulmonary valve replacement on arrhythmia propensity late after repair of tetralogy of Fallot. Circulation 2001; 103(20):2484–2494.

43. Wong KY, Venables AW, Kelly Mj, *et al.* Longitudinal study of ventricular function after the Mustard operation for transposition of the great arteries: A long term follow up. Br Heart J 1988; 60(4):316–323.

44. Fredriksen PM *et al.* Aerobic capacity in adults with various congenital heart diseases. Am J Cardiol 2001; 87(3):310–314.

45. Matthys D, De Wolf D, Verhaaren H. Lack of increase in stroke volume during exercise in asymptomatic adolescents in sinus rhythm after intraatrial repair for simple transposition of the great arteries. Am J Cardiol 1996; 78(5):595–596.

46. Musewe NN *et al.* Cardiopulmonary adaption at rest and during exercise 10 years after Mustard atrial repair for transposition of the great arteries. Circulation 1988; 77(5):1055–1061.

47. Ramsay JM, Venables AW, Kelly MJ, *et al.* Right and left ventricular function at rest and with exercise after the Mustard operation for transposition of the great arteries. Br Heart J 1984; 51(4):364–370.

48. Derrick GP *et al.* Failure of stroke volume augmentation during exercise and dobutamine stress is unrelated to load-independent indexes of right ventricular performance after the Mustard operation. Circulation 2000; 102(19, suppl 3):III154-III159.

49. Ohuchi *et al.* Comparison of the right and left ventricle as a systemic ventricle during exercise in patients with congenital heart disease. Am Heart J 1999; 137(6):1185–1194.

50. Van Son JA, Reddy VM, Silverman NH, *et al.* Regression of tricuspid regurgitation after two-stage arterial switch operation for failing systemic ventricle after atrial inversion operation. J Thorac Cardiovasc Surg 1996; III(2):342–347.

CHAPTER 14

The Left Ventricle in a Dual Chambered Circulation

Debra A. Dodd, MD, Ann Kavanaugh-McHugh, MD, & Thomas P. Graham, Jr., MD

Introduction

Today a wide variety of medical, interventional catheterization and surgical options are available for the management of congenital heart disease. For optimal care, it is crucial to determine who needs intervention, choose the correct intervention, and select the optimal timing for that treatment. In addition, we would like to be able to evaluate the success of these interventions so that we can modify procedures and continue to improve outcomes. The evaluation process involves assessment of multiple aspects of systemic ventricular function. For ductal dependent infants it is necessary to assess left ventricular size since the right ventricle may be needed to maintain adequate cardiac output. This is a major issue for most severe forms of left heart obstruction presenting at birth. For other lesions, a fairly simple measure of ventricular performance may suffice. There are numerous ways to measure this including shortening fraction, ejection fraction, stroke volume, and cardiac output. These are used as a surrogate measure for extent and/or velocity of shortening, or how much each muscle fiber contracts against a certain afterload, which is a measure of myocardial contractility.

These measures, however, vary greatly depending on the loading conditions of the myocardial fibers, specifically the preload and afterload on the heart itself. These shortening parameters may be most helpful in monitoring ventricular function after various interventions when loading conditions approach normal. However, most examples of unrepaired congenital heart lesions do not have normal loading conditions. Preload may be decreased (e.g. total anomalous pulmonary venous connection) or increased (e.g. ventricular septal defect), afterload may be decreased (e.g. D-transposition of the great arteries with intact ventricular septum) or increased (e.g. aortic stenosis). Monitoring of ventricular performance alone may not be optimal for these conditions. In many situations, such as those above, one would like to monitor intrinsic myocardial performance independent of loading conditions, that is, myocardial contractility. A number of indices have been developed which are less dependent on loading conditions but none is perfect. Most of these indices compare some measure of length or volume change to a measure of pressure, force, or stress. These are variations on the Frank–Starling principle of preload recruitable stoke work [1].

With yet other congenital lesions, it is not abnormal loading conditions that invalidate the use of the simpler measures of ventricular performance, but it is abnormal left ventricular geometry. Many of these indices make assumptions about left ventricular geometry that are not valid in the presence of potentially detrimental interactions with the pressure or volume overloaded right ventricle (e.g. pulmonary stenosis, Ebstein's anomaly). With other lesions the important questions may relate to the presence or absence of regional wall motion abnormalities (e.g. pulmonary atresia with coronary fistulae; anomalous left coronary artery from the pulmonary artery, D-transposition of the great arteries following arterial switch repair). While discussions of left ventricular performance generally focus on systolic performance, left ventricular dysfunction can be primarily systolic, diastolic, or a combination of both. Measures of diastolic dysfunction have been historically more difficult than that of systolic function. Finally, the presence of conduction delays on the electrocardiogram can alter left ventricular performance (e.g. Wolff–Parkinson–White syndrome; bundle branch block).

Many factors influence the method chosen for assessment of ventricular function. With congenital heart disease we also have to remember that our patients are often unable or unwilling to cooperate with personnel trying to perform the testing, and sedation or general anesthesia may be required for some procedures in children that would be done more easily and with less risk in the cooperative adult. Patient size and age are also an issue as the resolution or ability to gate with faster heart rates or respirations may be inadequate for some methodologies. Obese patients may have insufficient windows for imaging by ultrasound, necessitating use of another technique. Often the normal range for a given test may vary from infancy to adolescence. Also the frequency with which testing is anticipated may influence the index utilized. One must decide whether one wishes to perform a detailed, more invasive, and usually pro-

longed exam or whether one wishes to be able to repeat a faster, noninvasive measure on multiple occasions to monitor changes in function over time. Finally, in the patient undergoing cardiac catheterization for evaluation of other hemodynamic features of their disease, intracardiac testing may add little additional risk, whereas, noninvasive testing may be preferred in most other settings. All these issues must be considered when choosing a method to evaluate the left ventricle in a dual chambered circulation in the presence of congenital heart lesions. It is good to be familiar with the various modalities that have been validated and their limitations so that inappropriate application does not occur. Also it is common to use more than one index.

Assessment of systolic function

Ventricular size, ejection fraction, and mass

Left ventricular size, ejection fraction, and mass have been measured by angiography, radionuclide angiography, 2D echocardiography, magnetic resonance imaging (MRI), and 3D echocardiography, and normal values established for children (Table 14.1) [2–7]. Analyses for the first three methods make assumptions that the ventricle is

Table 14.1 Normal Childhood Values for Left Ventricular End-Diastolic Volume, Ejection Fraction and Mass Using Various Methods.

Investigator	Method	Age group	Left ventricular end-diastolic volume (ml/m²) mean ± SD	Ejection fraction (%) mean ± SD	Mass (g/m²) mean ± SD
Graham et al. [2]	Angiography	<2 years	42 ± 10^a	68 ± 5	96 ± 11
		>2 years	73 ± 11	63 ± 5	86 ± 11
Graham [3]		BSA<0.5m²	$74.3\,(\text{BSA})^{1.49a}$		
Mercier et al. [5]	2D Echocardiography	6 weeks–20 years	b	b	b
Parrish et al. [4]	RVG, rest	5–19 years	74 ± 13^c	62 ± 8^c	NA
	RVG, exercise		66 ± 20^c	71 ± 8^c	
Poutanen et al. [7]	3D Echocardiography	8–13 years	57.3	60.8 ± 1.8	61.8
Lorenz et al. [6]	MRI	7–20 years	67 ± 9		81 ± 13
Poutanen et al. [7]		8–13 years	54.2	59.1 ± 3.8	61.2

RVG, radionuclide ventriculography; MRI, magnetic resonance imaging; SD, standard deviation; NA, not applicable.
[a] LVEDV vs. BSA is nonlinear below BSA of 0.5 m², normal values for younger patients are best approximated by the formula given.
[b] No studies with absolute values, only correlations with angiographic values:

$$\text{LVEDV}_{echo} = 0.64\,\text{LVEDV}_{cath} + 3.9\ (r = 0.97)$$
$$\text{EF}_{echo} = 0.94\,\text{EF}_{cath} + 6.7\ (r = 0.91).$$

[c] Values are estimated from graphs.

elliptoid or conical. Magnetic resonance imaging and 3D echocardiographic analyses usually do not make any assumptions about ventricular shape, with volume calculated by summing the volumes of the cavities in contiguous slices. Mercier *et al.* demonstrated that 2D echocardiographic measurements of end-diastolic volume and ejection fraction correlate well with angiographic measurements, though echocardiography underestimates volume but not ejection fraction compared to angiography [5]. This error in volume measurements may be more pronounced in infants due to the slower acquisition rates of echocardiography which means that the true end-diastolic volume may not be recorded. Because of this difficulty, Parsons *et al.* demonstrated in neonates with aortic stenosis using 2D echocardiography, that a measure of maximal area alone on parasternal long axis view >2 cm^2 allowed one to identify those infants with aortic stenosis whose left ventricles should be adequate for dual circulation [8].

Assuming relatively normal preload and afterload, ejection fraction can be a simple estimate of myocardial performance. Ejection fraction (EF) is equal to:

$$EF = \frac{V_d - V_s}{V_d},$$

where V_d is end-diastolic volume and V_s is end-systolic volume. Therefore, this measurement has the same limitations as described above for measurement of ventricular volume. If wall thickness is measured, using the specific gravity of myocardium (1.05), left ventricular mass (LVM) can be calculated using the formula:

$$LVM = 1.05\,(V_{c+w} - V_c),$$

where V_{c+w} is the volume inclusive of the wall thickness and V_c is the chamber volume. The American Society of Echocardiography has published this formula for m-mode derived LV mass:

$$LV\ mass = 1.04^*\,[(LVEDD + LVPW_d + IVS_d)^3 - LVEDD^3],$$

where LVEDD is left ventricular end-diastolic diameter (cm), $LVPW_d$ is left ventricular posterior wall thickness (cm), and IVS_d is interventricular septal thickness (cm). All these methodologies offer useful information provided one recognizes that they are not necessarily equivalent.

Angiography has the disadvantage of being the most invasive method with the highest radiation exposure. At the other extreme, 2D echocardiography is noninvasive, with no radiation exposure, and has a short acquisition time and analysis time so that it can be done repetitively in the clinical setting. However, in some patients it is technically impossible to get adequate echocardiographic pictures for analysis. This occurs frequently in obese and older congenital heart patients. Radionuclide ventriculography has no "window" limitations, but does require an intravenous injection and limited radiation exposure. However, resolution may be inadequate in infants and small children. For magnetic resonance imaging (MRI), the major limiting factors have been access to the imaging machine, cost, and time required for acquisition and analysis. Faster acquisition speeds and automation of analysis are improving clinical utility [9]. MRI has the definite advantage that it can be used for analysis in congenital heart lesions with abnormal left ventricular geometry. Niwa *et al.* used MRI to measure ventricular volumes in children, aged 4 months to 8 years with morphologically abnormal left ventricles due to tetralogy of Fallot, double outlet right ventricle, D-transposition of the great arteries, and found the volumes and ejection fractions compared favorably with those measured by angiography [10]. However, the patient must be immobile during MRI acquisition and this may require anesthesia for the young child. Acar *et al.* demonstrated in children that ejection fraction measured by 3D echocardiography correlated well with results from radionuclide angiography [11]. 3D echocardiography has the potential advantages of quicker acquisition, less expense, and more portability than MRI, yet has the same advantage of not making assumptions about left ventricular geometry. Apfel *et al.* demonstrated that 3D echocardiographic measurement of left ventricular size and ejection fraction in the presence of a hypertensive RV compared well with the same measurement by MRI [12].

Velocity of circumferential shortening (VCF)

The velocity of circumferential shortening (VCF) is a measure of ventricular performance that can be obtained noninvasively. It is calculated by normalizing the change in left ventricular dimension (shortening fraction or SF) measured on m-mode tracings of the

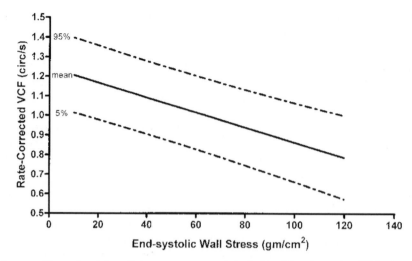

Figure 14.1 Diagram of the end-systolic wall stress vs. rate-corrected velocity of fiber shortening (VCF) relation for children >2 years. Linear regression with 5–95% confidence levels. Depressed contractile state (VCF$_c$ low for the level of σ_{es}) may be distinguished from situations in which contractility is normal (within 95% confidence lines) but afterload is increased. VCF$_c$ high for the level of σ_{es} is characteristic of an increased inotropic state. Based on current normative data, (Colan SD, personal communication).

left ventricle to the time over which the shortening occurs (left ventricular ejection time or LVET):

Mean velocity of circumferential shortening (VCF)
= SF/LVET

Ejection time can be measured from the aortic valve m-mode or on the pulse trace. Velocity of circumferential shortening is dependent on loading conditions.

Rate corrected velocity of circumferential shortening (VCF$_c$)

The velocity of circumferential shortening (VCF) can be corrected to a heart rate of 60 beats per min by dividing the ejection time by the square root of the RR interval to derive the rate-corrected velocity of circumferential fiber shortening:

$$VCFc = SF/ETc = \frac{(SF)(\sqrt{RR})}{ET}$$

This index is still dependent on loading conditions.

Index of ventricular systolic function

Colan *et al.* demonstrated that when VCFc is plotted against left ventricular end-systolic wall stress (a measure of afterload), the relationship is linear

and does not vary significantly with changes in preload or afterload but does change with inotropic stimulation [13]. Therefore, this appears to be a fairly good load-independent index of myocardial contractility. The slope of this linear relationship is constant above 2 years of age (Fig. 14.1), but below 2 years of age the slope becomes increasingly steeper [14]. That is, there is a progressive decrease in contractility from birth until approximately 2 years of age after which it remains fairly constant into adulthood. Normal values have been reported as absolute values for children over 2 years or by exponential equation over a wider age range (Table 14.2) [14,15].

Wall stress (σ) is the force exerted on the myocardium per unit area and is proportional to the intraluminal pressure (P) and the LV cavity dimension (D) and inversely proportional to the wall thickness (h):

$$\sigma = s^*PD/h$$

or more specifically for meridional wall stress is:

$$\sigma_{meridional} = [1.35(P)(D)]/\{(4)(h)[1 - h/D]\}$$

where σ is wall stress (g/cm^2), P is LV end-systolic pressure (mmHg), D is LV end-systolic dimension at aortic valve closure (cm), h is the LV end-systolic posterior wall thickness (cm), and 1.35 is the conversion factor from mmHg to g/cm^2 [13,16]. These

Table 14.2 Normal Childhood Values for Noninvasive Estimation of Left Ventricular Contractile State.

	Measure	Mean ± SD	Regression formula
Investigator		Franklin et al. [15]	Colan et al. [14]
Age of patients		2–12 years	7 days–19 years
	VCF (circ/s)	1.25 ± 0.15	
	VCFc (circ/s)	1.01 ± 0.11	$0.26(e^{-0.56 \times \text{Age}}) + 1.04$
	σ_m (g/cm2)	45.5 ± 12.4	$12.2(\text{Age}^{0.31}) + 20.4$
	σ_c (g/cm2)	114.5 ± 22.2	$13.3(\text{Age}^{0.32}) + 33.1$

VCR, velocity of circumferential fiber shortening; VCFc, rate-corrected velocity of circumferential fiber shortening; σ_m, endocardial end-systolic meridional wall stress; σ_c, endocardial end-systolic circumferential wall stress; SD, standard deviation; Age = age of patient in years.

calculations assume there is no regional variation in wall thickness or cavity dimension, the left ventricle is ellipsoid, and there is no regional variation in the phase of contraction. End-systolic meridional wall stress (σ_m) is defined as the load resisting long-axis shortening. Circumferential wall stress (σ_c) is defined as the load resisting short-axis shortening. Circumferential wall stress is more difficult to obtain as it requires measurement of the ventricular length, which is technically possible in only two-thirds of patients [14]. To perform these calculation, one needs: (1) m-mode trace with good septal endocardium and posterior wall endocardium and epicardium; (2) indirect arterial pressure waveform from carotid artery which is then calibrated with a cuff systolic and diastolic pressure, and end-systolic pressure is determined by interpolation of the pressure at the dicrotic notch, and (3) phonogram recording of the first high-frequency component of the aortic valve closure sound. These measurements will often require sedation in the small child or infant. A simpler method relying on the mean blood pressure rather than an end-systolic pressure also allows identification of children with abnormal contractility [17].

End-systolic elastance

An alternative measure of contractility is elastance and is generated from multiple pressure–volume loops at variable preload conditions. The limiting factor for use of this index clinically has been the difficulty in measuring ventricular volume. Chaturvedi et al. placed a conductance catheter and a pressure tipped catheter inserted through the left ventricular apex, with a snare on the inferior vena cava to vary preload, in 13 children undergoing open repair of simple congenital heart defects (atrial septal defect, double outlet right ventricle, aortic stenosis) and were able to generate good quality pressure–volume loops [18].

Time intervals

Systolic time intervals can be used to assess ventricular function. Ahmed et al. demonstrated a correlation between the ratio of preejection period (PEP) to left ventricular ejection time (LVET) and direct measurements of myocardial contractility ($+dP/dt$) obtained by invasive techniques in normal patients and in patients with myocardial disease [19]. With simultaneous aortic pulse trace and electrocardiogram, PEP is calculated by subtracting LVET (measured from onset of aortic pulse to dicrotic notch) from the total electromechanical systole (measured from the Q wave to the dicrotic notch). As ventricular function deteriorates, the PEP lengthens and the ejection time shortens, producing an increase in the ratio of preejection period to ejection time. While PEP and PEP/LVET are fairly independent of loading conditions, comparison of PEP between patients or groups is only valid in the absence of extramyocardial influences such as aortic valve disease, pulmonary hypertension, or shunt lesions. Also, conduction delays will prolong the PEP. To overcome the limitation of variable conduction time, some have recommended further subdivision of the PEP into electromechanical delay and the isovolumetric contraction time (ICT), with the latter being a potentially better index of contraction. Use of intervals in the clinical setting has been limited by the difficulty in measuring them accurately with the equipment available in the past. However, Doppler echocardiography has made measurement of isovolumetric contraction and relaxation easier.

Myocardial performance index (MPI) or Tei index

Tei *et al.* introduced a noninvasive Doppler-derived myocardial performance index that simplifies use of time intervals in the clinical setting by combining the measurement of isovolumetric contraction time and isovolumetric relaxation time [20]. Isovolumetric contraction time correlates with $+\mathrm{d}P/\mathrm{d}t$, an index of contractility; and isovolumetric relaxation time correlates with $-\mathrm{d}P/\mathrm{d}t$ and tau, indices of relaxation. This new measure of ventricular function, myocardial performance index (MPI or Tei index), correlates with noninvasive and invasive measures of left ventricular function.

$$\mathrm{MPI} = \frac{\mathrm{ICT} + \mathrm{IVT}}{\mathrm{ET}} = \frac{a - b}{b}$$

It is easily measured from mitral and aortic Doppler traces (Fig. 14.2). Because myocardial contractility and relaxation are energy dependent, myocardial dysfunction results in prolongation of the isovolumetric time intervals and an increase in the myocardial performance index. This index may be applicable to patients with abnormal left ventricular shape. This Doppler index was found to be more sensitive than mitral deceleration time or E/A ratio in the assessment of LV diastolic relaxation. The myocardial performance index for normal children is 0.35 ± 0.03 for the left ventricle, not significantly different than adults [21]. One limitation of the Doppler derived myocardial performance index is that the two intervals needed for calculation of myocardial performance index are measured sequentially and are less reliable in the presence of heart rate fluctuation, a common finding due to marked respiratory variation seen in many children. Discordant function due to conduction delays will affect most of these measurements even though individual fibers have good contractility.

Modified myocardial performance index (MPI) or Tei index by tissue Doppler imaging

Using tissue Doppler techniques, one can simultaneously measure contraction and relaxation velocities from the myocardium. Mitral annular velocities obtained from the apical 4-chamber view show three major distinctive waves: a positive wave toward the apex during systole (S) and 2 waves away from the transducer during diastole analogous to the aortic outflow trace and mitral inflow traces combined (Fig. 14.3). The first diastolic wave occurs during

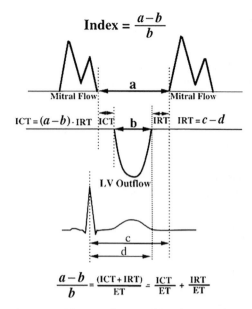

Figure 14.2 Schematic drawing of Doppler intervals. Myocardial performance index is calculated by measuring two intervals: a = interval between cessation and onset of mitral inflow, and b = ejection time (ET) of left ventricular outflow. Other available intervals include isovolumetric relaxation time (IRT) measured by subtracting interval d between R wave and cessation of left ventricular outflow from interval c between R wave and onset of mitral inflow. Isovolumetric contraction time (ICT) is obtained by subtracting isovolumetric relaxation time from $a-b$. Reprinted from [20] with permission from the American Society of Echocardiography.

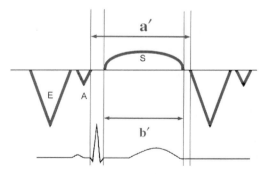

Figure 14.3 Schematic drawing of tissue Doppler intervals. E = early diastolic wave; A = late diastolic wave; S = systolic wave. Modified myocardial performance index is calculated by measuring two intervals: a' = interval between end and onset of mitral annular diastolic velocities, and b' = duration of the mitral annular systolic velocity. The modified MPI = $(a' - b'/b')$.

early filling (E), and the second corresponds to atrial contraction (A). Harada *et al.* showed in 46 children aged 5 days to 15 years that myocardial performance index could be calculated from tissue Doppler imaging (TDI) using the time interval between the end and the onset of mitral annular velocities during diastole (a') minus the duration of the S wave (b') divided by b' (i.e. ($a' - b'$)/b') and that this approximates the myocardial performance index obtained by conventional Doppler method (Fig. 14.3) [22]. Although the intervals measured by the tissue Doppler imaging were consistently longer than those measured by Doppler flow, the differences in myocardial performance index seen between 37 normal children and 9 children with heart disease were maintained with the myocardial performance index calculated by both techniques. This may be particularly useful as it eliminates error due to variation in heart rate over time, a common finding in children.

Assessment of diastolic function

From ventricular pressure recordings, several measures of ventricular relaxation have been widely utilized. An early measure was maximum rate of pressure decline ($-\mathrm{d}P\,\mathrm{d}t_{\mathrm{MAX}}$), but this is load dependent. The isovolumic fall in pressure is best approximated by an exponential curve, and the time constant describing this exponential fall in pressure (tau) is less load dependent than $-\mathrm{d}P/\mathrm{d}t_{\mathrm{MAX}}$. Time intervals have also been used to assess diastolic function, with isovolemic relaxation time (IRT) being used as a noninvasive measure of the rate of pressure decline. Isovolemic relaxation time is prolonged with impaired relaxation as it takes longer for the left ventricular pressure to reach left atrial pressure and mitral valve opening. Normal values for isovolemic relaxation time in children increase with age from 62 ± 10 ms for 3–8 year olds to 74 ± 13 ms for 13–17 year olds, and also vary with changes in heart rate [23]. However, conditions that increase left atrial pressure will also shorten isovolemic relaxation time.

Mitral and pulmonary vein Doppler patterns

Another noninvasive measure used to monitor diastolic function is the velocity of transmitral flow. With impaired relaxation, the rate of early ventricular filling (E wave velocity) is decreased, usually with compensatory increase in filling with atrial contraction

(A wave velocity). The E/A velocity ratio is decreased as a result. However, as diastolic ventricular function worsens with decreasing compliance, the patient will go through a period of "pseudonormalization" followed by an increase in E/A ratio and what is considered a restrictive inflow pattern (Fig. 14.4) [24]. When the pulmonary vein flow pattern is also considered, elevated left atrial pressure can be identified and pseudonormalization can be discriminated from normal inflow patterns. The transmitral flow pattern is also very dependent on preload, heart rate, and atrioventricular conduction interval. The E/A ratio for normal children over various heart rates has been reported, varying from approximately 3 at a heart rate of 50 down to 1.5 at a heart rate of 110 [23]. Since mitral flow measurements are so heart rate dependent they do vary significantly with age. In children, the relationship between the duration of the retrograde A wave in the pulmonary vein trace (PVAR) and the antegrade A wave in the mitral trace proved to be the most sensitive Doppler derived measure discriminating between normal patients and those with documented elevation of left ventricular end-diastolic pressure [23]. The duration of the retrograde A wave in the pulmonary vein trace lengthens and the mitral valve A wave duration decreases with increased ventricular end-diastolic pressure. In children, the ratio of the duration of the retrograde A wave in the pulmonary vein trace to the mitral valve A wave duration should be less than 1.2 and the difference between the duration of the retrograde A wave in the pulmonary vein trace and mitral valve A wave duration should be less than 29 ms.

Tissue Doppler

Tissue Doppler imaging is a new ultrasound technology that measures velocity of contraction and relaxation of the myocardium itself. Although information about both systolic (see myocardial performance index above) and diastolic function can be derived, this technique has gained popularity as a measure of diastolic function since alternatives are few. Mitral annulus motion is felt to reflect left ventricular volume changes since the apex is relatively fixed in the absence of severe abnormalities in ventricular geometry or severe regional wall motion abnormalities [25]. The rate of mitral annulus motion reflects rate of left ventricular volume change and is an indicator of systolic and diastolic function.

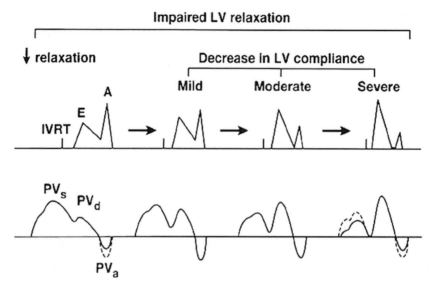

Figure 14.4 Schematic drawing of mitral inflow (upper) and pulmonary venous flow (lower) velocity during differenct stages of cardiac diseases. In most cardiac diseases, the initial diastolic filling abnormality is impaired myocardial relaxation. With mild to moderate decrease in left ventricular compliance and elevation of left atrial pressure, early rapid filling (E) and deceleration time return to normal, resulting in normalization of mitral inflow velocity pattern (pseudonormalization). With severe decrease in left ventricular compliance and marked elevation in left atrial pressure, early rapid filling (E) continues to increase along with shortening of IVRT, deceleration time, and A flow velocity. In purely impaired myocardial relaxation abnormality, pulmonary venous flow velocity has predominant systolic forward flow velocity (PV$_s$). With decrease in left ventricular compliance and increase in left atrial pressure, PVs component decreases and PV$_d$ component increases. With increase in left atrial pressure, PV atrial flow reversal velocity (PV$_a$) increases and the duration also becomes longer than the duration of mitral A flow velocity. Dashed lines represent variations seen at each stage. Reprinted from [24] with permission from the American Society of Echocardiography; as modified from Echocardiography, Vol. 9, Appleton CP and Hatle LK., The natural history of left ventricular filling abnormalities: assessment by two-dimensional and Doppler echocardiography, pg. 453, Copyright 1992, with permission from Blackwell Publishing.

In adults, this measurement has been demonstrated to be preload independent compared to mitral flow velocities which vary depending on the pressure gradient from left atrium to left ventricle [26]. Unlike mitral inflow velocities, annular velocity does not change significantly with alteration of preload with either saline infusion or nitroglycerin. Measurements are commonly done from the apical 4-chamber view, dividing each wall into thirds and measuring velocities in each segment, or measuring the velocity at the lateral mitral annulus. The pattern in each segment shows three major deflections, a positive deflection toward the apex in systole and two negative waves away from the apex in diastole, corresponding to the E and A waves of pulse Doppler (Fig. 14.3). Farias *et al.* showed in adults that both S and E myocardial velocities decrease steadily with worsening diastolic function independent of preload

compensation [27]. Pseudonormalization did not occur with tissue Doppler velocities as it did with mitral inflow patterns. They also showed that E myocardial velocity was the best single discriminator between normal adults and patients with diastolic dysfunction. Normal values for tissue Doppler in children have been reported (Table 14.3) [28–30]. The velocities decrease from base to apex for each wall, but the E/A ratio is constant. Harada *et al.* [28] did see an increase over age for E wave, E/A ratio, and S wave, whereas Kapusta *et al.* [29] did not see a significant change over age, and Swaminathan *et al.* [30] saw a slight decrease in A wave over age. While tissue Doppler can be measured from other views, the apical 4-chamber view gives the least intraobserver variability [29]. The use of this modality is only beginning to be explored in the population of patients with congenital heart disease.

Table 14.3 Normal Childhood Values for Tissue Doppler Velocities in Children Obtained from the Apical Four-Chamber View.

	Harada et al. [28] N = 48 7 days to 18 years mean ± SD	Kapusta et al. [29] N = 160 4 to 17.9 years mean (5th–95th percentiles)	Swaminathan et al. [30] N = 151 1 to 18 years mean ± SD
Left ventricle, basal			a
Peak E wave (cm/sec)	15.0 ± 4.1	17.6 (13.0–23.0)	18.5 ± 2.7
Peak A wave (cm/sec)	6.1 ± 1.7	5.5 (3.8–8.0)	7.3 ± 1.9
Peak E/A wave ratio	2.7 ± 1.0	3.3 (2.1–4.7)	
Peak S wave (cm/sec)	8.0 ± 2.4	9.7 (6.3–13.5)	9.6 ± 1.9
Interventricular septum, basal			
Peak E wave (cm/sec)	10.3 ± 2.7	14.3 (11.2–18.5)	
Peak A wave (cm/sec)	5.2 ± 1.4	5.8 (4.4–7.9)	
Peak E/A wave ratio	2.1 ± 0.6	2.5 (1.7–3.6)	
Peak S wave (cm/sec)	6.1 ± 1.7	8.1 (6.5–9.8)	

SD, standard deviation.

[a] Measurements taken at the lateral mitral annulus.

Evaluation of regional abnormalities

Evaluation of regional wall motion abnormalities is usually undertaken due to concerns about compromised myocardial perfusion and/or myocardial viability. Ischemia induces a state of hibernation in the myocardium characterized by persistent myocardial dysfunction with preserved viability. Whether myocardium is hibernating or is necrotic/scarred is an important issue when considering revascularization. The most commonly used methods for evaluation of perfusion and determination of viability include 2D echocardiography, myocardial perfusion imaging (thallium/sestamibi), and myocardial metabolic imaging (PET) with increasing sensitivity in the latter methods. Stress echocardiography improves on the early detection of perfusion abnormalities using this relatively less invasive method. A newer method, magnetic resonance imaging tagging, can give more detailed information about regional wall motion but is still limited in its clinical use.

Echocardiography/stress echo

Using 2D echocardiography, reduced diastolic wall thickness in an dyskinetic segment is usually indicative of scar, while preserved diastolic wall thickness in a hypokinetic or dyskinetic segment may represent viable myocardium. Stress echocardiography is a combination of 2D echocardiography and exercise/stress testing. Many investigators have demonstrated electrocardiographic changes and wall motion abnormalities associated with exercise in the presence of coronary artery disease. Berthe et al. were the first to perform dobutamine stress echocardiography, which is now the standard method for stress echocardiography [31]. With stress echocardiography one is assessing for inadequate myocardial perfusion by evaluating for new or worsened regional wall motion abnormalities induced by an increased inotropic state. The pediatric experience has been well reviewed [32].

Thallium-201 /technetium-99m sestamibi (MIBI) with single-photon emission CT (SPECT)

Uptake of thallium-201 (^{201}Tl) is a measure of both myocardial perfusion and viability [33]. Uptake involves an energy requiring metabolic pump, the sodium/potassium ATPase, which is present only in viable tissue. Technetium-99m Sestamibi is a synthetic lipophilic cationic myocardial perfusion agent that passively distributes across sarcolemmal and mitochondrial membranes and is primarily retained in the mitochondria [33]. A negative mitochondrial charge gradient is essential and this occurs only in viable myocardium. With both thallium-201 and Sestamibi, uptake is proportional to blood flow and, therefore, uptake will be decreased and viability may be underestimated in regions of low blood flow. Also, with these techniques there is sometimes difficulty in assessing the inferior wall due to scatter from sub-diaphragmatic activity [33].

Positron emission tomography (PET)

Positron emission tomography (PET) is known to ac-curately identify viable myocardium following my-ocardial infarction and is the standard for detec-tion of hibernation [33,34]. The superiority of this method over other nuclear imaging techniques is based on its high sensitivity and high spatial reso-lution. PET measures small amounts of radiophar-maceuticals labeled with positron-emitting radioiso-topes and the information obtained depends on the particular tracer injected. ^{13}N-ammonia ($^{13}NH_3$) is the most frequently used PET tracer and quanti-fies myocardial blood flow. 18F-fluorodeoxyglucose (FDG) uptake is closely linked to glucose uptake, which is increased in ischemic conditions due to a switch from fatty acid metabolism to glucose metabolism. Viable tissue is likely to be present if glu-cose uptake is preserved or increased despite low per-fusion, whereas, low glucose uptake and perfusion are suggestive of necrosis. ^{11}C-acetate is an alterna-tive tracer to determine viability and is a marker of regional oxygen consumption. Preservation of ox-idative metabolism is necessary for recovery of func-tion after revascularization. Thus, PET can provide information on perfusion and on metabolism which together aide in the determination of viability.

Myocardial tissue tagging

Newer methods with magnetic resonance imaging allow magnetic tagging of the myocardium itself [35,36]. With this technique the myocardium is presaturated in intersecting planes at the electro-cardiographic QRS immediately prior to scanning. The tagged myocardium appears as a grid within the myocardium for a very short period of time (less than one cardiac cycle). As systole progresses the tag becomes intrinsic to the myocardium and demon-strates motion of individual myocardial segments. This information can also allow calculation of my-ocardial regional strains. Use of this method in the clinical setting is limited by availability, acquisition speed, and analysis time, but may provide informa-tion on myocardial function previously only achiev-able by invasive placement of markers on the surface of the myocardium. It has been used to demonstrate wall motion abnormalities and regional strain asso-ciated with various congenital heart defects [36]. For optimal imaging, the patient must hold their breath for the time of acquisition, typically 16–20 cardiac cycles or 12–20 sec [35]. This makes this imaging technique less clinically relevant for the younger pe-diatric patient who cannot accommodate that re-quirement.

Examples of left ventricular assessment in specific congenital heart lesions

Decreased preload/total anomalous pulmonary venous connection

Patients with total anomalous pulmonary con-nection frequently presented with pulmonary ve-nous obstruction requiring emergent repair in the neonatal period. Typically these patients have enlarged right ventricles and small, underfilled left ventricles. Hammon et al. demonstrated a preoperative left ventricular end-diastolic volume (LVEDV) at 69 ± 7.5% of normal in the unobst-ructed patients and 70.1 ± 4.6% of normal in the obstructed patients [37]. The ejection fraction was mildly decreased at 50 ± 5% in the obstructed pa-tients. Left ventricular output was low at 2.1 ± 0.3L/(min·m^2) in the unobstructed patients and 1.6 ± 0.1 L/(min·m^2) in the obstructed patients. Although the majority of patients had abnormal left ventric-ular size and function preoperatively, this did not predict morbidity or mortality. Four of six patients with LVEDV <75% of predicted survived, including two with LVEDV of 50–52% of normal. In nine pa-tients undergoing cardiac catheterization both be-fore and after surgical repair, the left ventricular size increased from 75.1 ± 6.3% of normal before repair to 108 ± 8.2% of normal at late follow-up. Despite earlier concerns that a small left ventricle may play a role in the mortality and morbidity of this lesion, their data did not support this. Small left ventricular size and depressed left ventricular ejection fraction do not preclude successful repair in this group of pa-tients with low preload, and the ventricular size and function appear to normalize under normal loading conditions in late follow-up after surgical repair.

Increased preload/ventricular septal defect

The infant with a large ventricular septal defect (VSD) usually faces congestive heart failure. How-ever, the pathophysiology of their tachypnea and failure-to-thrive may be different than the adult with ischemic or dilated cardiomyopathy. Waggoner et al.

utilized m-mode echocardiography to study left ventricular function in 22 children with ventricular septal defects with a left-to-right shunt (Qp/Qs) of 2.5 (range 1.2 to 4.0) [38]. Systolic time intervals, velocity of shortening, and early diastolic lengthening remained normal, suggesting that ventricular contractility and relaxation were normal. The left ventricular shortening fraction was increased in patients with ventricular septal defects. Left ventricular mass was increased thus maintaining normal wall stress and radius/thickness ratio whether symptomatic or asymptomatic. Kimball *et al.* studied load-independent indexes of left ventricular systolic function and symptoms in 42 infants with ventricular septal defect [39]. Left ventricular performance (shortening fraction), preload (LV end-diastolic dimension), afterload (LV end-systolic wall stress), and contractility (the relation between velocity of circumferential shortening and wall stress) were measured by echocardiography. Preload was increased in patients with ventricular septal defect. No other index was different between controls, asymptomatic ventricular septal defect or symptomatic ventricular septal defect. Harada *et al.* compared transmitral Doppler E and A wave velocities with tissue Doppler mitral annular E and A wave velocities in children with ventricular septal defects [40]. They found no evidence of diastolic dysfunction. In contrast, Yoshikawa *et al.* looked at left ventricular shape, end-systolic wall stress to end-systolic volume index ratio, and left ventricular ejection fraction in children divided into small ($Qp/Qs < 1.5$), moderate (Qp/Qs 1.5−2), and large ($Qp/Qs > 2$) unoperated ventricular septal defects; postoperative patients with large preoperative shunts who underwent repair before 2 years of age; and a group of 27 control patients [41]. Left ventricular ejection fraction was slightly increased in the small shunt group, but remained normal in the moderate and large shunt group. Only the large shunt group had evidence of decreased contractility. The end-systolic wall stress to end-systolic volume index normalized in late follow-up of the large shunt patients operated on before two years of age. They conclude that decreased contractility was present preoperatively in children with large shunts, but was reversible in patents that underwent early repair of VSD. The findings in the patients with large VSD were similar to those in patients with decompensated mitral or aortic regurgitation. Studies suggest that the symptoms of heart failure associated with a large VSD in the infant may not always be secondary to depressed myocardial contractility/relaxation. This would have implications for optimal choice of medical therapy.

While there is a consensus that a large ventricular septal defect should be closed and a small ventricular septal defect may be left alone, the late consequences of a moderate size ventricular septal defect are less understood. Magee *et al.* studied a group of nine adolescents and young adults having restrictive ventricular septal defects with moderate size left-to-right shunts (median Qp/Qs 1.7, range 1.4−2.1) [42]. Left ventricular wall mass indexed to body surface area was significantly greater in subjects than in controls (102 ± 29 vs. 75 ± 13, $p < 0.016$). Left ventricular volumes were higher but did not reach statistical significance (91 ± 25 vs. 75 ± 16, $p = 0.1$). Left ventricular mass/volume ratios were normal. Indices of systolic function (LVEF; FS; VCFc) were preserved, or even slightly increased in patients with ventricular septal defect compared to controls. The E:A ratio was decreased but peak early filling normalized to mitral flow was not different, and other indices of relaxation were not different. Pacileo *et al.* studied 20 patients who had undergone surgical repair of ventricular septal defect either early (before 2 years) or late (after 2 years) [43]. The early repair group had a large shunt ($Qp/Qs = 3.1$) and the late group had a moderate size shunt ($Qp/Qs = 2.1$). At follow-up, the early repair group did not differ from controls with regard to left ventricular geometry (normalized volumes and mass for BSA, mass/volume and thickness/radius ratios), shape (long axis–short axis ratio), diastolic (mitral and pulmonary venous flow patterns), and systolic (fractional shortening and rate-corrected mean velocity of circumferential fiber shortening) function. The plot for rate-corrected mean velocity of circumferential fiber shortening to end-systolic stress was within the 95% confidence limits for normal, consistent with normal contractility. At follow-up, the patients undergoing late repair had persistently elevated left ventricular end-diastolic volume and mass, higher mass/volume ratio and reduced end-systolic stress. This suggests that increased preload over a prolonged period may have a detrimental effect on left ventricular contractility. The data are conflicting and the optimum management strategy for the child with a moderate size ventricular septal defect is still uncertain.

Decreased afterload/transposition of the great arteries

The operation of choice for D-transposition of the great arteries with intact ventricular septum is presently the arterial switch operation. However, if this congenital heart defect is diagnosed after the first few weeks of life, the left ventricle is deconditioned due to low afterload. The two-stage arterial switch operation has been utilized in this situation with the first stage being a pulmonary artery banding to induce ventricular hypertophy, prior to proceeding with the arterial switch operation as the second procedure. Boutin et al. compared systolic function after surgical repair in 19 infants undergoing the two-stage arterial switch operation (0.3 ± 0.2 years) with 33 patients undergoing one stage arterial switch operation (0.07 ± 0.09 years) [44]. Late global dysfunction was significantly more common in the two-stage infants compared to the one-stage infants. The only risk factor for poor outcome was rapid rate of appearance of hypertrophy following pulmonary artery banding. In these infants, the problem was not failure of the left ventricle to hypertrophy, it was too much hypertrophy too quickly. The rapidity with which the ventricle hypertrophied correlated with the LV:RV pressure ratio before arterial switch operation. This suggested that sudden, marked increases in afterload led to late myocardial dysfunction and placement of a looser pulmonary artery band or staged tightening of the band may be advantageous in this group of infants. Lacour-Gayet et al. performed the two-stage arterial switch operation in 22 patients (mean age 3.2 months) [45]. Their indication was age > 3 weeks, compressed left ventricular contour, and mainly a left ventricular mass < 35 G/m^2. They placed a loose pulmonary artery band with left ventricular pressure at 65% of systemic. They proceeded with the arterial switch operation when left ventricular mass was > 50 G/m^2 after a mean delay of 10 days (5 days to 6 weeks). Left ventricular retraining had to be discontinued in two patients and two patients died of noncardiac causes. In late follow-up, all 17 survivors where asymptomatic, on no medications, and had left ventricular shortening fraction of 39%. It appears that the deconditioned left ventricle can be retrained, at least in infants.

The two-stage arterial switch operation in association either with takedown of an atrial switch for older patients with D-transposition of the great arteries who had undergone either the Mustard procedure or Senning procedure, or with performance of an atrial switch operation for older patients with congenitally corrected transposition of the great arteries has been done as an alternative to heart transplantation in the patient with failure of the systemic right ventricle. In their series of 17 older children and adults requiring pulmonary artery banding for reconditioning of the left ventricle, Helvind et al. had poor outcome with the two young adults in the series [46]. Three patients failed pulmonary artery banding, including the two young adults who died. Left ventricular function following the arterial switch procedure was not reported for the rest of the patients in this study, so late function is not known. They suggest that the ability of the left ventricle exposed to prolonged low afterload, to be retrained with pulmonary artery banding may be limited by age.

Fogel et al. utilized MRI tagging to evaluate the deconditioned left ventricle in 11 adults with D-transposition of the great arteries after atrial switch operation [47]. These patients had altered elastic properties and abnormal wall motion, including less twisting motion of the left ventricle which may reflect altered orientation of myocardial fibers. What role these altered properties of ventricular function may play in the deconditioned ventricle, and how they change with retraining, is unclear.

Increased afterload/aortic stenosis and coarctation of the aorta

The fetus with left ventricular outflow tract obstruction utilizes the right ventricle to perform some of the work of systemic output. The result is a dilated right ventricle and a small left ventricle. However, after the ductus arteriosus closes the left ventricle must be able to support the entire systemic output. Thus, there exists a poorly defined left ventricular volume that is necessary for survival after aortic valvotomy in infants, and below which infants are better palliated with the Norwood procedure. Parsons et al. measured left ventricular volumes by angiography and long axis left ventricular area on 2D echocardiogram in 25 infants < 3 months of age undergoing surgical aortic valvotomy for congenital aortic stenosis [8]. A left ventricular end-diastolic volume index > 20 cc/m^2 and an absolute end-diastolic volume of > 4.5 cc was present in all survivors. Mean left ventricular end-diastolic volume in survivors was 43 cc/m^2 and in nonsurvivors was 11 cc/m^2. However, a noninvasive measurement, long-axis cross sectional area of <2 cm^2, was also an excellent predictor of surgical death. All five patients with measurements <2 cm^2 died, while among the 14 patients with cross sectional area >2 cm^2 there were two deaths. Rhodes et al. studied 65 infants with aortic stenosis preselected for presumed adequate left ventricular size undergoing valvotomy [48]. They compared 11 separate measurements of left ventricular inflow, outflow, volume, mass, and arch size with respect to outcome after attempted two-ventricle repair. Nine of the 11 parameters were significantly smaller in the group who died, but there was significant overlap between groups. Mortality was 100% in the 12 patients with two or more risk factors and 8% in the 31 patients with one or fewer risk factors. These risk factors were: mitral valve area $\leq$4.75 cm/m^2 or dimension of 1.1 cm in an infant with BSA of 0.2 m^2; aortic root area $\leq$3.5 cm/m^2 or diameter of 0.95 cm in an infant of 0.2 m^2; a left ventricular long axis to heart long-axis ratio $\leq$ 0.8; LV mass $\leq$ 35 g/m^2. The equation for the discriminating score was:

$$Score = 14.0\,(BSA) + 0.943\,(ROOT_i) + 4.78\,(LAR) + 0.157\,(MVA_i) - 12.03,$$

where BSA is body surface area, $ROOT_i$ is aortic root dimension indexed to body surface area, LAR is the ratio of the long-axis dimension of the left ventricle to the long-axis dimension of the heart, and MVA_i is the mitral valve area indexed to body surface area. A score of <-0.35 was predictive of death after two-ventricle repair.

Tani et al. looked at infants with coarctation of the aorta whose Rhodes score would have predicted the need for univentricular repair [49]. There were no early or late deaths. At late follow-up, 80% were asymptomatic and 20% had mild residual symptoms. In this patient population, the Rhodes score was not predictive of survival and infants with small left hearts underwent biventricular repair with excellent results. Schwartz et al. evaluated indices of left ventricular size in infants with multiple obstructive left heart lesions [50]. Presence of a moderate/large ventricular septal defect, unicommisural aortic valve, and hypoplastic mitral valve or left ventricle (z-score of < -2.0 or LV/RV long-axis ratio of <0.8) were independent predictors of poor outcome

after biventricular repair. However, 16 of 22 infants with hypoplastic left ventricle under this definition survived biventricular repair. Thus, determination of the adequacy of left ventricular size is also dependent on the specific associated anomalies present.

Outside the neonatal period, aortic stenosis usually presents with variable degrees of left ventricular hypertrophy. The hypertrophic response to pressure overload increases wall thickness and returns wall stress toward normal. Often the left ventricle appears hyperdynamic. Donner et al. demonstrated in 11 children with aortic stenosis (gradient 109 ± 43 mm Hg) that the ejection fraction (0.88 ± 0.08) was significantly higher than in normal subjects (0.64 ± 0.08), the mean velocity of fiber shortening was also higher (1.80 ± 0.35 circ/s) than in normal subjects (1.22 ± 0.35 circ/s), the left ventricular wall stress was reduced throughout the cardiac cycle in patients with aortic stenosis, and the end-systolic stress vs. end-systolic volume index ratio was unchanged [51]. This suggests that the ejection fraction is increased in the presence of normal contractility with decreased wall stress as though the ventricles had over responded in hypertrophy. Pacileo et al. demonstrated in 22 children (age 12.4 ± 5.6 years) with moderate aortic stenosis that left ventricular contractility (velocity of circumferential fiber shortening and meridional end-systolic stress relationship) and diastolic function (mitral flow indices) were normal [52]. Left ventricular hypertophy was not marked ($LVMI < 51$ g/m^2). However, despite normal functional indices in these children with moderate aortic stenosis, tissue acoustic characteristics were consistent with increased collagen deposition. The implication for this fibrosis in long-term follow-up is unclear.

Occasionally, children and adolescents with aortic stenosis will present with depressed ventricular performance and congestive heart failure. As aortic stenosis progresses, the ejection fraction is maintained at the expense of higher left ventricular end-diastolic pressure and volume according to the Frank–Starling mechanism. Once the maximal myocyte length is reached, the stiff ventricle resists further filling and any further progression in aortic stenosis will result in a fall in ejection fraction. However, myocardial contractility is preserved initially and function is still recoverable if the afterload is reduced. Jindal et al. looked at pediatric patients (5 to 18 years; mean 10.8 ± 4 years) with depressed left ventricular function due to aortic stenosis before and after aortic valvuloplasty [53]. The peak-to-peak systolic gradient decreased from 74.7 ± 30.8 to 33.9 ± 18.2 mmHg, and the echocardiographic left ventricular ejection fraction improved from 21.6 ± 5.4 to $31 \pm 6.5\%$ within 24 h. At late follow-up, the left ventricular ejection fraction had increased to normal, $59.4 \pm 11.4\%$. Thus, the depressed ventricular performance seemed due to increased afterload rather than depressed myocardial function as it normalized after valvuloplasty. Hofstetter et al. demonstrated similar findings in 16 infants undergoing valvotomy [54]. Eight of the sixteen had depressed ventricular function with wall motion abnormalities and evidence of ischemia on electrocardiogram, and four had myocardial infarction on intraoperative inspection. Postoperatively, all had normal or hyperdynamic function in late follow-up except for one infant with a small left ventricle who died with endocardial fibroelastosis at autopsy. Rubay et al. evaluated 24 patients (median age 10 years; range, 5 months to 27 years) who underwent the Ross procedure for congenital aortic stenosis or aortic insufficiency [55]. Left ventricular dimension normalized after one week and left ventricular mass reached a normal value after three months in all but two patients. These two patients had the more severely dilated ventricles prior to surgery and did not recover function. Thus, in most children, return of afterload toward normal with aortic valvuloplasty, valvotomy, or valve replacement will allow recovery of ventricular performance.

Right ventricular volume load/Ebstein's anomaly of the tricuspid valve

Abnormal left ventricular function has been recognized in Ebstein's anomaly. Saxena et al. studied the left ventricular function in eight patients older than 20 years with Ebstein's anomaly [56]. Each patient underwent 2D and Doppler echocardiography and radionuclide angiography. The motion of the ventricular septum was markedly paradoxical in all patients at the level of atrialized right ventricle and was flat or hypokinetic below the displaced tricuspid valve. Left ventricular wall motion was globally depressed in two patients. The resting left ventricular ejection fraction by radionuclide ventriculography varied from 28 to 71% (median 46%) and was abnormal in five patients. One patient died suddenly.

He had the ejection fraction of 28% and at autopsy he had extensive myocardial fibrosis of the left ventricle with normal coronary arteries. Hurwitz demonstrated significant left ventricular dysfunction in a group of 10 infants and children with Ebstein's anomaly and cardiorespiratory symptoms [57]. The left ventricular ejection fraction by radionuclide angiography was below normal in 7 of 10 patients (group value: 0.45 ± 0.13) compared to normal controls (0.68 ± 0.09). More importantly, an abnormal left ventricular ejection fraction was more predictive of death than the severity of right ventricular dysfunction. The ejection fraction in those who died was 0.34 to 0.39. Eidem et al. demonstrated in 45 patients with Ebstein's anomaly of the tricuspid valve that the left ventricular myocardial performance index was increased compared to controls even when function appeared normal and was even more abnormal if there was mild to moderate left ventricular dysfunction [58]. The right ventricular myocardial performance index did not correlate with the left ventricular myocardial performance index.

Right ventricular pressure load/valvar pulmonary stenosis

Sholler et al. studied left ventricular function in 25 infants with isolated valvar pulmonary stenosis (aged 1–24 months) [59]. They divided the patients into three groups, normal septal contour, abnormal septal contour only during early diasole, and abnormal septal contour during most of the cardiac cycle. These groups correlated with increasing right ventricular outflow tract gradient. Increasing pulmonary stenosis gradient was associated with smaller ventricular end-diastolic volume, decreasing left ventricular ejection fraction, lower cardiac output, and decreased early diastolic filling. Decreased early diastolic filling was felt to result from the fact that the most marked septal contour changes occur during this part of the cardiac cycle. They point out that a sphere has the largest volume for a given surface area, and distortion of the left ventricle away from a spherical shape will reduce the end-diastolic volume.

Thus, both volume overloaded and pressure overloaded right ventricles are associated with depressed left ventricular performance, in part due to changes in left ventricular shape, but also with potential contribution of other factors such as fibrosis, as seen in Ebstein's anomaly.

Regional wall motion abnormalities/anomalous left coronary artery from the pulmonary artery

Infants with anomalous left coronary artery from the pulmonary artery frequently present in infancy with severe, global left ventricular dysfunction. The severity of the dysfunction would suggest poor recovery following revascularization according to the adult literature. Azakie *et al*. reviewed the outcomes in 47 infants with anomalous left coronary artery from the pulmonary artery, who underwent repair by aortic reimplantation at a median age of 7.7 months [60]. Twenty percent presented in extremis and 80% in congestive heart failure. Operative survival was 92% and there were no late deaths. Echocardiographic left ventricular ejection fraction increased from $33 \pm 21\%$ preoperatively to $64 \pm 9\%$ postoperatively. Regional wall motion abnormalities were seen in 38% preoperatively and 9% postoperatively. Left ventricular ejection fraction and end-diastolic volumes had normalized by one year after surgery. Cochrane *et al*. evaluated 21 children at a median follow-up of 6.5 years after reimplantation of an anomalous left coronary artery [61]. Shortening fraction had increased from 19.6% preoperatively to 32.8% by one year after surgery. At a follow-up, ejection fraction by radionuclide angiography was $64 \pm 3\%$ at rest and $74 \pm 3\%$ with exercise. Treadmill endurance was normal in those old enough to exercise. Singh *et al*. utilized dynamic positron emission tomographic imaging (PET) in 11 patients after repair of anomalous left coronary artery from the pulmonary artery (median age 17 years). Echocardiographic ejection fraction was $63 \pm 6\%$ but 7 of 11 patients had septal hypokinesis. At rest perfusion in the distribution of the left coronary artery was mildly decreased compared to the right coronary artery. Exercise using a bicycle decreased further the relative perfusion in the distribution of the left coronary artery. Maximal oxygen consumption correlated with maximal left coronary flow during exercise, suggesting that limited myocardial flow reserve may play a role in the relative decrease in VO_2 in patients (23.9 ± 5.3) compared to controls (33.5 ± 3.5). Thus, while some residual perfusion defects do exist following repair of anomalous left coronary artery from the pulmonary artery, late ventricular performance and exercise tolerance are very good in the vast majority of these infants presenting such marked left ventricular dysfunction.

Summary

Assessment of left ventricular function usually begins with 2D echocardiography and measurement of shortening fraction, ejection fraction, and end-diastolic volume. If the patient has lesions associated with altered preload or afterload, velocity of circumferential shortening may allow discrimination between ventricular dysfunction secondary to the altered loading conditions and that due to depressed myocardial contractility. In the presence of regional wall motion abnormalities, or in lesions known to be associated with perfusion abnormalities, dobutamine stress ECHO or perfusion/metabolic scans may be indicated. If echocardigraphic windows are insufficient, radionuclide ventriculography or magnetic resonance imaging provide excellent alternative measures of ejection fraction and end-diastolic volume. 3D echocardiography has been utilized primarily in research, especially in children, and it is just emerging as a clinical tool. Its role is yet to be defined. Magnetic resonance tagging is presently still limited to research. And finally, the role of diastolic dysfunction in symptomatic heart failure in patients with congenital heart disease should not be underestimated, with echocardiography as the primary methodology utilized.

References

1. Glower DD, Spratt JA, Snow ND, *et al*. Linearity of the Frank–Starling relationship in the intact heart: The concept of preload recruitable stroke work. Circulation 1985; 71:994–1009.
2. Graham TP Jr, Jarmakani JM, Canent RV, *et al*. Left heart volume estimation in infancy and childhood: Reevaluation of methodology and normal values. Circulation 1971; 43:895–904.
3. Graham TP. Ventricular function. In Macartney FJ, ed, Congenital Heart Disease. MTP Press Limited, Lancaster, England, pp. 145–161, 1986.
4. Parrish MD, Graham TP, Jr, Born ML, Jones J. Radionuclide evaluation of right and left ventricular function in children: Validation of methodology. Am J Cardiol 1982; 49:1241–1247.
5. Mercier JC, DiSessa TG, Jarmakani JM, et al. Two-dimensional echocardiographic assessment of left ventricular volumes and ejection fraction in children. Circulation 1982; 65:962–969.
6. Lorenz CH. The range of normal values of cardiovascular structures in infants, children and adolescents

measured by magnetic resonance imaging. Pediatr Cardiol 2000; 21:37–46.

7. Poutanen T, Ikonen A, Jokinen E, *et al*. Transthoracic three-dimensional echocardiography is as good as magnetic resonance imaging in measuring dynamic changes in left ventricular volume during the heart cycle in children. Eur J Echocardiogr 2001; 2:31–39.

8. Parsons MK, Moreau GA, Graham TP *et al*. Echocardiographic estimation of critical left ventricular size in infants with isolated aortic valve stenosis. JACC 1991; 18:1049–1055.

9. Barkhausen J, Ruehm SG, Goyen M, *et al*. MR evaluation of ventricular function: True fast imaging with steady-state precession versus fast low-angle shot cine MR imaging: feasibility study. Radiology 2001; 219:264–269.

10. Niwa K, Uchishiba M, Aotsuka H, *et al*. Measurement of ventricular volumes by cine magnetic resonance imaging in complex congenital heart disease with morphologically abnormal ventricles. Am Heart J 1996; 131:567–575.

11. Acar P, Antonietti CM, Bonnet D, *et al*. Left ventricular ejection fraction in children measured by three-dimensional echocardiography using a new transthoracic integrated 3D-probe. Eur Heart J 1998; 19:1583–1588.

12. Apfel HD, Shen Z, Gopal AS, *et al*. Quantitative three dimensional echocardiography in patients with pulmonary hypertension and compressed left ventricles: comparison with cross sectional echocardiography and magnetic resonance imaging. Heart 1996; 76:350–354.

13. Colan SD, Borow KM, Neumann A. Left ventricular end-systolic wall stress-velocity of fiber shortening relation: a load-independent index of myocardial contractility. JACC 1984; 4:715–724.

14. Colan SD, Parness IA, Spevak PJ, *et al*. Developmental modulation of myocardial mechanics: Age- and growth-related alterations in afterload and contractility. JACC 1992; 19:619–629.

15. Franklin RCG, Wyse RKH, Graham TP, *et al*. Normal values for noninvasive estimation of left ventricular contractile state and afterload in children. Am J Cardiol 1990; 65:505–510.

16. Grossman W, Jones D, McLaurin LP. Wall stress and patterns of hypertrophy in the human left ventricle. J Clin Invest 1975; 56:56–64.

17. Karr SS, and Martin GR. A simplified method for calculating wall stress in infants and children. J Am Soc Echocardiogr 1994; 646–651.

18. Chaturvedi RR, Lincoln C, Gothard JWW *et al*. Left ventricular dysfunction after open repair of simple congenital heart defects in infants and children: quantiation with the use of a conductance catheter immediately after bypass. J Thorac Cardiovasc Surg 1998; 115:77–83.

19. Ahmed SS, Levinson GE, Schwartz CJ, *et al*. Systolic time intervals as measures of the contractile state of the left ventricular myocardium in man. Circulation 1972; 46:559–71.

20. Tei C, Nishimura RA, Seward JB, *et al*. Noninvasive Doppler-derived myocardial performance index: Correlation with simultaneous measurements of cardiac catheterization measurements. J Am Soc Echocardiogr 1997; 10:169–178.

21. Eidem BW, Tie C, O'Leary PW, *et al*. Nongeometric quantitative assessment of right and left ventricular function: myocardial performance index in normal children and patients with Ebstein anomaly. J Am Soc Echocardiogr 1998; 11:849–856.

22. Harada K, Tamura M, Toyono M, *et al*. Assessment of global left ventricular function by tissue Doppler imaging. Am J Cardiol 2001; 88:927–932.

23. O'Leary PW, Durongpisitkul K, Cordes TM, *et al*. Diastolic ventricular function in children: A Doppler echocardiographic study establishing normal values and predictors of increased ventricular end-diastolic pressure. Mayo Clin Proc 1998; 73:616–628.

24. Oh JK, Appleton CP, Hatle LK, *et al*. The noninvasive assessment of left ventricular diastolic function with two-dimensional and Doppler echocardiography. J Am Soc Echocardiogr 1997; 10:246–270.

25. Heimdal A, Stoylen A, Torp H, *et al*. Real-time strain rate imaging of the left ventricle by ultrasound. J Am Soc Echocardiogr 1998; 11:1013–1019.

26. Sohn DW, Chai IH, Lee DJ, *et al*. Assessment of mitral annulus velocity by Doppler tissue imaging in the evaluation of left ventricular diastolic function. JACC 1997; 30:474–480.

27. Farias CA, Rodriguez L, Garcia MJ, *et al*. Assessment of diastolic function by tissue Doppler echocardiography: Comparison with standard transmitral and pulmonary venous flow. J Am Soc Echocardiogr 1999; 12:609–617.

28. Harada K, Orino T, Yasuoka K, *et al*. Tissue Doppler imaging of left and right ventricles in normal children. Tohoku J Exp Med 2000; 191:21–29.

29. Kapusta L, Thijssen JM, Cuypers MHM, *et al*. Assessment of myocardial velocities in healthy children using tissue Doppler imaging. Ultrasound in Med Biol 2000; 26:229–237.

30. Swaminathan S, Ferrer PL, Wolff GS, *et al*. Usefulness of tissue Doppler echocardgiography for evaluating ventricular function in children without heart disease. Am J Cardiol 2003; 91:570–574.

31. Berthe C, Pierard LA, Hiernaux M, *et al*. Predicting the extent and location of coronary artery disease in acute myocardial infarction by echocardiography during

dobutamine infusion. Am J Cardiol 1986; 58:1167–1172.

32. Kimball TR. Pediatric stress echocardiography. Pediatr Cardiol 2002; 23:347–357.

33. Mari C and Strauss WH. Detection and characterization of hibernating myocardium. Nucl Med Commun 2002; 23:311–322.

34. Mesotten L, Maes A, Van de Werf F, et al. PET radiopharmaceuticals used in viability studies in acute myocardial infarction: a literature survey. Eur J Nucl Med 2002; 29:3–6.

35. Reichek N. MRI myocardial tagging. J Magn Reson Imaging 1999; 10:609–616.

36. Fogel MA. Assessment of cardiac function by magnetic resonance imaging. Pediatr Cardiol 2000; 21:59–69.

37. Hammon JW, Bender HW Jr., Graham TP Jr, et al. Total anomalous pulmonary venous connection in infancy. J Thorac Cardiovasc Surg 1980; 80:544–551.

38. Waggoner AD, Nouri S, Schaffer MS, et al. Echocardiographic evaluaton of left ventricular function, mass and wall stress in children with isolated ventricular septal defect. Texas Heart Inst J 1985; 12:163–170.

39. Kimball TR, Daniels SR, Meyer RA, et al. Relation of symptoms to contractility and defect size in infants with ventricular septal defect. Am J Cardiol 1991; 67:1097–1102.

40. Harada K, Tamura M, Yasuoka K, et al. A comparison of tissue Doppler imaging and velocities of transmitral flow in children with elevated left ventricular preload. Cardiol Young 2001; 11:261–268.

41. Yoshikawa M, Sato T. Left ventricular end-systolic wall stress to volume relationship before and after surgical closure of ventricular septal defect. Pediatr Cardiol 1987; 8:93–98.

42. Magee AG, Fenn L, Vellekoop J, et al. Left ventricular function in adolescents and adults with restrictive ventricular septal defect and moderate left-to-right shunting. Cardiol Young 2000; 10:126–129.

43. Pacileo G, Pisacane C, Russo MG, et al. Left ventricular mechanics after closure of ventricular septal defect: Influence of size of the defect and age at surgical repair. Cardiol Young 1998; 8:320–328.

44. Boutin C, Wernovsky G, Sanders SP, et al. Rapid two-stage arterial switch operation: Evaluation of left ventricular systolic mechanics late after an acute pressure overload stimulus in infancy. Circulation 1994; 90:1294–1303.

45. Lacour-Gayet F, Piot D, Zoghbi J, et al. Surgical management and indication of left ventricular retraining in arterial switch for transposition of the great arteries with intact ventricular septum. Eur J Cardiothorac Surg 2001; 20:824–829.

46. Helvind MH, McCarthy JF, Imamura M, et al. Ventriculo-arterial discordance: Switching the morphologically left ventricle into the systemic circulation after 3 months of age. Eur J Cardiothorac Surg 1998; 14:173–178.

47. Fogel MA, Gupta K, Baxter BC, et al. Biomechanics of the deconditioned left ventricle. Am J Physiol Heart Circ Physiol 1996; 271(40):H1193–H1206.

48. Rhodes LA, Colan SD, Perry SB, et al. Predictors of survival in neonates with critical aortic stenosis. Circulation 1991; 84:2325–2335.

49. Tani LY, Minich LL, Pagotto LT, et al. Left ventricular hypoplasia and neonatal aortic arch obstruction: Is the Rhodes left ventricular adequacy score applicable? J Thorac Cardiovasc Surg 1999; 118:81–86.

50. Schwartz ML, Gauvreau K, Geva T. Predictors of outcome of biventricular repair in infants with multiple left heart obstructive lesions. Circulation 2001; 104:682–687.

51. Donner R, Carabello BA, Black I, et al. Left ventricular wall stress in compensated aortic stenosis in children. Am J Cardiol 1983; 51:946–951.

52. Pacileo G, Calabro P, Limongelli G, et al. Left ventricular remodeling, mechanics, and tissue characterization in congenital aortic stenosis. J Am Soc Echocardiogr 2003; 16:214–220.

53. Jindal RC, Saxena A, Kothari SS, et al. Congenital severe aortic stenosis with congestive heart failure in late childhood and adolescence: Effect on left ventricular function after balloon valvuloplasty. Cathet Cardiovasc Intervent 2000; 51:168–172.

54. Hofstetter R, Zeike B, Messmer BJ, et al. Echocardiographic evaluation of systolic left-ventricular function in infants with critical aortic stenosis before and after aortic valvotomy. Thorac Cardiovasc Surgeon 1990; 38:236–240.

55. Rubay JE, Shango P, Clement S, et al. Ross procedure in congenital patients: Results and left ventricular function. Eur J Cardiothorac Surg 1997; 11:92–99.

56. Saxena A, Fong LV, Tristam M, et al. Left ventricular function in patients >20 years of age with Ebstein's anomaly of the tricuspid valve. Am J Cardiol 1991; 67:217–219.

57. Hurwitz RA. Left ventricular function in infants and children with symptomatic Ebstein's anomaly. Am J Cardiol 1994; 73:716–718.

58. Eidem BW, Tei C, O'Leary PW, et al. Nongeometric quantitative assessment of right and left ventricular function: Myocardial performance index in normal children and patients with ebstein's anomaly. J Am Soc Echocardiogr 1998;11:849–856.

59. Sholler GF, Colan SD, and Sanders SP. Effect of isolated right ventricular outflow obstruction on left ventricular function in infants. Am J Cardiol 1988; 62:778–784.

60. Azakie A, Russell JL, McCrindle BW, *et al.* Anatomic repair of anomalous left coronary artery from the pulmonary artery by aortic reimplantation: Early survival, patterns of ventricular recovery and late outcome. Ann Thorac Surg 2003; 75:1535–1541.

61. Cochrane AD, Coleman DM, Davis AM, *et al.* Excellent long-term functional outcome after an operation for anomalous left coronary artery from the pulmonary artery. J Thorac Cardiovasc Surg 1999; 117: 332–342.

CHAPTER 15

Blood Flow in the Normal and Diseased Aorta

Theresa Ann Tacy, MD

An understanding of flow dynamics in the normal and diseased aorta is essential to the study of the physiologic impact of many types of congenital heart disease. A review of blood flow in the normal and diseased aorta must be considered at several different levels. Aortic flow will be considered from the perspectives of (1) fluid dynamics of blood flow itself, (2) aortic wall mechanics, (3) the overall impact of these on the energetics of the cardiovascular system, (4) disease processes encountered in the pediatric population which impact arterial flow dynamics, such as an aortopulmonary shunts, or aortic coarctation, whereas others primarily affect the aortic wall, such as Marfan syndrome. Aortic flow patterns likely play a role in mechanotransduction of factors important to enthothelial function (and hence arterial wall properties). Aberrations in any of these factors will impact the hydraulic load presented to the heart. Thus, aortic flow is neither an independent nor isolated entity, but rather both composed of and affected by these various entities.

Understanding the impact of aortic flow abnormalities – regardless of the primary cause – is also essential to our evaluation of the aorta by either invasive or noninvasive means. Abnormal aortic wall mechanics impact the Doppler velocity assessment of coarctation severity and also affect the Doppler waveform pattern, which is also often used to subjectively assess the obstruction severity.

This chapter will review the basic concepts in fluid dynamics and solid mechanics, some methods used to characterize aortic flow in health and disease, and the effects of these flow dynamics from the cellular

level to a more global level of hydraulic load and efficient work expenditures.

Aortic fluid dynamics

Flow can be considered in either the spatial or the temporal realm (Fig.15.1). Cardiologists familiar with Doppler assessments of flow patterns are more accustomed to thinking of flow in the temporal realm, i.e. assessment of flow in one discrete region assessed over time by pulsed Doppler. In the discussion of flow development, the spatial realm of flow is considered, that is how flow particles form a velocity profile across the cross sectional area of the tube at one point in time.

We will begin the discussion of flow profile development by considering an example of steady, laminar flow in a simple, straight, rigid tube. Fluid enters this long tube from a large reservoir. At the entrance of the tube, the velocity profile is flat. As the flow moves away from this inlet, the velocity profile changes and begins to have curvature near the wall with a magnitude of zero at the wall. The center of the profile remains flat close to the inlet and continues to move as a mass. But as flow progresses distally, the fluid laminae close to the tube wall slide along successively more internal laminae. When all layers of flow are involved, an axisymmetric, parabolic flow profile is formed, and the flow is described as "fully developed." Fully developed flow represents a state in which regional flow rates are achieved which are necessary to maintain flow rate in that tube. Thus, no further flow acceleration occurs along the length of the tube after this point.

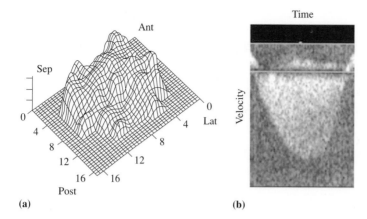

Time

Ant

Sep

(a)

(b)

Figure 15.1 Image A, an example of the digitized color Doppler velocity distribution in the LVOT illustrates a spatial velocity profile, which is a description of flow velocities over space at one point in time [72]. Image B is a spectral Doppler display, which is an example of a temporal velocity profile, describing the distribution of velocities over time, at one point in space.

Flow in the aorta is markedly different from the theoretical tube, different from the fact that at the entrance to the aorta significant skew already exists, to the fact that the flow is pulsatile. Fluid conditions, aortic geometry, wall compliance, and pulsatility can affect the flow profile in the aorta. The study of aortic flow is the study of pulsatile flow into a curved tube with large curvature. Flow in curved tubes comprises of both primary or axial flow patterns and secondary or helical flow patterns (Fig. 15.2). The axial flow component represents the vast majority of energy utilization, whereas helical flows are stable, low energy flow components that run oblique or counter to the axial flow, and are a seemingly unavoidable component of flow in curved tubes. Helical flow is enhanced as curvature is increased [1], and may play a role in minimizing aortic flow turbulence [2].

The curvature magnitude has a large impact on flow patterns; in flow models of steady flow in curved tubes skewing of the axial flow toward the outer wall is present, in addition to secondary flow. Once pulsatility is added, a skewing pattern toward the outer wall of curvature is seen in the ascending aorta, with shift toward the inner wall within the curve, and

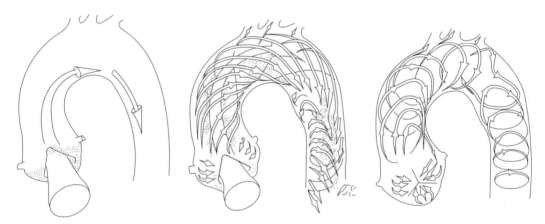

Figure 15.2 Schematic drawings to illustrate typical aortic arch flow development. A. Early systole: During acceleration, highest axial velocities begin along the shortest flow path, close to the inner curvature (cylindrical arrows). Axially directed flows through the remainder of the arch and its branches have not been drawn. B. Mid–to-late systole: The highest velocity stream migrates outward and secondary helical flows develop. Where streamlines separate from the inner wall of the distal arch, the separation zone is filled by oblique retrograde streamlines, curling back toward the viewer from the further wall. C. End systole: Combinations of rotational and recirculating secondary flows persist after aortic valve closure. The drawing is intended to indicate averaged streamlines, although instability of flow and beat-to-beat variation is likely at end systole [2].

shifting yet again toward the outer wall downstream. Thus, a truly parabolic profile is not formed at anytime, even at low frequencies. Significant skewing of the axial flow profile has been demonstrated in both modeling studies [1,3,4] as well as in vivo with magnetic resonance velocity mapping [5,6]. The ascending aortic flow velocity profile in normal children seems to be skewed rightward and anterior; and in the descending aorta, skew is more posterior [6].

Fluid dynamics and Doppler velocimetry

Many clinicians have become so accustomed to applications of Doppler velocimetry in the assessment of cardiac abnormalities that they have become alienated from the very principles of fluid dynamics upon which these assessments are based. These principles are reviewed in Chapter 2, so only brief mention will be made here.

Flow behaves according to several very basic principles, which form the bedrock upon which all further considerations of flow are built. The two principles most widely utilized by cardiologists are the principles of mass and energy conservation. Conservation of mass states that whatever mass that flows into a system must flow out, and is the basis of the continuity equation for determination of valve area. The conservation of energy states that the total energy flowing into the system is equal to that flowing out. However, exchanges in *types* of energy may occur, such as the conversion from potential to kinetic energy, which is the basis of the Bernoulli equation.

Fluid conditions impact the behavior of the fluid, and flow may be characterized as laminar, transitional, or turbulent. This characterization is based upon the balance of two forces, viscous and inertial. Whereas viscous forces (such as boundary effects) are those that tend to change the speed of fluid, inertial forces are those that maintain that speed (this seems counter to popular usage of this term, but inertial forces can either keep a structure in motion, or maintain its lack of motion). Flow conditions may be described by the Reynolds number, a dimensionless number which represents the ratio of inertial to viscous forces:

$$N_{Re} = \frac{\text{Inertial}}{\text{Viscous}}\text{forces} = \frac{\rho \overline{V} d}{\mu},$$

where ρ = fluid density, $\overline{V}$ = cross sectionally averaged fluid velocity, d = tube diameter, and μ = fluid viscosity. Low Reynolds numbers therefore

imply important viscous effects; high Reynolds numbers imply high inertial effects, which are associated with increased turbulence in the flow field. Laminar flow is organized; meaning flow lines are parallel and traveling at similar velocities. In turbulent flow, flow particles travel along the line of the tube, as well as in random pathways in other directions. In a Doppler pattern, laminarity is inferred when a narrow spectral envelope is present, indicating flow velocity similarity within the sampled region. In steady flow, a Reynolds number greater than 2000 generally indicates turbulent flow. Flow conditions impact the relationship between flow velocity and pressure drop. When the simplified Bernoulli equation is applied to flow of low Reynold's numbers (i.e. with viscous forces predominating), underestimation of the pressure gradient results, whereas in flow that has high Reynolds numbers (i.e. inertial forces predominating), overestimation results [7] (Fig. 15.3). Thus,

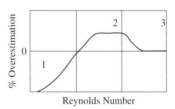

$$Re = \frac{\text{inertial forces}}{\text{viscous forces}}$$

$$\Delta P = \tfrac{1}{2}\rho\,(v_2^2 - v_1^2) + \frac{\text{viscous}}{\text{effects}} + \frac{\text{acceleration}}{\text{effects}}$$

$$\Delta P = 4\,v^2$$

Figure 15.3 Turbulent/viscous effects on pressure recovery. Reynolds number (Re) reconciliation of deleted terms and pressure recovery. The Reynolds number physically represents the ratio of inertial to viscous forces. Low Reynolds numbers therefore imply important viscous effects; high Reynolds numbers imply high inertial effects, which are associated with increased turbulence in the flow field. Therefore, when Doppler-predicted gradients using 4V2 are compared with overall catheter gradients, underestimation is observed at low Reynolds numbers (zone 1) because of deletion of the viscous term (compare with middle line, nonsimplified Bernoulli equation). With increasing Reynolds numbers, pressure recovery between the vena contracta and catheter position results in apparent overestimation (zone 2). Increasing Reynolds numbers are associated with increased turbulence and more nonrecoverable energy losses, which inhibit pressure recovery between the vena contracta and catheter, forcing the overestimation profile back toward zero (zone 3) [7].

it behooves the cardiologist to understand the flow conditions under which they are performing an assessment, to understand the errors inherent in application of the simplified Bernoulli equation at extremes of flow conditions.

Modeling studies of aortic flow (either by computational or *in vitro* methods) often measure conditions at peak flow and use steady conditions. In many cases this is both valid and useful, if the study is applicable to peak systole, which is considered a "pseudosteady" moment, with negligible accelerative forces. However, the effects of pulsatility are important to the understanding of flow conditions in the aorta.

Pulsatility is the repetition of a flow acceleration/deceleration cycle. Acceleration has a stabilizing effect on a flow field, whereas deceleration is destabilizing. These stabilizing/destabilizing periods are time-dependent developments, thus if there is a rapid heart rate, the stabilizing effect of acceleration may occur before the deceleration–dependent destabilization had chance to evolve. Over consecutive cardiac cycles, acceleration may cause relaminarization turbulence left over from a previous deceleration phase. Thus, in pulsatile flow the flow condition depends upon the pulse frequency, and this dependence is expressed in the Womersly number, which expresses the Reynolds number as a function of frequency:

$$N_W = \frac{d}{2}\sqrt{\frac{\rho\omega}{\mu}},$$

where ω = circular frequency of heart rate, d = vessel diameter, ρ = density of fluid, μ = fluid viscosity. The higher the heart rate, the higher the peak Reynolds number needed to create turbulent conditions. Animal studies indicate that a peak systolic Reynolds number of about 8000 would be required to cause turbulence in the ascending aorta of adult humans.

Aortic stenosis

A variety of physical factors and flow conditions impact the noninvasive assessment of aortic stenosis, including proximal aorta anatomy. One of the potential sources of discrepancy between catheter measured and Doppler estimated pressure gradients across a stenotic valve is the difference between instantaneous pressure drop predicted by the Doppler gradient and the peak to peak gradient usually assessed during heart catheterization. These peaks are slightly out of phase, yielding a lower difference compared to the instantaneous value. However, this phenomenon is not sufficient to explain Doppler overestimation, since comparison of simultaneous measures have also shown Doppler overestimation of pressure PIPG gradients [8].

The use of the simplified version of the Bernoulli equation is another potential source of error. The Bernoulli equation derives from the principle that energy is conserved. The acceleration of fluid across an obstruction (an increase in kinetic energy) is accompanied by a pressure drop (a decrease in potential energy). The Bernoulli equation states that the energy lost to a pressure drop across an orifice is related to energy gained in convective acceleration, flow acceleration (also called inertial effects), and in viscous friction. The energy gained in convective acceleration is that imparted to increasing the flow velocity across a stenotic orifice. Inertial effects relate to the energy required to accelerate fluid during ejection. During flow acceleration, some pressure is being expended to overcome inertia rather than being converted to kinetic energy. This effect is only during acceleration, during the valve opening. When we measure the peak pressure drop, flow acceleration is zero. Viscous losses arise from friction between neighboring fluid elements. In laminar flow, these losses will be minimal over the short length of most valve stenoses. Thus, dropping the acceleration and viscous terms when assessing the peak gradient across a discrete stenosis is a reasonable approach, and does not account for the discrepancies which have been observed between pressure drop and that predicted by velocity measures.

One possible source of error in gradient estimation can be attributed to pressure recovery effects. When flow accelerates into a stenotic orifice, the flow lines are converging and continue to converge beyond the stenotic orifice. At the point of maximal flow convergence (where the cross sectional area of flow is the smallest), the flow velocity is at the highest and pressure at the lowest. This very discrete region is termed the *vena contracta*. Beyond this region, flow lines expand again, the velocity decreases, and this energy is converted to potential energy, with a resultant increase in pressure. An assumption when using the peak Doppler gradient is that none of this pressure is "recovered." This would be the case if all the energy recovered from pressure drop across a stenosis were expended as viscous losses in turbulent eddies downstream to the vena contracta.

Fluid mechanics theory suggests that pressure recovery effects may be important to pediatric population. When flow is ejected into a larger receiving chamber, flow separation, vortex formation, and energy dissipation increase as viscous losses increase. With a smaller aorta, the pressure loss should decrease, creating greater pressure recovery since more energy is converted back to pressure (Fig. 15.4). In fact, the degree of pressure recovery can be predicted by the following equation [9]:

$$PR = 4v^2 2 \left(\frac{\text{AVA}_c}{\text{AoA}} \right) \left(1 - \frac{\text{AVA}_c}{\text{AoA}} \right)$$

Where AVA is the aortic valve area and AoA is ascending aorta cross sectional area. A recent study in the pediatric population demonstrated improvement in catheter gradient prediction when pressure recovery was estimated using the above equation [10].

When the aortic valve area is estimated using the continuity equation, operators should be aware that (1) they are estimating the area of the vena contracta and that (2) the area of the vena contracta, and its relation to the valve area varies with the flow characteristics proximal to the aorta. Specifically, flow convergence beyond the orifice is dependent upon convergence proximal to the orifice [11].

Fluid conditions also have an impact, and should be considered and their likely effects weighed when assessing valve gradients. One should always be mindful of situations that will lead to important viscous and inertial terms. In these situations, the use of the simplified Bernoulli equation is inappropriate. If viscous effects are significant, neglecting them will cause underestimation. These effects can become important in long segment stenoses such as complex subaortic obstruction, aortopulmonary shunts [12], and long segment aortic coarctation. On the other hand, turbulence is associated with gradient overestimation with the Doppler velocity applied to the simplified Bernoulli equation. These effects are more pronounced in fluids of low viscosity, such as the patient with a low hematocrit immediately post bypass.

Coarctation of the aorta

The condition of aortic coarctation is different from aortic stenosis due to a proximal reservoir of stored energy – the ascending aorta. The fact that the obstruction is preceded by a section of compliant aorta allows for potential storage of energy upstream, which is subsequently released during diastole, resulting in diastolic transcoarctation flow, and the "sawtooth" Doppler pattern typically seen in childhood coarctation. If the proximal aorta is stiff, all energy must be relayed across the coarctation in systole, without continued forward flow into diastole. The ability of this proximal chamber to accommodate energy affects the pressure gradient/Doppler velocity relationship as well as the Doppler waveform pattern. Decreased proximal aortic compliance leads to overestimation of the Doppler gradient [13]. This finding may be due to increased pressure recovery,

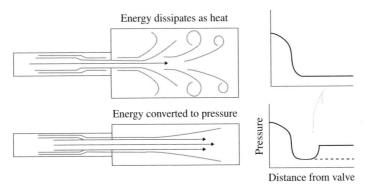

Figure 15.4 The magnitude of pressure recovery is determined by jet velocity, direction, and relative aortic valve area and ascending aorta area. Fluid mechanics theory suggests that pressure recovery effects may be greater in the pediatric population. Flow separation, vortex formation, and energy dissipation occur when flow is ejected into a larger receiving chamber. With a smaller aorta, the pressure loss should decrease, creating greater pressure recovery since flow is converted back to pressure.

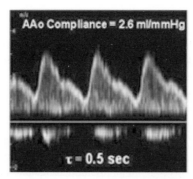 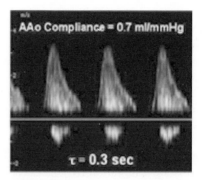

Figure 15.5 Doppler tracing of flow velocity across the aortic obstruction. For an aortic obstruction with a diameter of 8.7 mm, Cp of 0.7ml/mmHg, at a flow rate of 4 l/min, τ is 0.3 sec. When only the Cp is changed to 2.6 ml/mmHg, and all other parameters are held constant, (diameter of 8.7 mm, flow rate of 4 l/min), τ lengthens to 0.5 sec) [73].

which would enhance the conversion of potential energy to kinetic energy (not in storage of potential).

Investigators have related the magnitude of the antegrade diastolic flow to the severity of the lesion [14], however, fluid dynamic principles inform us that the rate of pressure decay within a vessel (and hence gradient decay across an obstructive outlet to that vessel) is determined largely by the wall compliance. Both *in vitro* modeling and computational models inform us that decreased proximal aortic compliance will result in a rapid decay in the proximal aortic pressure, reflected by Doppler as a rapid downstroke from the coarctation Doppler signal, thereby altering the typical "sawtooth" pattern, which is seen in the setting of a compliant ascending aorta (Fig. 15.5).

Local impact of aortic fluid dynamics

Aortic fluid conditions, flow profile, and pulsatility have effects on the aortic wall stress, which may influence various disease processes. The basic definition of stress is the intensity of force over an area. *Shear stress* exists because blood moves in layers, with flow in the middle of the vessel being more rapid than at the blood vessel interface. This type of stress is tangential to the axis of flow. *Fluid shear stresses* act on an element of fluid and are associated with turbulence and flow disturbance. These are often called Reynolds shear stresses, and have been measured in regions of valve stenosis and valve bioprostheses. In regions of high turbulence these stresses are elevated. These stresses are thought to be related to the development of poststenotic dilation, but not to the development of atherosclerosis.

Wall shear stress is the force acting in a direction parallel to a surface due to fluid passing over that surface. It is defined as the product of the slope of the velocity profile at the wall and the fluid viscosity. Laminar wall shear stress inhibits endothelial pro-atherogenic events, such as apoptosis [15], whereas endothelial cells exposed to high shear increase production of precursors to early atherosclerosis [16]. Higher wall shear has been demonstrated as a result of tube curvature, profile skew, and pulsatility itself. Wall shear stress triggers a variety of biochemical and physical changes in cell structure and function, including regulation of vascular tone and diameter, inflammatory responses, hemostasis, and vessel wall remodeling [17]. The complex three-dimensional flow development due to both curvature and pulsatility can be expected to have regions of high and low wall shear stress, which are probably the source and location of atherosclerotic plaque formation sites.

Shear stress also plays a role in endothelial basal NO production [18], which appears to be increased in response to high shear rates. In patients with hemodynamically significant atrial septal defect, large pulmonary blood flow with presumed high pulmonary endothelial shear, exhaled NO decreased immediately after transcatheter ASD closure [19].

Arterial mechanics

Thus far in this discussion of steady and pulsatile flow dynamics and shear we have been considering the environment within the aorta, i.e. the fluid itself and its local effects. Yet the arterial wall properties themselves impact arterial flow, hydraulic load, and overall physiology of the arterial system.

The mechanical properties of the arteries are determined by the structural components of the media, collagen and elastin. Elastin can be stretched up to 300% of its length without rupturing, and returns to its original state when released. Collagen fibers in contrast are stiffer and can handle much higher stressors than elastin fibers, but are much less extensible than elastin fibers. The blood vessel wall is thought to act in a biphasic manner with the elastin fibers, important to determining wall stiffness at low pressures; and collagen fibers, determining stiffness at high pressures. This biphasic behavior is one reason that arterial wall properties have a nonlinear relationship with distending pressure [20]. In addition, with age, elastin content decreases whereas collagen increases in human arteries, which is one reason why vascular stiffness increases with age [21]. Furthermore, while it is generally accepted that arterial changes with aging progressively impair arterial compliance, these changes do not occur in a uniform fashion in all arteries [22]. Collagen and elastin are linked by smooth muscle whose activity modulates the contribution of each to arterial stiffness, so measured stiffness is also impacted by smooth muscle tone [23].

The aortic wall is subjected to *radial stress* – due to force applied perpendicular to the aortic wall – in addition to the parallel forces which result in shear stress. This radial stress is due to aortic blood pressure associated with ventricular ejection, and must be balanced by a circumferential tensile stress in the vessel wall, or else vessel dilation or aneurysm formation will result. The law of LaPlace states that the tensile stress is inversely proportional to wall thickness and directly proportional to vessel radius: $\sigma = Pr/h$, where σ is the circumferential wall stress, P is the vessel pressure, h is the thickness of the vessel wall, and r is the radius of the vessel.

Since aortic wall properties vary with pressure, as well as with age, size, and location, no single number can describe the physical properties of a vessel. Due to the complex nature of the aortic wall, various methods have been developed to quantify arterial wall properties in both regional and global realms.

Regional measures of aortic wall properties

Many relatively simple methods have been utilized to quantify regional arterial wall properties, resulting in a plethora of studies describing abnormalities of regional wall properties (often termed "stiffness") in disease conditions. While these measures are easily performed, the simplicity of these measures limits their applicability and utility. For instance, they are only regional and do not describe global aortic wall properties. These measures are often pressure-dependent, so comparisons between groups should be performed at similar pressures. Comparison between different studies is often difficult due to nonuniformity in the measures performed, as well as the terminology used. This section is intended to be a brief overview of regional wall property measures.

Elastic modulus measures
Strain is a change in the length of a material and is expressed as a percent of the initial length. Stress and strain are related, a stress upon a material (i.e., pressure) will result in a change in the shape (diameter) and hence a strain, which is linear in many nonbiologic materials and nonlinear in arteries. The relation between stress and strain is expressed as an elastic modulus (Young's modulus is stress/strain). Peterson's modulus is a modification of Young's modulus (which depends on wall thickness measures, which are not readily available in *in vivo* measures).

Peterson's modulus =
  Pressure/strain elastic modulus = E_p
$$= \frac{(\Delta P)D_d}{\Delta D},$$

where D is the diastolic internal diameter, ΔD is the difference between systolic and diastolic internal diameters, and ΔP is the pulse pressure. This measure is limited by the assumptions inherent in its application, i.e. the arterial wall is linearly elastic and that the same percent change in diameter would be seen for a same pulse pressure but in a higher pressure range, which is not the case [24]. Peterson's modulus varies with age and pressure, thus any intergroup comparisons must take this into consideration.

The circumferential elastic modulus of the artery (E_q) can be estimated when the thickness of the vessel wall can be measured:

Circumferential elastic modulus = E_q
$$= \frac{(\Delta P)(r)(D)}{h(\Delta D)},$$

where D is the diastolic internal diameter, ΔD is the difference between systolic and diastolic internal diameters; ΔP is the pulse pressure, h the wall thickness, and r the wall radius. This method attempts to estimate average vessel wall stress using the law of LaPlace.

B index

In studies on excised vessels, a linear relation between the logarithm of relative pressure and the distention ratio was noted [25]. This has led to the application of the β index, which is the slope of the exponential function between the relative arterial pressure and the distension ratio of artery (the arterial diameter at a given pressure). This index characterizes, without pressure dependence, the entire deformation behavior of the vascular wall within the physiologic pressure range [26].

$$\beta = \frac{\ln \frac{P_s}{P_d}}{\frac{D_s - D_d}{D_d}}$$

where P_s is the systolic pressure, P_d is the diastolic pressure, D_s is the maximal vessel diameter, and D_d is the minimal vessel diameter.

The β index of both the ascending [27] and descending aorta has been shown to be *elevated* in patients with Marfan syndrome, in comparison to a control group. This seemingly paradoxical result is due to both the dilation of the aorta, as well as abnormal elastin fibers throughout the aorta, resulting in a stiffer vessel from childhood through adulthood.

Not surprisingly, patients with aortic coarctation have an elevated β index after successful repair [28], possibly due to increased collagen and decreased smooth muscle in proximal aorta compared with distal aorta [29]. This increased proximal aortic stiffness contributes to the findings of residual upper body hypertension and/or exercise induced hypertension despite adequate repair. The β index does vary with age, so comparison groups must be similar in this respect [30].

Pulse wave velocity

The arterial pressure waveform is derived from complex interactions of the LV stroke volume, the physical properties of the arterial tree, and the characteristics of the fluid of the system. At the time of ejection, a pressure wave is initiated that is propagated forward in the blood as well as by the aortic and arterial walls. The flow and pressure waves travel at different speeds. The normal peak velocity of flow into the ascending aorta is between 0.8–1.5 m/sec, whereas the pressure wave generated by ventricular ejection propagates through the arterial tree at a speed generally between 5–15 m/sec. This pressure wave velocity is determined by the elastic and geometric properties of the arterial wall and the blood density, and is elevated in stiffer vessels. The pressure wave is usually referred to as a "pulse wave," and the pulse wave velocity (PWV) is accepted as a valid estimate of arterial stiffness. The relationship between PWV and arterial properties is described by the Moens-Korteweg equation:

$$c = \sqrt{\frac{E h}{2 r \rho}},$$

where c is the velocity of the pulse wave, h the vessel thickness, r the radius of the vessel, ρ the density of blood, and E the elastic modulus of the vessel [31]. Note that the PWV is proportional to the square root of vessel stiffness, which would predict that the PWV is not particularly sensitive to changes in arterial stiffness.

As the pressure wave travels it accelerates blood flow along the arterial tree. Measuring a pulse wave is not the same as measuring flow velocity (as in Doppler ultrasound), but is accomplished by measuring the speed of flow propagation. Measuring the distance between two different sites in the arterial system and dividing that by the time between the onsets of the systolic flow wave at these two different sites determine the PWV. An alternative method is to measure the time between the onset of the QRS and the pulse onset at two separate sites, with the pulse wave transit time represented by the difference between these two time intervals. This can be done with applanation tonometry [32]. Doppler echocardiography [33]. and MRI with velocity mapping [34].

PWV has been shown to correlate with independently assessed cardiovascular risk scores [35], age, and systolic blood pressure [36]. PWV in 30 healthy children (11 ± 3 years) was 6.3 ± 1 m/sec [37]. Of note, age-related changes in PWV are more pronounced in the proximal aorta [38]. Several functional differences affect PWV values. For instance, since arterial stiffness varies as a function of pressure, there will be a direct correlation between blood pressure and PWV. In addition, heart rate may have an effect on PWV [39].

Manifestations of arterial stiffness

Wave reflections

The arterial pressure wave has two principal components, the initial forward wave generated by ventricular ejection and a reflected wave, which returns to the heart from peripheral sites. Potential wave reflection exists wherever there is a sudden change in compliance, or caliber, or configuration of the artery. Possible reflecting sites include branching points and high resistance arterioles. The high magnitude of the PWV causes it to travel rapidly to the periphery and return back to the ascending aorta early after reflection, within the same heart period in which it was generated. Reflected waves account for the markedly different pressure and flow contours observed in the ascending aorta, as a reflected pressure wave augments the incident pressure wave, yet diminishes the incident flow waveform [40].

There appears to be one major reflected wave in humans, and several studies have attempted to locate the region of the arterial tree wherein this reflection originates. However, it appears that this one wave represents the average of all reflecting sites in the vascular bed downstream [41]. The timing of the wave reflections is determined by the propagation properties of the arteries [42], as well as by blood pressure [43], age [44], and pharmacotherapy [45–48].

In healthy young adults the reflected wave returns to the ascending aorta after closure of the aortic valve, and so does not influence central systolic pressure [49], but does enhance diastolic coronary blood flow. However, with vascular stiffening, PWV and the amplitude of the reflected wave increase, such that the reflected wave arrives earlier and adds to (or augments) the central systolic pressure during ventricular ejection [50], resulting in a widened aortic pulse pressure and systolic hypertension, with resultant increased left ventricular afterload.

Augmentation index

High-fidelity recordings of aortic pressure demonstrate an inflection point that divides the pressure waveform into an early (P_i) and mid-to-late systolic peak (P_{pk}). The mid-to-late systolic peak is taken to be the result of the reflected wave returning from the peripheral site(s) causing an increase in pulse pressure and systolic pressure [32,51–55] This increase is the height of P_{pk} above P_i ($P_{pk} - P_i = dP$ in mmHg). The ratio of dP to the pulse pressure (PP) defines an augmentation index (dP/PP).

According to the shape of the aortic pressure wave and the dP/PP ratio, Murgo *et al.* [53–55] have divided patients into different subgroups. In young healthy individuals, the inflection point occurs after the systolic peak and the dP/PP ratio is less than 0.00, whereas in patients with systemic hypertension the P_{pk} occurs in late systole after a P_i and the dP/PP ratio exceeds 0.12. (Fig. 15.6).

With anti-hypertensive therapy in humans, changes in arterial pressure wave contour and impedance are usually due to a combination of effects on intensity and timing of wave reflections,

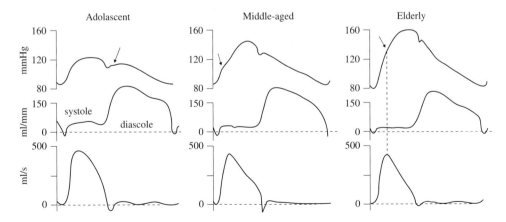

Figure 15.6 Schematic illustration showing pressure (top) and flow waves recorded in the ascending aorta (bottom) and coronary artery (middle) in normotensive subjects (adolescent, middle-aged, and elderly). In adolescents, the reflected pressure wave (beginning at the arrow) occurs in diastole and enhances coronary blood flow. With advancing age, the reflected wave arrives earlier, occurs in systole during ventricular ejection and causes a decrease in coronary blood flow. The deceleration phase of the flow wave is convex in adolescents, concave in middle aged, and linear in the elderly [31].

which can be evaluated using the above relations [51,56,57].

Compliance vs. stiffness

The classic definition of compliance is the change in blood volume given a change in blood pressure. Arterial compliance can be estimated by the use of vessel dimension instead of volume. In this pressure–dimension relation, compliance is represented by the slope of each point of the pressure–diameter (or radius) relation, and is a function of distending pressure. Thus, when discussing compliance one must clarify the distending pressure.

Total arterial compliance is difficult to assess because of the need to measure total arterial blood volume. For this reason, many indirect methods to estimate arterial compliance have evolved, such as diastolic pressure decay analysis, pulse wave velocity, augmentation index, pulse contour analysis, and Fourier transformation.

In the adult population, compliance of the large arteries may be decreased as a result of ageing, arterial hypertension, atherosclerosis, diabetes, and heart failure. In the pediatric population, abnormally low arterial compliance has been measured in children with Williams syndrome [58,59], and after successful coarctation repair [60]. Increased proximal aortic compliance is noted in Marfan syndrome and other connective tissue disorders, and is the main prelude to serious cardiovascular morbidity and mortality for these patients. Earlier identification of aortic wall abnormalities in these patients and response to therapy is also important. While the mechanisms of arterial compliance modulation are likely complex, recent trials suggesting that compliance is improved by drugs acting on vascular structure, or endothelial cell, or smooth muscle function increase the need for estimation of central aortic compliance in clinical settings.

Cardiovascular energetics

The arterial bed interacts with the input of blood flow from ventricular ejection to form characteristic flow and pressure waveforms. The Windkessel model of the arterial bed was formulated in an effort to understand how the properties of the aorta govern the aortic pressure response to an input of flow. If these effects are understood, then one can use the easily collected pressure waveforms to characterize these aortic properties. In the Windkessel concept of aortic function, the vascular bed is viewed as a single compartment with several properties governing the response of the compartment to an input of pulsatile flow.

The Windkessel model

The healthy proximal aorta serves as a compliant buffer to the pressure changes resulting from intermittent left ventricular ejection of blood. During systole the proximal aorta expands, creating a reservoir of energy that is expended in diastole to maintain pressure, forward flow, and coronary artery perfusion. This action of the arterial bed has been likened to the air-filled dome of an old fire engine that converted intermittent spurts of water from a pump to smooth flow, so that flow from the fire hose was almost continuous. The fire engine consisted of a pump and the air-filled dome served as the compliance component, and the fire hose represented the conduit function of the arterial system, the wall of the hose providing the recoil effect (contributing to inertance), and the nozzle introduced resistance. This model has persisted as a descriptor of the cushioning system of the arterial bed, as well as a basis for simplified models of the arterial tree. When one thinks of the arterial bed in terms of its elemental components, it can be thought of as being composed of 2–5 elements (Fig. 15.7). In the 2-element Windkessel model proposed by Hales in the early 1700s, vessel compliance and resistance characterize the systemic vasculature. A modification of this model takes into account inertance or proximal resistance in line between the input and the capacitance and resistive components. Inertance is due to the mass of the fluid and can be thought of as inertial effects encountered when accelerating fluid in a pipe.

This simplification of the arterial bed is essential for the development of *in vitro* and computational models of the arterial bed, and has contributed significantly to the understanding of the effects of the arterial system on the workload imposed upon the ventricle.

Diastolic pressure decay

In 1899, Otto Frank introduced a 2-element Windkessel in which the arterial tree is modeled as an elastic chamber with constant compliance and with a distal resistance. The decay time method assumes that diastolic pressure decays exponentially with a

Figure 15.7 A: Classic Windkessel model. R is total peripheral resistance and C is arterial compliance. B1: Modified windkessel. R is peripheral resistance, Z_0 is characteristic impedance, and C is arterial compliance. B2: Alternate configuration for the modified windkessel in panel B1; C1: Five-element model. L is inertance; $C = C1 + C2$; other symbols are as in B1. C2: Alternate configuration for the modified windkessel in panel C1 [74].

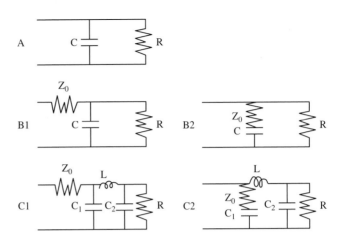

time constant that is the product of total arterial resistance and compliance [61]. Thus, if resistance is known, and the diastolic decay is fit to a monoexponential curve and the time constant measured, the compliance can be estimated. This relation of course assumes the exponential decay of diastolic pressure, and also does not account for the effects of wave reflections, taper, and other effects that may cause the diastolic pressure to deviate from the exponential. Other methods have been proposed using the diastolic pressure curve, which does not assume the decay function of the curve [61].

Pulse contour analysis

Another attempt to measure global arterial properties involves more detailed analysis of the pressure decay. Frank's description of the pressure decay included two components: wave reflection and exponential decay. Proponents of this method point out that consistent and predictable changes occur in the arterial pulse contour regardless of the site of measurement. The pulse contour analysis technique segments the total arterial compliance into large artery and small artery compliances. The large artery compliance is reflected by the exponential decay of the aortic pressure waveform, whereas the small artery compliance is reflected by fluctuations that represent wave reflections which are superimposed upon the basic shape of the pressure waveform [62]. With aging (decreased aortic compliance), the diastolic pressure decay becomes steeper and the waveform in early diastole has less amplitude, due to earlier reflection of the waves, resulting in summation of waveform in late systole. Changes in the pulse contour have been well described before significant augmentation of the systolic pressure becomes apparent [55].

Aortic input impedance analysis

Aortic flow and wall dynamics have long been understood to contribute to the workload of the ventricle. Ventricular afterload is indeed the external factors acting to oppose the shortening of muscle fibers and is often expressed as peak wall stress. However, if we instead say that afterload is opposition to flow, then the nature of forces opposing flow are quite different than those placed upon an isolated muscle fiber. The ventricle is not called upon to lift a weight but to move a viscous fluid into a viscoelastic arterial system. Thus, it is desirable to have some means of describing this system.

The pulsatile nature of the arterial system introduces phase relationships between pressure and flow that are similar to the relationship between voltage and current in an AC electric circuit. In a sinusoidally oscillating system containing proximal compliance (capacitance in the electrical model), peak pressure and flow are separated because of the alternating storage and discharge of the capacitance. Impedance is defined as a frequency-dependent description of opposition to pulsatile flow.

The description of impedance is in two parts. In a perfectly sinusoidal system, it is represented by (1) a modulus that represents the ratio of the peak amplitude pressure to the flow oscillation and (2) a phase angle that indicates the time difference between the sinusoidal pressure and flow [63]. The arterial pulse however is not sinusoidal, yet both the

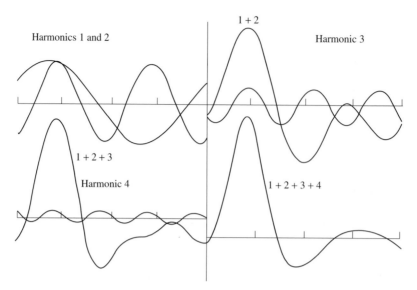

Figure 15.8 Harmonic waveform analysis. A complex waveform is seen in the lower left hand corner, comprising four simple sine waves, which are demonstrated in the other three panels. Each of these four waves can be described in terms of amplitude, frequency, and phase shift.

pressure and the flow waves *can* be mathematically dissected into a series of sinusoidal waves, each of which are described by a frequency, amplitude, and phase angle (Fig. 15.8). Thus, vascular impedance cannot be described by a single modulus or phase angle: rather, the circulatory pressure and flow must first be converted into their sinusoidal components and the impedance expressed as a spectrum of individual moduli and phase angles over the range of frequencies studied (generally to about 12 Hz).

The impedance modulus plot is characterized by a steep fall from its value at zero frequency (opposition to steady state flow or resistance, determined by frictional elements) followed by a relatively flat region above 2–3 Hz (Fig. 15.9). The steepness of the fall depends on the overall compliance of the vasculature; when compliance is low and the modulus fall is less steep, but when compliance is great, the fall is very steep and the impedance modulus approaches zero at a lower frequency [64]. The relatively steady region of the plot beyond 5 Hz is referred to as characteristic impedance (Z_c), which represents the opposition to pulsatile flow in the absence of wave reflections. In this region, inertial and elastic properties are being described. If measured at the aortic root, impedance is representative of the total systemic impedance and is termed "aortic input impedance" [65].

The data accrued by impedance assessment is useful for the characterization of hydraulic workload into steady and pulsatile components. O'Rourke used the ratio of pulsatile to total (pulsatile + steady) external left ventricular work to express the efficiency with which the vascular system accepts pulsatile flow from the heart, efficiency increasing as the ratio decreases and vice versa. The pulsatile workload is less than 10% under normal adult physiology and therefore, is usually neglected in estimations of workload because of its small contribution.

In hypertensive adults, the pulsatile work is increased [47,66]. When the pulsatile work is increased, the work performed by the ventricle is less efficient. The pulsatile workload is increased by early wave reflections, which can be caused by stiff arterial walls, compliance mismatch, as well as by a large pulse pressure.

Aortic flow considerations in postsurgical congenital heart disease

Aortopulmonary shunts

Placement of an aortopulmonary shunt (APS) results in many alterations of the aortic flow dynamics, which will now be considered. The flow profile within an aortopulmonary shunt has not been characterized *in vivo*, yet several computational models of

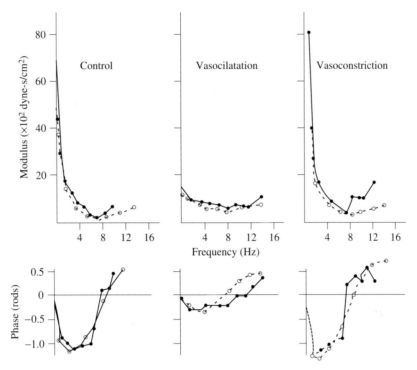

Figure 15.9 Experimentally determined values of impedance modulus (above) and phase (below) in the dog femoral artery (solid line) under control conditions, following intraarterial injection of acetylcholine (vasodilation), and after norepinephrine (vasoconstriction) [31].

steady flow into aortopulmonary shunts have proposed flow profile skew within the shunt [67,68]. Attempts at predicting pulmonary flow from the BTS Doppler velocity time integral (VTI) have not been very successful [68]. This is likely due to errors in both spatial mean velocity and temporal mean velocity estimations. When using Doppler VTI to estimate flow across a vessel or outflow tract, one assumes a flat velocity profile across the flow cross sectional area. If the velocity profile is skewed, errors in the spatial velocity profile assumptions lead to errors in flow rate estimation. Also, the VTI measurement assumes a relatively narrow range of instantaneous velocities, so that the peak velocity is representative of most instantaneous flow velocities. However, flow within an APS comprises a wide range of velocities. Tracing a peak velocity at each time will result in overestimation of the temporal velocity.

The connection between the high-resistance arterial circulation and the low-resistance pulmonary circulation results in a flow and pressure "run-off" from the systemic arterial bed. A large pulse pressure

in the aorta results, which interferes with the function of the proximal aorta, which is to "cushion" the effect of intermittent ventricular ejection and thereby minimize pulsatile work. This cushioning is accomplished by absorbing a proportion of the energy in systole and releasing it in diastole, resulting in peripheral blood flow smoothing and maintenance of diastolic pressure and flow.

The effect of these dynamics on aortic compliance and hydraulic load is intriguing, and the subject of recent investigations. In vitro investigations measuring pulsatile and steady work with aortic input impedance measures have established that the presence of an APS results in a higher workload to the ventricle, even when cardiac output is held constant. This was due to increased pulsatile losses, possibly due to the higher pulse pressure, or increased wave reflections.

It is widely understood that – in clinical practice – an APS increases the volume load returning to the heart. The LV output in juvenile lambs with an APS is twice as high as in age-related lambs without a shunt, and myocardial O2 consumption and coronary artery flow were also more than twice that of controls [69].

Norwood palliation of HLHS

Consideration of the hemodynamics of a reconstructed aortic arch after a Norwood procedure is daunting, due to the complex factors of the impact of abnormal anatomy, vessel compliance, APS connections, and potential arch obstruction on aortic blood flow. A recent study of a conceptual model of the Norwood circulation employed the Windkessel concept in an expanded fashion. In this method, the various components of the circulation (Neoaorta, Descending aorta, Proximal pulmonary artery, etc) are considered as separate Windkessel entities of either 2 or 3 elements. This model was helpful in predicting the response of systemic blood flow and pulmonary blood flow to changes in APS flow. The in vivo dynamics of the reconstructed aortic arch after a Norwood procedure and its recent modifications will undoubtedly be an area of intense investigation in the coming years.

The accurate diagnosis of aortic arch obstruction after a Norwood procedure is difficult [70]. The reconstructed proximal aorta is usually quite large, in comparison to descending aorta. This anatomy leads to difficulties in Doppler prediction of arch obstruction, for several reasons. Due to mass conservation, flow must accelerate as it flows from the large neoaorta to the native descending aorta, leading to elevations in descending aortic velocity that are not due to an obstruction. This can lead to over diagnosis of coarctation in the postoperative Norwood patient.

The opposite error can occur as well. A typical Doppler pattern of coarctation in an infant with low proximal normal arch compliance has a gradient that is greatest in systole, and that continues into diastole – often referred to as a "sawtooth" pattern. However, this pattern may be altered by the presence of an APS, and/or abnormal proximal arch compliance. The APS creates a low-resistance diastolic path for proximal aortic flow, thereby eliminating and in some cases even reversing diastolic descending aortic flow. If one waits for a sawtooth pattern to confirm the diagnosis of coarctation, obstruction will go unidentified.

The very definition of obstruction in this setting must be further explored, as one can envision enhanced and early wave reflections from both a compliance and size mismatch from neo- to descending aorta even in the best postoperative case. We do know that neoaortic arch size exceeds normal arch size, and that its growth parallels normal arch growth [71].

References

1. Naruse T, Tanishita K. Large curvature effect on pulsatile entrance flow in a curved tube: Model experiment simulating blood flow in an aortic arch. J Biomech Eng 1996; 118(2):180–186.
2. Kilner PJ, et al. Helical and retrograde secondary flow patterns in the aortic arch studied by three-directional magnetic resonance velocity mapping. Circulation 1993; 88(5 Pt 1):2235–2247.
3. Hamakiotes CC, Berger SA. Flow in curved vessels, with application to flow in the aorta and other arteries. Monogr Atheroscler 1990; 15:227–239.
4. Segadal L. Velocity distribution model for normal blood flow in the human ascending aorta. Med Biol Eng Comput 1991; 29(5):489–492.
5. Klipstein RH, et al. Blood flow patterns in the human aorta studied by magnetic resonance. Br Heart J, 1987; 58(4):316–323.
6. Fogel MA, Weinberg PM, Haselgrove J. Nonuniform flow dynamics in the aorta of normal children: A simplified approach to measurement using magnetic resonance velocity mapping. J Magn Reson Imaging 2002; 15(6):672–678.
7. Cape EG, et al. Turbulent/viscous interactions control Doppler/catheter pressure discrepancies in aortic stenosis. The role of the Reynolds number. Circulation 1996; 94(11):2975–2981.
8. Bengur AR, et al., Doppler evaluation of aortic valve area in children with aortic stenosis. J Am Coll Cardiol 1991; 18(6):1499–1505.
9. Niederberger J, et al. Importance of pressure recovery for the assessment of aortic stenosis by Doppler ultrasound. Role of aortic size, aortic valve area, and direction of the stenotic jet in vitro. Circulation 1996; 94(8):1934–1940.
10. Barker PC, et al. Comparison of simultaneous invasive and noninvasive measurements of pressure gradients in congenital aortic valve stenosis. J Am Soc Echocardiogr 2002; 15(12):1496–1502.
11. Gilon D, et al. Insights from three-dimensional echocardiographic laser stereolithography. Circulation 1996; 94(3):452–459.
12. Tacy TA, Whitehead KK, Cape EG. In vitro Doppler assessment of pressure gradients across modified Blalock-Taussig shunts. Am J Cardiol 1998; 81(10): 1219–1223.
13. Seifert BL, et al. Accuracy of Doppler methods for estimating peak-to-peak and peak instantaneous

gradients across coarctation of the aorta: An In vitro study. J Am Soc Echocardiogr 1999; 12(9):744–753.

14. Carvalho JS, *et al.* Continuous wave Doppler echocardiography and coarctation of the aorta: Gradients and flow patterns in the assessment of severity. Br Heart J 1990; 64(2):133–137.

15. Tsao PS, *et al.* Fluid flow inhibits endothelial adhesiveness. Nitric oxide and transcriptional regulation of VCAM-1. Circulation 1996; 94(7):1682–1689.

16. Silacci P, *et al.* Flow pulsatility is a critical determinant of oxidative stress in endothelial cells. Hypertension 2001; 38(5):1162–1166.

17. Davies PF, Flow-mediated endothelial mechanotransduction. Physiol Rev 1995; 75(3):519–560.

18. Fleming I, Busse R. Molecular mechanisms involved in the regulation of the endothelial nitric oxide synthase. Am J Physiol Regul Integr Comp Physiol 2003; 284(1):R1–12.

19. Tworetzky W. *et al.* Pulmonary blood flow alters nitric oxide production in patients undergoing device closure of atrial septal defects. J Am Coll Cardiol 2000; 35(2):463–467.

20. Lee RT, Kamm RD. Vascular mechanics for the cardiologist. J Am Coll Cardiol 1994; 23(6):1289–1295.

21. Buntin CM, Silver FH. Noninvasive assessment of mechanical properties of peripheral arteries. Ann Biomed Eng 1990; 18(5):549–566.

22. Van Merode T, *et al.* Different effects of ageing on elastic and muscular arterial bifurcations in men. J Vasc Res 1996; 33(1):47–52.

23. O'Rourke MF, *et al.* Clinical applications of arterial stiffness; definitions and reference values. Am J Hypertens 2002; 15(5):426–444.

24. Dobrin PB. Mechanical properties of arteries. Physiol Rev 1978; 58(2):397–460.

25. Hayashi K, *et al.* Stiffness and elastic behavior of human intracranial and extracranial arteries. J Biomech 1980; 13(2):175–184.

26. Kawasaki T, *et al.* Non-invasive assessment of the age related changes in stiffness of major branches of the human arteries. Cardiovasc Res 1987; 21(9):678–687.

27. Jeremy RW, *et al.* Relation between age, arterial distensibility, and aortic dilatation in the Marfan syndrome. Am J Cardiol 1994; 74(4):369–373.

28. Ong C, *et al.* Increased stiffness and persistent narrowing of the aorta after successful repair of coarctation of the aorta: relationship to left ventricular mass and blood pressure at rest and with exercise. Am Heart J 1992; 123:1594–1600.

29. Sehested J, Baandrup U, Mikkelsen E. Different reactivity and structure of the prestenotic and poststenotic aorta in human coarctation. Implications for baroreceptor function. Circulation 1982; 65(6):1060–1065.

30. Hirai T, *et al.* Stiffness of systemic arteries in patients with myocardial infarction. A noninvasive method to predict severity of coronary atherosclerosis. Circulation 1989; 80(1):78–86.

31. Nichols W, O'Rourke M. McDonald's Blood Flow in Arteries: Theoretical, Experimental and Clinical Properties, 4th edn. Arnold, London, 1998.

32. Kelly R, *et al.* Noninvasive registration of the arterial pressure pulse wave form using high-fidelity applanation tonometry. J Vasc Med Biol 1989; 1:142–149.

33. Cruickshank K, *et al.* Aortic pulse-wave velocity and its relationship to mortality in diabetes and glucose intolerance: An integrated index of vascular function? Circulation 2002; 106(16):2085–2090.

34. Groeninik M, *et al.* Changes in aortic distensibility and pulse wave velocity assessed with magnetic resonance imaging following beta blocker therapy in the Marfan syndrome. Am J Cardiol 1998; 82(2): 203–208.

35. Lehmann ED, *et al.* Relation between number of cardiovascular risk factors/events and non-invasive Doppler ultrasound assessments of aortic compliance. Hypertension 1998; 32:565–569.

36. Asmar R, *et al.* Assessment of arterial distensibility by automatic pulse wave velocity measurement: Validation and clinical application studies. Hypertension 1995; 26(3):485–490.

37. Tedesco MA, *et al.* Arterial distensibility and ambulatory blood pressure monitoring in young patients with neurofibromatosis type 1. Am J Hypertens 2001. 14(6 Part 1):559–566.

38. Rogers WJ, *et al.* Age-associated changes in regional aortic pulse wave velocity. J Am Coll Cardiol 2001; 38(4):1123–1129.

39. Lantelme P, *et al.* Heart rate: an important confounder of pulse wave velocity assessment. Hypertension 2002; 39(6):1083–1087.

40. O'Rourke MF, What is blood pressure? Am J Hypertens 1990; 3:803–810.

41. O'Rourke M. Arterial Function in Health and Disease. Edinburgh: Churchill Livingstone, 1982.

42. Yaginuma T, Cohn JN. Introduction to wave reflection, wave travel and changes with modification of geometric and physical parameters. J Hypertens Suppl 1992; 10(6):S71–72.

43. Ting C, *et al.* Arterial hemodynamics in human hypertension. J Clin Inves 1986; 78:1462–1471.

44. Avolio A. Ageing and wave reflection. J Hypertens Suppl 1992; 10(6):S83–86.

45. Kelly RP, *et al.* Nitroglycerin has more favourable effects on left ventricular afterload than apparent from measurement of pressure in a peripheral artery. Eur Heart J 1990; 11(2):138–144.

46. Ting C, *et al.* Arterial hemodynamics in human hypertension. Effects of adrenergic blockade. Circulation 1991; 84:1049–1057.

47. Ting C, *et al.* Arterial hemodynamics in human hypertension. Effects of angiotensin converting enzyme inhibition. Hypertension 1993; 22(6):839–846.

48. Elsheikh M, *et al.* The effect of hormone replacement therapy on cardiovascular hemodynamics in women with Turner's syndrome. J Clin Endocrinol Metab 2000; 85(2):614–618.

49. O'Rourke M, Kelly R, Avolio A, eds. The Arterial Pulse. Lea and Febiger, London, 1992.

50. Murgo J, Westerhof N. Arterial reflections and pressure waveforms in humans. In Yin F, eds., Ventricular/Vascular Coupling. Springer-Verlag, New York. pp. 140–158, 1987.

51. Kelly R, *et al.* Arterial dilatation and reduced wave reflection. Benefit of dilevalol in hypertension. Hypertension 14(1):14–21, 1989a.

52. Kelly R, *et al.* Noninvasive determination of age-related changes in the human arterial pulse. Circulation 80:1652–1659, 1989b.

53. Latham R, *et al.* Regional wave travel and reflection along the human aorta: A study with six simultaneous micromanometric pressures. Circulation 1985; 72:1257–1269.

54. Murgo J, *et al.* Manipulation of ascendiong aortic pressure and flow wave reflections with the Valsalva maneuver: relationship to input impedance. Circulation 1981; 63:122–132.

55. Murgo J, *et al.* Aortic input impedance in normal man: relationship to pressure wave forms. Circulation 1980; 62:105–116.

56. Yaginuma T, Avolio A, O'Rourke M. Effect of glyceryl trinitrate on peripheral arteries alters left ventricular hydraulic load in man. Cardiovasc Res 1986; 20:153–160.

57. Fitchett D, *et al.* Reflected pressure waves in the ascending aorta: effect of glyceryl trinitrate. Cardiovasc Res 1988; 66:323–326.

58. Aggoun Y, *et al.* Mechanical properties of the common carotid artery in Williams syndrome. Heart 2000; 84(3):290–293.

59. Salaymeh KJ, Banerjee A. Evaluation of arterial stiffness in children with Williams syndrome: Does it play a role in evolving hypertension? Am Heart J 2001; 142(3):549–555.

60. Aggoun Y, Sidi D, Bonnet D. Arterial dysfunction after treatment of coarctation of the aorta. Arch Mal Coeur Vaiss 2001; 94(8):785–789.

61. Liu Z, Brin KP, Yin FC. Estimation of total arterial compliance: An improved method and evaluation of current methods. Am J Physiol 1986; 251(3 Part 2):H588–600.

62. McVeigh GE, *et al.* Age-related abnormalities in arterial compliance identified by pressure pulse contour analysis: aging and arterial compliance. Hypertension 1999; 33(6):1392–1398.

63. Westerhof N, *et al.* Arterial impedance. In Hwang N, Gross D, Patel D, eds., Quantitative Cardiovascular Studies. University Park Press, Baltimore, p. 111, 1979.

64. O'Rourke M, Yaginuma T, Avolio A. Physiological and pathophysiological implications of ventricular/vascular coupling. AnnBiomed Eng 1984; 12(2):119–134.

65. Cohn J. Cardiac consequences of vasomotor changes in the periphery: Impedance and preload. In Fozzard H, ed. Raven Press, New York, p. 1525–1533, 1986.

66. Kelly RP, Tunin R, Kass DA. Effect of reduced aortic compliance on cardiac efficiency and contractile function of in situ canine left ventricle. Circ Res 1992; 71(3):490–502.

67. Whitehead K. Investigation of the hemodynamics of aortopulmonary shunts and the derivation of a relationship between the maximum shunt velocity and pressure drop. University of Pittsburgh, Ph.D., Engineering, biomedical, 1998.

68. Migliavacca F, *et al.* Calculating blood flow from Doppler measurements in the systemic-to-pulmonary artery shunt after the Norwood operation: A method based on computational fluid dynamics. Ultrasound Med Biol 2000; 26(2):209–219.

69. Bartelds B *et al.* Comparative effects of isoproteral and dopamine on myocardial oxygen consumption in conscious lambs with and without an aortopulmonary left to right shunt. J Am Coll Cardial 1998; 31(2): 473–481.

70. Fraisse A, *et al.* Accuracy of echocardiography for detection of aortic arch obstruction after stage I Norwood procedure. Am Heart J 1998; 135(2 Part 1):230–236.

71. Mahle WT, *et al.* Growth characteristics of the aortic arch after the Norwood operation. J Am Coll Cardiol 1998; 32(7):1951–1954.

72. Tsujino H, *et al.* Real-time three-dimensional color Doppler echocardiography for characterizing the spatial velocity distribution and quantifying peak flow rate in the left ventricular outflow tract. Ultrasound in Med Biol, 2001; 27(1):69–74.

73. Tacy TA, Baba K, Cape EG. Effect of aortic compliance on Doppler diastolic flow pattern in coarctation of the aorta. J Am Soc Echocardiogr 1999; 12(8):636–642.

74. Toy SM, Melbin J, Noordergraaf A. Reduced models of Arterial systems. IEEE Trans Biomed Eng 1985; 32(2):174–176.

CHAPTER 16

Blood Flow in Normal and Diseased Pulmonary Arteries

Brian D. Hanna, MD, PhD

Introduction

Pulmonary blood flow has a paramount role in gas exchange. The position of the pulmonary circuit within the influence of the respiratory pump determines many of the flow properties. In the normal physiological state, pulmonary blood flow occurs in a low pressure, high compliance system. Therefore, physiologic and anatomic perturbations have profound effects on pulmonary blood flow characteristics. The adaptation of pulmonary blood flow to the pathological changes of disease and postoperative anatomy involves changes in pulmonary physiology, autoregulation, and fluid dynamics.

The sole purpose of pulmonary blood flow is to bring the red blood cells within micron distances of alveolar gas for the longest time possible, thus enabling effective gas exchange. The anatomical structure of the pulmonary vascular circuit is adapted to this purpose and will be discussed. The effects of lung anatomy and respiratory physiology are important in determining total and regional pulmonary blood flow. These aspects are discussed in the context of the physiologically defined "lung zones of West" and the importance of "critical opening pressure."

The driving pressure for pulmonary blood flow and the overall pulmonary vascular resistance are low. For this reason, total and regional blood flow are determined predominantly by the above anatomical and physiological characteristics. However, the effects of bifurcations, turbulence, shear associated endothelial function, compliance, and impedance are phenomena that have special significance for pulmonary blood flow. Drawing from the derivations given in Chapters 3 and 14 for background, these

effects on pulmonary blood flow are discussed. Reference to these effects is made but the reader must refer to these chapters for precise definitions and derivations.

In the normal anatomic state, pulmonary blood flow is equal to systemic blood flow; however atrial, ventricular, and arterial communications change this relationship. The general issues of shunt calculations are discussed along with the specific effects of these three levels of shunt.

Ventricular outflow obstruction, branch pulmonary artery stenosis, and the general category of pulmonary hypertensive diseases affect total and regional pulmonary blood flow. This discussion focuses on fluid dynamics at the vascular bed but touches on etiology, diagnosis, and principles of therapy.

All surgical and catheter interventions for anatomical cardiovascular lesions must be considered to be palliative procedures. The natural history of many lesions includes pathology in total and regional pulmonary blood flow. Pulmonary valvar regurgitation, ventricular to pulmonary conduits, and aortopulmonary shunts are used as examples of our understanding of pulmonary flow and resistance.

Physiological considerations

The anatomy and histology of the pulmonary vessels

The pulmonary arterial tree arises as a series of bifurcations starting from the initial bifurcation on the main pulmonary artery into the right and left branch pulmonary arteries. The cross-sectional area of the vascular tree does not increase as the vessels run distally, so the cross-sectional area of the proximal branch pulmonary arteries is very representative of the total distal vascular bed. The central pulmonary arteries are considered elastic arteries with multiple elastic laminas [1]. The branching pattern follows that of the airway for the majority of the small pulmonary arteries; however, the so called supernumerary pulmonary arteries are smaller in caliber than conventional pulmonary arteries, arise with right angled branching, and run separately within the interstitum [2]. As the vessels become smaller there is a gradual reduction in the elastic content so that at the level of the lobular bronchioles the vessels are muscular. The precapillary arterioles and terminal bronchi enter the acinus where gas exchange takes place. The intraacinar arterioles are the first not to have internal lamina or a complete muscular layer; they divide into the network of extensively interconnected capillaries that surround the alveolus. The functional gas exchange unit, comprised of the single endothelial cell and the alveolar lining cell, is supported such that a maximum of capillary endothelium is exposed to the alveolus [3]. On the venous side the convergence of veins do not follow the bronchi but run in the intralobular and intersegmental septa back to the left atria.

Relation of pulmonary blood flow to ventilation

From clinical and pathophysiological points of view both total and regional pulmonary blood flow have important implications. Because of the expansile nature of the lung parenchyma and the low driving pressure from the right ventricle, there are significant changes in total and regional blood flow with changes in position and with the phases of respiration and the cardiac cycle. The relationship of flow to pressure and resistance is not static for pulmonary blood flow with several important determinants of total and regional pulmonary vascular resistance (Table 16.1).

Under normal physiologic states, gravity and the pressure relationships described by the "West Zones" have minimal effect on total pulmonary blood flow in the healthy lung [5]. Zone 1 rarely occurs unless there has been a decrease in P_{pa} or an increase in P_A as in hypovolemia and positive pressure ventilation, respectively. The pressure relationships found in Zones 2 and 3 govern the regional distribution of

flow. Zone 4 pathophysiology occurs only during abnormal elevation of P_{isf} as in pulmonary vein stenosis, mitral stenosis, or increased left ventricular diastolic pressure. These conditions are associated with production of more interstitial fluid than can be carried by the pulmonary lymphatics and this is the cause of the increased P_{isf}.

The effect of lung inflation on total pulmonary vascular resistance is significant. At lung volumes lower than FRC (functional residual capacity), precapillary arterioles can be completely occluded. To overcome this phenomenon the pulmonary pressure must exceed the critical opening pressure before flow occurs. The intraacinar vascular compression that occurs at total lung capacity is sufficient to double the vascular resistance seen at FRC [6]. However, during normal tidal breathing vascular resistance changes minimally with lung volume.

Pulmonary vascular resistance unexpectedly decreases with increases in pulmonary arterial pressures. Increased P_{pa} distends pulmonary resistance arterioles and recruits additional arterioles when the critical opening pressure is exceeded. The ability to recruit additional vessels is an important component of the pulmonary arterial bed to accommodate additional flow. The magnitude of this effect is a reduction in vascular resistance by 50% with a doubling in mean pulmonary arterial pressure [5]. This effect distorts the usual relationship of hydraulic resistance to the ratio of mean pressure drop to flow (Ohm's law) such that the predicted resistance change is less than expected for a change in either pressure or flow. Only at pulmonary blood flows in excess of four times the resting flow and pressures in excess of twice the normal does Ohm's law hold for total pulmonary resistance.

Hypoxic pulmonary vasoconstriction governs the ventilation to perfusion relationships within lobular units. Three to five terminal bronchi are associated with a single precapillary resistance arteriole and loss of ventilation to this unit is associated with active vasoconstriction and vessel closure. The exact mechanism by which this occurs has not been determined, although several dozen mediators have been eliminated. Extensive alveolar hypoxia (worse with hypercapnia) can cause a profound increase in total pulmonary vascular resistance and mean pulmonary arterial pressure and decrease in pulmonary blood flow. The response is not linear without an effect above a P_AO_2 of 100 mm Hg, minimal

Table 16.1 Determinants of Total and Regional Pulmonary Vascular Resistance.

Gravity	P_{pa} decreases 1 cm H_2O/cm of vertical distance
Relationship of P_{pa}, P_A, P_{pv}, and P_{isf} (West Zones [4])	West Zone 1: ventilation without perfusion occurs when gravity causes $P_{pa} < P_A < P_{pv}$. West Zone 2: perfusion is proportional to $P_{pa} - P_A$ and is independent of P_{pv} because $P_A > P_{pv}$. Also since P_A is not affected by gravity, flow increases in the more dependent parts of Zone 2. West Zone 3: perfusion is proportional to $P_{pa} - P_{pv}$ and is independent of P_A because $P_{pv} > P_A$. P_{pl} increases less with gravity than either P_{pa} or P_{pv}, therefore flow increases in the dependent parts of Zone 3. West Zone 4: perfusion is proportional to $P_{pa} - P_{isf}$ because P_{isf} pathologically has increased above P_{pv} [3]. Blood flow in Zone 4 is less that in Zone 3 because $(P_{pa} - P_{isf})$ of Zone 4 is less than $(P_{pa} - P_{pv})$ of Zone 3.
Lung inflation	Expands extraacinar large vessels and compresses intraacinar vessels. Small vessel resistance increases exponentially from residual volume (RV) to total lung capacity (TLC). Large vessel resistance decreases from RV to a minimum at TLV. Total resistance therefore has a parabolic relationship to lung volume: high at RV, lowest at functional residual volume, and highest at TLC
Pulmonary pressure	Increased flow causes an increase in P_{pa}, which both distends pulmonary arterioles and recruits more arterioles. Total pulmonary vascular resistance falls with increased flow: empirically, a threefold increase in flow is associated with a 33–50% reduction in resistance. However, once the flow increases over four times, all arterioles have been distended and recruited so that resistance changes as per Ohm's law (pressure/flow).
Alveolar gas mediated vasoconstriction	Hypoxic vasoconstriction is a hallmark of the pulmonary arterial tree. Alveolar P_{O2} is more efficacious in altering vascular tone than pulmonary artery blood gas composition. Intravascular P_{O2}, P_{CO2}, and pH are also components of the effect.
Flow- and pressure-related vascular remodeling	In the disease states of chronic hypoxia or increased pressure and flow related to cardiovascular shunt lesions, the small precapillary arterioles (<100 microns) become muscular. There is a concomitant increase in resistance and reduction in flow-related distensability. The supernumerary arteries are affected first in this process.

P_{pa}: Pulmonary artery pressure; P_A: alveolar pressure; P_{pv}: pulmonary vein pressure; P_{isf}: lung interstitial pressure; P_{pl}: intrapleural pressure.

vasoconstriction in the range of 80–100 mm Hg, and rapid vasoconstriction occurring around 70–80 mm Hg [5].

A word about pathologic muscularization of precapillary arterioles is needed. Remodeling of the pulmonary vascular bed occurs in the face of chronic hypoxia and in the clinical setting of pathologic pulmonary hypertension. This process occurs first with the supernumerary arterioles that are initially smaller than the conventional arterioles. Since a majority of the precapillary arterioles may be of this type, the lung rapidly loses its ability to accommodate increased flow. The bed becomes a high resistance, low capacitance system. Adaptation to stress and increased activity become impossible.

Fluid dynamics

The concepts addressed here have been well discussed in Chapter 2 and applied to the flow characteristics in the aorta in Chapter 14. Reference herein is made for completeness and where there is particular importance to pulmonary blood flow. Since the pulmonary circuit is a low pressure, high compliance system with vessels operating close to their critical closing and opening pressures, pressure loss down the circuit and pressure recovery become important concepts. In addition, alteration in the flow profile affects endothelial cell function with subsequent alteration in the production of local vasoactive mediators. These effects normally become more significant as flow increases with activity.

Geometry

The geometry of the pulmonary bed comprises a curved tube similar to the ascending aorta, and then a series of bifurcations and branch points; the conventional pulmonary vessels bifurcate with a subsequent increase in cross-sectional area, whereas the more numerous supernumerary vessels branch at 90° as smaller vessels leading to a reduction in cross-sectional area. The other important aspect of the pulmonary bed is the ability to dilate. As noted in Chapter 2, Poiseuille flow assumes steady laminar flow through a straight pipe of constant circular cross-sectional area. In the systemic arterial tree the estimated error in the equation caused by dispensability is roughly 10% [7], but with the vastly more distensible pulmonary arterial circuit the overestimation of flow by this equation is far greater.

The effect of curvature through the main pulmonary artery and the two proximal branch arteries would be distortion of the flow profile in a manner analogous to the ascending aorta [8]. The Dean number (Eq. 16.1) describes the effect of curvature on the transition to turbulent flow. The curvature of the left pulmonary artery is less dramatic than that of the right.

$$De = Re\sqrt{\left(\frac{r_{\text{cross section}}}{r_{\text{curvature}}}\right)} \qquad (16.1)$$

The bifurcations and branches within the pulmonary circuit have differing effects on down stream flow stability. The effect of bifurcation or branching on flow profile stability is proportional to the angle and is therefore more at branch points with 90° angles. This increases the wall shear stress on the inner wall, causes eddies, and separation along the outer wall. Wall shear stress is increased predominantly on the inner wall. An additional characteristic separates the branching supernumerary vessels from the conventional bifurcating vessels. The branching vessels have smaller cross-sectional area with each branch, whereas the bifurcating vessels have similar or increasing cross-sectional area [2]. In the case of

the branching vessels there is flow acceleration, less stability, and more pressure loss.

Turbulence

As described and defined previously, turbulence is the random fluctuation of flow when the inertial forces outweigh the viscous forces. As turbulence increases, there is increased wall shear stress both from the flow fluctuations and from a flattening of the velocity profile. The simplified Bernoulli equation governing the relationship of flow velocity to pressure drop, overestimates pressure gradients where turbulent flow predominates. The Womersley number best characterizes turbulence in the pulmonary circuit with pulsatile flow (Eq. 16.2).

$$\text{Womersley number } \alpha = \frac{d}{2}\sqrt{\frac{\rho\omega}{\mu}} \qquad (16.2)$$

where d is the vessel diameter, ρ the density, ω the frequency related to heart rate, and μ is the dynamic viscosity.

Shear effects and endothelial function

Shear stress increases with increased velocity in laminar flow and increases with the time average of the product of the velocity fluctuations in turbulent flow. High shear stress affects both the elements of blood and the vessel wall. Shear stress will also be affected by geometry in the regions of curvature, bifurcations, and branch points. Wall shear stress is increased in regions of flow separation, recirculation, and vorticity. Pathologic wall shear stress has been implicated in endothelial dysfunction, including inflammation, platelet activation and adherence, apoptosis, and local production of nitric oxide [9]. In the case of high flow and high pressure, the increased wall shear stress will be most significant at the branch points into the supernumerary vessels. This may explain why these vessels are the first to be occluded with the pathologic changes seen in pulmonary hypertension.

Pulmonary blood volume, compliance, and impedance

Pulmonary vascular resistance has been the gold standard for evaluation of the pulmonary vascular tree with the response to vasodilating medications used to estimate the ability to increase compliance with increased flow [10]. In the face of pathologic changes in vessel number, caliber, and vasoreactivity there is a reduced ability to increase pulmonary blood flow without an increase in pulmonary pressure or an increased pulmonary vascular resistance. However, resistance does not take into account the pulsatile nature of the pulmonary circuit where the distension of proximal vessels acts as an electrical capacitance. In addition, impedance, the frequency-dependent opposition to pulsatile flow, is an important characteristic of this viscoelastic vascular system that is not accounted by evaluation of the Ohm's law relationship. Development of electrical impedance tomography as a noninvasive technique to measure blood volume changes has allowed the evaluation of compliance changes throughout the cardiac cycle as well as with vasodilating maneuvers [11,12]. When this technique is expanded to include invasive pressure measurements, it may be possible to determine pulmonary capacitance and impedance.

Shunt lesions

General considerations

Shunt lesions are discussed here since the vast majority of pulmonary flow pathophysiology is related to increased pulmonary blood flow through shunt lesions. This discussion starts with measuring pulmonary blood flow and then a general description of the determinants of flow through shunt lesions. Finally, without strict anatomical description of the lesions there is a description of the individual determinants of shunt flow through atrial, ventricular, and arterial level shunts.

At catheterization, pulmonary blood flow is estimated based on the change in concentration of a known amount of an indicator. For thermodilution techniques, cold saline is the indicator and is injected into the right atrium and the temperature profile is determined by a distal temperature sensor in the pulmonary artery, thus maximizing mixing (see Eq. 16.3):

$$CO_{TD} = \frac{V_I\,(T_B - T_I)\left(S_I C_I / S_B C_B\right) 60\,(s/min)}{\int_0^\infty \Delta T_B\,(t)\,dt} \tag{16.3}$$

where CO_{TD} is the thermodilution cardiac output (L/min), V_I the volume of injectate (mL), and T_B, T_I, S_B, S_I, C_B, and C_I the temperature, specific gravity, and specific heat of blood and injectate, respectively.

Errors with this method occur when there is significant pulmonary and/or tricuspid regurgitation, when there is loss of indicator through a right-to-left shunt or incomplete mixing, as in a downstream left-to-right shunt, if there is excessive fluctuation of the blood temperature caused by the respiratory cycle, and lastly thermodilution will overestimate low cardiac outputs because the injectate warms up before it reaches the distal thermistor. Currently, in these situations determinations of pulmonary blood flow involve the Fick principle and oxygen as the indicator. Measurement of the consumption of oxygen is necessary for accuracy. However, oxygen consumption is frequently estimated from tables based on the age, sex, and heart rate of the subject. The Fick principle states that the oxygen consumption must equal the oxygen uptake by pulmonary blood (see Eqs. 16.4 and 16.5):

$$VO_2 = Q_P(C_{pv} - C_{pa}) \tag{16.4}$$

or

$$Q_P = \frac{VO_2}{(C_{pv} - C_{pa})} \tag{16.5}$$

where Q_P is the pulmonary blood flow (L/min), VO_2 the oxygen consumption (mL/min), and C_{pa} and C_{pv} the oxygen content of pulmonary arterial and venous blood, respectively (mL/L).

In the case of shunt lesions, it is possible to use the Fick principle to estimate the effective pulmonary blood flow and the shunt flow. Effective pulmonary blood flow (Q_{eff}), flow where mixed venous blood (mv: usually sampled in the superior vena cava) becomes fully saturated, is estimated by Eq. (16.6). The difference $Q_P - Q_{eff}$ is the shunt flow.

$$Q_{eff} = \frac{VO_2}{(C_{pv} - C_{mv})} \tag{16.6}$$

A clinically relevant term is the ratio of pulmonary blood flow to the systemic blood flow, $Q_P:Q_S$. Values of this ratio range from less than 1 for right-to-left shunts and up to 4–5 for large volume left-to-right shunts. With large left-to-right shunts C_{pa} approaches C_{pv} making the $Q_P:Q_S$ improbably large; convention sets the maximal reportable $Q_P:Q_S$ at 4–5. Since systemic blood flow is inversely proportional to $(C_{ao} - C_{mv})$, with C_{ao} the oxygen content of systemic arterial blood, Eq. (16.7) defines $Q_P:Q_S$ as

$$Q_P : Q_S = \frac{(C_{ao} - C_{mv})}{(C_{pv} - C_{pa})} \tag{16.7}$$

By echocardiography (and velocity-coded MRI), systemic cardiac output can be accurately determined; however, it is difficult to determine pulmonary blood flow accurately. Ventricular stroke volume is determined by integrating the velocity profile across the cross section of the ventricular outflow (see Eqs. 16.8 and 16.9).

$$Q = \int_{section} u \, dA \qquad (16.8)$$

where Q is the flow, u the velocity, and A the area.

$$SV = \frac{CSA \, V_M 60 \, (sec/min)}{1000 \, (cm^3/L)} \qquad (16.9)$$

where SV is the stroke volume (cardiac output = SV × heart rate), V_M the mean velocity which is calculated using the velocity–time integral of the spectral Doppler display, and CSA is the cross-sectional area.

For left ventricular stroke volume the mean velocity is taken at the aortic valve where the cross-sectional area does not change with ejection. For right ventricular stroke volume the architecture of the right ventricular outflow tract is complex and it is difficult to determine either the cross-sectional area or the area with any accuracy. The main pulmonary artery cross-sectional area can change by 2–18% with ejection [13]. Furthermore this equation is based on a known and measurable velocity profile across the measured cross-sectional area. The velocity–time integral is a rough estimate at best and inaccurate in the face of turbulent flow. For aortic flow measured at the aortic annulus, the correlation with invasive measurements can be as good as 0.97–0.99 [14]. For pulmonary flow measured at the pulmonary valve—with the CSA calculated from two orthogonal views—the correlation with invasive measurements is not as reliable [15].

The resistance of the shunt lesion and the balance of forces governing flow on either side of the lesion determine shunt flow. In essence blood travels along its usual path or deviates through the shunt, which increases total pulmonary blood flow. Poiseuille's law and Ohm's law define the resistance of the shunt lesion as being proportional to the size of the defect and the viscosity of blood (see Eqs. 16.10–16.12).

$$\text{Poiseuille's law } Q = \frac{\pi (P_i - P_o) r^4}{8 \eta l} \qquad (16.10)$$

where Q is the flow, P_i and P_o the inflow and outflow pressures, respectively, r the radius, η the viscosity, and l is the length.

Analogous to Ohm's law $Q = \Delta P / R$ (16.11)

where ΔP is the mean pressure drop and R is the hydraulic resistance.

$$R = \frac{P_i - P_o}{Q} = \frac{8 \eta l}{\pi r^4} \qquad (16.12)$$

Poiseuille's law assumes steady, nonpulsatile, laminar flow that may be appropriate in the case of atrial level shunts. Turbulent flow is usual for medium and small ventricular and arterial level shunts. In these cases Poiseuille's law underestimates the effects of inertial forces, and flow characteristics through a stenosis that increase the energy losses at high velocities, effectively decreasing the driving force for volume flow.

The primary driving force for volume flow across a shunt lesion can be a pressure gradient or an imbalance in the down-stream resistances and/or capacitances. In any specific lesion one or more of these terms is paramount as discussed below.

Atrial level shunts

Atrial septal defects do not have significant length so the resistance to flow is proportional only to the $(radius)^4$. Furthermore, the pressure gradient across the moderate to large defect is usually miniscule in the range of a few millimeters of mercury and often only during part of the cardiac cycle. Even with large defects volume flow is correlated to the instantaneous pressure gradient between the left and right atria [16]. The predominant factor that determines the pressure gradient is the ability of the ventricle to dilate and accept additional volume. The right ventricle is thinner and more compliant compared to the left ventricle and so during diastole the instantaneous difference between the ventricular compliances drives the volume flow from left to right. Furthermore, the respiratory cycle affects atrial septal defect flow, both in volume and direction. Left-to-right shunt is increased during increased intrathoracic pressure while right-to left shunt is decreased. The opposite occurs with the reduction in intrathoracic pressure as seen in inspiration. These effects are directly related to the effect of intrathoracic pressure on pulmonary and systemic venous return. Only if the right ventricle becomes hypertrophied and less compliant, secondary to high systolic pressures, will pulmonary artery pressure or resistance have an indirect effect on atrial level shunts.

Ventricular level shunts

Ventricular septal defects may have significant length if located within the muscular septum; however, most are found at the base of the heart and involve the thin membranous septum. The resistance to flow is therefore proportional to the (radius)^4. In restrictive defects (cross-sectional area $\leq$ aortic valve annulus) the driving force for flow is the instantaneous difference in pressure between the two ventricles. In the normal heart, right ventricular pressure is less than left ventricular pressure throughout the cardiac cycle. The restrictive nature of the defect guarantees that Ohm's law determines the right ventricular and pulmonary artery systolic pressures. However, when the defect is not restrictive (cross-sectional area $\geq$ aortic valve annulus) right ventricular and pulmonary artery systolic pressures are equal to the left ventricle and volume flow occurs in systole when both semilunar valves are open. Flow volume is determined by the instantaneous difference between pulmonary and systemic vascular resistances. As noted in Chapter 3 (Fig. 3.7 and Eq. 3.28), the proximal isovelocity surface area technique can be combined with Doppler interrogation to estimate volume flow through an orifice as in a VSD (Eq. 16.13).

$$Q_o = \left(4\pi r^2\right) u_r \qquad (16.13)$$

where Q_o is the flow rate at the orifice and r is the radial distance from the orifice at which the velocity, u_r, is measured. In this fashion, shunt flow added to systemic flow, determined accurately at the aortic valve annulus, will estimate pulmonary flow.

Increased systolic pressure, transmitted through the defect, is associated with a reduction in pulmonary vascular resistance and a further increment in flow. Eventually flow is limited by an increase in pulmonary vascular resistance, either on the basis of an increased P_{isf} associated with congestive failure, pressure, and flow-induced vasoconstriction or progressive pulmonary vascular occlusive disease.

Arterial level shunts

The patent ductus arteriosus connects the aorta at the level of the left subclavian artery to the pul-

monary tree, usually either at the bifurcation into left and right branch arteries or just leftward onto the proximal left pulmonary artery. The defect has length and the configuration of the defect is complex. Often the aortic end has a significant diverticulum that tapers to a much smaller pulmonary opening. The vast majority of these defects are restrictive to pressure so the pulmonary systolic and diastolic pressures are lower than in the aorta. Instantaneous flow is determined by the ratio of instantaneous pulmonary and systemic resistance. With a nonrestrictive defect the massive diastolic flow toward the pulmonary circuit can decrease systemic perfusion to the point of tissue ischemia and the aortic pulse pressure is increased. Because the position of the entrance is into the proximal pulmonary tree, shunt calculations for this lesion must rely on multiple, distal pulmonary artery samples. Doppler estimates of shunt flow are unreliable except in the case of the very short, nonrestrictive defect. In this situation the flow characteristics approach that of the similar, but more proximal aortopulmonary window.

Systemic to pulmonary collateral vessels include true bronchial arteries but also encompass abnormal vascular connections between systemic arteries and distal, intraparenchymal, pulmonary arteries. The vessels are often capable of transmission of significant pressure and flow to the distal pulmonary vasculature. However, by the very nature of the distal connections it is impossible to estimate the flow volume by the Fick principle. Regional inhomogeneities in flow and pressure exist and eventual vascular occlusive disease is possible.

Obstructive lesions

The obstructive lesions that significantly affect pulmonary blood flow affect not only the volume flow but also the flow profile. Obstruction can occur in complex lesions as in the right ventricular infundibulum, or severe and multiple peripheral pulmonary artery stenosis, or isolated lesions as in valvar pulmonary stenosis or isolated proximal branch pulmonary artery stenosis. Pathologic restriction and obstruction of the smallest vascular elements, precapillary arterioles, capillaries, and postcapillary venuoles, is associated with profound changes in pulmonary blood flow.

Right ventricular outflow tract obstruction

The right ventricular outflow tract obstruction (RVOT) is anatomically complex and dynamic throughout the cardiac cycle. From the origin of the infundibulum, the right ventricular inflow region the RVOT starts a long curve posteriorly to the pulmonary valve. In systole the full length of the RVOT contracts adding both volume and velocity to the ventricular stroke volume. In double chambered RV and tetralogy of Fallot the subvalvar obstruction occurs at the origin of the infundibulum thereby creating turbulent flow for the full length of the outflow tract out into the main pulmonary artery. As discussed in the previous chapters, the simplified Bernoulli equation, as used for Doppler evaluation of the pressure gradient over the RVOTO, overestimates the gradient in the face of turbulence. This explains the puzzling finding that the Doppler-estimated RVOT gradient can exceed the ventricular systolic pressure. Surgical excision of RVOTO often includes incision of the infundibular free wall as well as excision of the offending muscle bundles. Systolic contraction of the infundibulum is impaired; more so when graft material is needed to augment the RVOT. This structure can then act as a large capacitance sink for the kinetic energy of ventricular contraction.

Valvar pulmonary stenosis

Pure pulmonary valve stenosis rarely exists in isolation. The pressure load on the right ventricle rapidly leads to infundibular hypertrophy and stenosis. Estimates of pulmonary valve stenosis in the face of turbulence from subvalvar stenosis are inaccurate. The supravalvar region at the apex of the valvar commissure, the sinotubular junction, is often narrowed making the stenotic lesion longer. This is most often seen in dysplastic pulmonary valves as in Noonan's syndrome [17]. The fluid shear stresses from the turbulent flow are associated with poststenotic dilation, which is often more severe in the proximal pulmonary arterial tree than in the aorta because of the difference in wall composition. This is most striking in the case of tetralogy of Fallot with absent pulmonary valve, a lesion with severe pulmonary stenosis and regurgitation. The branch pulmonary arteries dilate to the extent that they interfere with the growth and development of the bronchi [18]. Treatment of pulmonary valve stenosis, either by catheter balloon dilation or surgical incision leads to significant valvar regurgitation and often does not relieve the stenosis completely [19].

Branch pulmonary artery stenosis

Isolated branch pulmonary artery stenosis is rare except as a postoperative finding. There can be a discrete stenosis when there is retention of ductal tissue within the pulmonary artery wall if the ductus arteriosus enters the branch pulmonary artery directly. Proximal pulmonary artery stenosis can be a feature of left pulmonary artery sling. William's syndrome is associated with proximal pulmonary artery stenosis, but more frequently there are also distal stenoses at subsequent bifurcations [20]. The effects of unilateral branch pulmonary artery stenosis are decreased distal growth on the side with reduced flow and dilation of the nonaffected side. Turbulent flow and poststenotic dilation is uncommon without increased proximal pressure, as in an associated nonrestrictive ventricular septal defect.

Treatment of isolated branch pulmonary stenosis is catheter balloon dilation [21]. This tears the intima and inner medial layers; however, without exposure to high pressure aneurysm formation is uncommon. Dilation of postsurgical lesions may not be optimal without the placement of an endovascular stent. This interferes with pressure wave propagation, wave reflection, and vascular capacitance. Unfortunately, separation, recirculation, and eddy formation increase the shear forces at each end of the stent. This is associated with neointimal hyperplasia and can result in stent narrowing. Careful dilation to match the caliber of the distal vessel limits these effects.

Multiple peripheral artery stenoses

Multiple peripheral arterial stenoses are seen in tetralogy of Fallot, often the worse cases are seen with absence of the main pulmonary artery and multiple aortopulmonary collateral vessels as the only source of pulmonary blood flow. William's syndrome and a similar form without the features of William's have severe stenoses at virtually every bifurcation. These diseases are associated with systemic or higher proximal pulmonary artery pressures and vessels with limited dispensability. Growth of distal vascular components is reduced. Treatment with catheter-based dilation is often associated with aneurysm formation from the elevated proximal pressure and the increased wall shear stress. Likewise surgical augmentation of proximal stenoses is also the site of aneurismal dilation, often to the extent that kinetic energy is lost in the massive capacitance.

Pulmonary hypertension

Outside of the cases where pulmonary pressure is elevated because of proximal obstructive lesions or unrepaired ventricular and/or arterial shunt lesions, elevated pulmonary pressures are the result of progressive alteration in the structure and number of precapillary arterioles, capillaries, or postcapillary venuoles. These are different pathologic and clinical diseases with very different etiologies, pathophysiology, and natural histories. However, proximal artery dilation is common to all etiologies.

By convention, the definition of abnormal pulmonary hypertension has two components: mean pulmonary artery pressure of greater than 25 mm Hg and pulmonary vascular resistance of >4 Wood units (mm Hg/(L min m^2). This defines a high pressure, low capacitance vascular bed. Increases in flow do not cause a decrease in resistance and there is both fixed vascular obstruction and reactive vasoconstriction. All forms of pulmonary hypertension should be expected to progress, although permanent clinical improvement with therapy is reported. Excellent reviews of these diseases are available [10, 22–25].

Arteriolar disease

Although the common final pathway for all pathologic pulmonary hypertensive diseases is arteriolar occlusion, this is the hallmark of primary pulmonary hypertension and Eisenmenger reaction. Initially there is muscularization of smaller and smaller arterioles until, associated with thrombosis, there is complete occlusion. Plexiform lesions develop around these occluded vessels and are the pathologic markers of the disease. Etiologic factors include a genetic component mapped to chromosome 2q 33, an abnormality in the structure of type II bone morphogenetic protein receptor, and environmental triggers, for example, flow and pressure in the case of Eisenmenger reaction [26]. Treatment with vasodilator therapy and anticoagulation is attempted and if there is reactivity then survival at 5 years can approach 95% [27,28].

Capillary disease

Alveolar Capillary dysplasia, otherwise known as misalignment of the pulmonary veins, is a rapidly progressive and lethal congenital disease of the capillary bed [29]. Pathologic evaluation demonstrates the pulmonary veins running with the arterial and bronchial structures, but the functional abnormality is at the level of the alveolar capillary membrane. Children present within weeks of birth both cyanotic and in low output failure. The predominant finding is suprasystemic pulmonary artery pressure and profound ventilation/perfusion mismatch. Most affected infants are diagnosed on postmortem and currently there is no effective treatment or palliative intervention short of urgent lung transplantation. Infrequently, an infant can be stabilized on inhaled nitric oxide, possibly because of an improvement in the ventilation–perfusion mismatch inherent to the disease. Systemic vasodilators have been consistently associated with a clinical deterioration.

Venous disease

Pulmonary veno-occlusive disease can be a progressive congenital disease or the result of an acquired disease possibly associated with viral infections [30,31]. The classic form involves occlusion of the postcapillary venuoles but a similar outcome occurs with unrepairable distal pulmonary vein stenosis, as in the result from obstructed anomalous pulmonary venous connection. Unlike the other two forms discussed above, pulmonary veno-occlusive disease presents with pulmonary edema, furthermore attempts at vasodilation can precipitate a profound clinical deterioration. Arteriolar vasoconstriction is protective and limits the flow to capillaries with obstructed venous return. Again inhaled agents, nitric oxide or prostacyclin, may stabilize the clinical situation long enough to allow lung transplantation.

Postoperative changes

Pulmonary regurgitation

Pulmonary regurgitation is a common finding after intervention for congenital heart disease. Currently, debate continues as to the significance of pulmonary regurgitation on long-term right ventricular function; however, there are clear effects on pulmonary blood flow and the ability to evaluate it. Initially pulmonary regurgitation increases the right ventricular stroke volume and this must be accommodated by distention of the proximal pulmonary arteries. The regurgitant fraction returns to the ventricle during diastole and the pulmonary diastolic pressure rapidly approaches the right ventricular pressure. Mean pulmonary pressure becomes dependent on the right ventricular diastolic function as opposed to down-stream resistance. In this case, the calculated pulmonary vascular resistance is falsely lowered. No method accurately assesses pulmonary vascular resistance or compliance in this situation; in fact, invasive evaluation cannot overcome the problem in determining a mean pulmonary artery pressure. However, it is theoretically possible to measure instantaneous pulmonary capillary blood flow using nitrous oxide uptake in a body plethysmograph simultaneously with pulmonary artery pressure [5]. In this manner, both instantaneous vascular resistance and vascular impedance could be determined [32]. I am not aware of this being accomplished in children; the advancement of our knowledge could be exceptional.

Right ventricle to pulmonary artery conduits
The surgical placement of right ventricle to pulmonary artery conduits presents a special case of altered pulmonary blood flow. Abnormalities in the architecture distort the flow profile, and calcification and destruction of the valve result in a point of obstruction and free regurgitation. The curvature of the conduit, altered velocity profile, increased wall shear stress, and turbulence are significantly worse the smaller the radius of the conduit. Inflammation and endothelial activation are the result [9]. This leads to calcification of homograph conduits and may explain why infants calcify homograph conduits in the pulmonary circuit faster than adults. Calcification of the conduit wall changes the ability of the pulmonary arteries to accommodate the stroke volume, increasing the hydraulic load on the ventricle and transmitting higher transmural pressure to more distal vessels. This in turn is associated with further muscularization and narrowing of small capacitance arterioles and eventually to an increase in overall vascular resistance.

Aortopulmonary surgical shunts
Initial palliation of congenital heart disease with pulmonary blood flow that is dependent on flow from the aorta can include the placement of an aortopulmonary shunt. The classic Blaylock–Taussig shunt comprised a connection of the subclavian artery to the branch pulmonary artery in an end to side fashion. The curvature of the shunt, the disturbed flow profile and the excessive flow with an increased pulse pressure all led to aneurismal dilation of the subclavian and pulmonary arteries. A fixed diameter tube graft interposed between these two arteries forms the modified form of this shunt. The appropriate diameter and length for the graft have been determined predominantly by experience. Smaller grafts are more susceptible to occlusion than the technical aspects would predict. The expected flow disturbances have been modeled [33] (see also Chapter 14). It should be expected that the increased shear stresses are involved in platelet activation and thrombosis of the small shunts. Additionally, growth of the pulmonary artery is often asymmetric, and depending on the flow pattern within the pulmonary artery, stenosis of the pulmonary artery is common.

Conclusion
Pulmonary blood flow occurs through a low pressure, high compliance vascular bed and is modified, both in volume flow and in velocity profile, by gravity, respiratory mechanics, and the geometry of the vascular bed. Critical opening pressure, flow-mediated decreases in vascular resistance, and a profound ability to constrict on exposure to hypoxemia are critical characteristics of the vascular bed that determine pulmonary blood flow in health and disease. Examples of pathologic high flow shunt lesions and low compliance obstructive lesions are discussed. There is a need to validate methods for determining the frequency-dependent measures of vascular compliance and impedance as well as methods to analyze instantaneous pulmonary blood flow and pressure relationships. Only in this way will it be possible to determine the effect of therapy and disease states on the determinants of total and regional pulmonary blood flow.

References
1. Gehr P, Bachofen M, Weibel ER. The normal human lung: Ultrastructure and morphometric estimation of diffusion capacity. Respir Physiol 1978; 32:121–140.
2. Elliott FJ, Reid L. Some new facts about the pulmonary artery and its branching pattern. Clin Radiol 1965; 16:193–198.
3. Weibel ER. Morphological basis of alveolar-capillary gas exchange. Physiol Rev 1973; 53:419–495.

4. West JB. Respiratory physiology—The essentials. Williams and Wilkins, Baltimore, 1979.

5. Pinsky MR. Determinants of pulmonary arterial flow variation during respiration. J Appl Physiol 1984; 56:1237–1245.

6. Weyman AE. Principles of flow. In: Weyman, AE, ed., Principles and Practice of Echocardiography. Lea and Febiger, Philadelphia, p 1335, 1994.

7. Hamakiotes CC, Berger SA. Flow in curved vessels, with application to flow in the aorta and other vessels. Monogr Atheroscler 1990; 15:227–239.

8. Davies PF. Flow-mediated endothelial mechanotransduction. Physiol Rev 1995; 73:519–560.

9. Widlitz A, Barst RJ. Pulmonary arterial hypertension in children. Eur Respir J 2003; 21:155–176.

10. Brown BH, Barber DC, Morice AH. Cardiac and respiratory related electrical impedance changes in the human thorax. IEEE Trans Biomed Eng 1994; 41:729–734.

11. Smit HJ, Vonk-Noordegraaf A, Marcus JT. Pulmonary vascular responses to hypoxia and hypercapnia in healthy volunteers and COPD patients measured by electrical impedance tomography. Chest 2003; 123:1803–1809.

12. Snider AR, Serwer GA. Echocardiography in pediatric heart disease. Mosby Year Book, St Louis, pp 21–133, 1990.

13. Lewis JF, Kuo LC, Nelson JG. Pulsed Doppler echocardiographic determination of stroke volume and cardiac output: Clinical validation of two new methods using the apical window. Circulation 1984; 70:425–431.

14. Valdez-Cruz LM, Horowitz S, Mesel E. A pulsed Doppler echocardiographic method for calculating pulmonary and systemic blood flow in atrial level shunts: Validation studies in animals and initial human experience. Circulation 1984; 69:80–86.

15. Levin AR, Spach MS, Boineau JP. Atrial pressure flow dynamics and atrial septal defects (secundum type). Circulation 1968; 37:476–488.

16. Noonan JA. Hypertelorism with Turner phenotype. A new syndrome with associated congenital heart disease. Am J Dis Child 1968; 116:373–380.

17. Pinsky WW, Gillette Pc, Duff DF. The absent pulmonary valve syndrome: Consideration of management. Circulation 1978; 57:159–162.

18. McCrindle BW. Independent predictors of long-term results after balloon pulmonary valvuloplasty. Circulation 1994; 89:1751–1759.

19. Beuren AJ, Schulze C, Eberle P. The syndrome of supravalvular aortic stenosis, peripheral pulmonary

stenosis, mental retardation and similar facial appearance. Am J Cardiol 1964; 13:471–483.

20. Kan JS, Marvin WJ Jr, Bass JL, Balloon angioplasty-branch pulmonary artery stenosis: Results from the valvuloplasty and angioplasty of congenital anomalies registry. Am J Cardiol 1990; 65:798–801.

21. Stuart RM. Primary Pulmonary Hypertension Executive Summary. The World Health Organization, Evian, France, pp. 1–27, 1998.

22. Barst RJ, Maislin G, Fishman AP. Vasodilator therapy for primary pulmonary hypertension in children. Circulation 1999; 99:1197–1208.

23. Gibbs JS. Recommendations on the management of pulmonary hypertension in clinical practice. Heart 2001; 86(Suppl I):i1–i13.

24. McLaughlin VV, Rich S. Severe pulmonary hypertension: critical care clinics. Crit Care Clin 2001; 17:453–467.

25. Rudarakanchana N, Trembath RC, Morrell NW. New insights into the pathogenesis and treatment of primary pulmonary hypertension. Thorax 2001; 56:888–890.

26. Barst RJ, Rubin LJ, McGoon MD, Survival in primary pulmonary hypertension with long term continuous intravenous prostacyclin. Ann Intern Med 1994; 121:409–415.

27. Clabby ML, Canter CE, Moller JH, Hemodynamic data and survival in children with pulmonary hypertension. J Am Coll Cardiol 1997; 30:554–560.

28. Boggs S, Harris MC, Hoffman DJ, Misalignment of pulmonary veins with alveolar capillary dysplasia: Affected siblings and variable phenotypic expression. J Pediat 1994; 124:125–128.

29. Rosenthal A, Vawter GF, Wagenvoorst CA. Intrapulmonary veno-occlusive disease. Am J Cardiol 1973; 31:78–83.

30. Voordes CG, Kuipers JRG, Elema JD. Familial pulmonary veno-occlusive disease: A case report. Thorax 1977; 32:763–766.

31. Westerhof N. Arterial impedance. In: Hwang N, Gross D, Patel D, eds., Quantitative Cardiovascular Studies. University Park Press, Baltimore, p 111, 1979.

32. Whitehead K. Investigation of the Hemodynamics of Aortopulmonary Shunts and the Derivation of a Relationship Between the Maximum Shunt Velocity and Pressure Drop. PhD Thesis, University of Pittsburgh, 1998.

33. West JB, Dollerry CT, Naimark A. Distribution of blood flow in isolated lung: Relation to vascular and alveoral pressures. J Appl Physiol 1964; 19:713–724.

CHAPTER 17

Considerations in the Single Ventricle

Mark A. Fogel, MD, FACC, FAAP

Introduction

The assessment of cardiac function and blood flow in patients with a single ventricle presents an enormous challenge to medical science. Apart from the fact that there are varied types of single ventricles, nearly all patients require either surgical reconstruction or heart replacement. In the staged surgical reconstruction leading to the Fontan procedure [1], the physiology varies from a volume-loaded ventricle to a volume-unloaded one, although even that is debatable at certain stages [2]. The systemic circulation also varies from one with a runoff lesion into the pulmonary circulation as in the Norwood Stage I reconstruction [3] (and the attendant perfusion abnormalities via a "steal" phenomenon from the coronary and gastrointestinal circulations) to one without a runoff lesion as in the final Fontan reconstruction [1]. In addition, in the systemic circulation, the aorta may or may not undergo an aortic to pulmonary anastomosis (e.g., Norwood stage I for hypoplastic left heart syndrome [3] versus a typical patient with tricuspid atresia with normally related great arteries respectively). Finally, the ability of the heart to pump blood to the systemic circulation and allow for passive flow into the lungs in the final stage of Fontan reconstruction is still poorly understood and optimizing this flow is continually discussed in the literature [4,5].

This chapter will discuss some of the issues behind ventricular function and blood flow as they relate to the single ventricle patient. A short background on the physiology of the single ventricle and the reconstructive surgery will be presented first. Many of these issues are unique to the single ventricle patient but are nevertheless critical to the understanding and care of the univentricular heart. Sometimes, as will be demonstrated, by examining these issues in single ventricles, unique insights into the functioning of the normal "dual-chambered" circulation can be obtained.

Background

As noted in Chapter 1 of this book, the detailed anatomy of ventricles in congenital heart disease, including functional single ventricles, are highly variable. Ventricular morphology can either be of the right ventricle (RV) or left ventricle (LV) type. Within these types, ventricles can either be of the D-loop variety or the L-loop variety, depending upon the particular geometry of the ventricle [6]. In addition, single ventricles can be either a true single ventricle or a "functional" single ventricle. A true single ventricle, rigorously defined in the segmental approach to congenital heart disease, is an atrioventricular valve to ventricle connection where both atrioventricular valves or a common atrioventricular valve enters one ventricle in the presence of only one sinus portion of the heart. A "functional" single ventricle can be any kind of ventricular arrangement (e.g., two ventricles with multiple large ventricular septal defects, straddling atrioventricular valve with hypoplasia of one ventricle, etc), where from a "functional" standpoint, the ventricle acts like a single pumping chamber and needs to be treated as such.

There is, however, a unifying anatomic and physiologic concept that allows a type of heart to fall under the rubric of "functional" single ventricle in studying ventricular function; only one usable ventricle is present to effectively pump blood while the other is hypoplastic or both ventricles are linked in such a way as separation of the circulations into two pumping chambers is impossible. As an associated abnormality in a number of cases, there can be obstruction to outflow or hypoplasia of one of the great vessels arising from the heart. Blood flow to the obstructed circulation is maintained in the newborn by one or all of the following routes: the patent ductus arteriosus, both great vessels arising from the usable ventricle with the pulmonary valve allowing just enough blood to enter the pulmonary circulation (e.g., double outlet RV and pulmonary stenosis [7]), or blood flow through a ventricular septal defect if one or both great vessels arises from the hypoplastic ventricle (e.g., tricuspid atresia with ventricular septal defect and pulmonic stenosis [8]). The goal of reconstructive surgery is to separate the systemic and pulmonary circulations allowing for passive blood flow into the pulmonary circulation while the functional single ventricle sustains flow to the systemic circulation. Surgical reconstruction is performed in stages, with changing physiology at each stage. Figure 17.1a shows the physiology of the normal circulation and Fig. 17.1b shows the physiology at all the three stages of reconstruction.

Prior to bidirectional superior cavopulmonary connection (BSCC)

At this stage, in some patients, no surgery may be necessary. Such as a patient with tricuspid atresia, normally related great arteries, and a ventricular septal defect [8], which allows adequate but restricted pulmonary blood flow. In this particular case, systemic venous return crosses an atrial septal defect, mixes with pulmonary venous return in the left atrium and LV, and gets pumped to the systemic circulation through the aorta and the pulmonary circulation via the ventricular septal defect. Other patients, such as in hypoplastic left heart syndrome, need immediate surgery. In this case, the LV and aorta are markedly hypoplastic and cannot support the systemic circulation alone. In this type of anatomy pulmonary venous flow crosses an atrial septal defect, mixes with systemic venous return in the right atrium and RV, and gets pumped to the pulmonary circulation as well as the systemic circulation (via antegrade flow in the patent ductus arteriosus). Since the patent ductus arteriosus is an unreliable source of blood flow, a Norwood Stage I procedure [3] is performed which involves

• transection of the main pulmonary artery and anastomosis with the hypoplastic aorta with homograft augmentation of the arch,
• atrial septectomy, and
• creation of a systemic to pulmonary artery shunt.

Some surgeons are now substituting an RV to pulmonary artery conduit [9,10] (so called Sano procedure) for the last bullet, which has the theoretical advantage of little diastolic runoff and better coronary perfusion than the classic Norwood stage I procedure. At this stage, whether surgical reconstruction is needed or not, the ventricle is volume overloaded since the single ventricle pumps blood to both the systemic and the pulmonary circulations in parallel (Fig. 17.1b, left).

BSCC

At approximately 6 months of age, once pulmonary vascular resistance has dropped adequately, the BSCC is performed, which come in various forms such as the hemiFontan procedure or the bidirectional Glenn procedure [2,11,12]. This creates a superior vena cava to pulmonary artery anastomosis with exclusion of the atrium (utilizing a patch) and ligation of the systemic to pulmonary artery shunt. The ventricle is thus volume unloaded because it does not have direct access to the pulmonary circulation (Fig. 17.1b, middle); instead, part of the systemic circulation's venous return (blood from the brain and upper body) is shunted into the lungs via the superior vena cava to pulmonary artery anastomosis. It is, however, not clear that it remains volume unloaded throughout the time the patient is in this physiology (see separate section below) [2]. Because only part of the systemic venous return enters the lungs, cardiac output is maintained at the expense of cyanosis. The rational for this intermediate procedure arose when it was noted that the ventricular wall thickness-to-chamber dimension ratio acutely increased when the Fontan procedure was performed without this step [2,11]. Tachycardia, low output, and hemodynamic deterioration were present after the Fontan procedure, suggesting ventricular compliance abnormalities. It was thought that the bidirectional superior cavopulomonary physiology would withstand the removal of the volume load and ventricular geometry changes much better since a substantial amount of the systemic venous return can fill the

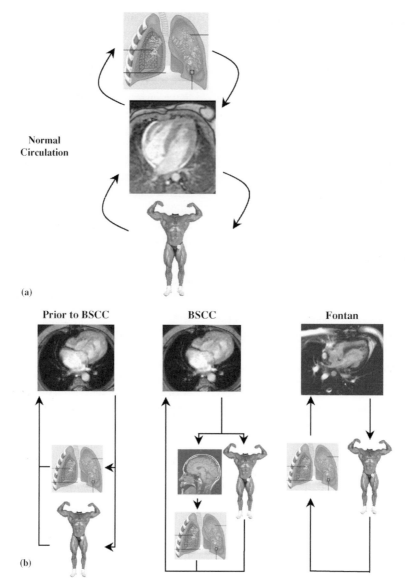

Figure 17.1 Diagrammatic representation of the different physiology at each stage of surgical reconstruction. (a) The normal circulation has two pumping chambers and the systemic and pulmonary circulations are in series with each other relative to the heart. (b) The single ventricle can undergo three stages of surgical reconstruction: Prior to the bidirectional superior cavopulmonary connection (BSCC), the single ventricle pumps to both systemic and pulmonary circulations in parallel (left). After BSCC, the single ventricle directly pumps only to the systemic circulation with blood from the brain and upper body supplying flow to the lungs as well (middle). After Fontan reconstruction, the circulations are in series again (right).

ventricle without first passing through the lungs. There is a form of BSCC that is definitely not volume unloaded—when there is an additional source of pulmonary blood flow left in place on purpose, such as forward flow through a stenotic pulmonary valve or a systemic to pulmonary artery shunt.

Fontan completion

Months later, at approximately 2 years of age, the circulations (with the possible exception of coronary venous flow) are separated by baffling inferior vena cava blood into the lungs (Fig. 17.1b, right). There are multiple ways to accomplish this including placement of a hemicylindrical polytetraflouroethe-lyne patch along the lateral wall of the atria or an extracardiac conduit from inferior vena cava to pulmonary artery. The "atriopulmonary connection," which has been used in certain kinds of functional single ventricles in the past, has fallen out of favor and is not used anymore. To maintain cardiac output, all blood must traverse the lungs by passive flow and at this stage the ventricle is volume unloaded. To improve outcome, a communication is purposely created between the systemic and pulmonary venous pathways (a "fenestration") to allow for right to left shunting when there is increased pulmonary vascular resistance. This allows for maintenance of the cardiac output at the expense of cyanosis, similar in concept to the bidirectional superior cavopulmonary connection. The fenestrations, in general, close on their own.

Ventricular function

Since the single ventricle undergoes various physiologic transformations over the course of two, if not three, surgeries, each stage will be considered in turn.

Prior to BSCC

Multiple factors are at play at this stage of single ventricle reconstruction and the major one is the volume load [2,11,13]. Since the single ventricle has direct access to both the systemic and pulmonary circulations, it must pump one cardiac output to the body and an additional amount of blood to the lungs and so the ventricle becomes volume overloaded (Fig. 17.1b, left). Other physiologic considerations are ventricular hypertrophy [2], systemic arterial desaturation, and the afterload as the systemic and pulmonary circulations are in parallel.

With the low-resistance pulmonary circulation and the much higher resistance systemic circulations in parallel, the resulting volume overload results in increased wall stress via Laplace's law with concomitant increases in myocardial hypertrophy to partially compensate for it. This increased wall stress increases myocardial oxygen demand in the setting of decreased systemic arterial oxygen saturation. In addition, alterations in the Starling curve characteristics [14] may lead to further cardiac dilation and even further increases in myocardial oxygen demand. As the volume overload is due to

the low-resistance pulmonary circuit in parallel with the systemic circulation, the physiology is similar to a systemic arterial–venous malformation; considerations should be given to the high output state, the potential for heart failure, and the neurohumoral changes associated with it.

This volume-loaded state may be exacerbated by atrioventricular valve insufficiency and much rarely by semilunar valve insufficiency. This may be a "primary" atrioventricular valve problem, such as in hypoplastic left heart syndrome, where the valve can be dysplastic, fused, or have shortened chordae [15]. It may also be a "secondary" problem as ventricular dilatation may enlarge the atrioventricular valve annulus resulting in increasing atrioventricular insufficiency, or it may be a combination of the two. Fifty to sixty percent of patients with hypoplastic left heart syndrome have tricuspid regurgitation preoperatively [15]. This aggravation of the volume load may have clinical consequences; indeed, presence and degree of tricuspid insufficiency in patients with hypoplastic left heart syndrome is one of the risk factors for outcome [15].

As mentioned earlier, a consequence of the volume load is the increased myocardial oxygen consumption required because of the greater wall tension given the larger cavity size and the increased work needed to pump this blood. This translates into increased coronary blood flow. In a study published in 1997 [12], the coronary blood flow of 22 patients with hypoplastic left heart syndrome and aortic atresia were studied by transesophageal echocardiography immediately prior to and after BSCC (i.e., change from volume-loaded to volume-unloaded state) and immediately prior to and after Fontan (i.e., volume-unloaded state). Two-dimensional imaging and Doppler interrogation of the retrograde flow of the native ascending aorta in patients with aortic atresia is a measure of flow into the coronary circulation as the native ascending aorta acts as the only conduit for coronary blood flow. Higher coronary blood flow (982 vs. 548 $cm^3/(min\,m^2)$), velocity time integral (20 vs. 12 cm), and peak velocity (96 vs. 51 cm/sec) were demonstrated in the preoperative BSCC than in postoperative BSCC or in the perioperative period of Fontan patients. This pattern of coronary flow is similar to the analogous physiology of aortic insufficiency [16,17]. In both hypoplastic left heart syndrome after Stage I Norwood reconstruction and aortic insufficiency, a volume load on the ventricle is imposed and a low systemic diastolic blood pressure is present (diastolic runoff secondary to flow into the ventricle in aortic insufficiency and flow into the pulmonary vascular bed via the systemic to pulmonary artery shunt in Stage I Norwood reconstruction).

Interestingly, in this study [12], flow changed from predominately systolic in preoperative BSCC to both systolic and diastolic after BSCC and in the perioperative Fontan period. In the normal LV, the majority of coronary blood flow occurs during diastole, while in the normal RV, flow is continuous throughout the cardiac cycle with systolic flow somewhat greater than diastolic flow. However, RV coronary flow changes to a more LV profile when RV pressure becomes systemic [17]. In patients with hypoplastic left heart syndrome, the RV is the systemic ventricle and it would be anticipated that it should mimic the coronary flow pattern in the normal LV, which is not the case in the preoperative BSCC. The flow pattern, again, is more consistent with the findings in aortic regurgitation, where coronary blood flow changes from predominantly diastolic to predominantly systolic with increasing degrees of aortic insufficiency [16,17].

The volume load on the univentricular heart has been implicated in neurohumoral changes, which may lead to the development of congestive heart failure. Brain and atrial natriuretic peptides are synthesized both in the atria and ventricles of the heart, released by myocardial stretch, and act as a diuretic with vasodilatory activity. They have emerged as markers of heart failure [18]. In a study comparing single ventricle patients prior to BSCC, after BSCC, and normal individuals, both brain and atrial natriuretic peptides were measured [19]. Patients prior to BSCC demonstrated a threefold increase in atrial natriuretic peptide over patients after BSCC and over normal controls. Similarly, a sevenfold increase was found in those patients with brain natriuretic peptide. Interestingly, these findings demonstrated elevated levels in the absence of qualitatively decreased ventricular shortening by echocardiography and may actually represent a precursor to heart failure.

Because of the uniqueness of the systemic and pulmonary parallel circulations in this physiology, mathematical models have been used to determine the optimal hemodynamic parameters to maximize oxygen delivery. Studies by Austin et al. [20] and Barnea et al. [21] were performed using this phys-

iologic setup with key variables such as cardiac output and pulmonary venous oxygen saturation. They provided a theoretical basis for optimization of the blood flow in patients prior to BSCC. Among the key findings were the following:

• The pulmonary to systemic flow ratio (Q_p/Q_s) vs. systemic oxygen availability curve is an upside down "U" shape, where (with increasing Q_p/Q_s) systemic oxygen delivery initially increases, reaches a peak, and then decreases (Fig. 17.2).
• Optimum Q_p/Q_s for systemic oxygen delivery is ≤1 (Fig. 17.2).
• As the cardiac output and pulmonary venous saturation increase, the optimal Q_p/Q_s decreases.

With the chronic volume overload, which has been documented by numerous techniques such as angiography [22], radionuclide assessment [22], echocardiography [23], and MRI [2], global ventricular performance parameters are different than those from normal hearts. A study using cardiac MRI documented an average ventricular output of 7.9 L/(min m^2), an end-diastolic volume of 104 cm^3/m^2, a ventricular mass of 171 g/m^2, and ejection fraction of 66%, in a cohort of these patients, which was significantly different from the volume unloaded Fontan stage [2]. Akagi et al. [22], by using angiography and radionuclide techniques, also found a significantly increased end-diastolic volume of 99 cm^3/m^2 when compared with controls but found a smaller ejection fraction (51–52%), ventricular output (4.8 L/(min m^2)), and ventricular mass (106 g/m^2) when compared with the MRI study. Three reasons why these studies may not produce similar results are as follows: (1) The cardiac MRI study was performed mostly on hypoplastic left heart syndrome patients, while the study by Akagi et al. [22] was performed on patients with many types of univentricular hearts, which were of the LV type. (2) The cardiac MRI study was performed on younger patients (mean age 5.7 months vs. 6.4 years). (3) The techniques were different and had different ways of calculating these global parameters. Age is an important consideration in this physiology; in a study using echocardiography, ejection fraction was found to be 59% for patients between 2 and 10 years, while it was 52% for patients >10 years [23]. End-diastolic volume and dimensions ranged from 245 to 283% and from 145 to 149% of normal, respectively [23].

In numerous studies, ventricular hypertrophy has been demonstrated to be present in patients prior to

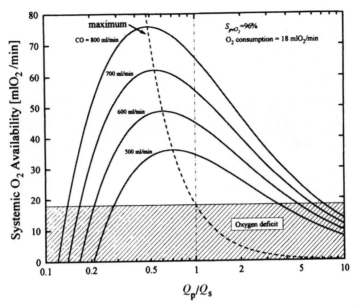

Figure 17.2 Mathematical model demonstrating optimal pulmonary to systemic flow ratio (Q_p/Q_s). Systemic oxygen (O_2) availability as a function of Q_p/Q_s for various levels of cardiac output (CO). S_{pvO_2} = percent oxygen saturation of pulmonary venous blood. From Barnea *et al.* [21] with permission.

BSCC, again, by various techniques [2,22,23]. This hypertrophy, as mentioned earlier, is a physiologic attempt to normalize wall stress because of the volume load. As a global measure of ventricular performance, hypertrophy plays an important clinical role in the univentricular heart. In a study using angiography, Seliem *et al.* found increased LV muscle mass preoperatively to be a significant risk factor for poor outcome in patients undergoing Fontan procedure from a pre-BSCC physiology [24] (during this period, BSCC was not routinely performed). Kirklin *et al.* found that even after Fontan, ventricular hypertrophy could be a significant risk factor for death [25].

The total heart volume (i.e., volume of both atria and ventricles) is a measure of the integrated function of the heart and should change little during the cardiac cycle (<5%) [26]. This phenomenon occurs by reciprocating volume changes in the atria and ventricles and minimizes the energy needed in moving extracardiac structures. Similarly, intracycle constancy of the center of mass motion is also true for that exact reason [27,28]. In a study published in 1992 [28], it was demonstrated by cardiac MRI that only 4 out of 10 patients prior to BSCC had total heart volumes vary by < 5% (threshold for normal individuals). Similarly, the center of mass of the entire heart significantly moved in the anteroposterior and superoinferior planes, all indicating that the volume-loaded single ventricle not only performs more volume work but also "wastes" energy by unnecessarily displacing extracardiac structures.

Regional ventricular function is also abnormal in the univentricular, volume overload physiology. After undergoing angiocardiography, 2 of 18 patients demonstrated regional wall motion abnormalities in a study by Akagi *et al.* [29]. In comparing regional walls of the univentricular heart in another quantifiable way, 13 patients prior to BSCC underwent myocardial tagging by cardiac MRI to assess strain and wall motion [30]. The inferior wall of this group of patients (11 out of 13 with hypoplastic left heart syndrome) demonstrated the largest compressive strain of all wall regions. In addition, both clockwise and counterclockwise wall motion was noted in the short axis of the ventricle (distinctly abnormal as the normal ventricle demonstrates uniform rotation in the short axis), meeting in an area of no twist, which demonstrated the greatest strain (Fig. 17.3).

As mentioned, a newer technique to provide blood flow to the lungs in patients requiring surgical reconstruction is the Sano procedure in which a ventricular to pulmonary artery conduit is created [9,10]. It is still unclear what effect the Sano operation will have on ventricular function or clinical outcome.

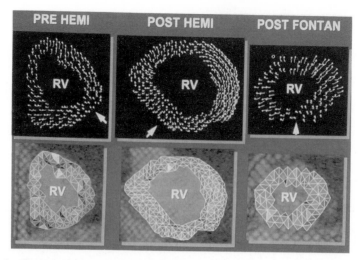

Figure 17.3 Regional wall motion (upper panels) and strain data (lower panels) of functional single right ventricles (RV) at various stages of Fontan reconstruction (from left to right panels: pre-hemiFontan (pre-Hemi), post-hemiFontan (post-Hemi), post-Fontan). Images are taken in short axis of the ventricle. Gray scale maps increased strain as dark regions and decreased strain as lighter regions. "Dots" represent starting point at end diastole and "tails" represent the subsequent systolic motion. Arrows point to the region of "transition zone" of no twist, with clockwise and counterclockwise regions on either side adjacent to the "transition zone." From Fogel *et al.* [30] with permission.

On the one hand, because there is no systemic to pulmonary artery shunt (which creates a "diastolic runoff" physiology), diastolic pressure is higher and, in theory, should provide better coronary perfusion. On the other hand, a ventriculotomy is performed, which could impact ventricular performance. Studies in the near future should sort out these effects.

BSCC

In general, at this stage, the ventricle is volume unloaded when compared to the previous stage. Unlike the ventricle prior to BSCC, after BSCC, there is no direct access to the pulmonary circulation from the univentricular heart. The ventricle pumps one cardiac output to the body and whatever percentage of flow goes to the brain and upper body gets channeled into the lungs via the superior vena cava and back to the heart via the pulmonary veins. Blood flow from the rest of the body enters the heart via the inferior vena cava (Fig. 17.1b, middle).

A number of studies have documented the decrease in ventricular volume immediately following surgery. Seliem *et al.* [11] demonstrated by echocardiography that immediately after BSCC reconstruction, ventricular end diastolic volume decreased by 33%. This was accompanied by an increased heart rate in 69% of patients. Other studies, also performed by echocardiography in the early postoperative period, demonstrated decreases from 20 to 25% in the end-diastolic volumes with preserved ejection fraction [31,32]. This can potentially have significant adverse clinical impact as well and affect ventricular function; for example, there have been reports of volume unloading by BSCC with resulting subaortic obstruction in patients with bulboventricular foramen caused by narrowing of that outlet [33].

Unfortunately, the question of decreased ventricular volumes after BSCC is not clear cut; there is some evidence to suggest that it does not occur in all patients or it may change during the course of BSCC physiology. In a cardiac MRI study, BSCC patients were studied for 6–9 months after surgery [2] and were found to have ventricular end-diastolic volumes of 123 cm^3/m^2, which was not statistically different from the patients prior to BSCC. In addition, cardiac index remained high at 6.5 L/(min m²) with an ejection fraction of 56%. Part of the reason for this may be a redistribution of blood flow, with increased perfusion to the brain to meet the needs of the pulmonary blood flow. Another reason may be the development of aortopulmonary collaterals, which have been shown to develop in 65% of patients, imposing a volume load on the ventricle [34].

In addition, a study Berman and Kimball bring into question whether it is only certain types of patients who benefit from volume unloading in BSCC [32]. In their study using echocardiography in the early postoperative period, they found a significant decrease in ventricular volumes in the overall study population. However, when they broke down the data by whether the patient had a pulmonary artery band versus a systemic to pulmonary artery shunt, they found no significant decrease in the subgroup with a pulmonary artery band. Further, patients with morphologic LVs did have a significant decrease in ventricular volumes postoperative, but those with morphologic RVs did not. In another study by Forbes *et al.* [35], patients who were >10 years of age also did not seem to benefit from volume unloading by BSCC and had a decreased ejection fraction, whereas patients <3 years of age had a decreased ventricular volume and a greater ejection fraction.

There are various reports on the effect of BSCC surgery with regard to ventricular mass. Cardiac MRI demonstrated no significant change in mass 6–9 months after surgery (202 g/m^2). However, Seliem *et al.* [11] demonstrated that immediately postoperative, there is only an 11–13% increase in ventricular wall thickness by echocardiography, which was not statistically significant. Forbes *et al.* demonstrated a significant decrease in ventricular mass after BSCC surgery, although this effect was seen only in patients >3 years of age [35].

Before the advent of the BSCC, the change in mass/volume during the volume unloading Fontan surgery was thought to play a major adverse role in outcome [2,11,24]. Indeed, Seliem *et al.* [24] found that the preoperative mass/volume was greater in the patients with a poor outcome than those with a good outcome after Fontan procedure (during this period of time, the BSCC was not routinely performed). It was thought that BSCC physiology would allow a substantial amount of the systemic venous return to fill the ventricle without first passing through the lungs and the single ventricle to tolerate the mass/volume change better. Seliem *et al.* [11] found that although insertion of the BSCC may improve clinical outcome, it did not change the mass/volume initially postoperative. They found a 103–111% increase in wall thickness-to-ventricular volume right after surgery. There is evidence that this increase in the mass/volume may "self-correct" as a cardiac MRI study showed no

difference in mass/volume between patients before and 6–9 months after BSCC surgery [2].

Similar to the work done on patients prior to BSCC, Santamore *et al.* created a mathematical model to optimize the pulmonary to systemic flow ratio after BSCC [36]. This provided a theoretical basis for optimization of the blood flow in patients after BSCC. Among the key findings were the following:
- As the superior to inferior vena cava flow ratio (Q_{SVC}/Q_{IVC}) increases, total body oxygen delivery and arterial and superior vena caval saturations increase.
- The Q_{SVC}/Q_{IVC} vs. lower body oxygen delivery and inferior vena cava oxygen saturation curves are in an upside down "U" shape, where (with increasing Q_{SVC}/Q_{IVC}) lower body oxygen delivery and inferior vena cava oxygen saturation initially increase, reaches a peak, and then decrease.
- As the percentage of lower body oxygen consumption increases, oxygen delivery and saturation decrease.
- For a given oxygen delivery, BSCC decreases the amount of cardiac output required.

Regional wall function in single ventricles change after BSCC surgery, although the pattern of wall twisting remained unchanged. Cardiac MRI [2] demonstrated that patients after BSCC had the smaller compressive strains and the largest heterogeneity of compressive strains in all four wall regions studied at two short axis slice levels when compared with patients prior to BSCC. However, similar to patients prior to BSCC, wall twisting around the short axis exhibited similar motion, that is to say there were regions of clockwise and counterclockwise twist meeting in an area of no twist (Fig. 17.3).

A hybrid circulation has also been created whereby the superior vena cava to pulmonary artery anastomosis is performed, excluding the right atrium from superior vena caval flow, but additional sources of pulmonary blood flow are left, such as a systemic to pulmonary artery shunt or antegrade flow from the ventricle such as in pulmonic stenosis [37]. This clearly adds another dimension to the physiology and places a volume load on the ventricle (it will not be discussed in this chapter because of space limitations).

Fontan

This final stage of single ventricle reconstruction completely separates the circulations. The Fontan operation has evolved over the years, which has had an impact on ventricular function. This section could be divided up into the following:

- Era prior to and after BSCC.
- Type of Fontan: (A) atriopulmonary, (B) lateral wall tunnel, (C) extracardiac conduit, or (D) miscellaneous forms.
- Heterotaxy vs. nonheterotaxy, etc.
- Fenestration vs. nonfenestrated Fontan.

The list could go on. This section will provide only an overview of ventricular function in the single ventricle after Fontan.

Prior to the BSCC era, Fontan reconstruction was the "volume unloading surgery" and placed the circulations in series rather than in parallel. In theory, the Fontan circulation should decrease ventricular size, wall stress, and hypertrophy. With the elimination of shunting to the low resistance pulmonary vascular bed, cardiac efficiency and peripheral perfusion should improve with normalization of sympathetic tone. However, by placing the circulations in series, the total resistance the ventricle faces should increase relative to the previous stage. In addition, it has been suggested that the noncompliant baffle attached to the ventricle may also increase afterload [2,28,30]. All these physiologic parameters will impact the ultimate ventricular performance of the single ventricle.

As a general rule, the altered mechanics in the single ventricle after Fontan can be summed up as follows: There is both systolic and diastolic myocardial dysfunction, altered venous and arterial hemodynamics impacting ventricular performance, conduction system trauma with ensuing arrhythmias, and valvar dysfunction.

Numerous studies have demonstrated that the single ventricle after Fontan has relatively low cardiac output [2,22,34] and diminished exercise capacity (see special chapter). The low cardiac output is the result of a number of altered states including elevated systemic vascular resistance [22] and abnormal venous mechanics.

A study by Senzaki et al. [37] compared the hemodynamics, impedance, and power in patients with single ventricle after Fontan, with the single ventricle after a systemic to pulmonary artery shunt and a normal dual chambered circulation. They separated out the pulsatile and nonpulsatile components of ventricular afterload and related these changes to ventricular vascular coupling. This was performed at rest and with dobutamine stress. The Fontan patient was found to have an elevation of both vascular resistance ("nonpulsatile" load on the ventricle) and the pulsatile component of ventricular afterload ("low-frequency impedance") at rest and with β-adrenergic stimulation, which was closely associated with decreased cardiac index. There was limited response to β-adrenergic stimulation in the Fontan patients. Both wave reflection and arterial compliance can contribute to low-frequency impedance and from this study, it was determined that wave reflections in the Fontan circuit was the major contributor to the increased ventricular afterload (Fig. 17.4). This seems to be unique to the Fontan circuit as this was not seen in single ventricle patients after systemic to pulmonary artery shunt. In addition, hydraulic power cost per unit of forward flow was 40% lower in the dual chambered circulation than the single ventricle circulation, which was attributed to the lack of a pulmonary pumping ventricle (Table 17.1). The conclusion was that Fontan physiology is associated with disadvantageous ventricular power and afterload profiles.

Another potential source of increased afterload in the Fontan patient is the noncompliant baffle in the atria. Atrial fibrillation has been known to restrict systolic atrioventricular valve plane motion toward the apex because of the loss of atrial compliance and to disrupt the constancy of total heart volume and center of mass [38,39]. A noncompliant baffle is attached to the atria in many types of Fontan hearts and could act in a manner similar to atrial fibrillation, disrupting normal cardiac mechanics. As evidence for this, a study performed by cardiac MRI measuring the constancy of total heart volume and center of mass in Fontan patients [28] demonstrated that a significant number of Fontan patients (71%) did not have constant total heart volume throughout the cardiac cycle, disrupted in part by baffle placement. In addition, when the heart's center of mass motion was broken down into orthogonal components, correlations existed between the lateral plane and the anteroposterior and superoinferior planes ($r^2 = 0.51 - 0.91$), presumably because these planes are linked by the lateral wall tunnel baffle sewn into the lateral and posterior walls of the atria. Differences in lateral motion between Fontan patients and patients before and after BSCC were demonstrated, regardless of whether the heart maintained constant total heart volume using two-factor analysis of variance.

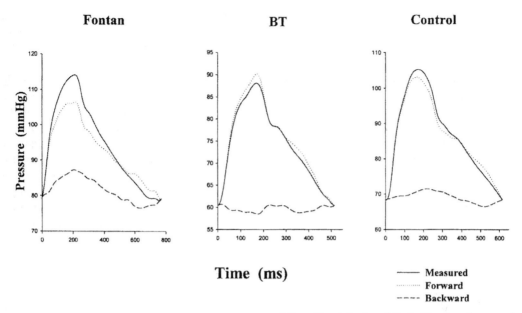

Figure 17.4 The effect wave reflection in Fontan patients. Forward (dotted lines), backward (dashed lines), and measured (solid lines) pressure wave forms in representative patients in the Fontan, Blalock Taussig (BT) shunt, and control group from [37]. Note the marked reflected wave in the Fontan group with minimal reflection in the other groups. From Senzaki *et al.* [37] with permission.

Complicating the issue of afterload is that of volume load. Although the Fontan ventricle is, in a strict sense, volume unloaded, certain factors may play into increasing the volume load on the heart. Atrioventricular and semilunar valve insufficiency is not uncommon. Indeed, a study by Cohen *et al.* found that 61% of patients who had hypoplastic left heart syndrome had neo-aortic insufficiency in a 21-year follow-up and 49% had progressed over time [40]. Another source of volume load on the ventricle are aortopulmonary collaterals, also found in BSCC patients. Triedman *et al.* observed by angiography that 30% of Fontan patients had these collaterals [34].

At the other side of the circulation, venous mechanics in the single ventricle patient after Fontan surgery is also altered and contributes to the overall detriment of cardiac efficiency. Kelly *et al.* demonstrated reduced venous capacitance in these patients with decreased pooling of blood in the legs as well [41]. There was increased venous tone which limits the ability to mobilize blood from the capacitance vessels, thereby impairing cardiac output. In addition, another study [42] demonstrated that after Fontan, there is a loss of the normal augmentation in portal venous flow that takes place with expiration. In addition, that there is elevated hepatic venous wedge pressure reflecting elevated splanchnic venous pressures (which is moderated by fenestration of the baffle).

These arterial and venous mechanical abnormalities may be related to elevated levels of circulating vasoactive substances after Fontan. In addition, these vasoactive substances may have direct effects on the single ventricle myocardium as well.

• A number of studies have documented an elevation of atrial natriuretic peptide after Fontan, which has multiple actions [43,44]. Atrial natriuretic peptide increases sodium excretion and promotes diuresis, decreases blood pressure and total peripheral resistance, and markedly inhibits rennin, aldosterone, and vasopressin secretion.

• An elevation of angiotensin II after Fontan has been documented [45], which is a potent vasoconstrictor, modulates vascular tone, glomerular and tubular function, and aldosterone secretion.

• An elevation of endothelin-1, which is a potent endothelium derived vasoconstrictor, is also elevated after Fontan [46]. Endothelin-1 is known to markedly elevate pulmonary vascular resistance, which becomes a major problem in Fontan patients as they depend upon passive blood flow into the lungs to maintain cardiac output (which is ameliorated, in part, but fenestration of the baffle, allowing right to

Table 17.1 Hemodynamics, Impedance, and Power in Single Ventricles and Controls.

	Fontan group	*BT group*	*Control group*
Hemodynamics			
Heart rate, bpm	130.6±22.2‡	135.1±17.2‡	122.7±19.7‡
CL_s, L/min per m^2	3.9±1.0*†‡	10.1±2.3*‡	7.7±1.5‡
Q_p/Q_s	1.0	1.32±0.56	1.0
AOP, mm/Hg			
Systolic	112.0±21.0‡	115.7±29.1‡	125.4±24.7‡
Diastolic	68.5±13.1	60.4±15.6*	78.2±17.3‡
Mean	88.0±15.2‡	86.7±21.8‡	101.0±17.2‡
Mean PAP, mm Hg	14.2±4.7‡	14.9±4.8	16.8±5.3‡
PVRI, dyne · s · cm^{-5} per m^2	165±49	131±39	124±30
dp/dt_{max}, mm Hg/s	2027±653*‡	2319±188‡	2558±443‡
$PWR_{max}/EDAI^{1.5}$, mW/cm^3	186±92*‡	201±80‡	227±103‡
EDAI, cm^2/m^2	8.4±2.5†‡	12.3±4.6*	8.1±2.6
EDP, mm Hg	5.8±2.9†‡	9.3±4.1*	7.4±2.4
Stiffness, mm/Hg/cm^2 per m^2	0.92±0.58	0.83±0.49	0.84±0.38
Impedance data			
Rt, dyne · s · cm^{-5} per m^2	2145±400*†	712±214*	1046±259
Zl, dyne · s · cm^{-5} per m^2	240±119*†	112±54	127±53
Zc, dyne · s · cm^{-5} per m^2	182±71*‡	110±44‡	98±34
Compliance, mL/mm Hg per m^2	0.94±0.39‡	1.03±0.17	1.03±0.37
Reflection factor	0.20±0.08*†	0.14±0.04	0.13±0.06
Hydraulic power			
Wm, mW/m^2	715±249*†‡	1965±805‡	1718±422‡
Wo, mW/m^2	95.2±17.4‡	149.0±94.3‡	113.3±64.0‡
Wt, mW/m^2	828±251*†‡	2398±799‡	1924±436‡
Wt/Cl, systemic	13.3±2.4	13.2±3.9	13.7±2.8
Wt/Cl, total	13.3±2.4*	13.2±3.9*	8.9±3.9

From Senzaki *et al.* with permission.

Note the 40% power drop in the Fontan group. AOP = ascending aortic pressure; BT = Blalock–Taussig shunt; CI = cardiac index; CI_s = cardiac output from systemic ventricle; cm = centimeter; dp/dt_{max} = maximum rate of ventricular pressure rise; EDAI = indexed end diastolic area; EDP = end diastolic pressure; L = liters; m = meters; min = minute; mL = milliliters; mm Hg = millimeters of mercury; mW = milliwatts; Q_p/Q_s = Pulmonary to systemic flow ratio; PAP = pulmonary artery pressure; PWR_{max} = preload adjusted maximum ventricular power; RpI = indexed pulmonary vascular resistance; Rt = total vascular resistance; Wm = mean power; Wo = oscillatory power; Wt = total power; Zc = characteristic impedance.

* $p < 0.05$ vs control.

† $p < 0.05$ vs BT group.

‡ $p < 0.05$ vs baseline.

left shunting to maintain cardiac output at the expense of cyanosis).

• There is little data in the literature on the circulating levels of tumor necrosis factor alpha, a known myocardial depressant, after Fontan procedure. One study in 16 patients showed no significant increase in these levels in these patients [47]; however, it has been suggested that intramyocardial tumor necrosis factor, which does not correlate with circulating levels in adults, is more important.

These major external factors (there are others) combine with intrinsic myocardial factors (see below discussion on ventricular–ventricular interaction)

to decreased rest and exercise ventricular performance. At rest, average cardiac index in Fontan patients generally range from 2.4 to 3 L/(min m^2) [2,22,34] and ejection fraction range from 50 to 56% [2,22,48] even 10 years after surgery. In the immediate postoperative period, wall thickness increases [49]; however, this does not persist nearly 2 years after Fontan completion as the ventricular mass (120 g/m^2) [2] by MRI falls much below the other stages of surgical reconstruction. This is clinically important data as ventricular hypertrophy is associated with increased risk of death after Fontan [25]. This trend continues as at 10 years after Fontan completion, myocardial mass was found to be 75 g/m^2 by MRI—not significantly different from a normal control group [48].

Ventricular wall stress, shape, and other systolic indices of ventricular performance in Fontan patients have been strongly associated with age of operation [23]. With increasing age (>10 years), patients with single LVs after Fontan repair had a greater end-systolic wall stress than those patients who were repaired at 2–10 years of age. The same held true for and other indices of ventricular function such as fractional shortening, velocity of circumferential fiber shortening, and ejection fraction which were not better than the palliated group who did not have a Fontan operation or BSCC. As a matter of fact, fractional shortening, velocity of circumferential fiber shortening, and ejection fraction were all negatively correlated with age of operation ($r = -0.41$ to -0.54, $P < 0.01$). However, age of operation >10 years was associated with a more normal ventricular ellipsoidal shape than age of operation between 2 and 10 years.

Similar to global measures of ventricular performance, regional ventricular wall function is also abnormal in patients after Fontan reconstruction. By cardiac MRI [30], both the superior and inferior walls near the base in short axis demonstrated increased compressive strains (hyperfunctioning) compared to other wall regions in patients (mostly hypoplastic left heart syndrome) who had undergone Fontan completion around 2 years of age. In general, strain was greater near the base than the apex. Endocardial compressive strain was less than epicardial strain, which is opposite the normal human LV.

Besides strain abnormalities, regional wall motion abnormalities are also present. Akagi et al. [29] found 11 out of 25 patients with tricuspid atresia after Fontan completion, at an average age of 6.5 years, to have hypokinesia of various wall regions. By cardiac MRI [30], in short axis, the greatest radial systolic motion was found in the superior wall although there was paradoxical inferior wall systolic motion (Figs. 17.3 and 17.5). From a rotational standpoint, in short axis, there were wall regions of counterclockwise and clockwise twist meeting in a zone of no twist, which demonstrated the greatest compressive strains similar to other stages of reconstruction (Fig. 17.3). It is interesting to note that the hypoplastic LV in patients with hypoplastic left heart syndrome demonstrated little contraction and basi-cally got "pulled along for the ride" by the septal wall of the RV (Fig. 17.5).

Not only is systolic function impaired, but a number of studies have documented impaired diastolic function as well. Akagi et al. [22] measured diastolic filling time, peak filling rate, and time to peak filling rate using radionuclide techniques in patients with mostly single LV morphology (some with single RV morphology were mixed in as well) after Fontan. Diastolic filling time was longer and the time to peak filling rate was shorter in patients after Fontan than prior to Fontan. Peak filling rate was smaller in Fontan patients than in a control group of patients with a normal two-ventricle circulation. Cheung et al. [50] performed echocardiographic serial diastolic assessment at a mean of 2.8 and 11.4 years after Fontan surgery. They demonstrated that isovolumic relaxation time was significantly longer and E wave deceleration time, E and A wave velocities, and E:A velocity ratio were reduced compared to normal both early and late after the procedure. The mean z score of the isovolumic relaxation time and E wave deceleration time decreased significantly (+2.50 to +1.24, $P = 0.002$ and −1.69 to −2.4, $P = 0.03$, respectively) during follow-up.

Other considerations in studying single ventricular function

Evaluation of single ventricle function is complex not only because of the bizarre shapes of hearts but also because of the variety of types of hearts that can be labeled as single ventricle and the various types of surgical reconstruction that are currently used. This complicates the current framework of studying single ventricle function with regard to the stage of reconstruction. As mentioned in the Background section of this chapter and in Chapter One, intrinsic ventricular geometry can be D- or L-looped, the ventricle can be of RV or LV morphology, or it can be a true single ventricle or "functional" single ventricle. Indeed, studies such as Ohuchi et al. [51] demonstrate that single ventricular morphology is related to exercise capacity, atrioventricular valve regurgitation, hypoxia, and impaired heart rate response with exercise. In terms of surgery:

• a fenestration (communication between systemic and pulmonary venous pathways) may or may not be present in the Fontan reconstruction,

• prior to BSCC, pulmonary blood flow can be from a systemic to pulmonary artery shunt, an RV to

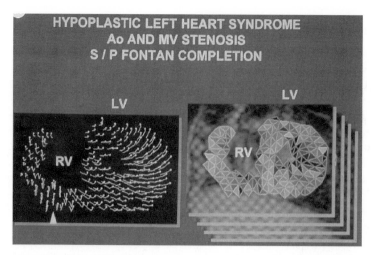

Figure 17.5 Wall motion in hypoplastic left heart syndrome. Images are taken in the ventricular short axis. Wall motion data is on the left and strain data is on the right. Gray scale maps increased strain as dark regions and decreased strain as lighter regions. "Dots" represent starting point at end diastole and "tails" represent the subsequent systolic motion. Arrows point to the region of "transition zone" of no twist, with clockwise and counterclockwise regions on either side adjacent to the "transition zone." Note the paradoxical inferior wall motion of the right ventricle (RV) and how the hypoplastic left ventricle (LV) gets "pulled along for the ride" with the septal wall. Ao = aortic, MV = mitral valve, S/P = status post. From Fogel *et al.* [30] with permission.

pulmonary artery conduit, or via the main pulmonary artery with pulmonic stenosis, and
• the Fontan baffle could be extracardiac, lateral wall tunnel, etc.
All these variations could, in some way, affect ventricular function.

Coronary blood flow, which obviously affects ventricular function, can be compromised in patients with single ventricles. One example is hypoplastic left heart syndrome, which has been demonstrated in numerous studies to have an abnormal coronary artery morphology [52–54]. Another example is pulmonary atresia with intact ventricular septum, which must sometimes undergo single ventricle reconstructive surgery. Coronary cameral fistulae as well as the so-called "RV-dependent coronary circulation" may exist in these lesions, with effects on ventricular function.

A very important consideration in single ventricle function is ventricular–ventricular interaction. Numerous investigators have demonstrated that the normal RV and LV do not act independently of each other and that ventricular–ventricular interaction occurs [55–59]. The mechanism of ventricular interdependence is the mechanical coupling of the ventricles and is demonstrated by a contribution of the LV to RV pressure generation and the

RV to LV pressure generation. Some investigators have attributed this relationship to the interventricular septum but others, noting that the myocardium forms an anatomic continuum around both chambers, have suggested that the free walls may also affect the contralateral ventricle independent of septal bulging. In single ventricles, there is by definition, no second ventricle to augment ventricular function and this absence may adversely affect ventricular mechanics and ultimately the long-term viability of the single ventricle. A comparison of ventricular mechanics in single ventricles to the mechanics in a dual-chambered circulation has been studied by cardiac MRI and regional function delineated [60,61].

In summary, the study of single ventricular function in aggregate was presented in this section under the framework of stages of reconstruction. However, there are numerous complicating factors that play a role in determining ventricular function and teasing out differences among these will be a difficult task for future research.

Blood flow

Some blood flow considerations have already been discussed in the previous section to explain the volume loading of the single ventricle prior to BSCC

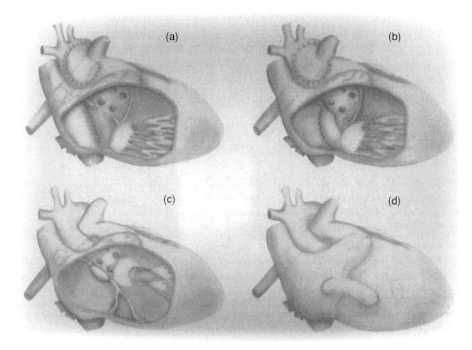

Figure 17.6 A few of the multiple types of Fontan connections. Four types of Fontan connections are represented: (a) Total cavopulmonary connection, (b) left atrium to right sided atrioventricular valve baffle with superior vena caval connection to the pulmonary arteries (not used anymore), (c) atriopulmonary connection (not used anymore), and (d) right atrium to right ventricle conduit (generally not used anymore).

as well as optimization of blood flow in patients prior to or at the BSCC stage. A great deal of literature has been generated on blood flow in Fontan patients because of the "passive" flow of blood into the lungs (because of space limitations, the majority of the discussion herein will focus only on this stage and on the systemic venous pathway).

Flow in the systemic venous pathway

As stated previously, the systemic venous pathway has had many incarnations over the years (Fig. 17.6). Various types include
• Total cavopulmonary connection, where the inferior and superior vena cavae are connected directly to the pulmonary arteries (Fig. 17.6). The inferior vena cava may be connected directly to the pulmonary arteries via a
  ○ baffle using the lateral wall of the atria or
  ○ conduit that is intracardiac or extracardiac (extracardiac conduits may be either a straight cylindrical tube or may use the epicardial surface of the atria).

• In cases of interrupted inferior vena cava with azygous continuation, a baffle is placed connecting hepatic veins to the pulmonary artery–superior vena cava junction.
The superior vena cava(e) is/are connected directly to the pulmonary arteries. In some instances, if there is a left superior vena cava that connects to a coronary sinus, instead of ligating and dividing the left superior vena cava and connecting it to the left pulmonary artery, a baffle may be created to anastomose the coronary sinus to the inferior portion of the inferior vena cava–right pulmonary artery baffle (generally not performed).
• Atriopulmonary connection, where the atria are anastomosed to the pulmonary arteries, used in cases of right sided atrioventricular valve atresia (not used anymore).
• Left atrium to right sided atrioventricular valve baffle with superior vena caval connection to the pulmonary arteries (not used anymore).
• Right atrium to right ventricle conduit (generally not used anymore).

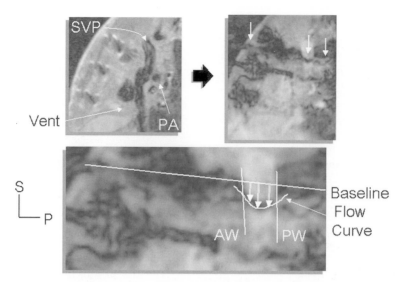

Figure 17.7 Bolus tagging in the systemic venous pathway. The top-left image is a spin-echo sagittal view of the systemic venous pathway (SVP). The top-right image is a cine MRI performed with bolus tagging in the superior vena cava in the same plane as the top-left image. A linear black "tag" is placed on the chest wall, spine, and the superior vena cava. Movement of blood by cardiac (with electrocardiographic triggering) as well as respiratory (with respiratory gating) mechanisms can be observed using this technique. The bottom image is a zoom of the top-right image demonstrating how the images are analyzed—by tracing the anterior (AW) and posterior walls (PW) of the vessel, the flow curve, and the original tag position (baseline). Distance the blood has moved can be measured (double arrows) and since the time between blood tagging and image generation is known, velocity and flow can be calculated.

The nature of flow in the systemic venous pathway

There has been much discussion in the past on the nature of flow in the systemic venous pathway of Fontan patients. One perplexing question concerns the driving force behind "passive" flow into the lungs without a pulmonary pumping chamber to generate pressure. Most investigators agree that it is a combination, to some degree, of negative intrathoracic pressure during inspiration and either directly or indirectly, of the systemic ventricle's contraction, relaxation, and motion [62–69]. However, the degree to which all these factors contribute to this passive flow is debatable. During the cardiac cycle, there are reports of either atrial contraction [67,68], ventricular systole [62,63,67–69], or ventricular diastole [62,63,69] determining this flow. These factors were noted to be different, depending upon whether or not the patient had an atriopulmonary Fontan connection or a total cavopulmonary connection [67–70]. In addition, the respiratory component is thought to be a major component by some [64,66] and to play a more minor role by others [62].

Clearly, the dependence of pulmonary blood flow in Fontan physiology is not wholly based on respiration because a Fontan patient on a respirator receiving positive pressure ventilation would not survive. It is also clearly not wholly cardiac dependent [62,71]. Part of the problem stems from how to define "cardiac" and "respiratory" dependency. In one study by cardiac MRI using bolus tagging [62], flow in the systemic venous pathway was imaged both triggered to the cardiac cycle and gated to the respiratory cycle at end-inspiration and end-expiration (Fig. 17.7). If there were no component of flow in synchrony with the cardiac cycle (i.e., if it was soley respiratory controlled), then a study triggered to the cardiac cycle would demonstrate similar images at all cardiac phases. Similarly, if there were no component of flow in synchrony with the respiratory cycle (i.e., if it was soley cardiac controlled), then a respiratory-gated study would demonstrate similar images at end-inspiration and end-expiration. Both types of studies demonstrated different images during the cardiac cycle and the respiratory cycle. Since the cardiac and respiratory cycles occur at the same time, flow dependency in this project was defined as the percent change in flow during imaging triggered to the cardiac cycle (or gated to the respiratory cycle) as a fraction of the sum of flow changes noted during *both* cardiac triggering and respiratory gating. Using this definition, it was determined that nearly 70% of flow was cardiac dependent, with the rest of the flow being respiratory dependent. Maximum flow occurred during late systole–early diastole (second quarter of the cardiac cycle) with the slowest flow occurred during diastasis in the third quarter of the cardiac cycle.

A significant amount of flow occurred in ventricular systole in this cardiac MRI study, which is consistent with other studies in the literature, performed in both atriopulmonary and total cavopulmonary connections. Studies by Nakazawa *et al.* [72] and DiSessa *et al.* [69] suggested that atrial relaxation may contribute to this. Nakazawa *et al.* found that as the right atrium relaxed, rapid forward flow was found in the inferior and superior vena cava. Qureshi *et al.* [68] demonstrated by Doppler echocardiography that pulsatile flow occurred during ventricular systole, implying an "active" mechanism. Frommelt *et al.* [63] noted a correlation of pulmonary artery flow with biphasic left atrial pressure suggesting both an active and passive mechanism, they further suggested that even with impaired ventricular relaxation in Fontan hearts, the forward flow is maintained during diastole. Hagler *et al.* [73] found a significant amount of flow in late systole–early diastole by Doppler echocardiography, and Giannico *et al.* [70] demonstrated systolic forward flow (although less than diastolic forward flow, which they stated was the predominant determinant of flow), but neither speculated on the mechanism.

There are a number of investigators who have quantified the amount of flow during respiration in various ways in atriopulmonary and total cavopulmonary connections [62,64,66]. Penny *et al.* [64] elegantly demonstrated the difference in flow between inspiration and expiration using Doppler echocardiography combined with simultaneous readings by respirometer, ECG, and phonocardiogram. They found forward flow during inspiratory cardiac cycles was 35% higher than during expiratory ones. Redington *et al.* [74] even suggested that pulmonary blood flow was "critically" dependent on changes in intrathoracic pressure in their study using Doppler echocardiography. During Valsalva maneuvers, they found blood flowed either away from the lungs (brief Valsalva) or no spontaneous blood flow and during sustained Valsalva, a "low velocity pulsatile pulmonary flow" which coincided with ventricular systole.

Minimizing the amount of energy loss in the systemic venous pathway is important in optimizing cardiac energetics [75,76]. de Leval *et al.* [76] have

suggested that forming the systemic venous pathway in the Fontan reconstruction as a cylindrical tube minimizes energy losses and creates a uniform flow pattern. In the cardiac MRI study utilizing bolus tagging in the cylindrical tube type of systemic venous pathway [62], it was demonstrated that the tag did not "break up" during both cardiac triggering and respiratory gating studies (Fig. 17.7). The tag created by the bolus technique is very sensitive to turbulent flow and if chaotic or nonlaminar flow was present, it would disperse or disintegrate in the image. This confirmed the laminar nature of flow in the total cavopulmonary connection. In addition, in this study [62], by direct visualization of the velocity profile, it was noted that the flow is nearly uniform in the center of the systemic venous pathway in this type of Fontan connection during both cardiac-triggered and respiratory-gated flow images.

"Passive" flow in the systemic venous pathway, as noted, has a cardiac component associated with it. It would be hypothesized from this finding that blood would not be continuously flowing at a steady rate but rather would vary in relation to the cardiac cycle. Indeed, this has been demonstrated by the cardiac MRI study previously discussed [62] and other MRI studies [71]. In addition, there is a vast literature by Doppler echocardiography which has also confirmed this finding, [63,68–70] although there are varying reports on the Doppler spectral morphology of the interrogated flow. A study by Houlind *et al.* [77] utilized a combination of cardiac catherization data and cardiac MRI flow information to measure pressures as well as calculate a "pulsatility" index in the systemic venous pathway. They found that this index (the higher the index the greater the pulsatility) was greatest in the middle of the lateral wall tunnel, lowest in the superior vena cava, and "intermediate" in the branch pulmonary arteries. They noted that "flow and pressure waveforms were biphasic with maxima in atrial systole and late ventricular diastole."

Power loss a computational fluid dynamics
Power loss
An interesting study on power loss and how laminar flow in the systemic venous pathway was performed *in vitro* by Sharma *et al.* [5]. They studied the geometry of the pathway using glass models based on *in vivo* cardiac MRI geometric data and visualized flow with Amberlite particles recorded on video (Fig. 17.8). They used offsets of the caval connection by fractions of the superior vena caval diameters with

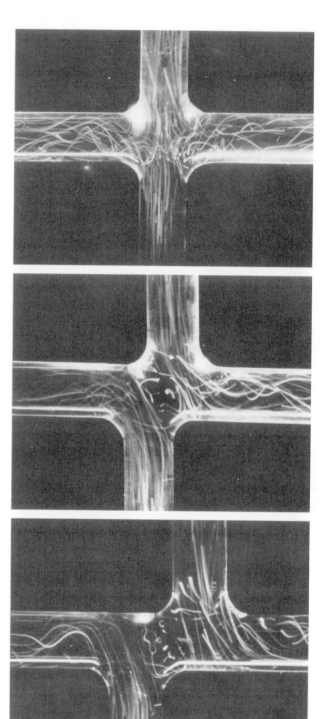

Figure 17.8 *In vitro* glass flow models of the Fontan circulation. Still photographs of glass models created to simulate the systemic venous pathway of the Fontan circulation. The three images are of 0 (top), 0.5 (middle), and 1.0 (bottom) superior vena caval diameter offsets (see text) with a 60:40 right/left pulmonary artery flow ratio. Amberlite particles were used to visualize the flow patterns. Note the turbulent flow at the cross with "0" offset the relatively more uniform flow with a "1-diameter" offset. From Sharma *et al.* [5] with permission.

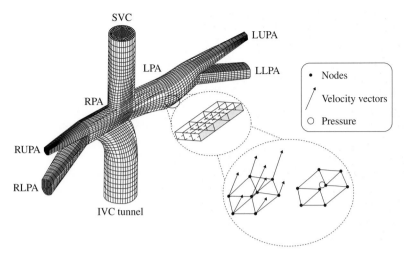

Figure 17.9 Computational fluid dynamic model of Fontan pathway. This is a diagram of the finite element model mesh of a total cavopulmonary connection pathway. The mesh deforms during flow modeling. Insets show an eight-node finite element with locations for velocity vectors and pressure. From de Leval *et al.* [76] with permission.

various flow rates in the branch pulmonary arteries. They found that when the Fontan baffle connects inline with the superior vena cava, energy losses were double the losses of the 1 and 1.5 times diameter offset, which had minimal energy losses. By direct visualization of flow, this power loss was a result of the "chaotic" pattern seen at the zero offset. In addition, they found that energy savings were more evident at an equal split of flow between right and left pulmonary arteries and that energy losses increased with increased total flow. Of course, this *in vitro* model does not entirely mimic the *in vivo* situation, especially since the compliance of *in vivo* materials are no similar to the rigid glass used, but it does provide a basis for future investigation.

Computational fluid dynamics

The issue of elucidating how blood flows in the systemic venous pathway and designing it in such a way as to optimize this flow has been studied by complex modeling using computational fluid dynamics (CFD) based on finite element techniques (Fig. 17.9) [76,78,79]. These calculations depend upon the Navier–Stokes equations and the goal of the model is to predict velocity, pressure, and flow as a function of time and position. In one study by de Leval *et al.* [76], the CFD model was used to determine flow and energy dissipation with various offsets of superior vena cava and the Fontan baffle, similar to the *in vitro* work of Sharma *et al.* [5]. They found that the best flow distribution to right and left lungs (55% to right, 45% to left) occurred with an Fontan baf-

fle anastomosis of 0.5–0.7 cm toward the right pulmonary artery, which unfortunately corresponded to the maximal energy dissipation. In an attempt to correct this, they altered the geometry of the model by enlarging the Fontan baffle (2.5 cm) and moving it alongside the pulmonary artery and "angling" the Fontan baffle toward the right pulmonary artery (by 17°); this resulted in minimal energy loss with a right to left pulmonary artery flow ratio ~1. The ability to "design" the geometry of the systemic venous pathway to optimize blood flow and minimize energy loss is a powerful use of CFD.

The validation of CFD modeling was undertaken in single ventricle patients after Fontan by Migliavacca *et al.* [80], who used cardiac MRI anatomic information to build the CFD model and velocity mapping to validate the model (Fig. 17.9). A number of assumptions were built into the CFD model including the absence of vessel wall compliance and respiratory variation. Nevertheless, there was good agreement between the CFD model and MRI *in vivo* data. They even went so far as to state that CFD models of the total cavopulmonary connection based on preoperative anatomy could be used to predict postoperative hemodynamics.

CFD modeling is not confined to the Fontan operation in single ventricles. Migliavacca and coworkers [81] published CFD modeling on the Norwood Stage I circulation with regard to shunt size, vascular resistance, and heart rate. Highlights of their simulations demonstrated (1) larger shunts diverted an increased portion of cardiac output to the lungs and away from the body, (2) systemic vascular resistance exerted a greater hemodynamic effect than did pulmonary vascular resistance, (3) systemic arterial oxygenation was affected little by heart rate, (4) venous oxygen saturation and delivery was more tightly linked than the arterial equivalent, and (5) a Q_p/Q_s of 1 was optimal (which is similar but not quite the same as the two studies by Austin *et al.* [20] and Barnea *et al.* [21] mentioned previously). Migliavacca *et al.* [82] even used CFD modeling in conjunction with Doppler flow measurements to quantify shunt flow in these patients and proposed a simple formula to perform these calculations with.

The BSCC has also been the subject of CFD modeling. A number of CFD models have been created based on patients with a BSCC with an additional source of pulmonary blood flow such as pulmonic stenosis. Pennati *et al.* [83] used mathematical modeling in these patients, both pre- and postoperatively, and varied the amount of pulmonary outflow obstruction from 50 to 100% (i.e., a pure BSCC). They found that the percentage of blood flow to the right lung was heavily affected by the flow competition. Migliavacca *et al.* [84] used cardiac catheterization and angiography data to base their CFD model on and found that hemodynamics in the pulmonary artery were greatly affected by the forward flow through the native pulmonary valve. Pulsatility, noted in the pulmonary arteries, did not increase superior vena cava pressure excessively. In addition, Migliavacca *et al.* [85] performed CFD analysis on varying degrees and shape of native pulmonic stenosis in BSCC patients and noted that a tighter stenosis can lead to flow to the left lung reaching 70%. The most intense jets to the left pulmonary artery occurred with discrete pulmonary stenosis of 75%. Flow in the right pulmonary artery was nearly steady because of the damping effect of the caval flow.

All these mathematical models and optimization of flow in Fontan patients are predicated on the knowledge of the caval contribution of flow to each lung, to systemic venous return, and the relative flow to each lung. A cardiac MRI study [4], using presaturation tagging to "label" blood from each cava, was performed on 10 single ventricle patients with lateral wall tunnel Fontans to determine just those parameters (Fig. 17.10). It was demonstrated that 60% of superior vena caval blood flowed into the right pulmonary artery and 67% of inferior vena caval blood flowed toward left pulmonary artery (i.e., superior vena caval blood was directed to the right

pulmonary artery and inferior vena cava blood was directed toward left pulmonary). The inferior vena cava contributed 40% to total systemic venous return in these approximately 2 year olds and the distribution of blood to each lung was nearly equal.

Arterial flow in Fontan patients

Up till now, the discussion has been limited to the systemic venous pathway. Because of space limitations, a lengthy discussion of the arterial side of single ventricle reconstruction (e.g., aortic to pulmonary artery anastomosis) cannot be undertaken. However, to give the reader a feel for the kinds of issues on this side of the circulation, a study published in 1997 will be mentioned [86]. Using cardiac MRI and bolus tagging, velocity profiles in aortas of 9 patients who had undergone the Fontan procedure without aortic reconstruction were compared to aortas in 13 patients who had undergone both the Fontan procedure and an aortic to pulmonary anastomosis (Fig. 17.11). This was performed at the levels of the ascending and descending aorta in the center of the vessel. A "flat" profile in the nonreconstructed ascending aorta was visualized, while an anterior "skew" to the velocity profile was found in the reconstructed ascending aorta. In these reconstructed aortas, there were higher flows anteriorly, took longer to reach maximum velocity and was less "plug" flow like than the aortas without an aortic to pulmonary anastomosis. Regardless of whether aortic reconstruction was present, the descending aorta displayed velocity profiles (at various phases of systole) skewed posteriorly. The study concluded that an aortic to pulmonary anastomosis alters the aortic velocity profile, which may be detrimental to cardiac energetics as evidenced by the longer time to reach maximum velocity and the diminished similarity to plug flow.

Conclusion

The study of ventricular function and blood flow in single ventricle patients is an extremely complex evaluation because of numerous factors including the variability in the types of single ventricles as well as reconstructive techniques. Much progress has been made in understanding the complicated pumping action of the heart and how blood moves in this physiology but much more needs to be accomplished. With advancements in imaging and other techniques, it is clear that the next 33 years

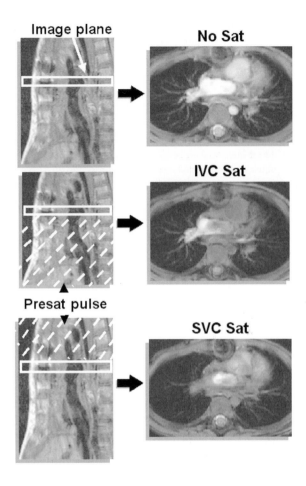

Figure 17.10 Determination of caval contribution of flow to the branch pulmonary arteries in Fontan patients. The left images are spin-echo sagittal images through the Fontan baffle. The axial imaging plane used to perform cine MRI (right images) is designated by the open box. Hatched lines represent the placement of a presaturation pulse (presat pulse) (sat). The resulting cine without a sat (upper panels), sat placement on the inferior vena caval (IVC) flow (middle panels), and sat placement on the superior vena caval (SVC) flow (lower panels) are shown. Note the uniform signal in the top-right panel to the branch pulmonary arteries when no saturation is used (top right). When blood coming from the IVC is saturated (and therefore becomes black on the image), the signal in blood heading toward the left pulmonary artery is diminished more than that of blood heading toward the right pulmonary artery (middle right). When blood coming from the SVC is saturated, the signal in blood heading toward the right pulmonary artery is diminished more than that of blood heading toward the left pulmonary artery (lower right).

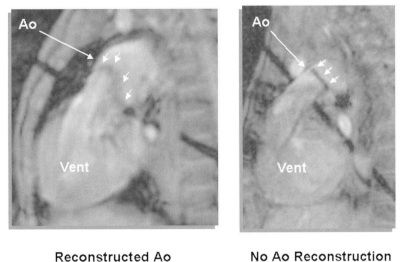

Figure 17.11 Velocity profiles in reconstructed (left) and normal (right) ascending aortas (Ao). Representative images in mid-systole utilizing bolus tagging demonstrate an anterior skew to the velocity profile (arrows) in reconstructed Ao and a flat profile in the normal Ao. Note the original position of the tag on the chest wall and spine. From Fogel *et al.* [86] with permission.

of research in this area will be as interesting as the past 33 years since the first report of Fontan reconstruction.

References

1. Fontan F, Baudet E. Surgical repair of tricuspid atresia. Thorax 1971; 26:240–248.

2. Fogel MA, Weinberg PM, Chin AJ, *et al.* Late ventricular geometry and performance changes of functional single ventricle throughout staged Fontan reconstruction assessed by magnetic resonance imaging. J Am Coll Cardiol 1996; 28(1):212–221.

3. Norwood WI, Lang P, Hansen D. Physiologic repair of aortic atresia—hypoplastic left heart syndrome. N Engl J Med 1983; 308:23–26.

4. Fogel MA, Weinberg PM, Rychik J, *et al.* Caval contribution to flow in the branch pulmonary arteries of Fontan patients using a novel application of magnetic resonance presaturation pulse. Circulation 1999; 99:1215–1221.

5. Sharma S, Goudy S, Walker P, *et al.* In vitro flow experiments for determination of optimal geometry of total cavopulmonary connection for surgical repair of children with functional single ventricle. J Am Coll Cardiol 1996; 27:1264–1269.

6. Van Praagh R. Terminology of congenital heart disease. Glossary and commentary. Circulation 1977; 56:139–143.

7. Sondheimer HM, Freedom RM, Olley PM. Double outlet right ventricle: Clinical spectrum and prognosis. Am J Cardiol 1977; 39:709.

8. Edwards JE, Burchell HB. Congenital tricuspid atresia: A classification. Med Clin North Am 1949;33:1117–1196.

9. Sano S, Ishino K, Kawada M, *et al.* Right ventricle-pulmonary artery shunt in first-stage palliation of hypoplastic left heart syndrome. J Thorac Cardiovasc Surg 2003; 126:504–510.

10. Pizarro C, Malec E, Maher KO. Right ventricle to pulmonary artery conduit improves outcome after Stage I Norwood for hypoplastic left heart syndrome. Circulation 2003; 108(suppl II):II-155–II-160.

11. Seliem MA, Baffa JM, Vetter JM, *et al.* Changes in right ventricular geometry and heart rate early after Hemi-Fontan procedure. Ann Thorac Surg 1993; 55:1508–1512.

12. Fogel MA, Rychik J, Vetter J, *et al.* Effect of volume unloading surgery on coronary flow dynamics in patients with aortic atresia. J Thorac Cardiovasc Surg 1997; 113:718–727.

13. Pasque MK. Fontan hemodynamics. J Cardiac Surg 1988; 3:45–52.

14. Alyono D, Ring WS, Anderson MR, *et al.* Left ventricular adaptation to volume overload from large aortocaval fistula. Surgery 1984; 96:360.

15. Weinberg PM, Peyser K, Hackney JR. Fetal hydrops in a newborn with hypoplastic left heart syndrome: Tricuspid valve stopper. J Am Coll Cardiol 1085; 6:1365–1369.

16. Kinsanuki A, Murayama T, Matsushita R, *et al.* Transesophageal Doppler echocardiographic assessement of left coronary blood flow velocity in chronic aortic regurgitation. Am Heart J 196; 131:101–106.

17. Hongo M, Goto T, Watanabe N, *et al.* Relation of phasic coronary flow velocity profile to clinical and hemodynamic characteristics of patients with aortic valve disease. Circulation 1993; 88:953–960.

18. Muders R, Kromer EF, Griese DP, *et al.* Evaluation of plasma natriuretic peptides as markers for left ventricular dysfunction. Am Heart J 1997; 134:442–449.

19. Wahlander H, Westerlind A, Lindstedt G, *et al.* Increased levels of brain and atrial natriuretic peptides after the first palliative operation, but not after a bidirectional Glenn anastomosis, in children with functionally univentricular hearts. Cardiol Young 2003; 13:268–274.

20. Austin EH, Santamore WP, Barnea O. Balancing the circulation in hypoplastic left heart syndrome. J Cardiovasc Surg 1994; 35:137–139.

21. Barnea O, Austin EH, Richman B. Balancing the circulations: Theoretic optimization of pulmonary/systemic flow ratio in hypoplastic left heart syndrome. J Am Coll Cardiol 1994; 24:1376–1381.

22. Akagi T, Benson LN, Green M, *et al.* Ventricular performance before and after Fontan repair for univentricular atrioventricular connection: Angiographic and radionuclide assessment. J Am Coll Cardiol 1992; 20:920–926.

23. Sluysmans T, Sanders SP, van der Velde M, *et al.* Natural history and patterns of recovery of contractile function in single left ventricle after Fontan operation. Circulation 1992; 86:1753–1761.

24. Seliem M, Muster AJ, Paul MH, *et al.* Relation between preoperative left ventricular muscle mass and outcome of the Fontan procedure in patients with tricuspid atresia. J Am Coll Cardiol 1989; 14:750–755.

25. Kirklin JK, Blackstone EH, Kirklin JW, *et al.* The Fontan operation. Ventricular hypertrophy, age and date of operation as risk factors. J Thorac Cardiovasc Surg 1986; 92:1049–1064.

26. Hoffman EA, Ritman EL. Invariant total heart volume in the intact thorax. Am J Physiol 1985; 249:H883–H890.

27. Hoffman EA, Rumberger J, Dougherty L. A geometric view of cardiac "efficiency." J Am Coll Cardiol 1989; 13:86A.

28. Fogel MA, Weinberg PW, Fellows KE, *et al.* Magnetic resonance imaging of constant total heart volume and center of mass in patients with functional single ventricle before and after staged Fontan procedure. Am J Cardiol 1993; 72:1435–1443.

29. Akagi T, Benson LN, Williams WG, *et al.* Regional ventricular wall motion abnormalities in tricuspid atresia after the Fontan procedure. J Am Coll Cardiol 1993; 22:1182–1188.

30. Fogel MA, Gupta KB, Weinberg PW, *et al.* Regional wall motion and strain analysis across stages of Fontan reconstruction by magnetic resonance tagging Am J Physiol Heart Circ Physiol 1995; 269(38):H1132–H1152.

31. Lemes V, Ritter SB, Messina J, *et al.* Enhancement of ventricular mechanics following bidirectional superior cavopulmonary anastomosis in patients with single ventricle. J Cardiac Surg 1995; 10:119–124.

32. Berman NB, Kimball TR. Systemic ventricular size and performance before and after bidirectional cavopulmonary anastomosis. J Pediatr 1993; 122:S63–S67.

33. van Son JA, Falk V, Walther T, *et al.* Instantaneous subaortic outflow obstruction after volume reduction in hearts with univentricular atrioventricular connection and discordant ventriculoarterial connection. Mayo Clin Proc 1997; 72:309–314.

34. Triedman JK, Bridges ND, Mayer JE, *et al.* Prevalence and risk factors for aortopulmonary collateral vessels after Fontan and bidirectional Glenn procedures. J Am Coll Cardiol 1993; 22:207–215.

35. Forbes TJ, Gajarski R, Johnson GL, *et al.* Influence of age on the effect of bidirectional cavopulmonary anastomosis on left ventricular volume, mass and ejection fraction. J Am Coll Cardiol 1996; 28:1301–1307.

36. Santamore WP, Barnea O, Riordan CJ, *et al.* Theoretical optimization of pulmonary-to-systemic flow ratio after a bidirectional cavopulmonary anastomosis. Am J Physiol 1998; 274:H694–H700.

37. Senzaki H, Masutani S, Kobayashi J, *et al.* Ventricular afterload and ventricular work in Fontan circulation. Comparison with normal two-ventricle circulation and single ventricle circulation with Blalock-Taussig shunt. Circulation 2002; 105:2885–2892.

38. Hoffman EA, Ritman EL. Law of constant volume disrupted by atrial fibrillation. Fed Proc 1986; 45: 776.

39. Hoffman EA. Constancy of total heart volume: An imaging approach to cardiac mechanics. In: Sideman S, Beyer R, eds., Imaging Measurements and Analysis of the Heart. Hemisphere Publishing, New York, pp. 3–19, 1991.

40. Cohen MS, Marino BS, McElhinney, *et al.* Neo-aortic root dilation and valve regurgitation up to 21 years after staged reconstruction for hypoplastic left heart syndrome. J Am Coll Cardiol 2003; 42:533–540.

41. Kelley JR, Mack GW, Fahey JT. Diminished venous vascular capacitance in patients with univentricular hearts after the fontan operation. Am J Cardiol 1995; 76:158–163.

42. Hsia TY, Khambodkone S, Redington AN, *et al.* Effects of respiration and gravity on infradiaphragmatic venous flow in normal and Fontan patients. Circulation 2000; 102: III77–III82.

43. Stewart JM, Seligman KP, Zeballos G, *et al.* Elevated atrial natriuretic peptide after the Fontan procedure. Circulation 1987; 76:III77–III82.

44. Hiramatsu T, Imai Y, Takanashi Y, *et al.* Hemodynamic effects of human atrial natriurectic peptide after modified Fontan procedure. Ann Thorac Surg 1998; 65:761–764.

45. Hjortdal VE, Stenbog EV, Ravn HB, *et al.* Neurohormonal activation late after cavopulmonary connection. Heart 2000; 83:439–443.

46. Hiramatsu T, Imai Y, Takanashi Y, *et al.* Time course of endothelin–1 and adrenomedullin after the Fontan procedure. Ann Thorac Surg 1999; 68:169–172.

47. Mainwaring RD, Lamberti JJ, Hugli TE. Complement activation and cytokine generation after modified Fontan procedure. Ann Thorac Surg 1998; 65:1715–1720.

48. Eiken A, Fratz S, Gutfried C, *et al.* Hearts late after Fontan operation have normal mass, normal volume and reduced systolic function. J Am Coll Cardiol 2003; 42:1061–1065.

49. Chin AJ, Franklin WH, Andrews BA, *et al.* Changes in ventricular geometry early after Fontan operation. Ann Thorac Surg 1993; 56:1359–1365.

50. Cheung YF, Penny DJ, Redington AN. Serial assessment of let ventricular diastolic function after Fontan procedure. Heart 2000; 83:420–424.

51. Ohuchi H, Yasuda K, Hasegawa S, *et al.* Influence of ventricular morphology on aerobic exercise capacity in patients after the Fontan operation. J Am Coll Cardiol 2001; 37:1967–1974.

52. Baffa JM, Chen SL, Guttenberg ME, *et al.* Coronary artery abnormalities and right ventricular histology in hypoplastic left heart syndrome. J Am Coll Cardiol 1992; 20:350–358.

53. Sauer U, Gittenberger- de Groot AC, Geishauser M, *et al.* Coronary arteries in the hypoplastic left heart syndrome. Histopathologic and histometrical studies and implications for surgery. Circulation 1989; 80(Suppl I):II68–II76.

54. O'Connor WN, Cash JB, Cottrill CM, *et al.* Ventriculo-coronary connection in hypoplastic left heart: An autopsy microscopic study. Circulation 1982; 66:1078–1086.

55. Feneley MP, Gavaghan TP, Baron DW, *et al.* Contribution of left ventricular contraction to the generation of right ventricular systolic pressure in the human heart. Circulation 1985; 71:473–480.

56. Santamore WP, Lynch PR, Heckman JL, *et al.* J App Physiol 1976; 41:925–930.

57. Brinker JA, Weiss JL, Lappe DL, *et al.* Leftward septal displacement during right ventricular loading in man. Circulation 1989; 61:626–633.

58. Santamore WP, Constantinescu M, Vinten-Johansen J, *et al.* Alterationsin left ventricular compliance due to changes in right ventricular volume, pressure and compliance. Cardiovasc Res 1988; 22:768–776.

59. Santamore WP, Constantinescu M, Minczak BM, *et al.* Contribution of each ventricular wall to ventricular interdependence. Basic Res Cardiol 1988; 83:424–430.

60. Fogel MA, Weinberg PM, Fellows KE, *et al.* A study in ventricular–ventricular interaction: Single right ventricles compared with systemic right ventricles in a dual chambered circulation. Circulation 1995; 92(2):219–230.

61. Fogel MA, Weinberg PM, Gupta KB, *et al.* Mechanics of the single left ventricle: A study in ventricular–ventricular interaction, II. Circulation 1998; 98:330–338.

62. Fogel MA, Weinberg PM, Hoydu A, *et al.* The nature of flow in the systemic venous pathway in Fontan patients utilizing magnetic resonance blood tagging. J Thorac Cardiovasc Surg 1997; 114:1032–1041.

63. Frommelt PC, Snider AR, Meliones JN, *et al.* Doppler assessment of pulmonary artery flow patterns and ventricular function after the Fontan operation. Am J Cardio 1991; 68:1211–1215.

64. Penny DJ, Redington AN. Doppler echocardiographic evaluation of pulmonary blood flow after the Fontan operation: the role of the lungs. Br Heart J 1991; 66:372–374.

65. Lane S, Daubeney P, Walsh K, *et al.* Seizure activity causing loss of cardiac output after a Fontan operation. Arch Diseases Childhood 1995;72:62–63.

66. Penny DJ, Hayek Z, Redington AN. The effects of positive and negative extrathoracic pressure ventilation on pulmonary blood flow after the total cavopulmonary shunt procedure. Int J Cardiol 1991; 30:128–130.

67. Miura T, Matsuda H, Nakano S, *et al.* Assessment of pulmonary blood flow after total cavopulmonary shunt operation and the modified Fontan procedure for univentricular heart. J Cardiol 1998; 18:837–844.

68. Qureshi SA, Richheimer R, McKay R, *et al.* Doppler echocardiographic evaluation of pulmonary artery flow after modified Fontan procedure: Importance of atrial contraction. Br Heart J 1990; 64:272–276.

69. DiSessa TG, Child JS, Perloff JK, *et al.* Systemic venous and pulmonary arterial flow patterns after Fontan's procedure for tricuspid atresia or single ventricle. Circulation 1984; 70:898–902.

70. Giannico S, Corno A, Marino B, *et al.* Total extracardiac right heart bypass. Circulation 1992; 86:II110–II117.

71. Rebergen SA, Ottenkamp J, Doornbos J, *et al.* Postoperative pulmonary flow dynamics after Fontan surgery: Assessment with nuclear magnetic resonance velocity mapping. J Am Coll Cardiol 1993; 21:123–131.

72. Nakazawa M, Nakanishi T, Okuda H, *et al.* Dynamic of right heart flow in patients after Fontan procedure. Circulation 1984; 69:306–312.

73. Hagler DJ, Deward JB, Tajik AJ, *et al.* Functional assessment of the Fontan operation: Combined M-mode, two-dimensional and Doppler echocardiographic studies. J Am Coll Cardiol 1984; 4:756–764.

74. Redington AN, Penny D, Shenebourne EA. Pulmonary blood flow after total cavopulmonary shunt. Br Heart J 1991; 65:213–217.

75. de Leval MR, Kilner P, Gewillig M, *et al.* The total cavopulmonary connection: A logical alternative to atriopulmonary connection for complex Fontan operations. J Thorac Cardiovasc Surg 1988; 96:682–695.

76. de Leval MR, Dubini G, Migliavaci F, *et al.* Use of computational fluid dynamics in the design of surgical procedures: Application to the study of competitive flows in cavopulmonary connections. J Thorac Cardiovasc Surg 1996; 111:502–513.

77. Houlind K, Stenbog EV, Sorensen KE, *et al.* Pulmonary and caval flow dynamics after total cavopulmonary connection. Heart 1999; 81:67–72.

78. Migliavaci F, de Leval MR, Dubini G, *et al.* Computational fluid dynamic simulations of cavopulmonary connections with an extracardiac lateral conduit. Med Eng Phys 1999; 21:187–193.

79. Migliavacca F, Kilner PJ, Pennati G, *et al.* Computational fluid dynamic and magnetic resonance analyses of flow distribution between the lungs after total cavopulmonary connection. IEEE Trans Biomed Eng 1999; 46:393–399.

80. Milgliavacc F, Kilner PJ, Pennati G, *et al.* Computational fluid dynamic and magnetic resonance analyses of flow distribution between the lungs after total cavopulmonary connection. IEEE Trans Biomed Eng 1999; 46:393–399.

81. Migliavacca *et al.* Am J Physiol Heart Circ Physiol 2001; 280:H2076–2086.

82. Migliavacca *et al.* Ultrasound Med Bio. 2000; 26:209–219.

83. Pennati G, Migliavacca F, Dubin G, *et al.* A mathematical model of circulation in the presence of the bidirectional cavopulmonary anastomosis in children with a univentricular heart. Med Eng Phys 1997; 19:223–234.

84. Migliavacca F, de Leval MR, Dubini G, *et al.* A computational pulsatile model of the bidirectional cavopulmonary anastomosis: The influence of forward flow. Trans ASME 1996; 118:520–528.

85. Migliavacca F, Dubini G, Pietrabissa R, *et al.* Computational transient simulations with varying degree and shape of pulmonic stenosis in models of the bidirectional cavopulmonary connection. Med Eng Phys 1997; 19:394–403.

86. Fogel MA, Weinberg PM, Hoydu A, *et al.* Effect of surgical reconstruction on flow profiles in the aorta using magnetic resonance blood tagging. Ann Thorac Surg 1997; 63:1691–1700.

CHAPTER 18

Exercise Performance in Fontan Patients

Stephen Paridon, MD

Exercise Capacity

By all the usual standards of exercise performance, the exercise capacity in subjects with the Fontan physiology is significantly impaired when compared to an age and sex matched healthy population. Studies on exercise performance have shown maximal oxygen consumption (max VO_2) and maximal work rates for the Fontan population to range between approximately 50–60% of that predicted for healthy subjects. This corresponds to a max VO_2 of approximately 15–30 mL/(kg min) [1].

The reasons for these wide ranges are several. The populations being studied are quite heterogeneous for age at testing, underlying cardiac diagnosis, and type of surgeries performed. The age of surgery is also an important consideration. Recent studies that have assessed the effects of early surgical procedures to reduced volume loads on the single ventricle have suggested that this approach may improve exercise capacity. Mahle *et al.* have reported max VO_2 as high as 38 mL/(kg min) in a subpopulation of preadolescent Fontan subjects who had undergone early surgical volume unloading of their ventricles (Table 18.1) [2].

Measurements of physical working capacity show degrees of impairments similar to max VO_2. This is true regardless of the type of ergometry used in the exercise testing. The work rates have usually been about 60% of those measured in the healthy population [1].

Few data are available for submaximal measurements of exercise performance, but these also show significant impairment. Measurements of the VO_2 at the anaerobic threshold (VAT) show this to occur at about 60–65% of the max VO_2. This ratio is very similar to the ratio of VAT to max VO_2 observed in healthy children. This would indicate a similar degree of impairment for VAT and max VO_2 in the Fontan population [3].

Other studies assessing initial oxygen uptake with the onset of exercise and oxygen debt have also shown subjects with Fontan physiology to be impaired compared to both healthy subjects, as well as subjects with other types of congenital heart lesions. The response to exercise of oxygen uptake in the Fontan population maybe 75% delayed compared to healthy matched subjects. This delayed response results in a significantly increased oxygen debt with any activity [4,5].

Reasons For Decreased Exercise Performance

Stroke volume

The primary reason for decreased exercise performance in the Fontan physiology is an inability to augment stroke volume with exercise. Figure 18.1 shows the changes in cardiac output, stroke volume, and heart rate during exercise in a study by Gewilleg *et al.* [6]. In this study, two subpopulations with superior and inferior exercise performance were identified. As can be seen from Fig. 18.1, the significant difference between the two groups is the ability to augment and maintain stroke volume during exercise.

Although failure to augment and maintain stroke volume is clearly the major limiting factor in Fontan exercise performance, the cause of this failure is far from clear. Studies suggest that the Fontan physiology has similarities to that seen in congestive heart failure with structurally normal hearts. Markers of heart failure such as brain and atrial natriuretic

Table 18.1 Affects of Age at Ventricular Volume Unloading on Exercise Performance.

		Age at volume unloading		
	Entire group (n = 46)	>2 years (n = 22)	<2 years (n = 24)	p^a
HRmax (beats/min)	155.9 ± 21.0	157.5 ± 17.8	154.0 ± 24.3	NS
VO_2max (mL/(min kg))	32.3 ± 8.9	26.3 ± 7.5	37.9 ± 5.9	<0.001
VO_2max (% predicted)	76.1 ± 21.1	62.5 ± 17.9	88.6 ± 24.1	<0.001
O_2 saturation (%)	94.0 ± 2.9	93.3 ± 3.3	94.6 ± 2.3	NS
RER	1.05 ± 0.10	1.07 ± 0.09	1.04 ± 1.0	NS
FEV_1 (% predicted)	78.8 ± 15.6	75.6 ± 16.4	81.9 ± 14.3	NS
FVC (% predicted)	77.7 ± 16.9	75.1 ± 15.6	80.3 ± 18.1	NS
Breathing reserve (%)	19.2 ± 8.1	18.7 ± 8.6	19.8 ± 7.6	NS
VE (% predicted)	78.7 ± 19.8	83.9 ± 16.1	74.1 ± 18.3	NS

From Mahle *et al.* [2] with permission.

^{a} Comparison between the two groups of patients volume-unloaded at > 2 y and <2 y.

FVC: Functional vital capacity; FEV_1: Forced expiratory volume at 1 sec.; HRmax: Maximum heart rate; NS: Not significant; RER: Respiratory exchange ratio; VO_2max: Oxygen uptake at peak exercise; VE: Minute ventilation.

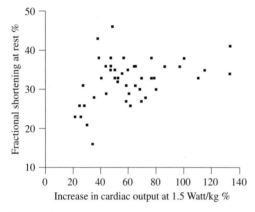

Figure 18.1 The relationship of echocardiographic fractional shortening and increase in cardiac output during exercise in subjects after the Fontan operation. Note that except at very low fractional shortening there is no relationship between the two measurements. From Gewillig *et al.* [6] with permission.

peptides (BNP and ANP) are both significantly elevated in the Fontan populations. Norepinephrine response during exercise is also abnormal [7,8]. Despite these markers suggesting abnormal ventricular function, systolic function in the Fontan physiology is usually preserved. Except in severe cases, exercise performance does not appear to correlate with resting measurements of systolic function. Figure 18.2, also from the study by Gewilleg et al. [6], shows that there is no correlation between cardiac output and echocardiographic shortening fraction. These data

suggest that in the typical subject with Fontan physiology the inotropic state is not the limiting factor in the ability to maintain stroke volume [6].

The above findings have led to increasing study of the pulmonary vascular bed and diastolic function during exercise. The lack of a ventricular pumping chamber in the pulmonary circuit has several consequences during exercise. Firstly, there is less of a pressure gradient across the pulmonary bed. In order to maintain adequate filling of the systemic ventricle, the pulmonary vascular resistance must fall sufficiently to maintain increased flow across the pulmonary bed. Obstruction to blood flow at any point in the pulmonary bed will be poorly tolerated. Secondly, the Fontan physiology results in the systemic and pulmonary circuit being arranged in series rather than in parallel. One of the consequences of this arrangement is that the systemic ventricle must pump across the combined resistance of both vascular beds. Studies that have compared exercise performance in different types of Fontan anatomy have generally shown improved performance with the total caval pulmonary connection (TCPC) rather than the atrial pulmonary connection (APC). The reason for the improved performance appears to be due to the improved hemodynamic efficiency of the systemic venous flow through the pulmonary bed in the TCPC versus the APC. This appears to be more pronounced at submaximal levels of exercise [9].

The other requirement to maintain low total resistance across the pulmonary circuit is a highly

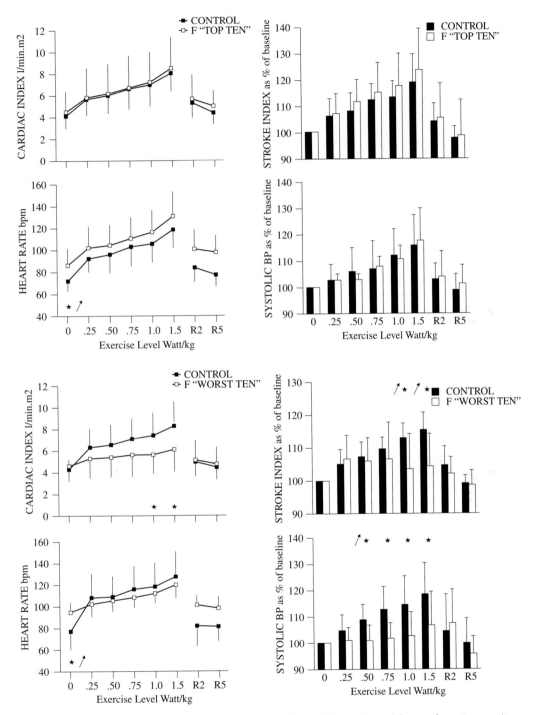

Figure 18.2 Measurements of cardiac performance in two populations with superior and decreased exercise capacity following the Fontan operation. Note the fall in stroke volume and failure to increase cardiac output in the impaired group when compared to healthy age matched control subjects. From Gewillig *et al.* [6] with permission.

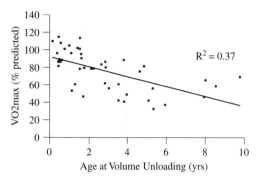

Figure 18.3 Plot of the max VO_2 (percentage predicted) versus the age at ventricular volume unloading. The solid line represents the regression line for the 46 study patients. VO_{2max} = maximal oxygen consumption. From Mahle *et al.* [2] with permission.

compliant systemic ventricle. High compliance and low diastolic filling pressures will result in a larger net transpulmonary gradient. This would suggest that those interventions that result in improved diastolic function should result in improved exercise performance. Ventricular volume unloading appears to be such a circumstance. Volume unloading at a young age appears to result in improved diastolic function. Figure 18.3 shows the relationship of max VO_2 to the age of ventricular volume unloading [2]. This figure shows improved exercise performance as function of the age at volume unloading. Table 18.1 shows the data from the same study demonstrating the superior performance of those subjects who underwent early as oppose to late ventricular volume unloading.

Chronotropic Response

The significance of chronotropic impairment in limiting cardiac output in the Fontan physiology is unclear. Most subjects who have undergone exercise testing show a moderate degree of chronotropic impairment. However, the correlation between maximal heart rate and maximal cardiac output and maximal VO_2 has generally been poor. As can be see in Table 18.1 and Fig. 18.1, heart rate response to exercise was very similar in groups with both superior and impaired max VO_2 and cardiac output [2,6]. Studies involving artificial pacing of Fontan subjects during exercise are very limited, but have also failed to demonstrate a significant improvement in aerobic capacity by increased chronotropy [10].

These findings are interesting since VO_2 during exercise is very closely correlated with heart rate in normal cardiac physiology. This would suggest that a significantly different cardiac physiology is at work during exercise in the Fontan subjects. In Fig. 18.1 note that for the poorly functioning Fontan subjects, stroke volume actually falls in mid-to-high work rates. One possible explanation for this finding may be that at higher heart rates diastolic filling time becomes inadequate to allow the necessary filling to maintain preload for the ventricle. In these circumstances, higher heart rates do not result in greater cardiac output and there is little physiologic advantage to superior chronotropic response. The "optimal" heart rate response of the Fontan physiology needs much more research especially the need to study the best pacing strategies for this physiology.

Physiologic Adaptation to Exercise

The lack of a pulmonary ventricle results in several physiologic adaptations to exercise in the Fontan population. Some of these adaptations appear to reflect a limited ability to increase cardiac output. Others reflect the type of Fontan repair. Rosenthal *et al.* compared exercise physiology in two groups of Fontan subjects with TCPC and APC anatomy [9]. The APC group tended to have lower stroke volumes compared to the TCPC group for a given work rate and VO_2. The APC group compensated for this decreased stroke volume by increasing arterial–venous oxygen difference as a way of maintaining oxygen consumption.

In the same study, the TCPC subjects tended to have a higher respiratory rate and a lower tidal volume for any given minute ventilation when compared with the APC subjects. The authors suggested that this might be a physiology adaptation that improved pulmonary blood flow by increasing the negative intrathoracic pressure during exercise. This theory is supported by studies of negative pressure ventilation augmenting cardiac output following the Fontan surgery [11]. Interestingly, this respiratory difference tended to disappear at higher work rates; this would suggest that there is perhaps like heart rate, an "optimal" breathing pattern during exercise resulting in the most efficient pulmonary augmentation of blood flow. More studies are clearly needed to assess the role of the pulmonary contribution to cardiac output in the Fontan physiology.

References

1. Paridon S. Exercise physiology and capacity. In: Rychik, Wernovsky, G, eds., Hypoplastic Left Heart Syndrome. Kluwer, Boston, MA, 2003.

2. Mahle WT, Wernovsky G, Bridges ND, *et al.* Impact of early ventricular unloading on exercise performance in preadolescents with single ventricle fontan physiology. JACC, 1999; 34(5):1637–1643.

3. Wasserman K, Hansen JE, Sue DY, *et al.* Principles of Exercise Testing and Interpretation, secondary edition. Lea & Febiger, Philadelphia, 1994.

4. Mocellin R, Gildein P. Velocity of oxygen uptake response at the onset of exercise: A comparison between children after cardiac surgery and healthy boys. Ped Cardiol 1999; 20:17–20.

5. Gildein P, Mocellin R, Kaufmehl K. Oxygen uptake transient kinetics during constant-load exercise in children after operations of ventricular septal defect, tetralogy of fallot, transposition of the great arteries, or tricuspid valve atresia. Am J Cardiol 1994; 74:166–169.

6. Gewillig MH, Lundstrom UR, Bull C, *et al.* Exercise responses in patients with congenital heart disease after Fontan repair: Patterns and determinants of performance. J Am Coll Cardiol 1990; 15:1424–1432.

7. Ohuchi H, Tasato H, Sugiyama H, *et al.* Responses of plasma norepinephrine and heart rate during exercise in patients after Fontan operation and patients with residual right ventricular outflow tract obstruction after definitive reconstruction. Pediatr Cardiol 1998; 19:408–413.

8. Ohuchi H, Arakaki Y, Hiraumi Y, *et al.* Cardiorespiratory response during exercise in patients with cyanotic congenital heart disease with and without a Fontan operation and in patients with congestive heart failure. Int J Cardiol 1998; 66:241–251.

9. Rosenthal M, Bush A, Deanfield J, *et al.* Comparison of cardiopulmonary adaptation during exercise in children after the atriopulmonary and total cavopulmonary connection Fontan procedures. Circulation 1995; 91:372–378.

10. Paridon SM, Karpawich PP, Pinsky WW. Effects of Rate responsive pacing on exercise performance in the postoperative univentricular heart. PACE 1993; 16:1256–1262.

11. Shekerdemian LS, Bush A, Shore DF, *et al.* Cardiopulmonary interactions after Fontan operations. Augmentation of cardiac output using negative pressure ventilation. Circulation 1997; 96:3934–3942.

CHAPTER 19

Considerations in Intensive Care

Meryl S. Cohen, MD

Abnormal myocardial performance is common in children with congenital heart disease (CHD) and is observed frequently in the intensive care unit (ICU) setting. Although technical and medical advances in ICU care have been associated with a significant improvement in survival for children with CHD, ventricular dysfunction remains one of the most common causes of morbidity and mortality in this population of patients. Ventricular dysfunction has a very broad definition that may include abnormal contractility (in the setting of abnormal or normal myocardium), abnormal relaxation or compliance, abnormal loading conditions, and disturbances of electrical activation of the myocardium. This chapter will describe methods to assess ventricular systolic and diastolic performance for children in the ICU setting, describe the group of patients with CHD that are at risk for the development of ventricular dysfunction, and discuss low cardiac output syndrome. Mechanical methods of treatment of ventricular dysfunction in the ICU will also be covered.

Assessment of left ventricular systolic performance in the ICU

Systole begins with the electrical activation of the myocardium (the QRS complex on the electrocardiogram). During early systole, the ventricular pressure increases with contraction of the muscle fibers, but aortic pressure remains higher than left ventricular pressure. Thus, there is no change in the ventricular volume (isovolumic contraction). This period is then followed by ventricular ejection, when the ventricular pressure exceeds the aortic pressure and the aortic valve opens. Blood then flows across the aortic valve and ventricular volume decreases. Closure of the aortic valve marks the end of systole.

Echocardiography is the most accurate, portable, noninvasive tool to assess ventricular systolic performance in the intensive care setting. The most commonly used methods in determining systolic performance are the shortening fraction (SF) and ejection fraction (EF) (see Table 19.1). Normal SF falls within the range of 28–40% (mean of 36%) and the mean EF is generally 60–65%, but depends on method of volume calculation that is used [1–3]. SF and EF are independent of age and heart rate; both methods give the practitioner a facile, accurate, and reproducible assessment of systolic pump function. Overall systolic ventricular function depends on contractility (intrinsic properties of the myocardium), preload (myocardial fiber length), afterload (force the myocardial fibers must overcome to shorten), and left ventricular mass [4,5]. Since EF and SF depend on these factors, they do not identify the cause of ventricular dysfunction. In addition, there are several caveats in the performance of SF and EF. These measurements are accurate only in patients with systemic, ellipsoid-shaped left ventricles and since they are measured in only one plane, they are not sensitive to regional wall motion disturbances. If there is paradoxical septal wall motion (as can be seen with right ventricular volume overload, right ventricular hypertension, and ischemic ventricular septal disease), SF calculation will significantly underestimate ventricular performance. Assessment of cardiac blood flow by ejection velocity, acceleration of flow, or velocity time integral have the advantage of being independent of ventricular geometry [6,7]. However, they are dependent on the loading conditions, contractility, and heart rate. Other indices of ventricular systolic performance can determine the relative effects of loading conditions and contractility on the myocardium. Although these methods

Table 19.1 Echocardiographic Indices of Ventricular Performance.

SF(%)	$\dfrac{\text{(Left ventricular end-diastolic dimension)} - \text{(Left ventricular end-systolic dimension)}}{\text{(Left ventricular end-diastolic dimension)}}$
EF(%)	$\dfrac{\text{(Left ventricular end-diastolic volume)} - \text{(Left ventricular end-systolic volume)}}{\text{(Left ventricular end-diastolic volume)}}$
Vcf_c	$\dfrac{\text{(Left ventricular end-diastolic dimension)} - \text{(Left ventricular end-systolic dimension)}}{\text{(Left ventricular end-diastolic dimension)} \times \text{(Left ventricular ejection time)}}$
	where ejection time $= \dfrac{\text{Left ventricular ejection time}}{\text{Square root of R-R interval}}$
ESWS	$\dfrac{\text{(End-systolic pressure)} \times \text{(Radius)}}{\text{Wall thickness}}$
MPI	$\dfrac{\text{(Time from closure to opening of atrioventricular valve)} - \text{(Ventricular ejection time)}}{\text{Ventricular ejection time}}$

SF: Shortening fraction; EF: ejection fraction; Vcf_c: heart rate corrected mean velocity of circumferential fiber shortening; ESWS: End-systolic wall stress; MPI: Myocardial performance index.

can be performed in the ICU, many are not feasible because of conditions necessary for measurements, time constraints, and invasive technique. For example, dP/dt, a measure of the rate of change of left ventricular pressure with time, can be calculated in children but only if there is mild (not greater) mitral regurgitation [8]. The velocity of fiber shortening estimates the rate of change of left ventricular circumference and can be corrected for heart rate (VCF$_c$) (Table 19.1). VCF$_c$, a preload-independent measure, can be performed only on a left ventricle with normal geometry [9]. End-systolic wall stress (ESWS) is a measure of afterload in ventricular performance (Table 19.1) [10]. Meridional wall stress is most frequently used in analysis because it is easiest to measure. Colan and colleagues reported that the linear, inverse relationship between VCF$_c$ and ESWS measures contractility of the ventricle and is preload independent [11]. To some degree, the relationship of VCF$_c$ to ESWS changes with age; the slope of the relationship appears to be steeper in younger infants and normalizes to adults levels by 3 years of age [12,13] Unfortunately, accurate measurement of ESWS requires a carotid pulse tracing and phonocardiogram as well as M-mode echocardiography. These recordings are technically difficult to perform in small children and particularly in the ICU setting where patients often have intracardiac lines, pacing wires and in some cases, open chests in the immediate postoperative period. Automated border detection by echocardiography is a newer method of assessment of ventricular performance that uses continuous detection of myocardial tissue to measure ventricular cavity area [14]. Although this method is feasible in the ICU, it requires two-dimensional images of extremely good quality (often difficult to obtain in the postoperative period).

Other, more precise measures of ventricular performance require invasive techniques such as placement of conductance catheters in the left ventricle. These catheters inserted directly through the apex of the left ventricle measure the instantaneous relationship between pressure and volume throughout the cardiac cycle [15,16]. While these measures may provide accurate information about ventricular performance, maintaining a catheter in the apex of the left ventricle carries significant risks and may cause scarring [17]. Therefore, in addition to standard monitoring of venous filling pressure and arterial blood pressure, SF and EF by echocardiography remain the standard method of assessing left ventricular systolic performance in the ICU. Serial echocardiographic assessment of ventricular dysfunction may be integral to the management of critically ill children on inotropic support. It is therefore important to use the same method when evaluating the same patient at different time points.

Congenital heart defects associated with left ventricular systolic dysfunction

Left ventricular systolic dysfunction is seen with higher frequency in certain congenital heart lesions. In general, significant changes in preload, afterload, or contractility that result from open heart surgery puts patients at risk for diminished systolic performance. For example, increased preload is seen in patients with significant residual ventricular septal defects (VSD) after tetralogy of Fallot repair. Although these patients have a VSD prior to surgery, the flow is predominantly from the right ventricle into the aorta. Once the right ventricular outflow tract is repaired, a residual VSD causes increased flow to the left ventricle and thus increased demand at a time when the ventricle is recovering from injury (cardiopulmonary bypass). Valvuloplasties and valve replacements are another group of operations where there is higher risk for the development of left ventricular dysfunction. Mitral regurgitation, for example, can be seen in association with such cardiac defects as common atrioventricular canal, cleft mitral valve, mitral valve prolapse, and anomalous left coronary artery from the pulmonary artery. Significant mitral regurgitation results in increased preload to the left ventricle and decreased afterload as the blood empties into the left atrium. Although well tolerated for long periods of time in children, the chronic volume overload gradually leads to impairment of left ventricular function and irreversible myocardial damage [18]. It is often a challenge to determine the ideal timing for mitral valvuloplasty or replacement, because left ventricular dysfunction may not become evident until after surgery. Repair of mitral regurgitation results in a significant acute increase in afterload to the left ventricle. This phenomenon along with the ill effects of cardiopulmonary bypass often result in left ventricular dysfunction after repair. As a result, mitral valvuloplasty and replacement continue to have a relatively high morbidity and mortality when compared to other congenital heart surgeries, particularly in children less than 2 years old [19,20]. Surgical intervention for aortic valve disease can also be associated with left ventricular dysfunction in the postoperative period, particularly if repair or replacement of the valve is required in the newborn period. Critical aortic stenosis (ductal dependency of the systemic circulation) is often seen in association with left ventricular dysfunction and congestive heart failure [21]. The left ventricular systolic performance fails because of significant pressure overload from the diminutive aortic orifice. Although surgical- or catheter-directed intervention to relieve the aortic obstruction is the treatment of choice if the left ventricle is of adequate size, balloon dilation or aortic valvotomy can result in the development of aortic insufficiency [22]. This new volume load on an already injured left ventricle is often tolerated quite poorly and these infants

may be quite ill after such a procedure. Intervention for aortic stenosis in later infancy or childhood tends to have better outcome because the left ventricle has responded over time to the pressure load by developing hypertrophy [23]. Children who undergo surgical intervention for isolated aortic insufficiency (such as those with bicuspid aortic valve) may, similar to those with mitral regurgitation, have left ventricular dysfunction that is unmasked after repair [24]. Hence, patients who have systemic atrioventricular or semilunar valve repair or replacement require diligent observation, particularly in the first 24–48 h after surgery, for evidence of low cardiac output and/or left ventricular dysfunction.

Some surgical procedures for CHD may negatively impact the coronary circulation, particularly those operations that require coronary artery manipulation. The coronary arteries are transferred to the neoaorta in the arterial switch operation for transposition of the great arteries (TGA) and in the Ross procedure for aortic valve disease. Recent reports suggest that some coronary variations in TGA including single coronary anatomy and in particular coronaries that take an intramural course are associated with left ventricular dysfunction and increased risk of sudden death after arterial switch operation [25]. Coronary insufficiency can also be seen after coronary reimplantation to the aorta for anomalous left coronary artery from the pulmonary artery [26]. Other surgical interventions where coronary blood flow may become compromised include tetralogy of Fallot (if the left anterior descending coronary artery crosses the right ventricular outflow tract), mitral valve surgery (sutures are in close proximity to the circumflex artery), and repair of single coronary lesions.

Assessment of right ventricular systolic performance in the ICU

The right ventricle has a complex geometric shape that changes dramatically with contraction. Developing an index of right ventricular systolic performance has posed a challenge for pediatric cardiologists. The importance of such a measure is clear because right ventricular dysfunction is common in many forms of CHD. Volume analysis can be performed using three-dimensional echocardiographic techniques and MRI [27,28]. However, these methods are not always feasible in an ICU patient. MRI is presently not portable and difficult to perform on a ventilated, critically ill patient. Heusch *et al.* recently reported that three-dimensional echocardiographic volumetric analysis of the right ventricle could not be accurately performed on 66% of the pediatric patients in their cohort [28]. The dP/dt (mean rate of rise of ventricular pressure) of the right ventricle can be measured if there is mild tricuspid regurgitation [29]. Yet, as with left ventricle dP/dt, the value may be erroneous if tricuspid regurgitation is more than mild. One of the most facile methods for assessing global right ventricular performance (including systolic and diastolic performance) is the myocardial performance index (MPI, also known as Tei index) [30]. This method uses Doppler echocardiography or M-mode to measure the ratio of isovolumic contraction and relaxation time to ventricular ejection time and is independent of geometry (Table 19.1). Some have reported that right ventricular MPI is insensitive to preload and afterload [31,32]. However, others have questioned the reliability of MPI particularly in the setting of pulmonary insufficiency—an almost universal finding after repair of tetralogy of Fallot and other similar lesions [33]. A recent study by Mahle *et al.* found that the MPI in those with single right ventricles was significantly higher compared to normal subjects and that ejection time was shorter, suggesting less efficient ventricular mechanics [34]. Other new innovative echocardiographic techniques are being validated in the pediatric population. Automated border detection to assess ventricular pressure–area relationship has been validated for assessment of right ventricular contractility [35]. Although MPI and automated border detection may be accurate indices of right ventricular performance, it is clear that there is no gold standard measurement. The most common method used at present is subjective assessment of right ventricular shortening on two-dimensional echocardiography or angiography. This method is quick and easy to perform, particularly with user experience, but is clearly flawed with regard to interobserver variability and reproducibility.

Congenital heart defects associated with right ventricular dysfunction

Right ventricular systolic dysfunction may occur in the immediate postoperative period after repair of right-sided obstructive cardiac lesions. Repair of such lesions as tetralogy of Fallot, truncus arteriosus, and double outlet right ventricle usually includes augmentation of the right ventricular outflow tract with transannular patch or conduit placement to assure unobstructed flow from the right ventricle to the pulmonary artery. An incision in the right ventricle is performed, which may alter the compliance and systolic performance of the right ventricle. In addition, patients with these lesions are often left with pulmonary insufficiency (the pulmonary valve leaflets are often removed or the conduit is nonvalved), which results in a sudden volume load to the right ventricle. Patients with single right ventricles (e.g., hypoplastic left heart syndrome (HLHS)) are at particularly high risk for the development of ventricular dysfunction. The Norwood operation for HLHS and other single ventricle lesions requires anastomosis of the diminutive ascending aorta (frequently with aortic atresia) to the pulmonary artery [36]; when the aorta is severely hypoplastic, the coronaries may "kink" during the operation causing right ventricular dysfunction due to coronary insufficiency [37]. Bartram *et al.* found that 27% of infants with HLHS who died after Norwood procedure had impaired coronary perfusion [38]. Right ventricular dysfunction may occur prior to surgical intervention as well. Up to 30% of infants with HLHS present in cardiovascular collapse as a result of ductal constriction or closure [39]. Right ventricular dysfunction and tricuspid regurgitation result from poor perfusion to the coronary circulation as the ductus closes. In single ventricle physiology such as HLHS, the ventricle supports both the systemic and pulmonary circulations and thus has limited ability to meet increased demands such as fever, infection, anemia, or sudden blood loss all common complications after open-heart surgery.

Assessment of diastolic dysfunction in the ICU

Isovolumic relaxation, the period after the aortic valve closes but before the left atrial pressure exceeds the left ventricular pressure, marks the initiation of diastole. Ventricular filling begins when the mitral valve opens. Early in diastole, ventricular filling is augmented by ventricular relaxation (E wave on Doppler); later in diastole, the atrium contracts so that there is a second period of filling (A wave on Doppler). Diastolic performance encompasses the complex relationships of several myocardial properties including ventricular relaxation, elastic recoil, passive filling and suction, atrial contractility, and the impact of external tissues such as the pericardium [40]. Detailed discussion of diastolic performance is out of the scope of this chapter. However, diastolic dysfunction is quite common in the pediatric ICU setting.

Doppler echocardiographic analysis of blood flow is typically used to detect abnormalities of diastolic performance in children with CHD. In general, inflow patterns across the atrioventricular valves are used to assess diastolic filling. There are two peak velocities that occur during diastole including the E wave (rapid ventricular filling) and the A wave (atrial contraction) [41]. In normal adults, the peak E wave is larger than the peak A wave. A variety of indices have been developed to detect diastolic abnormalities including E/A ratio, diastolic time intervals, deceleration rate of early diastolic flow, peak and mean ventricular filling rates, and Doppler area fractions [42]. In addition, the pulmonary venous flow pattern (particularly reversal of flow) has been used to assess for abnormal relaxation of the left ventricle [43]. Tissue Doppler is used to assess abnormal mitral annulus motion [43]. While these measures may be useful in certain clinical settings, many factors, including age, heart rate, respiratory patterns, ventilatory support, and loading conditions, impact diastolic filling particularly in critically ill children. Cardiac catheterization provides additional information; elevated ventricular end-diastolic pressure and atrial pressure (without distal atrioventricular valve stenosis) indicate diastolic dysfunction. Unfortunately, serial assessment by this method is too invasive. In the adult population, ICU management often includes placement of a catheter in the pulmonary artery with intermittent measurements of pulmonary capillary wedge pressures (giving an estimate of left atrial pressure and thus left ventricular end-diastolic pressure). This method carries a much higher complication rate in children and therefore is generally utilized only in older children and young adults.

Congenital heart defects associated with diastolic dysfunction

Physical signs of diastolic dysfunction include hepatomegaly (from increased right atrial pressure), gallop rhythm (from diminished ventricular

compliance and augmented atrial contraction), and end organ edema. With severe left ventricular diastolic dysfunction, pulmonary edema may occur. Diastolic dysfunction typically develops in children with conditions that result in increased afterload. For example, systemic arterial hypertension is associated with impaired left ventricular filling likely secondary to diminished compliance [44]. Similar disturbances of mitral inflow have been found in children with hypertrophic cardiomyopathy [45] and left-sided obstructive lesions such as aortic stenosis [46]. Diastolic dysfunction can also be seen in right-sided obstructive lesions such as pulmonary atresia/critical pulmonary stenosis or tetralogy of Fallot. Although the etiology of this dysfunction is unclear, it is likely related to the increased mass of the ventricles and/or subendocardial ischemia as a response to the pressure overload [47]. Myocardial edema may occur as a result of diastolic dysfunction. Complex surgical interventions require long periods of cardiopulmonary bypass and in some cases, circulatory arrest; capillary leak occurs in various organs of the body, including the heart, leading to diminished ventricular compliance and diastolic dysfunction.

Diastolic dysfunction is also common after the Fontan procedure for single ventricle lesions. Prior to the era of staging with the bidirectional cavopulmonary shunt, it was common to observe significant morbidity and mortality after Fontan operation, including recalcitrant pleural and pericardial effusions, ascites, electrolyte abnormalities, and low cardiac output. Echocardiographic assessment in these patients often revealed a ventricle with diminished volume and relaxation abnormalities but good systolic performance. The single ventricle with an aortopulmonary shunt develops increased mass in order to pump to both circulations. The Fontan operation significantly alters the physiology so that the single ventricle now pumps exclusively to the systemic circulation, and is thus "volume unloaded." The increased mass does not regress immediately; therefore, the mass-to-volume ratio increases dramatically with the Fontan [48]. By staging the Fontan with the interim bidirectional cavopulmonary shunt, the single ventricle adapts over time to the changes in volume with an adequate output to the body via the inferior vena cava.

While diastolic dysfunction after cardiac surgery is relatively easy to identify, treatment is extremely difficult and remains primarily supportive. Modified ultrafiltration, which removes excess fluid that has accumulated at the end of a surgical procedure, has been associated with improved outcome after cardiac surgery [49]. In children undergoing Fontan operation, pleural effusions are less likely to develop if modified ultrafiltration is performed [49]. Once in the ICU, maneuvers to increase ventricular filling in a noncompliant ventricle include lowering the heart rate to increase filling time (with beta blockade or amiodorone), volume expansion, and assuring atrioventricular electrical conductance. In tetralogy of Fallot and other lesions with right ventricular hypertrophy the foramen ovale is left patent at the time of repair. This allows for right-to-left shunting across the atrial septum, thus augmenting cardiac output while the right ventricle adapts [50]. Although some inotropic medications have effects on diastolic performance, there is no exclusively lusotropic medication. Inotropic medications may have some effects on diastole but primarily improve systolic ventricular function (digoxin, dopamine, dobutamine, epinephrine), provide afterload reduction (phosphodiesterase inhibitors), and help reverse end organ edema (diuretics). Detailed discussion of inotropic medications is covered in elsewhere in the book.

Low cardiac output syndrome in the ICU

Low cardiac output is often the end result of ventricular systolic dysfunction and occurs in approximately 25% of infants and children following congenital heart surgery [51]. Patients with low cardiac output are at higher risk for early postoperative death as well as complications such as renal dysfunction and prolonged intubation. Physical signs of low cardiac output include tachycardia, hypotension, decreased urine output, and metabolic acidosis. Wernovsky *et al.* reported that infants with transposition of the great arteries had a reduction in cardiac output (measured by thermodilution technique) and a rise in both pulmonary and systemic vascular resistance 6–18 h following the arterial switch operation, with subsequent improvement by 24 h [51]. Several studies report a similar trend of decreased cardiac output after surgery for other congenital heart defects as well [52,53], even in simple lesions such as primum or secundum atrial septal defects [16].

Patients with single ventricle lesions and in particular HLHS are at relatively high risk for the development of low cardiac output after surgical intervention. Arterial pO_2 and oxygen saturation have been used in the ICU setting to roughly estimate the Q_p/Q_s in patients with HLHS and other shunted single ventricle lesions. However, these measures do not adequately identify all patients at risk for low systemic oxygen delivery. Moreover, the oxygen saturation can be in normal range in the face of low cardiac output. Accurate calculation of Q_p/Q_s requires a measure of the mixed venous saturation. Hence, ICU management of single ventricle patients now often includes placement of a catheter in the superior vena cava to give a more accurate means of determining cardiac output and systemic oxygen delivery [54]. Identification of low cardiac output early allows for urgent interventions such as initiation of inotropic support, thus avoiding the sudden negative events that are frequently seen in the first few days after palliation. Tweddell *et al.* recently reported significantly improved survival of infants with HLHS undergoing Norwood procedure if continuous monitoring of the superior vena cava oxygen saturation was performed [55].

Several medical and mechanical techniques have been developed to help augment cardiac output in the immediate postoperative period. Some of these cardioprotective therapies occur in the operating room. Modified ultrafiltration immediately following cardiopulmonary bypass has been shown to improve left ventricular performance in children [56]. Aprotinin, a medication used in the operating room to reduce blood loss after cardiac surgery, has recently been found to have some beneficial effects on cardiac performance as well. Wippermann *et al.* reported that children receiving aprotinin after intracardiac surgery were less likely to require inotropic support than those receiving placebo [57]. Once in the ICU, inotropic support is commonly used in infants and children who have had open-heart procedures. A recent multicenter clinical trial by Hoffman and colleagues revealed that prophylactic use of milrinone (a phosphodiesterase inhibitor) reduces the risk of low cardiac output after congenital heart surgery [58]. Others have used the α-blocker phenoxybenzamine to improve systemic oxygen delivery after the Norwood procedure [59]. Low cardiac output that persists after the immediate postoperative period tends to occur in patients with prolonged periods of cardiopulmonary bypass and/or circulatory arrest (therefore more complicated intracardiac operations), inadequate myocardial protection, large ventricular incisions, evidence of ventricular dysfunction prior to surgical intervention, significant residual lesions, or disruption of coronary perfusion. On rare occasions, low cardiac output occurs for unclear reasons. In extreme circumstances, mechanical circulatory support may be required for a period of time after cardiac surgery.

Mechanical circulatory support

Mechanical circulatory support has been utilized in pediatric patients in the ICU for severe ventricular failure after cardiac surgery (including those who cannot be weaned from cardiopulmonary bypass at the time of surgery), cardiac arrest as a form of resuscitation, and bridging to cardiac transplantation with variable but improving success [60–62]. Various mechanical support systems are now available for pediatric patients including the older more widely used extracorporeal membrane oxygenation (ECMO) (Fig. 19.1) and the newer ventricular as-

sist devices (VAD) including centrifugal and pulsatile systems [60]. ECMO generally includes peripheral cannulation via the femoral or cervical vasculature with support of both the cardiac output (via nonpulsatile flow) and oxygenation. Trained personnel are required to run ECMO systems 24 hours a day. VAD systems can support one or both ventricles but have no oxygenator. They can generally be managed by the nursing staff in the ICU, allow the patient some mobility (if portable), and provide support for longer periods of time (particularly the systems with pulsatile flow). Although recent advances in VAD systems (i.e., implantable devices, portability) have emerged for the adult population, many of these devices are still too large for safe use in neonates. VAD systems have generally been used in children with primary left ventricular dysfunction such as those with cardiomyopathy, myocarditis, or ischemic injury to the left ventricle [61,62]. In contrast, ECMO is more appropriate for infants and young children who require cardiopulmonary support (i.e., pulmonary hypertension, hypoxemia)

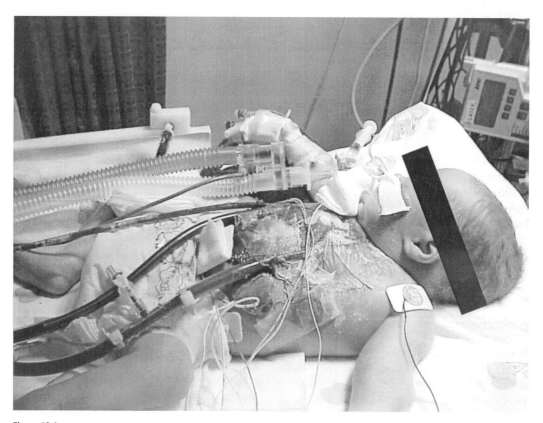

Figure 19.1

Table 19.2 ECMO and VAD Uses in Pediatric Population.

	ECMO	VAD
Hypoxemia, pulmonary hypertension	+	
Anomalous left coronary		+
Peripheral cannulation (i.e. femoral, carotid)	+	
Left ventricular decompression		+
Biventricular support in infancy	+	
Diminished trauma to blood elements		+
Requires less anticoagulation		+

From Duncan [59] with permission.

(see Table 19.2). Most recently, rapid resuscitation ECMO circuits have become available, which are more portable than previous systems and are housed in the ICU. These circuits are used for patients with cardiac arrest who do not respond within 10–20 min of medical resuscitation [61].

Survival after ECMO or VAD support has improved significantly over the past decade and may depend on the reason support was initiated. Duncan *et al.* recently reported that 40% of cardiac patients on ECMO and 41% of those on VAD systems survived to hospital discharge [63]. The primary risk factors for death in the total cohort was ventricular dysfunction for greater than 72 h after initiation of mechanical support. Indication for ECMO and type of cardiac defect did not appear to impact on survival and the complication rate for the ECMO and VAD groups did not differ significantly [63]. Other risk factors for poor outcome have been identified in association with mechanical support, including renal failure, prolonged cardiopulmonary resuscitation prior to initiation of support [64], initiation of ECMO in the operating room, or initiation at greater than 50 h after surgery and single ventricle physiology [65]. Children with a primary diagnosis of myocarditis have a higher survival rate (ranging from 58 to 80%) than other groups requiring mechanical support [66,67]. In fact, mechanical support may impart some protective effects on the heart with myocarditis because many patients who successfully wean from support recover ventricular function and ultimately do not require cardiac transplant [60].

Use of ECMO and VAD can be associated with serious complications and therefore should only be used in life-threatening situations. With both systems, indwelling prosthetic material increases the risk of serious infections. In addition, both systems require

some degree of anticoagulation; children are therefore at risk for the development of stroke and/or intracranial hemorrhage. Damage to the vessels that are cannulated may cause long-term peripheral vascular insufficiency. Once removed, the scar tissue in the ventricle from the VAD systems may become a nidus for long-term ventricular dysfunction and arrhythmias. A recent study by Ibrahim *et al.* identified 37 survivors of mechanical support (both ECMO and VAD), followed for more than 4 years. Moderate to severe neurologic impairment was seen in more than 60% of those who had been on ECMO in contrast to 20% of those who had been on VAD support [68]. The ECMO group had a higher number of critically ill newborns, which may in part explain these results. Certainly, the long-term neurologic outcome of patients who have required mechanical support remains to be seen.

Conclusions

Assessment of ventricular function is critical to the management of pediatric patients with cardiac disease in the ICU setting. Ventricular dysfunction and associated low cardiac output remain the primary cause of morbidity and mortality in children with CHD and significantly prolongs the length of stay in the ICU. Despite this, significant strides have been made in ICU care for children with CHD and survival for most lesions has overwhelmingly improved over time. Future efforts should be directed toward developing more reliable methods of assessing right ventricular performance, better lusotropic agents to treat diastolic dysfunction, and more portable mechanical support systems for neonates and infants. In the future, cardiologists will likely be able to predict whether individual children are at risk for the development of ventricular dysfunction and low cardiac output (based on genetic predisposition) in order to anticipate and possibly prevent the deleterious effects of such events.

References

1. Gutgesell HP, Paquet M, Duff DF, *et al.* Evaluation of left ventricular size and function by echocardiography: Results in normal children. Circulation 1977; 56:457–462.

2. Schiller NB. Two-dimensional echocardiographic determination of left ventricular volume, systolic function, and mass: Summary and discussion of the 1989 recommendations of the American Society of Echocardiography. Circulation 1991; 84(suppl I): I280–I287.

3. Silverman NH, Ports TA, Snider AR, *et al.* Determination of left ventricular volume in children: Echocardiographic and angiographic comparisons. Circulation 1980; 62:548–557.

4. Reichek N, Wilson J, St John Sutton, *et al.* Noninvasive determination of left ventricular end systolic stress: Validation of the method and initial application. Circulation 1982; 65:99–108.

5. Weber KT, Janicki JS, Hunter WC, *et al.* The contractile behavior of the heart and its functional coupling to the circulation. Prog Cardiovasc Dis 1982; 24:375–400.

6. Stein PD, Sabbah HN. Ventricular performance measured during ejection. Studies in patients of the rate of change of ventricular power. Am Heart J 1976; 91:599–606.

7. Harrison MR, Clifton GD, Berk MR, *et al.* Effect of blood pressure and afterload on Doppler echocardiographic measurements of left ventricular systolic function in normal subjects. Am J Cardiol 1989; 64:905–908.

8. Chen C, Rodriquez L, Lethor JP, *et al.* Continuous wave Doppler echocardiography for noninvasive assessment of left ventricular dP/dt and relaxation time constant from mitral regurgitant spectra in patients. J Am Coll Cardiol 1994; 23:970–976.

9. Nixon JV, Murray RG, Leonard PD, *et al.* Effect of large variations in preload on left ventricular performance characteristics in normal subjects. Circulation 1982; 65:698–703.

10. Borow KM, Green LH, Grossman W, *et al.* Left ventricular end-systolic stress-shortening and stress-length relations in human. Normal values and sensitivity to inotropic state. Am J Cardiol 1982; 50:1301–1308.

11. Colan SD, Borow KM, Neumann A. The left ventricular end-systolic wall stress-velocity of fiber shortening relation: A load independent index of myocardial contractility. J Am Coll Cardiol 1984; 4:715–724.

12. Kimball TR, Daniels SR, Khoury P, *et al.* Age-related variation in contractility estimate in patients ≤20 years of age. Am J Cardiol 1991; 68:1383–1387.

13. Colan SD, Parness IA, Spevak PJ, *et al.* Developmental modulation of myocardial mechanics: Age- and growth-related alterations in afterload and contractility. J Am Coll Cardiol 1992:19:619–629.

14. Gorcsan J III, Morita S, Mandarino WA, *et al.* Two-dimensional echocardiographic automated border detection accurately reflects changes in left ventricular volume. J Am Soc Echocardiogr 1993; 6:482–489.

15. Cassidy SC, Teitel DF. The conductance volume catheter technique for measurement of left ventricular volume in young piglets. Pediatr Res 1992; 31:85–90.

16. Chaturvedi RR, Lincoln C, Gothard JWW, *et al.* Left ventricular dysfunction after open repair of simple congenital heart defects in infants and children: Quantitation with the use of a conductance catheter immediately after bypass. J Thorac Cardiovasc Surg 1998; 115:77–83.

17. Colan SD, del Nido PJ. Editorial: Left ventricular dysfunction after open repair of simple congenital heart defects in infants and children. J Thorac Cardiovasc Surg 1998; 115:74–76.

18. Murakami T, Nakazawa M, Nakanishi T, *et al.* Prediction of postoperative left ventricular pump function in congenital mitral regurgitation. Pediatr Cardiol 1999; 20:418–421.

19. Lorier G, Kalil RA, Barcellos C, *et al.* Valve repair in children with congenital mitral lesions: Late clinical results. Pediatr Cardiol 2001; 22:44–52.

20. Erez E, Kanter KR, Isom E, *et al.* Mitral valve replacement in children. J Heart Valve Dis 2003; 12:25–29.

21. Gundry S, Behrendt D. Prognostic factors in valvotomy for critical aortic stenosis in infancy. J Thorac Cardiovasc Surg 1986; 92:747–754.

22. Justo RN, McCrindle BW, Benson LN, *et al.* Aortic valve regurgitation after surgical versus percutaneous balloon valvotomy for congenital aortic valve stenosis. Am J Cardiol 1996; 77:1332–1338.

23. Witsenburg M, Cromme-Dijkhuis A, Frohn-Mulder IME. Short and midterm results of balloon valvuloplasty for valvular aortic stenosis in children. Am J Cardiol 1992; 69:945–950.

24. Jin XY, Pepper JR, Gibson DG, *et al.* Early changes in the time course of myocardial contraction after correcting aortic regurgitation. Ann Thorac Surg 1999; 67:139–145.

25. Pasquali SK, Hasselblad V, Li JS, *et al.* Coronary artery pattern and outcome of arterial switch operation for transposition of the great arteries: A meta-analysis. Circulation 2002; 106:2575–2580.

26. Sauer U, Stern H, Meisner H, *et al.* Risk factors for perioperative mortality in children with anomalous origin

of the left coronary artery from the pulmonary artery. J Thorac Cardiovasc Surg 1992; 104:696–705.

27. Vogel M, Gutberlet M, Dittrich S, *et al.* Comparison of transthoracic three-dimensional echocardiography with magnetic resonance imaging in the assessment of right ventricular volume and mass. Heart 1997; 78:127–130.

28. Heusch A, Rübo J, Krogmann ON, *et al.* Volumetric analysis of the right ventricle in children with congenital heart defects: Comparison of biplane angiography and transthoracic 3-dimensional echocardiography. Cardiol Young 1999; 9:577–584.

29. Anconina J, Danchin N, Selton-Suty C, *et al.* Noninvasive estimation of right ventricular dP/dt in patients with tricuspid valve regurgitation. Am J Cardiol 1993; 71:1495–1497.

30. Tei C, Dujardin KS, Hodge DO, *et al.* Doppler echocardiographic index for assessment of global right ventricular function. J Am Soc Echocardiogr 1996; 9:838–847.

31. Eidem BW, O'Leary PW, Tei C, *et al.* Usefulness of the myocardial performance index for assessing right ventricular function in congenital heart disease. Am J Cardiol 2000; 86:654–658.

32. Ishii M, Eto G, Tei C, *et al.* Quantitation of the global right ventricular function in children with normal heart and congenital heart disease: A right ventricular myocardial performance index. Pediatr Cardiol 2000; 21:416–421.

33. Abd El Rahman MY, Abdul-Khaliq H, Vogel M, *et al.* Value of the new Doppler-derived myocardial performance index for the evaluation of right and left ventricular function following repair of tetralogy of Fallot. Pediatr Cardiol 2002; 23:502–507.

34. Mahle WT, Coon PD, Wernovsky G, *et al.* Quantitative echocardiographic assessment of the performance of the functionally single right ventricle after the Fontan operation. Cardiol Young 2001; 11:399–406.

35. Ochai Y, Morita S, Tanoue Y, *et al.* Use of transesophageal echocardiography for postoperative evaluation of right ventricular function. Ann Thorac Surg 1999; 67:146–153.

36. Norwood WI, Lang P, Castaneda AR, *et al.* Experience with operations for hypoplastic left heart syndrome. J Thorac Cardiovasc Surg 1981; 82:511–519.

37. Abdullah MH, Van Arsdell GSV, Hornberger LK, *et al.* Precoronary stenosis after stage 1 palliation for hypoplastic left heart syndrome. Ann Thorac Surg 2000; 70:2147–2149.

38. Bartram U, Grunenfelder J, Van Praagh R. Causes of death after the modified Norwood procedure: A study of 122 postmortem cases. Ann Thorac Surg 1997; 64:1795–1802.

39. Freedom RM, Benson LN. Hypoplastic left heart syndrome. In: Emmanouilides GC, Riemenschneider TA, Allen HD, Gutgesell HP, eds., Heart Disease in Infants, Children, and Adolescents Including the Fetus and Young Adult. William and Wilkins, Baltimore, MD, pp 1133–1153, 1995.

40. Penny DJ. The basics of ventricular function. Cardiol Young 1999; 9:210–223.

41. Kitabatake A, Inoue M, Asao M, *et al.* Transmitral blood flow reflecting diastolic behavior of the left ventricle in health and disease: A study by pulsed Doppler technique. Jpn Circ J 1982; 46:92–102.

42. Snider RA, Serwer GA, Ritter SB. Methods of obtaining quantitative information from the echocardiographic examination. In: Snider RA, Serwer GA, Ritter SB, eds., Echocardiography in Pediatric Heart Disease. Mosby-Year Book, Inc. St. Louis, MO, pp. 133–234, 1997.

43. Nagueh SF, Lakkis NM, Middleton KJ, *et al.* Doppler estimation of left ventricular filling pressures in patients with hypertrophic cardiomyopathy. Circulation 1999; 99:254–261.

44. Snider AR, Gidding SS, Rocchini AP, *et al.* Doppler evaluation of left ventricular diastolic filling in children with systemic hypertension. Am J Cardiol 1985; 56:921–926.

45. Gidding SS, Snider AR, Rocchini AP, *et al.* Left ventricular diastolic filling in children with hypertrophic cardiomyopathy: Assessment with pulsed Doppler echocardiography. J Am Coll Cardiol 1986; 8:310–316.

46. Meliones JN, Snider AR, Serwer GA, *et al.* Pulsed Doppler assessment of left ventricular diastolic filling in children with left ventricular outflow obstruction before and after balloon angioplasty. Am J Cardiol 1989; 63:231–236.

47. Lorell BH, Grossman W. Cardiac hypertrophy: the consequences for diastole. J Am Coll Cardiol 1987; 9:1189–1193.

48. Wernovsky G, Bove EL. Single ventricle lesions. In: Chang AC, Hanley FL, Wernovsky G, Wessel DL, eds., Pediatric Cardiac Intensive Care. William and Wilkins, Baltimore, MD, pp. 271–287, 1998.

49. Gaynor JW. Use of modified ultrafiltration after repair of congenital heart defects. Semin Thorac Cardiovasc Surg Pediatr Card Surg Ann 1998; 1:81–90.

50. Spray TL, Wernovsky G. Tetralogy of Fallot. In: Chang AC, Hanley FL, Wernovsky G, Wessel DL, eds., Pediatric Cardiac Intensive Care. William and Wilkins, Baltimore, MD, pp 257–265, 1998.

51. Wernovsky G, Wypij D, Jonas RA, *et al.* Postoperative course and hemodynamic profile after the arterial switch operation in neonates and infants: A comparison of low-flow cardiopulmonary bypass and circulatory arrest. Circulation 1995; 92:2226–2235.

52. Burrows FA, Williams WG, Teoh KH, *et al.* Myocardial performance after repair of congenital cardiac defects in infants and children. J Thorac Cardiovasc Surg 1988; 96:548–56.

53. del Nido P, Mickle DAG, Wilson GJ, *et al.* Evidence of myocardial free radical injury during elective repair of tetralogy of Fallot. Circulation 1987; 76(suppl): V174–V179.

54. Rossi AF, Sommer RJ, Lotvin A, *et al.* Usefulness of intermittent monitoring of mixed venous oxygen saturation after stage 1 palliation for hypoplastic left heart syndrome. Am J Cardiol 1994; 73:1118–1123.

55. Tweddell JS, Hoffman GM, Mussatto KA, *et al.* Improved survival of patients undergoing palliation of hypoplastic left heart syndrome: Lessons learned from 115 consecutive cases. Circulation 2002 106(suppl I):I82–I89.

56. Davies MJ, Nguyen K, Gaynor JW, *et al.* Modified ultrafiltration improves left ventricular systolic function in infants after cardiopulmonary bypass. J Thorac Cardiovasc Surg 1998; 115:361–370.

57. Wippermann CF, Schmid FX, Eberle B, *et al.* Reduced inotropic support after aprotinin therapy during pediatric cardiac operations. Ann Thorac Surg 1999; 67:173–176.

58. Hoffman TM, Wernovsky G, Atz, AM, *et al.* Efficacy and safety of milrinone in preventing low cardiac output sundrome in infants and children after corrective surgery for congenital heart disease. Circulation 2003; 107:996–1002.

59. Tweddell JS, Hoffman GM, Fedderly RT, *et al.* Phenoxybenzamine improves systemic oxygen delivery after the Norwood procedure. Ann Thorac Surg 1999; 67:161–168.

60. Duncan BW. Mechanical circulatory support for infants and children with cardiac disease. Ann Thorac Surg 2002; 73:1670–1677.

61. Duncan BW, Ibrahim AE, Hraska V, *et al.* Use of rapid-deployment extracorporeal membrane oxygenation for the resuscitation of pediatric patients with heart disease after cardiac arrest. J Thorac Cardiovasc Surg 1998; 116:305–311.

62. Del Nido PJ, Armitage JM, Fricker J, *et al.* Extracorporeal membrane oxygenation support as a bridge to pediatric heart transplantation. Circulation 1994; 90(part 2):II66–II69.

63. Duncan BW, Hraska V, Jonas RA, *et al.* Mechanical support in children with cardiac disease. J Thorac Cardiovasc Surg 1999; 117:529–542.

64. Aharon AS, Drinkwater DC, Churchwell KB, *et al.* Extracorporeal membrane oxygenation in children after repair of congenital cardiac lesions. Ann Thorac Surg 2001; 72:2095–2102.

65. Kulik TJ, Moler FW, Palmisano MA, *et al.* Outcome-associated factors in pediatric patients treated with extracorporeal membrane oxygenator after cardiac surgery. Circulation 1996; 94(suppl II):II63–II68.

66. ECMO Registry Report. Extracorporeal Life Support Organization, Ann Arbor, 1999.

67. Duncan BW, Bohn DJ, Atz AM, *et al.* Mechanical circulatory support for the treatment of children with acute fulminant myocarditis. J Thorac Cardiovasc Surg 2001; 122:440–448.

68. Ibrahim AE, Duncan BW, Blume ED, *et al.* Long-term follow-up of pediatric cardiac patients requiring mechanical circulatory support. Ann Thorac Surg 2000; 69:186–192.

PART IV

Ventricular Function and Blood Flow in Specific Categories

CHAPTER 20

Considerations in Catheter Interventions

Michael Cheung, MB, CHB, MRCP(UK) & Lee Benson, MD, FRCP(C), FSCAI

Introduction

Advances in the field of interventional catheterization have allowed increasing numbers of congenital heart defects to be addressed nonsurgically, with complex lesions frequently being managed through combined catheter–surgical treatment algorithms. Catheter techniques can be broadly grouped into those that create or close septal defects, dilate valves and vessels, or occlude vessels. The future prospect of potentially replacing valves, redirecting blood flow with stent grafts, and fetal interventions adds exciting new avenues to transcatheter therapy. With these advances, however, the ability to intervene must be tempered by consideration of the short- and long-term consequences of such therapies.

It is now possible to modulate conditions that induce ventricular dilation, hypertrophy, or disturbances of blood flow across valves and within vessels. Although the hemodynamic benefits of occluding left-to-right shunts due to atrial and ventricular septal defects are obvious, even in the absence of immediate compromise of surrounding structures due to device impingement, the long-term consequences of a fixed rigid structure within the cardiac septae are uncertain. In this regard, use of large devices in small children must be done with caution. In this chapter we will examine a variety of different clinical conditions as paradigms of hemodynamic disturbances and their catheter-based management. However, detailed descriptions of the technical aspects of each procedure are beyond the scope of this chapter [1].

Aortic stenosis

First reported in 1984, balloon dilation has become the initial treatment of choice for valvar stenosis in

childhood. Based upon local experience and expertise, however, surgical therapy continues to play an important role in management. Clearly, the best approach remains controversial, and differs according to age group. With increasing knowledge, experience, and refinements in techniques and patient selection this approach is becoming an integral component of management algorithms.

Ventricular function

The hypertrophic response to left ventricular outflow tract obstruction is reportedly better tolerated in children compared to adults, with the compensatory changes resulting in decreased end-systolic wall stress [2] and supernormal ejection performance. This is in contrast to adults with acquired aortic stenosis who have normal or increased systolic wall stress resulting in either normal or subnormal contractile performance. In a study by Assey et al. [3], left ventricular wall stress was found to be lower in congenital aortic stenosis when compared to age matched normal subjects or adults with acquired stenosis. Indeed, with time, there was no tendency for patients with congenital stenosis to revert to an adult pattern. Such observations suggest a fundamental difference in the hypertrophic response to pressure overload when the stenosis originates at birth, compared with that of acquired disease. How this influences outcomes after intervention may be a fruitful area for research. There must, however, intuitively be a limit to how long this form of compensation may continue before irreversible changes in myocardial function and structure ensue [4,5].

The report of the Second Joint Natural History Study of patients with valvar aortic stenosis [6] advised that patients with an initial gradient of

<25 mm Hg could be followed medically, having a 21% chance of requiring an intervention in the subsequent 25 years. Of patients with an initial gradient ≥50 mm Hg, there was a 71% chance of eventual intervention, and this group was at increased risk of sudden death due to presumed ventricular arrhythmias. Patients with gradients between 25 and 49 mm Hg had a 41% chance of requiring intervention due to increasing lesion severity. For this latter group, the authors recommended medical follow-up, in view of the potential for inducing aortic regurgitation with intervention [7]. Overall estimated 25-year survival probability was 85 ± 2% for the 457 patients in the original cohort from the First Joint Natural History Study [8]. This compares favorably with an expected 25-year survival of 96% for individuals of a similar age and sex, obtained from the survival distribution of the US white population in 1970.

The indications for intervention are summarized in the guidelines from the American College of Cardiology and American Heart Association for the management in adolescents and young adults [9]. Intervention is advised in symptomatic patients with a catheter peak-to-peak systolic gradient ≥50 mm Hg; if asymptomatic, with a gradient ≥60 mm Hg, if the catheter peak-to-peak systolic gradient was ≥50 mm Hg and new electrocardiographic ST or T wave changes at rest or during exercise developed, or if the peak-to-peak systolic gradient was >50 mm Hg and the patient was taking part in competitive sport. Other authors have suggested an isolated peak-to-peak systolic gradient of >50 mm Hg as an absolute indication for intervention in children [10]. It is, however, impractical to frequently monitor aortic gradients through catheterization. In this regard, echocardiographic Doppler flow measurements have supplemented hemodynamic assessment. However, echocardiography measures the peak instantaneous gradient across the valve, and unlike pulmonary valve stenosis, the peak instantaneous gradient has no relationship to the peak-to-peak gradient because of the contour of the waveforms. Furthermore, while measured as the standard for determination of severity (from the natural history studies), the peak-to-peak gradient is a nonphysiological quantity, and the peak aortic and left ventricular pressures occur at different times during the cardiac cycle. To address this inequity, Beekman

et al. [11] described a regression equation, derived from a multivariate analysis, to estimate peak-to-peak gradients across the aortic valve, and which requires only the determination of the pulse pressure and mean gradient. Lima and colleagues [12] from our laboratory validated the echocardiographic measurement of mean aortic gradient and correlated the estimate to simultaneously measured peak-to-peak gradients in children with aortic stenosis. The formula employed is [11]

Peak-to-peak gradient (mm Hg) = 6.04 +
   1.4 (mean gradient) − 0.4 (pulse pressure)

We use this formula to calculated peak-to-peak aortic gradients, directly applying the results to clinical practice.

Following relief of stenosis by balloon dilation, left ventricular remodeling occurs relatively slowly. Shim *et al.* [13] calculated left ventricular mass, indexed to body surface area, from M-mode echocardiographic measurements taken from patients before and after balloon dilation. Those with residual gradients of >50 mm Hg or more than mild aortic regurgitation were excluded. The authors reported that statistically significant reductions in left ventricular mass did not occur until the second year (average 19 ± 3 months) following a successful procedure. Comparative adult data, in contrast, shows that most mass regression occurs within 6 months (of valve replacement). As the majority of patients following balloon dilation are left with a mild residual gradient, this discrepancy is not entirely unexpected.

The long-term effects of mild to moderate aortic regurgitation, which may develop following balloon intervention, are unclear in this age group, particularly in the newborn or infant. Justo *et al.* [14], from our unit, studied 187 patients managed surgically or by catheter intervention and compared the incidence of aortic regurgitation in follow-up. These authors reported a similar incidence, severity, and rate of progression of regurgitation following either procedure. The rate of progression of left ventricular dilation after dilation of the aortic valve in childhood is influenced not only by the presence of left ventricular hypertrophy (increased cell size) but by hyperplasia (increased cell numbers) also. It appears that the youngest of patients with congenital aortic stenosis requiring intervention present a different myocardial substrate and respond very differently to the intervention when compared to adults [7,15]. As such, the influence of myocardial adaptation to pressure overload impacts tolerance and response to the sequelae of intervention [16].

Technical considerations

Data from the Valvuloplasty and Angioplasty of Congenital Anomalies (VACA) registry reported independent predictors of immediate results from 630 balloon dilation procedures for aortic stenosis [17]. The median age at intervention was 6.8 years (range 1 day to 18 years) and the mean peak-to-peak pressure gradient was 69 ± 24 mm Hg prior to dilation. Suboptimal outcomes in this series included 1 or more of the following: Failure to complete or perform the procedure, a residual gradient of ≥ 60 mm Hg, a residual left ventricular-to-aortic pressure ratio of ≥ 1.6, or the occurrence of mortality or major morbidity. Major morbidity included severe arterial vascular complications, cardiac or vascular perforation, valve avulsion, cardiac tamponade, stroke, or the production of severe aortic regurgitation. Using these criteria 17% of procedures resulted in a suboptimal outcome.

As expected, the size of the balloon relative to aortic valve annulus had important implications for the success of the procedure. Undersized balloons were associated with increased risk for residual obstruction, with a balloon-to-aortic valve ratio of 0.9:1.0, giving optimal results. Counter intuitively perhaps, the use of oversized balloons was also associated with inadequate relief. This was postulated to represent a subset of valves, which could not be dilated with any size of balloon, in particular, those with thickened dysplastic leaflets and a small annulus. The presence of more than trivial aortic regurgitation prior to intervention and the use of oversized balloons were significantly associated with the development of greater degrees of aortic regurgitation following dilation. While annulus diameter is the variable used to choose an appropriate balloon size, it appears to be the balloon circumference, which is critical to the success of the procedure. For aortic stenosis, balloons of diameters identical to or slightly smaller than the diameter of the valve (and therefore similar to the annular circumference) are generally chosen. Several operators [18,19] have proposed simultaneous double balloon techniques, where the annulus is stretched into an oval configuration. This allows continued (albeit reduced) forward flow between the balloons through the aortic valve during the dilation, in part maintaining cardiac output, but more importantly stabilizing the balloon across the valve. This issue of balloon motion across the valve due to systolic ejection frequently leads to repeated inflation–deflation cycles before the balloon appropriately straddles the valve. This to-and-fro motion is also thought to result in a higher incidence of leaflet rupture or prolapse and resultant regurgitation. In this regard, several authors have suggested the use of intravenous adenosine (500 mg/kg) to induce transient (about 5 sec) atrioventricular block allowing an inflation–deflation cycle during the asystolic period [20].

In choosing balloon pairs, a circumference equivalent to the undisturbed annulus circumference is calculated [21]. For example, if the annular diameter was 25 mm, then two balloons whose paired circumference would be equivalent to a 25 mm diameter circle are chosen. This may be any number of balloon diameter combinations, creating a symmetrical or asymmetrical oval. In this example combinations could be a 20 and 10 mm, 18 and 12 mm, or two 15 mm balloons. A rule of thumb suggested by Mullins *et al.* [18] was the use of any combination of balloon diameters whose sum is equivalent to the annulus diameter times 1.2.

The VACA registry reported transection of the femoral or iliac artery in 2% of procedures, across all age groups. In the neonatal population, Egito *et al.* [22] reported that of 20 patients undergoing dilation from the femoral artery all had loss of the arterial pulse, with restoration in 35% after thrombolysis. At mid-term follow-up (mean age 4 ± 2 years, range 2–8 years) the femoral pulse remained absent in 9 children, albeit without any discrepancies in leg length. The same group reported that freedom from reintervention was 64% at 8 years. In view of these experiences, some centers have proposed alternative approaches to positioning the balloon across the aortic valve. Borghi *et al.* [23] recently reported their experience of using a surgical cut down on the right carotid artery. At a mean follow-up of 4 ± 2 years after dilation in 17 children, the right carotid artery was patent by Doppler flow studies. The arterial cannulation site was detectable by ultrasound in 5 children, despite the absence of flow disturbances on flow assessment. Although asymptomatic, 1 of the children showed mild obstruction to flow and a 35% reduction in vessel diameter.

Several institutions, using femoral venous access and a transseptal entry to the left heart, have favored an antegrade approach. Clearly, this approach avoids arterial complications, and its proponents also cite better balloon positioning and the reassurance that the wire has gone through the hemodynamic orifice, in contrast to the potential of valve leaflet perforation with the retrograde approach [24]. In a study comparing retrograde to antegrade approaches in 26 neonates, although efficacy in relief of stenosis was comparable, the occurrence of more severe aortic regurgitation with an antegrade approach was considered to be due to unrecognized valve leaflet perforation [25]. Additionally, mortality in the retrograde group was significantly greater. The two groups were not directly comparable, however, with the patients in the retrograde group being recruited from an earlier era in the development of transcatheter intervention techniques and some may not have been biventricular repair candidates using today's criteria [26]. A further modification of the antegrade approach using a femoral vein to femoral artery loop technique by way of a transseptal approach has also been described, allowing for improved balloon control [27]. Additional approaches include the right brachial artery or transumbilical (artery or vein) approaches, the latter primarily used in the neonate.

Neonatal aortic stenosis

Neonates with aortic stenosis constitute a unique cohort of patients, both in terms of physiology and response to treatment. In the presence of a closed arterial duct and normal ventricular function, the gradient required for intervention is as in the older child. However, with depressed ventricular function or duct-dependent systemic blood flow, gradients *per se* are misleading, and intervention is based upon clinical presentation, the morphological assessment of ventricular form, and function and aortic valve morphology (annular diameter, valve thickness, and mobility). This patient group has consistently shown more complications related to intervention and a higher requirement for reintervention; as such, neonates are generally considered separately when results of therapy are assessed. Analysis of data from the Second Joint Natural History Study, for those patients <2 years of age,

identified this cohort as having a higher mortality from therapy (primarily surgical at the time) [6], as did the data from VACA registry [17].

Despite the demonstrated efficacy of transcatheter techniques, there continues to be centers employing surgical valvotomy as the initial treatment choice for valvar aortic stenosis. Alexiou *et al.* [28] from Southampton, United Kingdom, recently reported results of open surgical valvotomy in 97 consecutive patients from 1979 through 2000. Neonates comprised 26 patients of the cohort, and the operative mortality for the newborns was 8%, which compares favorably with the 8% mortality reported by McCrindle [17] for children <3 months of age. Following surgical valvotomy, the Southampton group reported that for the whole patient population, residual or recurrent stenosis occurred in 17 patients and severe regurgitation in 8 patients. Data from the Congenital Heart Surgeons Society [29] in part lends support for this approach in the neonate, at least in the short term. In a study of 110 neonates, although the median residual systolic gradient was significantly greater following surgical valvotomy, the incidence of important aortic regurgitation was found to be higher (18 vs. 3%) following balloon dilation, although this difference was not statistically significant between groups. The mean balloon to aortic valve ratio in this study was 0.99 ± 0.13, perhaps accounting for the relatively higher incidence of significant regurgitation.

The right ventricular outflow tract

Abnormalities of blood flow through the right ventricular outflow tract are commonly encountered in children with congenital heart defects, and obstructive lesions such as valvar pulmonary stenosis are now readily managed by interventional catheterization. There are also increasing numbers of long-term survivors of surgical repair, such as tetralogy of Fallot, who must cope with the sequelae of chronic pulmonary regurgitation and associated right ventricular dilation. Additionally, such patients with pulmonary artery stenosis may also benefit from transcatheter–catheter techniques. New equipment and techniques, such as the cutting balloon, percutaneous pulmonary valve implantation, and radiofrequency-based perforation of atretic valves, may allow greater numbers of this population to be treated in the catheter laboratory.

Pulmonary stenosis

The generally accepted indication for intervention in valvar pulmonary stenosis is a gradient of ≥ 50 mmHg from echocardiographic assessment (peak instantaneous gradient), in the setting of a normal cardiac output. Unlike valvar aortic stenosis, the pulmonary artery waveform is relatively flat through systole and the ventricular trace is triangular shaped, such that the peak-to-peak and peak instantaneous gradients are very close, if not identical. In the setting of neonatal critical pulmonary stenosis, however, this must be tempered by consideration of patency of the arterial duct, the competence of the tricuspid valve, and right ventricular contractile performance. Relief of valvar obstruction usually results in rapid improvement of any associated systolic dysfunction; however, diastolic impairment may take longer to resolve. Indeed, there are patients following successful relief of critical obstruction, who require pharmacological maintenance of ductal patency to provide an adequate pulmonary blood flow due to reduced right ventricular compliance, excluding those patients with anatomical chamber hypoplasia or inflow or persistent outflow tract obstructive lesions. Regression of right ventricular hypertrophy and ventricular enlargement is the rule, given an adequate timeline, with the induced pulmonary regurgitation potentially enhancing this evolution. Flow through the right ventricle may be aided with the use of β-blockade if there is dynamic outflow tract obstruction. Whether the effect is due to the drugs' negative inotropic or chronotropic actions has not been determined. These therapies are unsuccessful in a small percentage of patients and systemic-to-pulmonary shunts may be required to palliate intractable cyanosis.

In this clinical setting, several authors have suggested the placement of endovascular stents to support the arterial duct, avoiding surgical shunt placement or prolonged prostaglandin infusions [30,31]. However, early experience with this approach noted early and at times rapid in-stent stenosis, in addition to the technical difficulties in placement with the first- or second-generation stent designs. The normal biology of ductal tissue requires normally quiescent luminal endothelial cells and medial smooth muscle cells [32] to migrate into the subendothelial space, forming intimal mounds, which coalesce and occlude the vessels lumen. As such, these metal implants, while maintaining the lumen initially, do not alter the aggressive inherent mechanism of closure. Recently, drug-eluting stents (e.g., serolimus) have been found to alter the biology of smooth muscle cell migration retarding (or eliminating) the mechanism responsible for in-stent stenosis in coronary arterial vessels [33]. Whether such implants will similarly decrease the closure of ductal tissue is still under investigation.

Although problematic early after intervention, the diastolic dysfunction observed in these patients may be advantageous in the long term. In a study of flow patterns in patients with severe pulmonary stenosis [34], antegrade diastolic flow in the main pulmonary artery coincident with atrial contraction and present throughout the respiratory cycle (detected by Doppler echocardiography) was considered a marker of diastolic dysfunction. In this situation, the noncompliant right ventricle acts as a conduit during atrial systole, demonstrating restrictive physiology. Additional studies have shown that restrictive right ventricular physiology in patients after repair of Fallot's tetralogy may be protective against the deleterious effects of long-term pulmonary regurgitation, such as malignant ventricular arrhythmias, impaired exercise tolerance, or sudden death [35,36]. Whether this is an issue in the setting of isolated pulmonary stenosis, addressed early, has not been defined.

Pulmonary regurgitation

There are recent and very exciting reports of the potential for percutaneous transcatheter insertion of valved stents in the pulmonary position, to address the effects of pulmonary regurgitation [37,38]. Clinical trials of this procedure in children are underway and the results of these are awaited. Because of the limited expansion ratio of the stent, implants have been limited to 18–20 mm diameter outflow tracts, primarily right ventricle to pulmonary artery conduits. Early efficacy has been demonstrated with an increase in pulmonary artery diastolic pressure from 9 ± 3 to 13 ± 3 mmHg with little or no stenosis [38]. While the mechanism of pulmonary insufficiency is related to the lack of valvular support after previous interventions or a surgically enlarged annulus, the origin of the regurgitant volume, until recently, was poorly defined. Using magnetic resonance techniques, Yoo and colleagues from the Hospital for Sick Children [39] have determined, in the majority of children with pulmonary regurgitation, that the largest percentage of the regurgitant stroke volume originates from the left pulmonary artery. As such, it is interesting to speculate that unilateral percutaneous valve implants may significantly reduce the regurgitant volume, allowing even those patients (the majority in adults) with an aneurysmal outflow tract dimension to benefit from percutaneous valve implantation.

Other transcatheter techniques are presently employed in the management of patients with pulmonary regurgitation. Repaired tetralogy of Fallot represents a commonly encountered model of chronic pulmonary regurgitation, albeit in conjunction with the confounding variable of ventriculotomy in many. Within this patient cohort the effects of pulmonary artery stenosis on the degree of pulmonary regurgitation have recently been demonstrated [40]. Using conductance catheter methods with integrated micromanometers, pulmonary regurgitation was assessed from generated pressure–volume loops under conditions of either increased airway pressure or unilateral pulmonary artery stenosis. The maneuver of transient inflation of a balloon in a branch pulmonary artery (simulating branch pulmonary artery stenosis) was associated with a significant increase in the regurgitant volume from 27 to 37%, ($P < 0.05$) with an increase in end-systolic pressure from 69 to 79 mm Hg ($P < 0.05$). One patient had branch arterial stenosis addressed with stent implantation, with a reduction in the pulmonary regurgitant fraction from 38 to 24%. Attention to branch pulmonary stenosis by transcatheter techniques, such as balloon dilation or stent implantation, could therefore be of benefit to those patients through potential reductions in the degrees of regurgitation. In this regard, Rhodes *et al.* [41] demonstrated significant exercise impairment in tetralogy of Fallot patients with branch pulmonary artery stenosis because of ventilation–perfusion mismatch. Improvement in exercise performance after vessel enlargement is an anticipated but yet an unproven finding.

Pulmonary valve atresia with intact ventricular septum

Pulmonary atresia with intact ventricular septum (PA-IVS) is an infrequent but enigmatic disorder with significant morphological heterogeneity [42]. In the absence of a right ventricular dependent coronary circulation, decompression of the right ventricle (RV) is a component of a treatment algorithm, which attempts to salvage the right heart as a component of a biventricular or so-called $1^1/_2$ ventricular repair. An alternative to primary surgical decompression strategies is the use of percutaneous laser or radiofrequency-assisted perforation of the atretic valve and subsequent balloon dilation. A recent study from our unit reviewed the clinical outcomes and morphological changes to the tricuspid valve and right ventricle after a percutaneous perforation and balloon dilation strategy.[42a]

Between 1992 and 2000, 30 patients with PA-IVS underwent attempted percutaneous valve perforation and balloon dilation of the pulmonary valve. Longitudinal echocardiographic measurements of the tricuspid valve diameter, right ventricular length, and area were recorded. Z scores were calculated according to published formulae. Perforation was achieved in 27 patients. In 14 patients a modified Blalock–Taussig shunt was performed between 2 and 24 days after valve dilation. There were 3 early and 2 late deaths. In survivors, after a follow-up time of 1–87 months, 16 patients had a biventricular circulation, 3 a $1^1/_2$-ventricle circulation, and 1 patient had univentricular palliation with a Fontan operation. Four patients are awaiting further palliation (current status: modified Blalock–Taussig shunt, $n = 1$, or bidirectional cavopulmonary connection, $n = 3$). While the tricuspid valve and right ventricle grew, there was no significant change of the Z scores suggesting that there was no "catch-up" growth.

Percutaneous balloon valvotomy appears an effective treatment strategy for patients with PA-IVS provided that there is a patent infundibulum and a lack of a right ventricular dependant coronary circulation. Despite the observation that right heart growth does not increase with body growth in early follow-up, it appears adequate to maintain a biventricular circulation in many patients.

Other studies

Transcatheter approaches to opening the atretic pulmonary valve in PA-IVS are a relatively recent technical advance, applied to a relatively rare lesion and hence the lack of large patient numbers and follow-up [43–48]. Data addressing the growth of RV structures (tricuspid valve, chamber dimensions) in patients achieving a biventricular circulation using this strategy have not been analyzed previously.

Surgical repair for the neonate with PA-IVS is associated with a high morbidity, a 1-year mortality of 52%, and a 4 years survival of 64% from a recent multicenter surgical study [49]. In a highly selective patient population, 98% survival can be achieved. Final stage surgery for these patients incorporates all potential circulations including a biventricular or $1\frac{1}{2}$-ventricle repair or univentricular palliation. While reasonable survival can be achieved with a biventricular repair as shown in a recent retrospective series by Sano *et al.* [50] in 72% of patients (critical pulmonary stenosis with suprasystemic right ventricular pressures and pinhole patency of the pulmonary valve $n = 6$, pulmonary atresia $n = 19$), Mishima *et al.* [51] observed progressive dilation of the right atrium in their patients leading to the development of arrhythmias. The choice of treatment algorithm depends upon the estimated adequacy of the RV to cope with systemic venous return, the size of the tricuspid valve, and the status of the coronary arteries. In the presence of adequate right heart structures surgical strategies have generally required the creation of a modified Blalock–Taussig shunt in the newborn period to maintain pulmonary artery blood flow in addition to a RV outflow tract reconstruction, leading to a biventricular or $1\frac{1}{2}$-ventricle circulation. In the presence of inadequate right heart anatomy or coronary artery anomalies, patients are managed with staged procedures leading to a univentricular circulation. Prediction of RV growth based upon RV size or tricuspid valve diameter at presentation has not been reproduced by all authors, however.

Clearly there are benefits and disadvantages to a catheter-based approach, compared to a surgical strategy, in patients who will eventually require a univentricular repair. In a recent editorial, Cheatham [52] suggested that as long as there was a tripartite RV and a well-formed infundibulum, a tricuspid valve annulus ≥ 11 mm and membranous atresia of a pulmonary valve with an annulus ≥ 7 mm, transcatheter therapy should be performed. However, no supportive data for these recommendations were given. Our intervention was not predicated upon predefined anatomical measurements, only the presence of a patent tract to the valve plate and the absence of RV dependent coronary blood flow.

While the intervention can be achieved without thoracotomy or cardiopulmonary bypass,

complications include potential vascular occlusion, cardiac perforation with possible tamponade, and rhythm disturbances, all of which are in general self-limiting. Primary transcatheter valvotomy strategy permits (as does surgery) forward flow through the RV outflow tract early in life, which may encourage pulmonary artery growth and with acquired pulmonary insufficiency potential RV growth. Ovaert *et al.* [53] noted from their review of valve perforation and dilation in PA-IVS ($n = 5$) resulting in a biventricular circulation, an increased tricuspid valve diameter over time, with a positive relationship toward a higher tricuspid/mitral valve diameter ratio. In this regard, Hanséus *et al.* [54] showed for patients managed with a surgical algorithm that newborns with a very hypoplastic RV almost always had normalized values for RV size after 52 months (range 18–87 months). The best chamber growth was achieved in patients who underwent RV outflow reconstruction in the neonatal period.

There is debate as to the best method to assess RV size and its adequacy for a biventricular repair as well as how to monitor growth of the chamber and valve. As noted by Ovaert *et al.* [53] normal tricuspid valve growth might not be necessary for an RV competent circulation, to maintain the pulmonary circulation, and its initial size, only a weak indicator of outcome. The irregular topology of the RV in patients with PA-IVS confounds techniques to evaluate chamber anatomy and approaches used for chamber size calculations. An indirect assessment was proposed by Minich *et al.* [55] using a tricuspid/mitral valve ratio of >0.5 as a predictor for a successful biventricular repair. The question was raised whether the initial size of the RV was significant in defining the treatment algorithm, particularly as it was difficult to estimate its size or volume. In patients achieving a biventricular circulation from our data series, the tricuspid valve Z score was lower than in patients with other management formats, whereas RV length and Z scores were not that different between the groups and indeed well below normal [56].

The central question therefore is whether there is appropriate anatomical criteria to select patients, for a particular treatment algorithm. With the diverse spectrum of morphologies seen in this disorder, it is difficult to predict, at time of presentation, whether the RV will have the potential for accommodating systemic blood return. Underscored by our data, management of newborns with

PA-IVS has changed. Only those patients with very diminutive right-sided structures, a severely attenuated infundibulum, or coronary artery anomalies were not considered as candidates for catheter-based valvotomy.

Also shown in this dataset, there was little catch up growth of RV structures over time, apart from the RV area, which showed an initial decrease, followed by more stable development. There was, however, enlargement of the tricuspid valve and RV length, which paralleled normal. Despite apparently inadequate right heart size, a biventricular repair was achievable in 53% of patients. This suggests that a "normal" sized right heart is not required to maintain a normal pulmonary blood flow at rest with an acceptable right atrial pressure. Do some of these patients develop restrictive right heart physiology as in Fallot's tetralogy? (Interesting question to address in longer-term follow-up.)

The requirement of a shunt following successful RV decompression varies amongst clinical units. In children born in Sweden with PA-IVS between 1980 and 1999 when transcatheter management was not available, a systemic to pulmonary shunt was created in 93% of patients [57], whereas the number of shunts constructed in our institution in this population was 46%. While 44% of the patients undergoing a successful interventional valvotomy did not require a surgical shunt procedure in one series, 84% of the patients reported by Alwi *et al.* [58] achieved a biventricular circulation without a shunt. Initially, in our unit, a shunt was offered with failure of the first attempt at weaning prostaglandins, but more recently a policy has evolved, allowing the patients a longer time period to accommodate and improve right ventricular compliance. Persistent forward and regurgitant flow through the opened pulmonary valve may allow the right ventricle to adapt to the circulation and potentially grow, although a "normal" size may not be reached.

The impact of prenatal diagnosis of pulmonary atresia with intact ventricular septum for potential intrauterine or catheter-based postnatal management is an intriguing avenue to pursue, based upon these postnatal observations [59]. Finally, in those patients, who after RV decompression, persist with an inadequate RV inflow or chamber to achieve a biventricular or $1^1/_2$-ventricle circulation, the reduction in RV pressure remains advantageous in the univentricular circulation. A low RV pressure allows

for a nonisometrically contracting chamber and eliminates the development of subaortic stenosis [60].

In conclusion, percutaneous balloon valvotomy appears effective in palliation and in achieving a RV circulation in a selected population with PA-IVS. The technique can be considered as an alternative to surgical intervention in patients with PA-IVS with a patent infundibulum, without a RV-dependant coronary circulation.

The univentricular circulation

With increasing numbers of survivors of the Fontan procedure reaching their teenage years, the long-term complications of this treatment strategy are becoming evident [61]. In this regard, interventional cardiac catheterization plays an important role in management algorithms of patients with either a functional or an anatomical single ventricle prior to, and following, palliation.

Left-to-right shunting

The incidence of systemic-to-pulmonary collaterals has been reported to range between 42 and 71% prior to Fontan completion [62,63]. At longer-term follow-up after the procedure, the reported incidence is approximately 20–30% [62,64]. Understandably, detection of these vessels is dependent on the extent to which they are sought. For example, a change of protocol at one catheterization laboratory to include routine selective angiography was associated with an increase in the detection of collaterals from 25 to 71% [63]. At the Hospital for Sick Children, our practice is to selectively inject subclavian and internal mammary arteries in addition to the descending aorta in all patients undergoing preparatory Fontan catheterization studies.

The hemodynamic effect of these vessels is to increase the volume load on the ventricle, the extent of flow estimated to amount to 8% of cardiac output [65] and up to 55% of the pump flow returning by way of the pulmonary veins [66]. The immediate and longer-term consequences of a slight increase in left atrial pressure in the Fontan circuit have a greater effect on flow than in a biventricular circulation. Furthermore, such collaterals, if they have distal anastomosis to the pulmonary arteries (within the hilum), result in competitive flow, which may affect central pulmonary artery growth. Finally, the potential to increase pulmonary artery pressure may have implications for pulmonary vascular resistance and long-term function of the Fontan circuit. There is, however, little data to help in deciding which collaterals are significant and which are not. Most would agree that a single origin collateral, which when selectively injected with contrast, densely opacifies the pulmonary circulation (arteries or veins), should be occluded. However, this assessment is qualitative, depending upon nonphysiological variables such as rate of injection (hand or power), catheter size and position, and contrast opacity. Additionally, the presence of such vessels should be suspected when washout of contrast is observed during pulmonary artery angiography.

There have been conflicting reports as regards the management of these collateral vessels. Patients with systemic-to-pulmonary collaterals undergoing Fontan completion have been shown to have more chronic pleural effusions [67] and higher mortality [66]; thus occlusion of these vessels prior to surgery would seem a logical approach. In contrast McElhinney et al. [63] showed that such vessels were not associated with a higher incidence of prolonged effusions after surgery and did not correlate with poorer outcomes. Despite these observations, these authors advised that "significant" collaterals should be embolised to optimize haemodynamics in the postoperative period and the longer term. Our own bias is to aggressively search for these vessels by selective angiography. Large vessels, >2 mm in diameter, with a single orifice, prompt, and dense opacification of the pulmonary circulation when selectively injected, are embolised. The vast majority being amenable to coil occlusion. We subscribe to the view that this approach may contribute to a smoother course after surgery.

Right-to-left shunts
These may commonly present as systemic-venous to pulmonary-venous collaterals, baffle leaks or fenestrations deliberately created within the Fontan circuit. While the presence of a right-to-left shunt will lead to systemic desaturation, there may also be benefits associated with their presence. Since the first reports of surgical fenestration of the Fontan circuit for those patients at increased risk [68,69], this modification has become common practice. Such fenestrations provide a route by which cardiac output can be maintained in the presence of an increased systemic venous pressure within the Fontan circuit.

Furthermore, the development and ease of catheter fenestration closure techniques is increased its application largely obviating the need for a surgically placed snare [69].

Major fluctuations in the systemic venous pressure within the Fontan circuit have their most dramatic impact in the immediate postoperative period. Late after surgery, however, most patients gradually become more restricted in activities due to the cyanosis than gain benefit from the fenestration. Closure of fenestrations in suitable patients leads to an increase in systemic saturation, decreased cardiac output, increased pressure within the Fontan circuit, and improved growth [70]. Despite concerns in some earlier reports, patients with hypoplastic left heart syndrome have shown the same hemodynamics after fenestrated Fontan surgery and also following fenestration closure [71]. A significant number of fenestrations may close spontaneously (20–30%), so the optimal timing of closure is unclear. Similarly, the optimum device (umbrella, plug or coil) has yet to be defined.

Not all patients will tolerate fenestration closure. Hemodynamic criteria for fenestration closure include an increase in arterial saturation without a significant concomitant drop in systemic blood pressure or increase in Fontan baffle pressures. Suitability may be assessed by balloon test occlusion of the surgical defect, acquiring a haemodynamic profile. Generally, systemic venous pressure and arterial oxygen saturation are monitored and arteriovenous oxygen content difference (C_{ao2}, C_{vo2}) calculated [64]. If oxygen consumption can be measured, cardiac output (Q_s), systemic oxygen transport (SOT; $Q_s \times C_{ao2}$) and oxygen extraction (($C_{ao2} - C_{vo2})/(C_{ao2})$; ($V_{o2}$/SOT)) additionally calculated.

Complete separation of the systemic and venous circulations by elimination of shunting is accomplished at the expense of a decreased Q_s and oxygen delivery, despite improved levels of arterial oxygenation. Hijazi and colleagues [72] studied 14 patients shortly after surgery (median 32 days), before and after test occlusion. Mixed venous saturation, oxygen consumption, and right atrial pressure did not change while systemic saturation rose, left atrial pressure, cardiac output, and systemic oxygen transport fell, and oxygen extraction increased. Indeed, cardiac output fell an average of 24%, while aortic saturation and oxygen content increased by approximately 13%. This increase in saturation was insufficient to balance the fall in cardiac output and systemic oxygen delivery fell. As oxygen consumption in this study did not change before and after test occlusion, the patients compensated for the decrease in oxygen delivery by an increase in oxygen extraction. As such, acute fenestration closure resulted in decreased oxygen availability to the peripheral tissues and heart. Closure of the fenestration thus eliminates the right-to-left shunt and minimizes the risk of a paradoxical embolus and stroke, but this is achieved at the expense of a reduced cardiac output and systemic oxygen delivery and may decrease cardiac reserve.

If a patient has more than a 30% reduction in cardiac output associated with a significant increase in right atrial pressure (>4 mm Hg), the patient should not undergo permanent closure [72]. Angiographic assessment of the baffle circulation to determine the presence of anatomic obstruction, pulmonary artery distortion, or stenosis and the presence of aortopulmonary collaterals further supplements the catheterization assessment, particularly if an elevated systemic venous pressure is present. Other criteria for permanent fenestration closure used by Bridges et al. [64] include a right atrial pressure of <18 mm Hg during test occlusion, an increase in the arteriovenous oxygen difference of <33%, or a right atrial saturation of >40% [64].

Bridges and colleagues [64] additionally investigated whether the results of the hemodynamic assessment could predict later functional status, and if the catheterization procedure would further affect patient management. The hemodynamic responses to test occlusion were qualitatively similar to those of Hijazi et al. [72]. When comparing baseline measurements, patients that responded unfavourably to fenestration closure had higher systemic venous pressures, and lower arterial oxygen saturations than the favourable responders. However, was overlap between groups [64]. Furthermore, the catheter study identified a number of patients who had branch pulmonary artery stenosis and aortopulmonary collaterals requiring intervention. Systemic venous pressure measured prior to intervention was slightly higher in those patients with these additional lesions (13 vs. 11 mm Hg, $P < 0.01$). Also identified was a significant association of right atrial pressure in predicting subsequent functional class, a higher right atrial pressure reducing the likelihood of being in functional Class 1, those with a right atrial pressure

of <16 mm Hg more likely to be in Class 1. It was also noted that baseline systemic venous pressure (before test occlusion) did not predict the response (i.e., <16 mm Hg) with test occlusion.

The decision to close a fenestration, in those patients with a favourable response, was based on the assumption that the benefits from a high oxygen saturation outweigh the lower cardiac output and increased systemic venous pressure that ensues. Adolescents and adults with persistent cyanosis are typically more symptomatic, with headaches, reduced concentration, parasthesiae, fatigue, and myalgia. There is the additional risk as noted above of paradoxical emboli. As such, fenestration closure is favoured when the hemodynamics are reasonable.

This approach to assessment is successful in the majority of cases, although occasionally, hemodynamics may deteriorate following fenestration closure in apparently otherwise suitable patients. Senzaki and colleagues [73] reported 2 patients with suitable hemodynamic responses to test occlusion based on changes in central venous pressure and cardiac output. One of the patients, however, developed symptoms of heart failure following closure. At follow-up catheterization, there was no apparent difference in ventricular performance based on hemodynamics at rest. Challenge by atrial pacing and dobutamine, however, elicited markedly different responses in the 2 patients. The patient with symptoms of heart failure showed a blunted force–frequency and relaxation–frequency response to increases in heart rate. Furthermore, the same patient showed a comparatively depressed contractile response to dobutamine challenge when assessed by end-systolic pressure-area measurements during transient caval occlusion.

It is unclear which patients require more detailed assessment; however, the approach relying on basic hemodynamics would seem to be adequate in the vast majority of patients. Indeed, in a long-term study (median follow-up 3.4 years) of 154 patients following device closure of Fontan fenestration, clinical decompensation was rare, affecting 4.5% of the cohort [70]. In this study, there were 2 deaths, both patients having undergone fenestration closure within a month of surgery. One patient developed congestive failure 2.5 years after surgery and died with poor ventricular function following unexpected cardiac arrest associated with a ventricular arrhythmia. The second patient having undergone a fenestrated Fontan procedure at 10 years of age, developed progressive aortic incompetence and left ventricular dysfunction resulting in congestive symptoms and acute decompensation with a pericardial effusion 8 years after surgery. Two further patients decompensated; one with chronic ascites and the other with protein losing enteropathy. Patients that decompensated were significantly more like to have undergone fenestration closure earlier in the postoperative period.

Late fenestration for post-Fontan complications after surgery

Despite huge improvements in early survival following the Fontan procedure, late complications such as the development of the chronic pleural effusions, low cardiac output, and protein losing enteropathy persist. These may in part be explained by the inherently disadvantageous circulation a Fontan patient has, with decreased ventricular power and increased afterload profiles, limiting reserve capabilities [74].

As noted above, some surgically created fenestrations close spontaneously and some patients present with late problems after device closure. In this regard, there have been reports of patient improvement following creation of a communication within the Fontan circuit to reestablish the right-to-left shunt. This procedure can now be readily accomplished using catheter techniques regardless of the type of Fontan circulation.

Rychik et al. [75] reported their findings in 9 Fontan patients undergoing surgical creation of fenestration at a postoperative interval ranging from 3 to 81 months after surgery. Four patients had chronic effusions and 5 had protein-losing enteropathy. Improvement was observed in 6 patients with resolution of effusions ($n = 3$) and protein-losing enteropathy ($n = 3$) within 6 weeks of surgery. A recurrence of effusions with spontaneous closure of the fenestration was reported in one of the patients, which again resolved after refenestration. The patients with resolved protein losing enteropathy remained symptom free 2 years after fenestration creation. In a later study of patients with protein-losing enteropathy, Rychik reported abnormal Doppler flow patterns in the superior mesenteric artery of Fontan patients compared with normals [76]. Within the Fontan group, those with protein-losing enteropa-

thy showed patterns consistent with significant further elevation of mesenteric vascular resistance.

Other authors have also reported low cardiac output to be an important factor in protein-losing enteropathy [77] and it is likely that increased resistance to flow within the mesenteric bed is a compensatory mechanism. The cause of protein-losing enteropathy and chronic pleural effusions remains uncertain; however, the creation of fenestrations does seem to be beneficial in some patients. In a study of the flow patterns in the hepatic veins and inferior caval vein, Hsia et al. [78] noted significantly less retrograde flow in the hepatic vein of patients with a fenestrated total cavopulmonary connection compared with those who were nonfenestrated. The combination of this and increased cardiac output following creation of a fenestration may partly underlie the improvement seen in these patients.

Transcatheter completion of the Fontan circuit

This exciting prospect is quickly becoming a reality with reports of procedures in patients following initial animal studies. The potential opportunity to avoid a further operation in patients with a bidirectional cavopulmonary anastomosis has obvious implications for patient morbidity and workload. Different approaches have been proposed but essentially rely upon a transcatheter method to establish continuity between the inferior caval vein and pulmonary circulation. The insertion of a ring mounted membrane at the junction of the oversewn superior caval vein and pulmonary arteries at the time of surgery, which can be perforated and dilated with a covered stent to establish flow and complete the Fontan circulation, is one approach being investigated in our unit. Although improvements in surgical techniques have greatly reduced the morbidity and mortality associated with Fontan completion following a bidirectional cavopulmonary anastomosis, this promising technique may allow further reduction in perioperative complications.

Coarctation of the aorta

Since the first report of surgical repair of coarctation in 1945, it has become evident that the condition is not simply an isolated, discrete mechanical obstruction within a blood vessel that is correctable by surgery. Patients with "successfully repaired" coarctation remain at risk of developing hypertension, and premature cardiovascular disease with its attendant morbidity and mortality. In addition to surgery, treatment options now include balloon dilation and stent insertion; indeed, catheter intervention has become the method of first choice in the setting of recoarctation. As described below, although of benefit, even complete abolition of the pressure gradient does not correct the vascular abnormalities associated with aortic coarctation. As such, this must be considered in the long-term management of patients following "successful repair" regardless of technique of intervention.

Hemodynamic changes in patients following coarctation repair

It has been well described that despite surgical success, there are persistent vascular abnormalities intrinsic to the vessel wall in addition to those at the site of surgical scar. Theoretical modeling of even minimal stenosis within a distensible vessel with pulsatile flow has shown marked flow disturbances and alterations of wall shear stress [79]. With vasodilation and increased flow (by 50%) the vortex circulation in the poststenotic region has been predicted to induce shear stress up to five times greater than basal levels. Interestingly, with vasodilation, wall shear stress in diastole is even greater than the systolic peak.

In a study of 13 patients undergoing balloon dilation of coarctation, Xu et al. [80] measured indices of aortic wall stiffness, distensibility, and compliance at various levels relative to the site of stenosis. Luminal dimensions were measured using intravascular ultrasound and aortic pressures by fluid filled catheters. Measurements were made in the aortic segments proximal, distal, and at the site of coarctation before and after dilation. The mean gradient across the coarctation for the group was 33 ± 10 mm Hg and age ranged from 5 months to 16.5 years. The stiffness ß index of the coarctation segment and the proximal aorta were significantly greater than that of the distal segment. Distensibility of the coarctation segment and proximal aorta were significantly less than that of the distal segment. Following balloon dilation the mean residual gradient was 10 ± 9 mm Hg and intravascular ultrasound showed the presence of an intimal flap in all patients. The stiffness ß index did not change significantly in any of the three segments and distensibilty of the proximal and coarcted segments were unchanged. As such, the abnormal proximal aortic stiffness may

be a strong contributing factor in the development of late hypertension after repair.

A noninvasive study of normotensive patients following coarctation repair, who had arm–leg blood pressure gradient of <20 mm Hg has also shown a significantly increased stiffness ß index for the transverse aorta [81]. Furthermore, univariate analysis showed that aortic stiffness did not significantly correlate with residual aortic narrowing. As expected, left ventricular mass index significantly correlated positively with residual aortic narrowing.

Further evidence for abnormal upper body vasculature has been described by the vascular dysfunction in response to flow-mediated dilation and sublingual nitroglycerin in patients after coarctation repair [82]. Brachial artery responses were significantly impaired in comparison to controls, whereas there were no significant differences in posterior tibial artery response to the same challenge. Pulse wave velocities of the brachial-radial and femoral-dorsalis pedis tracts were also examined in order to measure arterial stiffness. Similarly, there were significant differences in the stiffness of the upper limb arteries, but not those of the lower limb, in comparison with controls. Interestingly, age at surgical repair was significantly related to brachial-radial pulse wave velocity, but not to brachial responses to flow-mediated dilation or nitroglycerin. It appears, therefore, that early repair is associated with preservation of the arterial elasticity but endothelial reactivity remains abnormal. As expected, left ventricular mass index significantly correlates with residual arch gradient.

Patients following repair have also been shown to have increased left ventricular contractile function based on endocardial indices of contractility [83,84]. Although the validity of endocardial indices in the setting of ventricular hypertrophy has been questioned, analysis of midwall shortening and end-systolic fibre stress, has also demonstrated enhanced contractility [85]. Even though the increased contractile performance could be partly attributable to the intrinsic vessel abnormalities described above, the midwall shortening indices were only significantly elevated compared to controls in those patients with a residual arm–leg blood pressure gradient of >15 mm Hg.

Balloon dilation

Angioplasty acts by tearing the vessel wall, with disruption of the wall layers. Intimal and medial lesions are more likely to be detected by transesophageal echocardiography or intravascular ultrasound than by angiography. Sohn *et al.* [86] reported their findings in 17 patients following balloon dilation of an aortic coarctation. A minor flap or dissection was defined as a thin mobile membrane extending into the wall over no more than a quarter of the circumference of the aorta on ultrasonography. Those more extensive were considered to be major lesions. Intravascular ultrasound detected major dissections in 14 and minor lesions in 2 patients. In comparison, angiography detected lesions in only 8 of the 17 patients. Repeated examination of 6 patients with major dissections at follow-up catheterization by intravascular ultrasound showed persistent major lesions in 2, a decrease to minor lesions in 2, and the remaining 2 showed only scarring without intimal flaps.

The incidence of true aneurysm formation ranges from 5 to 14% in recent reports of balloon angioplasty for aortic coarctation. Considering that the time taken for the completion of the healing process is lengthy and persistent hemodynamic changes noted, even in those patients with only minimal gradients, the incidence may increase with longer follow-up. However, at present, with 15 years follow-up this does not appear to be the case.

Restenosis

Although balloon angioplasty mostly results in immediate and successful relief of obstruction, restenosis can occur. The incidence in older children with native coarctation is approximately 10%. Long-term follow-up of up to 12 years after angioplasty for re-coarctation showed 72% of patients to be free of further intervention [87]. Various investigators have identified risk factors for restenosis, as being hypoplasia of the isthmus [88,89] and also the absolute size of the coarctation segment [88]. Less predictable factors include elastic recoil or unfavorable scarring following the previous angioplasty. For these reasons, stent implantation as an alternative mode of therapy in appropriate patients has been gaining favor.

Stent implantation

The use of endovascular stents in coarctation was first reported in the early 1990s [90]. There have now been several recent reports of large numbers of patients having undergone stent implantation with short-term follow-up.

Stent implantation in older patients results in excellent immediate relief of stenosis with a slight increase in gradient at follow-up. In a study of 54 patients (mean age 22 ± 9 years range 8–49 years), follow-up gradients, where available, had increased from a mean of 5 ± 8 immediately after implantation to 7 ± 10 mm Hg at a mean of 25 months [91]. Similar results were reported in a slightly older patient group (mean age 30 ± 13 years) with mean immediate gradient after stenting of 3 ± 5 mm Hg and a mean gradient of 4 ± 8 mm Hg at a mean follow-up of 2 years. Marshall *et al.* [92] reporting their findings in 33 patients with median age of 14 years (range 5–60 years), showed that gradients increased from 4 mm Hg (range 0–30 mm Hg) to 14 mm Hg (range 0–76 mm Hg) at a median of 7 months in those that were recatheterized.

De Lezo *et al.* [93] reported their findings in 48 patients with a mean age of 14 ± 12 years, though of interest, they ranged from 1 month to 45 years. Thirty patients were available for follow-up at a mean 25 months after implantation. Although immediate gradient relief was achieved in all with a reduction from 42 ± 12 mm Hg to 3 ± 4 mm Hg, at restudy, the mean gradient had risen to a mean of 14 ± 11 mm Hg. Of note, restenosis in 3 of the 5 children treated <2 years of age was due to significant neointimal proliferation producing a mean gradient of 37 ± 3 mm Hg. Intimal in-growth was noted to be mainly located focally, at either the inflow or outflow of the stent, suggesting disruption of blood flow in these areas. Nevertheless, restenosis does not appear to be a significant clinical problem, and in a number of patients may be addressed with further dilation.

Although the immediate and short-term efficacy in reduction of gradients has been demonstrated, the hemodynamic consequences of a rigid segment due to the stent implantation are uncertain. In a porcine model of stent implantation in an otherwise normal aorta, there was no significant difference in aortic pulse wave, maximum velocity of flow or stiffness index ß, between those animals with 3 cm long stents and controls, when restudied at a median of 7 weeks following implantation using ultrasonic crystals in the aorta [94]. Interestingly, using the augmentation index as a measure of the degree of wave reflection, it was noted that following stenting, there was no significant difference between groups. However, using an absolute induction angiometer, *in situ* measurements of changes of vessel diameter have shown an immediate decrease in mean vessel compliance in the stented segment [95]. In this study, as early as 1 week after the procedure, some of the stented arteries were noncompliant. Postmortem examination showed reduced compliance to be associated with a periadventitial fibrous reaction around the stented vessels. Although neither of these studies are exact models of stenting of coarctation it could be inferred that at least in the short term, the resulting changes in vessel compliance do not appear to significantly disrupt blood flow. Caution is advised when concluding the effects of stenting on the aortic wall. Loss of exposure to the normal pulsatile changes in vessel diameter alters the phenotype of vascular smooth muscle and connective tissue, increasing apoptosis, which may result in aneurysm formation [96].

Transcatheter relief of stenosis

Relief of stenosis using transcatheter techniques does not affect the intrinsic vessel abnormalities present in coarctation patients [80]. There is, however, still obvious benefit to relief of important obstruction and most would advise that patients with resting gradients of >20 mm Hg, or upper body hypertension warrant intervention. Whether lesser degrees of obstruction should also be addressed and by which means is less clear. Theoretically, there may be a lower limit of obstruction below which no significant additional benefit is gained when the intrinsic compliance abnormalities are taken into account. Small but significant reduction in left ventricular end-diastolic pressure has, however, been shown in a group of patients undergoing stent implantation for coarctation with a median baseline gradient of 25 mm Hg (range 15–90 mm Hg) [92]. Left ventricular end-diastolic pressure at a median of 7 months (range 3–46 months) after stenting had decreased from median 17 mm Hg (range 10–24 mm Hg) to median 14 mm Hg (range 5–24 mm Hg)($P = 0.002$).

Summary

The intrinsic arterial abnormalities in the upper body following surgical repair appear to be less severe with younger age at the time of operation. Patients have enhanced contractility and left ventricular mass compared with the normal population. Midwall indices of ventricular contractile performance are significantly elevated in those patients with a residual arm–leg blood pressure gradient of >15 mm Hg. Even though catheter intervention is unable to improve the vascular dysfunction of the proximal arterial tree, abolition of residual stenosis has been shown to improve the elevated end-diastolic pressures seen even in patients with relatively mild resting gradients. Although stent implantation has been shown to successfully reduce gradients, there are residual flow disturbances with a stent in place. Whether the presence of a rigid segment within a distensible vessel and a pulsatile flow will have detrimental effects in the long term are unclear; however, the prospect of biodegradeable stents in the future may negate this concern.

References

1. Lock KE, Keane JF, Perry SB, eds. Diagnostic and Interventional Catheterization in Congenital Heart Disease, 2nd edn. Kluwer, Amsterdam, 1999.
2. Borow KM, Colan SD, Neumann A. Altered left ventricular mechanics in patients with valvular aortic stenosis and coarctation of the aorta: Effects on systolic performance and late outcome. Circulation 1985; 72(3):515–522.
3. Assey ME, Wisenbaugh T, Spann JF Jr, et al. Unexpected persistence into adulthood of low wall stress in patients with congenital aortic stenosis: Is there a fundamental difference in the hypertrophic response to a pressure overload present from birth? Circulation 1987; 75(5):973–979.
4. Denslow S. Constraints on cardiac hypertrophy imposed by myocardial viscosity. J Appl Physiol 2000; 89(3):1022–1032.
5. Aoyagi T, Fujii AM, Flanagan MF, et al. Transition from compensated hypertrophy to intrinsic myocardial dysfunction during development of left ventricular pressure-overload hypertrophy in conscious sheep. Systolic dysfunction precedes diastolic dysfunction. Circulation 1993; 88(5, pt 1):2415–2425.
6. Keane JF, Driscoll DJ, Gersony WM, et al. Second natural history study of congenital heart defects. Results of treatment of patients with aortic valvar stenosis. Circulation 1993; 87(2 suppl):I16–I27.
7. Perloff JK, Warnes CA. Challenges posed by adults with repaired congenital heart disease. Circulation 2001; 103(21):2637–2643.

8. Wagner HR, Ellison RC, Keane JF, *et al.* Clinical course in aortic stenosis. Circulation 1977; 56(1 Suppl):I47–I56.

9. Bonow RO, Carabello B, de Leon AC Jr, *et al.* Guidelines for the management of patients with valvular heart disease: Executive summary. A report of the American College of Cardiology/American Heart Association Task Force on Practice Guidelines (Committee on Management of Patients with Valvular Heart Disease). Circulation 1998; 98(18):1949–1984.

10. Lock KE, Keane JF, Perry SB, eds. Diagnostic and Interventional Catheterization in Congenital Heart Disease, 2nd edition, Kluwer, Amsterdam, pp. 151–178, 1999.

11. Beekman RH, Rocchini AP, Gillon JH, *et al.* Hemodynamic determinants of the peak systolic left ventricular-aortic pressure gradient in children with valvar aortic stenosis. Am J Cardiol 1992; 69(8):813–815.

12. Lima VC, Zahn E, Houde C, *et al.* Non-invasive determination of the systolic peak-to-peak gradient in children with aortic stenosis: Validation of a mathematical model. Cardiol Young 2000; 10(2):115–119.

13. Shim D, Michelfelder EC, Lee KJ, *et al.* Effect of balloon aortic valvuloplasty of congenital aortic stenosis in children in regression of left ventricular mass. Am J Cardiol 2001; 87(7):916–919.

14. Justo RN, McCrindle BW, Benson LN, *et al.* Aortic valve regurgitation after surgical versus percutaneous balloon valvotomy for congenital aortic valve stenosis. Am J Cardiol 1996; 77(15):1332–1338.

15. Perloff JK. Normal myocardial growth and the development and regulation of ventricular mass. In: Perloff JK, Child JS, eds., Congenital Heart Disease in the Adult, 2nd edn. Saunders, Philadelphia, 1998.

16. Starling MR, Kirsh MM, Montgomery DG, *et al.* Mechanisms for left ventricular systolic dysfunction in aortic regurgitation: Importance for predicting the functional response to aortic valve replacement. J Am Coll Cardiol 1991; 7(4):887–897.

17. McCrindle BW. Independent predictors of immediate results of percutaneous balloon aortic valvotomy in children. Valvuloplasty and angioplasty of congenital anomalies (VACA) Registry Investigators. Am J Cardiol 1996; 77(4):286–293.

18. Mullins CE, Nihill MR, Vick GW III, *et al.* Double balloon technique for dilation of valvular or vessel stenosis in congenital and acquired heart disease. J Am Coll Cardiol 1987; 10(1):107–114.

19. Beekman RH, Rocchini AP, Crowley DC, *et al.* Comparison of single and double balloon valvuloplasty in children with aortic stenosis. J Am Coll Cardiol 1988; 12(2):480–485.

20. De Giovanni JV, Edgar RA, Cranston A. Adenosine induced transient cardiac standstill in catheter interventional procedures for congenital heart disease. Heart 1998; 80(4):330–333.

21. Yeager SB. Balloon selection for double balloon valvotomy. J Am Coll Cardiol 1987; 9(2):467–468.

22. Egito ES, Moore P, O'Sullivan J, *et al.* Transvascular balloon dilation for neonatal critical aortic stenosis: Early and midterm results. J Am Coll Cardiol 1997; 29(2):442–447.

23. Borghi A, Agnoletti G, Poggiani C. Surgical cutdown of the right carotid artery for aortic balloon valvuloplasty in infancy: Midterm follow-up. Pediatr Cardiol 2001; 22(3):194–197.

24. Peuster M, Fink C, Schoof S, *et al.* Anterograde balloon valvuloplasty for the treatment of neonatal critical valvar aortic stenosis. Catheter Cardiovasc Interv 2002; 56(4):516–520.

25. Magee AG, Nykanen D, McCrindle BW, *et al.* Balloon dilation of severe aortic stenosis in the neonate: Comparison of anterograde and retrograde catheter approaches. J Am Coll Cardiol 1997; 30(4):1061–1066.

26. Rhodes LA, Colan SD, Perry SB, *et al.* Predictors of survival in neonates with critical aortic stenosis. Circulation 1991; 84(6):2325–2335.

27. Hosking MC, Benson LN, Freedom RM. A femoral vein-femoral artery loop technique for aortic dilation in children. Cathet Cardiovasc Diagn 1991; 23(4):253–256.

28. Alexiou C, Chen Q, Langley SM, *et al.* Is there still a place for open surgical valvotomy in the management of aortic stenosis in children? The view from Southampton. Eur J Cardiothorac Surg 2001; 20(2):239–246.

29. McCrindle BW, Blackstone EH, Williams WG, *et al.* Are outcomes of surgical versus transcatheter balloon valvotomy equivalent in neonatal critical aortic stenosis? Circulation 2001; 104(12, suppl 1):I152–I158.

30. Schneider M, Zartner P, Sidiropoulos A, *et al.* Stent implantation of the arterial duct in newborns with duct-dependent circulation. Eur Heart J 1998; 19(9):1401–1409.

31. Gibbs JL, Uzun O, Blackburn ME, *et al.* Fate of the stented arterial duct. Circulation 1999; 99(20):2621–2625.

32. Clyman RI, Tannenbaum J, Chen YQ, *et al.* Ductus arteriosus smooth muscle cell migration on collagen: Dependence on laminin and its receptors. J Cell Sci 1994; 107(pt 4):1007–1018.

33. Marx SO, Marks AR. Bench to bedside: The development of rapamycin and its application to stent restenosis. Circulation 2001; 104(8):852–855.

34. Redington A, Penny D, Rigby M, *et al.* Antegrade diastolic pulmonary arterial flow as a marker right ventricular restriction after complete repair of pulmonary atresia with intact septum and critical pulmonary valve stenosis. Cardiol Young 1992; 2: 382–386.

35. Gatzoulis MA, Balaji S, Webber SA, *et al.* Risk factors for arrhythmia and sudden cardiac death late after repair of tetralogy of Fallot: A multicentre study. Lancet 2000; 356(9234):975–981.

36. Carvalho JS, Shinebourne EA, Busst C, *et al.* Exercise capacity after complete repair of tetralogy of Fallot: Deleterious effects of residual pulmonary regurgitation. Br Heart J 1992; 67(6):470–473.

37. Bonhoeffer P, Boudjemline Y, Saliba Z, *et al.* Transcatheter implantation of a bovine valve in pulmonary position: A lamb study. Circulation 2000; 102(7):813–816.

38. Bonhoeffer P, Boudjemline Y, Qureshi SA, *et al.* Percutaneous insertion of the pulmonary valve. J Am Coll Cardiol 2002; 39(10):1664–1669.

39. Kang, IS, Redington AR, Benson LN, *et al.* Differential regurgitation in branch pulmonary arteries after repair of tetralogy of Fallot: A phase-contrast cine magnetic resonance study. Circulation 2003; 107(23): 2938–2942.

40. Chaturvedi RR, Kilner PJ, White PA, *et al.* Increased airway pressure and simulated branch pulmonary artery stenosis increase pulmonary regurgitation after repair of tetralogy of Fallot. Real-time analysis with a conductance catheter technique. Circulation 1997; 95(3):643–649.

41. Rhodes J, Dave A, Pulling MC, *et al.* Effect of pulmonary artery stenoses on the cardiopulmonary response to exercise following repair of tetralogy of Fallot. Am J Cardiol 1998; 81(10):1217–1219.

42. Freedom RM. The morphologic variations of pulmonary atresia with intact ventricular septum: Guidelines for surgical intervention Pediatr Cardiol 1983; 4(3):183–188.

42a. Humpl T, Soderberg B, McCrindle B W et al. Percutaneous balloon valvotomy is pulmonary atresia with intact ventricular septum: impact on patient case. Circulation 2003; 108(7): 826–832.

43. Hausdorf G, Schneider M, Schirmer KR, *et al.* Interventional high frequency perforation and enlargement of the outflow tract of pulmonary atresia. Z Kardiol 1993; 82(2):123–130.

44. Hausdorf G, Schulze-Neick I, Lange PE. Radiofrequency-assisted "reconstruction" of the right ventricular outflow tract in muscular pulmonary atresia with ventricular septal defect. Br Heart J 1993; 69(4):343–346.

45. Rosenthal E, Qureshi SA, Chan KC, *et al.* Radiofrequency-assisted balloon dilatation in patients with pulmonary valve atresia and an intact ventricular septum. Br Heart J 1993; 69(4):347–351.

46. Justo RN, Nykanen DG, Williams WG, *et al.* Transcatheter perforation of the right ventricular outflow tract as initial therapy for pulmonary valve atresia and intact ventricular septum in the newborn. Cathet Cardiovasc Diagn 1997; 40(4):408–413.

47. Gibbs JL, Blackburn ME, Uzun O, *et al.* Laser valvotomy with balloon valvoplasty for pulmonary atresia with intact ventricular septum: Five years' experience. Heart 1997; 77(3):225–228.

48. Gournay V, Piechaud JF, Delogu A, *et al.* Balloon valvotomy for critical stenosis or atresia of pulmonary valve in newborns. J Am Coll Cardiol 1995; 26(7):1725–1731.

49. Hanley FL, Sade RM, Blackstone EH, *et al.* Outcomes in neonatal pulmonary atresia with intact ventricular septum. A multiinstitutional study. J Thorac Cardiovasc Surg 1993; Mar;105(3):406–427.

50. Sano S, Ishino K, Kawada M, *et al.* Staged biventricular repair of pulmonary atresia or stenosis with intact ventricular septum. Ann Thorac Surg 2000; 70(5):1501–1506.

51. Mishima A, Asano M, Sasaki S, *et al.* Long-term outcome for right heart function after biventricular repair of pulmonary atresia and intact ventricular septum. Jpn J Thorac Cardiovasc Surg 2000; 48(3):145–152.

52. Cheatham JP. To perforate or not to perforate-that's the question . . . or is it? Just ask Richard! Cathet Cardiovasc Diagn 1997; 42(4):403–404.

53. Ovaert C, Qureshi SA, Rosenthal E, *et al.* Growth of the right ventricle after successful transcatheter pulmonary valvotomy in neonates and infants with pulmonary atresia and intact ventricular septum. J Thorac Cardiovasc Surg 1998; 115(5):1055–1062.

54. Hanseus K, Bjorkhem G, Lundstrom NR, *et al.* Cross-sectional echocardiographic measurements of right ventricular size and growth in patients with pulmonary atresia and intact ventricular septum. Pediatr Cardiol 1991; 12(3):135–142.

55. Minich LL, Tani LY, Ritter S, *et al.* Usefulness of the preoperative tricuspid/mitral valve ratio for predicting outcome in pulmonary atresia with intact ventricular septum. Am J Cardiol 2000; 85(11):1325–1328.

56. Powell AJ, Mayer JE, Lang P, *et al.* Outcome in infants with pulmonary atresia, intact ventricular septum, and right ventricle-dependent coronary circulation. Am J Cardiol 2000; 86(11):1272–1274, A9.

57. Ekman Joelsson BM, Sunnegardh J, Hanseus K, *et al.* The outcome of children born with pulmonary

atresia and intact ventricular septum in Sweden from 1980 to 1999. Scand Cardiovasc J 2001; 35(3):192–198.

58. Alwi M, Geetha K, Bilkis AA, *et al.* Pulmonary atresia with intact ventricular septum percutaneous radiofrequency-assisted valvotomy and balloon dilation versus surgical valvotomy and Blalock Taussig shunt. J Am Coll Cardiol 2000; 35(2):468–476.

59. Kohl T, Szabo Z, Suda K, *et al.* Fetoscopic and open transumbilical fetal cardiac catheterization in sheep. Potential approaches for human fetal cardiac intervention. Circulation 1997; 95(4):1048–1053.

60. Freedom RM. Subaortic obstruction and the Fontan operation. Ann Thorac Surg 1998; 66(2):649–652.

61. Freedom RM, Hamilton R, Yoo SJ, *et al.* The Fontan procedure: Analysis of cohorts and late complications. Cardiol Young 2000; 10(4):307–331.

62. Triedman JK, Bridges ND, Mayer JE Jr, *et al.* Prevalence and risk factors for aortopulmonary collateral vessels after Fontan and bidirectional Glenn procedures. J Am Coll Cardiol 1993; 22(1):207–215.

63. McElhinney DB, Reddy VM, Tworetzky W, *et al.* Incidence and implications of systemic to pulmonary collaterals after bidirectional cavopulmonary anastomosis. Ann Thorac Surg 2000;69(4):1222–1228.

64. Bridges ND, Lock JE, Mayer JE Jr, *et al.* Cardiac catheterization and test occlusion of the interatrial communication after the fenestrated Fontan operation. J Am Coll Cardiol 1995; 25(7):1712–1717.

65. Salim MA, Case CL, Sade RM, *et al.* Pulmonary/systemic flow ratio in children after cavopulmonary anastomosis. J Am Coll Cardiol 1995; 25(3):735–738.

66. Ichikawa H, Yagihara T, Kishimoto H, *et al.* Extent of aortopulmonary collateral blood flow as a risk factor for Fontan operations. Ann Thorac Surg 1995; 59(2):433–437.

67. Spicer RL, Uzark KC, Moore JW, *et al.* Aortopulmonary collateral vessels and prolonged pleural effusions after modified Fontan procedures. Am Heart J 1996; 131(6):1164–1168.

68. Bridges ND, Lock JE, Castaneda AR. Baffle fenestration with subsequent transcatheter closure. Modification of the Fontan operation for patients at increased risk. Circulation 1990; 82(5):1681–1689.

69. Laks H, Pearl JM, Haas GS, *et al.* Partial Fontan: Advantages of an adjustable interatrial communication. Ann Thorac Surg 1991; 52(5):1084–1094.

70. Goff DA, Blume ED, Gauvreau K, *et al.* Clinical outcome of fenestrated Fontan patients after closure: The first 10 years. Circulation 2000; 102(17):2094–2099.

71. Lloyd TR, Rydberg A, Ludomirsky A, *et al.* Late fenestration closure in the hypoplastic left heart syndrome: Comparison of hemodynamic changes. Am Heart J 1998; 136(2):302–306.

72. Hijazi ZM, Fahey JT, Kleinman CS, *et al.* Hemodynamic evaluation before and after closure of fenestrated Fontan. An acute study of changes in oxygen delivery. Circulation 1992; 86(1):196–202.

73. Senzaki H, Naito C, Masutani S, *et al.* Hemodynamic evaluation for closing interatrial communication after fenestrated Fontan operation. J Thorac Cardiovasc Surg 2001; 121(6):1200–1202.

74. Senzaki H, Masutani S, Kobayashi J, *et al.* Ventricular afterload and ventricular work in Fontan circulation: Comparison with normal two-ventricle circulation and single-ventricle circulation with Blalock-Taussig shunts. Circulation 2002; 105(24):2885–2892.

75. Rychik J, Rome JJ, Jacobs ML. Late surgical fenestration for complications after the Fontan operation. Circulation 1997; 96(1):33–36.

76. Rychik J, Gui-Yang S. Relation of mesenteric vascular resistance after Fontan operation and protein-losing enteropathy. Am J Cardiol 2002; 90(6):672–674.

77. Mertens L, Hagler DJ, Sauer U, *et al.* Protein-losing enteropathy after the Fontan operation: An international multicenter study. PLE study group. J Thorac Cardiovasc Surg 1998; 115(5):1063–1073.

78. Hsia TY, Khambadkone S, Redington AN, *et al.* Effect of fenestration on the sub-diaphragmatic venous hemodynamics in the total-cavopulmonary connection. Eur J Cardiothorac Surg 2001; 19(6):785–792.

79. Cavalcanti S. Hemodynamics of an artery with mild stenosis. J Biomech 1995; 28(4):387–399.

80. Xu J, Shiota T, Omoto R, *et al.* Intravascular ultrasound assessment of regional aortic wall stiffness, distensibility, and compliance in patients with coarctation of the aorta. Am Heart J 1997; 134(1):93–98.

81. Ong CM, Canter CE, Gutierrez FR, *et al.* Increased stiffness and persistent narrowing of the aorta after successful repair of coarctation of the aorta: Relationship to left ventricular mass and blood pressure at rest and with exercise. Am Heart J 1992; 123(6):1594–1600.

82. de Divitiis M, Pilla C, Kattenhorn M, *et al.* Vascular dysfunction after repair of coarctation of the aorta: Impact of early surgery. Circulation 2001; 104(12, suppl 1):I165–I170.

83. Pacileo G, Pisacane C, Russo MG, *et al.* Left ventricular remodeling and mechanics after successful repair of aortic coarctation. Am J Cardiol 2001; 87(6):748–752.

84. Kimball TR, Reynolds JM, Mays WA, *et al.* Persistent hyperdynamic cardiovascular state at rest and during exercise in children after successful repair of coarctation of the aorta. J Am Coll Cardiol 1994; 24(1):194–200.

85. Gentles TL, Sanders SP, Colan SD. Misrepresentation of left ventricular contractile function by endocardial indexes: Clinical implications after coarctation repair. Am Heart J 2000; 140(4):585–595.

86. Sohn S, Rothman A, Shiota T, *et al.* Acute and follow-up intravascular ultrasound findings after balloon dilation of coarctation of the aorta. Circulation 1994; 90(1):340–347.

87. Yetman AT, Nykanen D, McCrindle BW, *et al.* Balloon angioplasty of recurrent coarctation: A 12-year review. J Am Coll Cardiol 1997; 30(3):811–816.

88. Rao PS, Koscik R. Validation of risk factors in predicting recoarctation after initially successful balloon angioplasty for native aortic coarctation. Am Heart J 1995; 130(1):116–121.

89. Fletcher SE, Nihill MR, Grifka RG, *et al.* Balloon angioplasty of native coarctation of the aorta: Midterm follow-up and prognostic factors. J Am Coll Cardiol 1995; 25(3):730–734.

90. O'Laughlin MP, Perry SB, Lock JE, *et al.* Use of endovascular stents in congenital heart disease. Circulation 1991; 83(6):1923–1939.

91. Ledesma M, Alva C, Gomez FD, *et al.* Results of stenting for aortic coarctation. Am J Cardiol 2001; 88(4):460–462.

92. Marshall AC, Perry SB, Keane JF, *et al.* Early results and medium-term follow-up of stent implantation for mild residual or recurrent aortic coarctation. Am Heart J 2000; 139(6):1054–1060.

93. Suarez de Lezo J, Pan M, Romero M, *et al.* Immediate and follow-up findings after stent treatment for severe coarctation of aorta. Am J Cardiol 1999; 83(3):400–406.

94. Pihkala J, Thyagarajan GK, Taylor GP, *et al.* The effect of implantation of aortic stents on compliance and blood flow. An experimental study in pigs. Cardiol Young 2001; 11(2):173–181.

95. Back M, Kopchok G, Mueller M, *et al.* Changes in arterial wall compliance after endovascular stenting. J Vasc Surg 1994; 19(5):905–911.

96. Kollum M, Kaiser S, Kinscherf R, *et al.* Apoptosis after stent implantation compared with balloon angioplasty in rabbits. Role of macrophages. Arterioscler Thromb Vasc Biol 1997; 17(11):2383–2388.

CHAPTER 21

Pharmacology and Ventricular Performance

Stanford Ewing, MD, FAAP, FRCP(C)

Introduction

Ventricular performance is a combination of systolic and diastolic performance and both exhibit congestive symptoms when significant dysfunction is present. Although classic thinking has focused on systolic performance, isolated diastolic dysfunction (with normal systolic function) has now been well recognized as cause of congestive symptoms. More than one third of adult patients with congestive symptoms have isolated diastolic dysfunction and results in a significant increase in morbidity and mortality [1]. Comparable studies are not available in pediatric patients. The pharmacology for augmentation of ventricular performance has made remarkable progress in the last 15–20 years. Multiple factors have been studied in the evaluation of ventricular function and have helped guide pharmacologic treatment.

Ventricular systolic performance is determined by four major factors and includes heart rate (HR), force/frequency; preload (preL), the Frank–Starling relationship, force/volume; afterload (afterL), force/impedance; and contractility. Exceeding the physiologic limits of the cardiac myofibril/sarcomere unit in relation to any one of these factors will result in a negative effect on performance. Although each factor in isolation will alter systolic performance, there is some interdependence between these factors [2]. HR, preL, and contractility are all directly proportional and afterL is inversely proportional to ventricular performance. As a result, any pharmacologic agent that increases HR, preL, and/or contractility and/or decreases afterL will augment ventricular performance.

Ventricular diastolic performance is determined primarily by ventricular myocardial relaxation and compliance. The clinical signs consist of evidence of congestive heart failure (CHF) and may or may not have associated abnormal ventricular systolic performance. Ventricular relaxation is dependent on the rapid uptake of intracellular calcium into the sarcoplasmic reticulum (SR). Any pharmacologic agent that augments this uptake will improve the diastolic ventricular performance. Ventricular compliance is determined by both passive and active elasticity. Hypertrophic cardiomyopathy, whether postoperative or congenital, remains a dominant lesion in pediatrics where there is disturbance of diastolic performance [3].

For further details, the reader is referred to the introductory chapter on the basic science of ventricular function (Chapter 2). This chapter will focus on the pharmacology available to treat abnormal ventricular performance.

Receptors and ventricular performance

Various receptors are present in the myocardium, the systemic vascular bed, and the pulmonary vascular bed and act as portals for most of the pharmacologic agents used to improve ventricular performance. The most important exception to this rule is in the use of inhaled nitric oxide (iNO), which diffuses through the tissues to enter the pulmonary vascular smooth muscle cells where direct stimulation of guanylate cyclase takes place. The following paragraphs give brief descriptions of α-adrenergic, β-adrenergic, dopaminergic, and G protein linked receptors.

The α-adrenergic receptors are present in both α_1 and α_2 subtypes. The α_1 receptors are exclusively postsynaptic and are present in both peripheral vascular smooth muscle and the myocardium. Stimulation causes peripheral vasoconstriction (increases afterL) and increases central cardiac inotropy. The α_2 receptors are both presynaptic and postsynaptic. Presynaptic stimulation decreases norepinephrine (NE) release causing vasodilation (decreases afterL), whereas postsynaptic stimulation decreases coronary blood flow.

The β-adrenergic receptors are present in both β_1 and β_2 subtypes. The β_1 receptor predominates in the myocardium and stimulation causes increased inotropy and chronotropy. The β_2 receptor predominates in the periphery and stimulation causes both vasodilation and bronchodilation.

The dopaminergic (DA) receptors are present in both DA_1 and DA_2 subtypes. DA_1 receptors are postsynaptic located in the kidneys and stimulation results in renal vascular dilation and subsequent increased urine output. DA_2 receptors are located in the postganglionic sympathetic nerves and stimulation results in decreased NE release and subsequent splanchnic vasodilation.

The largest group of cell surface receptors are the G protein linked receptors that are involved in signal transduction of cardiac cells with β-adrenergic, muscarinic cholinergic innervated, and adenosine receptors. These G proteins link to several intracellular enzymes to activate a cellular response. Atrial natriuretic peptide (ANP), produced primarily by the atria as a result of stretch, has been shown to bind to a G protein linked receptor, natriuretic peptide-A. This binding stimulates production of cyclic guanosine 3'-5' monophosphate (cGMP), which subsequently activates cGMP-dependent protein kinase with natriuresis and peripheral vascular smooth muscle relaxation (both venous and arteriolar vasodilation) [4]. In addition, human brain natriuretic peptide (hBNP), produced primarily by the ventricles, uses the same receptor with similar effects. Both peptides are proportionately increased in CHF, and elevated hBNP serum levels can detect and are more sensitive in predicting ventricular systolic and diastolic dysfunction and LVH. Infusion of exogenous, recombinant hBNP (nesiritide, Natrecor) in CHF patients has demonstrated decreases in all of the following pressures: right atrial, pulmonary arterial, pulmonary capillary wedge, and mean systemic arterial. Cardiac index, urine volume, and urine sodium excretion all increased in these patients without adverse neurohumoral activation [5].

Heart rate and ventricular performance

The relationship of the HR to ventricular performance is known as the force/frequency curve and is also known as the Treppe or Bowditch effect. Within physiologic limits, an increase in HR augments the force of ventricular contraction and conversely, a decrease in HR diminishes the force of ventricular contraction. The speculative mechanism favors that with an increase in HR there is repetitive Ca^{2+} entry and increased cytosolic Ca^{2+} is made available for contraction. Optimal contractile force with isometric contraction is seen at HRs of 150–180 bpm, maintained for relatively short periods of time. In diseased cardiac muscle or hearts with no "reserve," an increase in HR produces little augmentation or may actually diminish the force of ventricular contraction [6]. Tachycardias and bradycardias outside physiologic limits can lead to the following problems.

Tachycardic cardiomyopathy

Incessant tachycardias, occurring more than 20% of the time, will generally decrease ventricular performance. The mechanisms are felt to be decreased coronary perfusion and decreased ventricular filling, both from a shortened diastolic time, despite the positive effect of the force/frequency curve. Pathologic rates have a wide variation from a slow ectopic atrial tachycardia with 1:1 conduction and ventricular rates in the 130 bpm to a rapid reentrant tachycardia with variable conduction and ventricular rates from 150 to 300 bpm. Clinically, there is decreased cardiac output with signs of CHF. The time to onset of clinical symptoms is proportional to the ventricular rate. Examples of this time to onset is seen in permanent junctional reciprocating tachycardia (PJRT) often with HRs in the 170 bpm where clinical symptoms evolve over a period of weeks to months, in contrast to incessant reentrant tachycardia with HRs of 250–300 bpm in neonates where clinical symptoms evolve over a few hours to 1–2 days. Resolution of the tachycardia by spontaneous conversion, medical therapy, or invasive interventional pathway ablation will reverse the decreased ventricular performance to a normal profile. The medical and interventional therapies are discussed in Chapter 19, "Considerations in Intensive Care." See related discussion in Fetal Ventricular Performance and Pharmacologic Agents Section.

Bradycardic cardiomyopathy

Incessant bradycardias, at rates below physiologic limits, will also decrease ventricular performance. The mechanism is felt to be inadequate cardiac output as a result of having reached the upper limit of Frank–Starling curve (fixed stroke volume) in combination with an inadequate heart rate. Therapy consists of increasing the heart rate via various strategies and is further discussed in Chapter 19.

Preload and ventricular performance

The term preload (preL) is defined as the length to which a muscle is stretched prior to contraction and is represented by the Frank–Starling relationship or the force/volume curve. Within physiologic limits, a diastolic increase in muscle fiber length or stretch increases myocardial force of contraction. In the intact heart, a diastolic increase in muscle fiber length translates to an increased ventricular diastolic volume and fiber tension prior to contraction. Thus, increased preL is directly proportional to (increased) stroke volume and cardiac output. For practical purposes, these increases in fiber length and tension

can be estimated by increases in end-diastolic volumes and pressures. In the clinical setting, end-diastolic venous pressures are commonly substituted and used to estimate preL. Although there are limitations in this approach, these pressures do represent the physiology in a given clinical situation. In general, when there is significant elevation of preL, congestive symptoms result and the pharmacologic therapy is directed at lowering the increased preL.

Currently, two standard approaches have been utilized to lower excessive preL, increased diuresis and venodilation. To increase diuresis, pharmacologic stimulation of renal blood flow with "renal dose" dopamine and diuretics are common clinical practices. In addition, natriuretic peptides increase diuresis, with recombinant hBNP available for infusion. To increase venodilation, various drugs have been used that act as venodilators, either alone or in combination with arteriolar dilation. These drugs include nitrovasodilators (nitroglycerin and nitroprusside, see Table 21.1), angiotension-converting enzyme (ACE) inhibitors (see Table 21.2), angiotensin receptor blockers (see Table 21.3), and natriuretic peptides.

Nitroglycerin: Nitroglycerin is used primarily in the postoperative patient and remains commonly

Table 21.1 Pulmonary Vasodilators (i.v.).

Agent - i.v.	Dose	Route	Comments	Mechanism
Prostacyclin (PGI2) (epoprostenol) (Flolan)	2 ngm/(kg min) increase q 2wks by 2 ngm/(kg min) max 160 ngm/(kg min)	Cont. infusion via CADD pump	Tachyphylaxis titrate to effect	Increases cAMP
PGE1 (Alprostadil, others)	0.0125–0.1 mcg/(kg min) high dose (>0.1–0.4 mcg/(kg min))	Cont. infusion cont. infusion	Minimizes side effects rarely maximizes side effects	Used primarily for ductal patency
Milrinone (Primacor)	0.25–1 mcg/(kg min)	Cont. infusion	Initial bolus 25–75 mcg/kg (over 60 min) intraop-higher doses tolerated	PDE III inhibitor/ cAMP
Amrinone lactate (Inocor)	5–10 mcg/(kg min)	Cont. infusion	Initial bolus 750 mcg/kg (0.75 mg/kg)	PDE III inhibitor/ cAMP
Nitroprusside (Nipride, others)	0.1–5 mcg/(kg min) 0.1–1 mcg/(kg min infant)	Cont. infusion Cont. infusion	Both sys/pulm vasodilator	Increases cGMP/NO
Nitroglycerin (Nitro-bid, others)	0.5–20 mcg/(kg min)	Cont. infusion	Both sys/pulm vasodilator	Increases cGMP/NO

Table 21.2 Angiotensin Converting Enzyme (ACE) Inhibitors.

Drug	Dosages, all oral	Dosage interval	Comment
Captopril (Capoten)	infants: 0.1–0.5 mg/(kg dose), 2–3x/day (max to 4 mg/(kg day po)) child: 0.1–2 mg/(kg dose), 2–3x/day teen: 6.25–25 mg/dose, 2–3x/day	2–3 divided doses	max 150 mg/day
Enalapril (Vasotec)	0.08 mg/(kg dose), 1–2x/day po (1–4 mg/(kg day) po)	1–2 divided doses	max 40 mg/day
Lisinopril (Prinivil, Zestril)	1–4 mg/(kg day) po	1 dose	max 40 mg/day
Ramipril (Altace)	1–2 mg/(kg day) po	1–2 divided doses	max 20 mg/day
Trandolapril (Mavik)	1–4 mg per day po	1 dose	max 4 mg/day

used. The mechanism of action is to stimulate the production of NO, which results in increased production of cGMP and causes primarily venodilation. This decreases both atrial and ventricular filling pressures with reduced pulmonary venous and arterial pressures. At standard doses, there is little effect on systemic vascular resistance (SVR) or pressure. Indications for use include abnormally elevated systemic and pulmonary preL and venous congestion and should be used with caution in patients with low preL.

Nitroprusside: Nitroprusside also works via the endothelial induction of NO, is primarily used in the postoperative patient, and is commonly used to reduce abnormally elevated LV preL. Nitroprusside acts as a balanced arteriolar and venous vasodilator and reduces SVR and pulmonary vascular resistance (PVR) and atrial pressures and increases cardiac output. Metabolism is via nonenzymatic RBC conversion to cyanide, which is converted to thiocyanate by the liver enzyme, rhodanase. Toxicity involves cyanide accumulation and causes metabolic acidosis and methemoglobinemia. Cyanide and thiocyanate levels should be appropriately monitored in liver or renal dysfunction, respectively. Nitroprusside is contraindicated during active ischemia as an increase in mortality has been noted.

ACE inhibitors: ACE inhibitors act as balanced arteriolar and venous vasodilators through inhibition of the conversion of angiotensin I to angiotension II. This conversion is performed primarily, but not exclusively, by the pulmonary vascular endothelium. In addition, ACE inhibitors block the breakdown of bradykinin and substance P, both vasodilators that are felt to be the etiology of the chronic cough associated with ACE inhibitors. Angiotensin II is the final circulating protein of the renin–angiotensin system and is a potent vasoconstrictor and also inhibits aldosterone production. The combined effects result in decreased preL and afterL and have made them standard theray in CHF. Several ACE inhibitors are available (see Table 21.2) and vary primarily in dosing strength and frequency. Combined usage of ACE inhibitors with potassium supplementation or potassium sparing diuretics is not advised because of the risk of hyperkalemia. All are oral preparations that facilitate outpatient management therapy.

Table 21.3 Angiotensin II Receptor Blockers.

Drug	Dose, all oral	Dose interval	Comment
Candesartan (Cilexetil, Atacand)	8–32 mg per day po	in 1 dose	adult dosages
Eprosartan (Teveten)	400–800 mg per day po	in 1–2 divided doses	adult dosages
Irbesartan (Avapro)	150–300 mg per day po	in 1 dose	adult dosages
	6–12 yrs, 75–150 mg/day po	in 1 dose	pediatric dosages
Losartan (Cozaar)	25–100 mg per day po	in 1–2 divided doses	adult dosages
Telmisartan (Micardis)	40–80 mg per day po	in 1 dose	adult dosages
Valsartan (Diovan)	80–320 mg per day po	in 1 dose	adult dosages

Angiotensin Receptor Blockers: Angiotensin II is the final circulating protein of the renin–angiotensin system and is a potent vasoconstrictor. Two receptors are known: AT_1 and AT_2. The initial receptor blocker was losartan, which blocks the binding of angiotensin II to type 1 (AT_1) receptors [7]. Because of the specificity of this receptor blockade, there is no disturbance in bradykinin or substance P metabolism. Losartan is rapidly absorbed from the GI tract and has a half-life of 1.5–2.5 h. The principle metabolite is active and has a half-life of 6–9 h. Metabolism is via the cytochrome P450 system. Neither cough nor angioedema has been described with the receptor blockers in contrast to the ACE inhibitors. Modest increases in serum potassium have been reported but do not require drug stoppage. The receptor blockers and ACE inhibitors are contraindicated during pregnancy.

Both the angiotensin receptor blockers and ACE inhibitors appear equally effective in reducing preL and afterL; however, receptor blockers tend to increase mortality when compared to ACE inhibitors in adult patients with CHF. It has been suggested that future cornerstone therapy will consist of using a combination of a receptor blocker and an ACE inhibitor in patients with CHF for additive effects [8].

Natriuretic Peptides: Both ANP and hBNP, produced as a result of stretch, have been shown to bind to the same G protein linked receptor, natriuretic peptide-A, activating cGMP-dependent protein kinase with natriuresis and peripheral vascular smooth muscle relaxation (both venous and arteriolar vasodilation with dominant venous component) [4]. Both peptides are proportionately increased in CHF, and elevated hBNP serum levels can detect and are more sensitive in predicting ventricular systolic and diastolic dysfunction and LVH. Infusion of exogenous, recombinant hBNP (nesiritide, Natrecor) in CHF significantly decreases preL on both sides of the heart. Cardiac index, urine volume, and urine sodium excretion are all increased without adverse neurohumoral activation [5]. Currently at Children's Hospital of Philadelphia, we are routinely assessing hBNP serum levels in our cardiac patients with pulm htn and CHF. Anecdotally, elevated levels have been proportional to the severity of pulm htn and RV failure in these patients. We are establishing a protocol for using recombinant hBNP in selected patients with pulm htn and CHF.

Others: Neutral endopeptidase (which degrade natriuretic peptides) inhibitors, α_1 antagonists (e.g. prazosin), and centrally acting α_2 agonists (e.g. clonidine) have limited applications for reducing preL in pediatrics and will not be discussed here.

Afterload and ventricular performance

Left ventricular afterload

Left ventricular afterload (LV afterL) can be defined as the sum of forces opposing cardiac performance during LV contraction. This sum of forces is most accurately defined as vascular impedance that measures opposition to flow in pulsatile systems and includes vessel elastance and distal wave reflections. Vascular resistance, which measures opposition to flow in nonpulsatile systems, is much easier to calculate and therefore used to estimate LV afterL [9]. Resistance is measured as the mean pressure difference across a vascular bed divided by the flow. Using Poiseuille's Law, vascular resistance (R) is also equated to blood viscosity (μ), vessel length (L), vessel radius (r), and constants by the following formula:

$$R = \frac{8\mu L}{\pi r^4}$$

The SVR is determined primarily by the caliber of the peripheral arteriolar vessels and small changes have a large logarithmic effect. The net vascular caliber of these vessels is determined by the cumulative ratio of the opposing forces of vasoconstriction and vasodilation via receptors and direct cellular response. These receptors include α adrenergic (vasodilation and vasoconstriction), β_2 adrenergic (vasodilation and bronchodilation), dopaminergic (vasodilation), and endothelin (vasoconstriction and vasodilation). The receptors are located in various systemic vascular beds and includes skin, cerebral, renal, splanchnic, skeletal muscle and coronary. In addition, systemic autacoids, including prostaglandins, thromboxane, and leukotrienes, use receptors with vascular regulatory functions but are beyond the scope of this chapter and will not be discussed.

In general, the systemic vascular impedance and resistance trend in the same direction and are inversely proportional to LV performance [9]. The best estimate of SVR is LV end systolic wall stress (discussed later in this chapter). Pharmacologic manipulation of the SVR to maximize LV performance has become an important area of therapy and research.

Right ventricular afterload
Right ventricular afterload (RV afterL) can be defined as the sum of forces opposing cardiac performance during RV contraction. The same comments above regarding vascular impedance and resistance apply to the pulmonary vessels. The PVR is determined by the caliber and number of pulmonary arteriolar vessels. In fetal lesions where displacement of the lungs results (e.g., congenital diaphragmatic hernia or pleural effusion) in a markedly decreased pulmonary vascular bed may be evident at the time of delivery. Following birth, in these lesions, even maximum dilation of all recruitable pulmonary vessels may result in severe pulm htn and elevated afterL from an inadequate vascular bed. The net vascular caliber of these vessels is determined by the cumulative ratio of the opposing forces of vasoconstriction and vasodilation via receptors and direct cellular response. These receptors include β_2 adrenergic (bronchodilation), endothelin (vasoconstriction and vasodilation), and prostacyclin (vasodilation). In addition, other autacoids, including other prostaglandins, thromboxanes, and leukotrienes, use receptors with pulmonary vascular regulatory functions but are beyond the scope of this chapter and will not be discussed. Currently, receptor antagonists of these other autacoids that induce pulmonary vasoconstriction are not being used in the standard therapy of pulm htn.

In general, the PVR and resistance trend in the same direction and are inversely proportional to ventricular performance. Direct measurement of the PVR in the cardiac catheterization laboratory remains the gold standard but can be estimated by echocardiographic techniques (see Ventricular Function Evaluation section in this chapter). Various pathologic conditions affect the pulmonary vessels postnatally to elevate the PVR. Pharmacologic manipulation to decrease PVR and maximize RV performance has become an important area of therapy and research.

Systemic vasodilation and LV performance

Many disease states in pediatric cardiology result in increased LV afterL, decreasing LV performance. These can be due to structural lesions that re-

quire surgical intervention or abnormal peripheral vasoconstriction that is amenable to medical therapy. The above noted peripheral receptors are of paramount importance in maintaining systemic vascular tone and can be therapeutically manipulated to maximize LV performance. Two major therapeutic strategies have been used to decrease SVR: intravenous (i.v.) and oral.

Intravenous therapy for systemic vasodilation
Intravenous (i.v.) therapy has been a mainstay for hospitalized patients and remains a gold standard. The half-lives of PDE III inhibitors and nitroprusside are short and require continuous infusions for effect.

Phosphodiesterase III (PDE III) Inhibitors: Milrinone has emerged as the preferred PDE III inhibitor as a result of being a selective inhibitor with fewer side effects. Milrinone acts through the induction of cAMP and results in increased cAMP mediated Ca^{2+} uptake by the sarcoplasmic reticulum and dilates both arterioles and veins. The conversion of cAMP to AMP is catalyzed by PDE III and centrally decreases inotropy and peripherally decreases vascular smooth muscle relaxation. Inhibition of this conversion maintains higher levels of cAMP and therefore increases both inotropy and smooth muscle relaxation (vasodilation). This combination of effects has made milrinone very effective in the postoperative state (see Practical Clinical Question 1 below).

Nitroprusside: Nitroprusside works via the endothelial induction of NO, is primarily used in the postoperative patient, and is commonly used to reduce LV afterL. Nitroprusside acts as a balanced arteriolar and venous vasodilator and reduces SVR, PVR, and atrial pressures and increases cardiac output. See discussion above for details.

Natriuetic Peptides: Both ANP and hBNP stimulate production of cGMP, activating cGMP-dependent protein kinase with natriureis and peripheral vascular smooth muscle relaxation arteriolar [4]. Infusion of exogenous, recombinant hBNP (nesiritide, Natrecor) in CHF patients decreases in mean systemic arterial pressure and increases cardiac index, urine volume, and urine sodium excretion without adverse neurohumoral activation [5]. See discussion above on receptors and preL for more detailed description. Protocols are being established for using recombinant hBNP in patients to decrease systemic afterL and to improve ventricular performance and cardiac output.

Oral therapy for systemic vasodilation

Oral therapy for increased systemic afterL has improved both inpatient and outpatient therapy for patients. Powerful inhibitors and receptor blockers have joined the β-blockers in decreasing systemic afterL (see Tables 21.2 and 21.3).

ACE Inhibitors: ACE inhibitors act as balanced arteriolar and venous vasodilators. The mechanism of action and side effects are detailed above. The combined actions result in decreased SVR and systemic pressure. Tissue production of angiotensin II is speculated to be important for local control of blood flow. Clinical indications include excessive afterL (not due to fixed renal artery stenoses), significant AV valve insufficiency, and CHF.

Angiotensin Receptor Blockers: As a result of a final common pathway, angiotensin receptor blockade is felt to be superior to ACE inhibition. The initial receptor blocker was losartan, which blocks the binding of angiotensin II to type 1 angiotensin II (AT-1) receptors [7]. Receptor blocker mechanisms, metabolism, and side effects are described above. Both the receptor blockers and ACE inhibitors appear equally effective in afterL reduction [10].

β-Blockers: See discussion below for the use of β-blockers to improve ventricular performance, especially in association with CHF.

Others: Other agents are known to have systemic vasodilation effects. These include hydralazine (potassium channel agonist, i.v./i.m., po), clonidine (central acting α_2 adrenergic agonist, po), prazosin/phentolamine (α_1 adrenergic receptor antagonists, po, i.m./i.v.), and calcium channel blockers (po). These agents have all been overshadowed by the i.v. or oral therapies (see above) and are uncommonly used in pediatric cardiology at this time.

Conclusion

Both i.v. and oral therapies have been developed that allow improved manipulation to decrease LV afterL with improved ventricular performance.

Pulmonary vasodilation and right ventricular performance

With constriction of the pulmonary vascular bed, abnormal increases in pulmonary artery pressure and PVR occur leading potentially to decreased RV performance and/or RV failure. Various strategies have evolved over the last 20 years to target vasodilation of this bed. Pulmonary vasobiology has stimulated the

Table 21.4 Therapeutic Manipulation of RV Afterload.

General therapy for increased pulmonary
vascular resistance
Oxygen support to maintain normal arterial PO_2
Ventilatory support to maintain eucarbia/hypocarbia
Bicarbinate infusion to maintain normal pH
Diuretics
Bronchodilators
Inotropes to increase contractility
Specific vasodilators
Prostaglandins
Calcium channel blockers
Endothelin receptor blockers
ACE inhibitors
$\beta2$ receptor agonists
Nitric Oxide replacement therapy
Nitric Oxide endothelial stimulators
Nitric Oxide breakdown inhibitors

development of new therapies in the successful treatment of congenital heart disease and increased RV afterL. The lungs are the only organ to receive and process the entire cardiac output and offer many strategies for medical therapy. General therapy of pul htn is listed in Table 21.4. Three major delivery strategies have been utilized to decrease PVR: i.v., oral, and inhalational. Failure of medical therapy may indicate an irreversible, fixed pulmonary vascular obstruction, or LV dysfunction.

Intravenous therapy for pulmonary vasodilation

Intravenous (i.v.) therapy has included evaluation in the catheterization lab with i.v. infusion peripherally or directly into the pulmonary artery, with various agents, including adenosine triphosphate (ATP), acetylcholine (Ach), tolazoline, phosphodiesterase III (PDE III) inhibitors, and prostacyclin (PGI2). i.v. therapy with the nonspecific agents, PGE1, nitroglycerin, and nitroprusside, has been overshadowed with pulmonary specific agents (see Table 21.1).

Phosphodiesterase III (PDE III) Inhibitors: Milrinone acts through the induction of cAMP and increases both inotropy and smooth muscle relaxation. When infused intravenously at catheterization, both pulmonary and systemic vasodilation result with a half-life of 2–4 h. In one study of 10 pediatric patients with significant postcardiopulmonary bypass pulm htn (all had repair of TOF), there was a significant reduction in the pulmonary to systemic pressure ratio, using standard milrinone i.v. dosaging [11]. Combinations of i.v. or inhaled milrinone with other i.v. or inhaled pulmonary vasodilators have shown additive effects. Delivery via inhalation is felt to be associated with less systemic hypotension [12–14].

Prostacyclin (PGI$_2$) : Prostacyclin (PGI$_2$, epoprostenol) is a well-known vasodilator and is generally given by intravenous drip. The parent substrate is arachidonic acid, which undergoes enzymatic conversion by cyclooxygenase-1 to prostaglandin G$_2$(PGG$_2$). Further peroxidase enzyme activity converts PGG$_2$ to PGH$_2$, which is subsequently converted via prostacyclin synthetase to PGI$_2$. PGI$_2$ is produced primarily by the vascular endothelium where prostacyclin synthetase is concentrated and then released to diffuse into the surrounding smooth muscle. PGI$_2$ binds to an inositol phosphate receptor where G protein activation increases cAMP, causing vasodilation. PGI$_2$ is approximately five times more potent than PGE$_2$ in causing vasodilation and is not inactivated to a major extent during passage through the lungs. PGI$_2$ is hydrolyzed nonenzymatically with a half-life of ~3 min. Additionally, increased levels of PGI$_2$ inhibit platelet aggregation. A potent stimulator for PGI$_2$ production is increased endothelial shear stress. Potent inhibitors of PGI$_2$ production include both aspirin and nonsteroidal antiinflammatory agents that decrease PGI$_2$ levels via cyclooxygenase inhibition [15].

At the Children's Hospital of Philadelphia, continuous infusion of PGI$_2$ has been successfully used in pulm htn for afterL reduction to improve RV performance and cardiac output. Hinderliter *et al.* reported a large multicenter trial of 81 patients with primary pulm htn and showed a significant response with the addition of 12 weeks of i.v. PGI$_2$ to conventional therapy. Echocardiographic follow-up showed beneficial effects on RV size, interventricular septal position, and tricuspid insufficiency velocity [16].

Natriuetic Peptides: Both ANP and hBNP cause natriureis and peripheral vascular smooth muscle relaxation [4]. Infusion of exogenous, recombinant hBNP (nesiritide, Natrecor) in CHF patients has demonstrated decreases in right atrial, pulmonary arterial, and pulmonary capillary wedge pressures [5]. We are attempting to establish a protocol for using recombinant hBNP in patients to decrease RV afterL.

Oral therapy for pulmonary vasodilation

Oral therapy for increased RV afterL has added significantly to the medical armamentarium for pulm htn. The calcium channel blocker nifedipine has the longest experience and demonstrated some success. The addition of both sildenafil and bosentan (see Table 21.5) for manipulation of PVR has been shown to effectively reduce RV afterL and increase RV performance.

Calcium Channel Blockers, Nifedipine: Oral therapy has included nifedipine, from the dihydropyridine

Table 21.5 Pulmonary Vasodilators (Oral).

Agent, oral	Dose	Route	Comments	Mechanism
Sildenafil citrate (Viagra)	2–16 mg/(kg day), initial dose 0.25 mg/kg (max 12.5 mg), then 0.5–2 mg/(kg dose) (max 100 mg)	po/ng divided q 3–6 h	25 mg tab dissolved in 5 mL sterile H$_2$O (5 mg/mL, for infants), CHOP protocol, titrate to effect	PDE V inhibitor
Bosentan (Tracleer)	Child: >6 yrs, start 31.25 mg bid; after 1 month, 62.5 mg bid teens: start 62.5 mg bid; after 1 month, 125 mg bid	po divided bid po divided bid po divided bid po divided bid	Only ET receptor blocker approved for pulm htn	Non selective ETa/ETb receptor blocker
Nifedipine (Adalat, Procardia, and others)	0.1–0.5 mg/(kg dose) q 8 h; max 20 mg q 8 h	po divided tid	Modest effect	Inhibition of slow Ca^{2+} nflux

ET: Endothelin; ETT: endotracheal tube; PDE: phosphodiesterase; pulm htn: pulmonary hypertension.

class of Ca^{2+} channel blockers and has dominant vasodilation effects. The decreased pulmonary artery pressures result from arteriolar vasodilation. This effect is mediated through inhibition of calcium influx through voltage-dependent slow channels in the sarcolemmal cell membrane, decreasing the amount of cytoplasmic Ca^{2+} available for smooth muscle vasoconstriction. Uses of nifedipine include acute and chronic therapy of systemic hypertension, prophylaxis of high altitude pulmonary edema, and pulm htn.

Following absorption from the gastrointestinal tract, there is considerable first past clearance in passing through the hepatic circulation. Metabolism is via the liver CYP 450 3A3/4 and the inactive metabolites are then excreted by the kidney. Systemic hypotension is infrequent and there is no appreciable effect on lipids. Grapefruit juice with dosing increases bioavailability and effects and nifedipine may increase levels of cyclosporine and digoxin. Nifedipine has been shown to have modest effects in dilating the pulmonary vascular bed and offers oral therapy in an outpatient setting. Depression of myocardial contractility precludes use in patients with severely decreased myocardial function.

Phosphodiesterase V (PDE V) Inhibitors, Sildenafil: Recent evaluations with oral PDE V inhibitors, including sildenafil, have shown good vasodilation properties. PDE V catalyzes the metabolism of cGMP and therefore inhibition increases the levels of both cGMP and NO, increasing vasodilation. Studies of the human forearm have shown that not only do increased levels of cGMP alone cause vasodilation but that this increased cGMP, increases the effect of cAMP-mediated vasodilation through inhibition of PDE III. The effect is additive when agents are used that further increase cAMP levels [14]. Animal studies have confirmed PDE V inhibition has an additive pulmonary vasodilation effect when combined with Ino [17].

Endothelin (ET) Receptor Blockers, Bosentan: ETs are a group of 21 aminoacid peptides, ET1, ET2, ET3, and ET4 isoforms that exhibit vasoactive and cell proliferation properties (and others that will not be discussed here). The endothelins are formed in the endothelium, smooth muscle cells, cardiac myocytes, mesangial cells, and by some cellular blood components, including leukocytes and macrophages. The precursor molecule is preproendothelin, a 203 aminoacid peptide, which is cleaved by furin

convertase to big ET, a 38 aminoacid peptide. A group of endothelin converting enzymes (ECEs), a chymase, and a nonECE metalloprotease cleave big ET to form the 4ET isoforms. The ECEs have been shown to be located in endothelial and smooth muscle cells, cardiac myocytes, and macrophages. ECEs are not selective for ETs and also hydrolyze bradykinin (vasodilator), substance P (vasodilator), and insulin. Once formed, ET is released primarily abluminally, away from the vascular lumen, to act on the smooth muscle layer, suggesting paracrine properties. Autocrine feedback regulates synthesis. Stimuli for ET production include exercise, hypoxia, pulsatile vascular stretch, increased shear stress, and decreased pH. Inhibitors for ET production include NO, prostacyclins, atrial natriuretic peptides, and estrogens.

There are two major receptors for the ETs found in mammals, which have opposing effects: ETa and ETb. The ETa receptors mediate vasoconstriction, cell proliferation, cell adhesion, and thrombosis and are located primarily in the smooth muscle cells. The ETb receptors mediate vasodilation via the release of NO and prostacyclin and the inhibition of ECE1 expression and are located primarily on the endothelial cell surface. Affinity varies for the two receptors: ETa receptors have > 100-fold higher affinity for ET1 and ET2, and ETb receptors have equal affinity for all four ET isoforms. Age differences are also noted for receptor affinity of exogenously administered ET1. In fetal and newborn pulmonary circulation, ET1 causes vasodilation (dominant ETb affinity) in contrast to juvenile and adult models where pulmonary vasoconstriction is noted (dominant ETa affinity) [18].

As a result of multiple enzymatic pathways for the formation of the dominant ET1, the usefulness of blocking ECE1 and the subsequent formation of ET1 is limited. As a result, emphasis has concentrated on more than 50 experimental compounds for blockade of the two major receptors, ETa and ETb, either alone or in combination. Drugs that selectively block ETa have been more successful in reducing vasoconstriction and cell proliferation. In addition, with this selective blockade, hypercholesterolemia induced endothelial dysfunction is restored [19,20].

The ET receptor blocker currently used in pediatric cardiology is bosentan, a nonselective ETa/ETb receptor blocker. Bosentan has been shown to improve symptoms, exercise capacity, and hemodynamics in patients with pulm htn. Several recent studies have evaluated the effects of bosentan on ventricular function and the pulmonary vascular bed. In a piglet model, bosentan was seen to abolish the pulmonary intimal hypertrophy resulting from shunt-induced pulmonary overcirculation and activation of the ET system [21]. In a placebo controlled study involving 85 patients with pulm htn, bosentan improved echocardiographic-derived cardiac output, LV early diastolic filling, RV systolic function and led to a decrease in RV dilation and an increase in LV size [22]. In a follow-up study of 29 patients with pulm htn treated for more than 1 year with bosentan, *Sitbon et al.* found improved hemodynamics and exercise tolerance [23]. In addition to an improvement in modified New York Heart Association (NYHA) functional class, the drug was well tolerated. Finally, a recent study evaluating the pharmacokinetics, safety, and efficacy in pediatric patients with pulm htn showed similar dosing results compared to healthy adults and resulted in hemodynamic improvement [24].

Inhalational therapy for pulmonary vasodilation

Inhalational (i) therapy represents targeted effective therapy in the treatment of increased RV afterL. Standard inhalational therapy with supplemental oxygen to maintain normal saturations and ventilation to maintain normocarbia continue to be cornerstones for therapy in pulm htn. With the addition of iNO and other agents usually given by the i.v. route, inhalational therapy has become the therapy of choice for many pediatric diseases involving increased RV afterL. These agents (see Table 21.6) appear to be additive when combined with both i.v. and oral therapy.

Oxygen: Inhaled supplementary O_2 is a potent pulmonary vasodilator and at concentrations of 100% is used to test the "reactivity" of the pulmonary vasculature in the catheterization lab.

Prostacyclin (PGI$_2$): Although usually given by continuous i.v. infusion for pulmonary effects, recent reports of iPGI$_2$ have demonstrated good results in refractory pulm htn in adults post cardiopulmonary bypass [12] and in persistent pulm htn of the newborn [25]. IPGI$_2$ minimized the systemic side effects seen with continuous i.v. infusion and no tolerance developed. In addition, Haraldsson *et al.* showed significant additive affects of iPGI$_2$ and imilrinone in 11 postoperative cardiac patients with pulm htn and elevated PVR. Again, no decrease in SVR or mean arterial pressure was noted with inhalational delivery [12].

Milrinone: Although usually given by continuous i.v. infusion for pulmonary effects, the above trial involving postoperative cardiac surgical patients with pulm htn showed that both imilrinone and iPGI2 have potent selective pulmonary vasodilation with no change in systemic BP. Both were administered via routine nebulizer techniques during mechanical ventilation with invasive monitoring to evaluate changes in pulmonary artery pressures and afterL. The vasodilation effect of both was additive and prolonged compared to iPGI2 alone [12].

Nitric Oxide: iNO has been available for many years now and is a very potent pulmonary vasodilator. NO has been shown to be identical to "endothelium-derived relaxing factor" (EDRF) and normally requires an intact pulmonary vascular endothelium for production. The cellular substrate for NO production is L-arginine (from the urea cycle), which is

Table 21.6 Pulmonary Vasodilators - Inhalational (i).

Agent (i)	Dose	Route	Comments	Mechanism
Nitric oxide (NO) (Inomax)	5–40 ppm	ETT/nasal cannula	by cont. flow	endothelial replacement therapy
Prostacyclin (PGI2) (Flolan)	20–100 ngm/kg/min	cont. nebulizer	by cont. flow	increases cAMP
Milrinone (Primacor)	0.25 mg/ml, 0.5 mg/ml, and 1 mg/ml	intermittent nebulizer	adult dosages in postop hearts with pulm htn additive effect with iPGI2 (10 mcg/ml)	PDE III inhibitor
			no effect on systemic BP	increases cAmP

Table 21.7 Inotropic Agents, Digoxin Dosaging.

Agent	i.v. Dose		po Dose		Comments
Digoxin	Total dig dose (TDD)		Total dig dose (TDD)		Inhibits Na/K ATPase
(Lanoxin)	preemie	15 mcg/kg	preemie	20 mcg/kg	TDD u. divided as
	full term	20 mcg/kg	full term	30 mcg/kg	1/2–time 0
	<2 yrs	30–40 mcg/kg	<2 yrs	40–50 mcg/kg	1/4–time 8 h
	2–10 yrs	20–30 mcg/kg	2–10 yrs	30–40 mcg/kg	1/4–time 16 h
	>10 yrs	8–12 mcg/kg	> 10 yrs	10–15 mcg/kg	
	Maintenance per day		Maintenance per day		
	preemie	3–4 mcg/kg	preemie	5 mcg/kg	u. divided bid
	full term	6–8 mcg/kg	full term	8–10 mcg/kg	start time 24 h
	<2yrs	8–9 mcg/kg	<2yrs	10–12 mcg/kg	
	2–10 yrs	6–8 mcg/kg	2–10 yrs	8–10 mcg/kg	
	>10 yrs	2–3 mcg/kg	>10 yrs	2.5–5 mcg/kg	

enzymatically converted by NO synthase (NOS) to give NO with citrulline as a byproduct. NO diffuses to the underlying smooth muscle and activates guanylate cyclase, increasing intracellular cGMP from GTP, which results in vascular smooth muscle relaxation. Acetycholine (Ach) works via muscarinic receptors on the endothelial cell surface to release NO and subsequently the above cascade. When lung injury limits or stops native endothelial NO production, replacement therapy via inhalation has been shown to be very effective.

Although delivery of iNO via an endotracheal tube is preferred, delivery via nasal cannula or mask has also been shown to be effective in patients with pulm htn [26]. Doses currently used at Children's Hospital of Philadelphia include preemie/NB doses up to 20 ppm, weaning to 15, 10, 5, 3, 2, 1, and off based on clinical and echo data. Metabolism of iNO is rapid via uptake into red cells where it combines with hemoglobin (Hgb) to form nitrosylHgb. The latter is further broken down to metHgb and nitrates. At the above iNO dosages, toxicity is rare and routine serum monitoring of metHgb and nitrate levels has therefore been abandoned. Other potential side effects of iNO include epithelial injury, surfactant inactivation, and inhibition of platelet adhesion.

Conclusion

Standard oxygen and ventilatory therapy continue to be cornerstones for the treatment of pulm htn. With the addition of powerful inhalational agents, combined with oral and i.v. agents (see Practical Clinical Question 2), significant progress has been made in treating many pediatric cardiology disease states associated with abnormally increased RV afterL.

Contractility and ventricular performance

Inotropic agents augment the line of contractility, shifting the endsystolic points on the pressure volume loop upward and to the left. Various agents are given to improve contractility and include digoxin, catecholamines, and noncatecholamines. The available catecholamines include both endogenously and synthetically produced agents. In general, these agents work through increasing cAMP and the subsequent available Ca^{2+} for contraction, improving ventricular systolic performance. There are new experimental agents that increase the Ca^{2+} sensitivity of the cardiac myocytes directly, also improving ventricular performance [27] but have no pediatric application at this time. The following agents are highlighted for their use in pediatric cardiology.

Digoxin

Digoxin is a member of the cardiac glycoside family and the dominant agent used in pediatric cardiology (see Table 21.7). The shorter half-life (34 h) and primary metabolism via renal excretion (unchanged) are advantages that favor its use over digitoxin. Oral bioavailability is 72% and peak serum levels occur 30–90 min after an oral dose. Digoxin works as an inotrope by inhibition of the sarcolemmal $Na^+–K^+$ ATPase pump (binds to the α subunit), which exchanges $3Na^+$ for $2K^+$ and pumps Na^+ out of the

Table 21.8 Catecholamines and NonCatecholamines Dosaging.

Agent	Dose		Comment
Dopamine (Dopastat, others)	3–20 mcg/(kg min)		Splanchnic and renal vasodilator at low dose. vasoconstriction at >10
Dobutamine (Dobutrex)	3–20 mcg/(kg min)		Primarily β_1, modest β_2
Epinephrine (Adrenalin, others)	0.05–1 mcg/(kg min)s		α, β_1, β_2 β_2 decreased at high dose
Norepinephrine (Levophed, others)	0.05–2 mcg/(kg min)		Strong α, moderate β_1 no β_2
Isoproterenol (Isuprel, others)	0.05–2 mcg/(kg min)		Strong/equal β_1 and β_2 no α
Milrinone (Primacor)	50 mcg/kg load over 10 min maintenance: 0.25–1 mcg/(kg min)		PDE III inhibitor via cAMP β_1 and β_2
Amrinone (Inocor)	Neonates: 750 mcg/kg load over 3 min maintenance, 3–5 mcg/(kg min) infant-adult: 750 mcg/kg load over 3 min maintenance: 5–10 mcg/(kg min)	Max dose 10 mg/kg/day	PDE III inhibitor via cAMP β_1 and β_2

cell and K^+ into the cell. This inhibition results in lower extracellular Na^+ (higher intracellular Na^+), which subsequently increases intracellular Ca^{2+} via a negative effect on the Na^+–Ca^{2+} exchanger, which is high capacity exchange of three extracellular Na^+ for one intracellular Ca^{2+}. This increased Ca^{2+} available to the contractile proteins results in augmented contractility. Digoxin also has a positive direct effect on vagal tone to the heart resulting in a decreased SA node rate and decreased AV conduction through the AV node. Additional effects are speculated to stabilize membranes, inhibit sympathetic tone, and decrease SVR. As a result of these effects, digoxin continues to be of use for CHF even when echocardiographic data indicates normal systolic pump function.

Measurement of serum digoxin levels is most informative for compliance and absorption, although endogenous digoxin like immunoreactive substances may contribute to falsely elevate serum levels. In the face of normal renal and hepatic function and normal dosaging, routine serum level monitoring is *not* recommended. Evaluation of the clinical response and ECG monitoring is preferred and more informative. ECG therapeutic effects include repolarization changes with lengthening of the PR interval and toxic effects include conduction abnormalities with variable degrees of heart block and ectopy. Digoxin-induced ventricular arrhythmias and ectopy are uncommon in children in contrast to adults.

Catecholamines

Catecholamines are either naturally occurring (dopamine, norepinephrine, epinephrine) or synthetic (dobutamine, isoproterenol) agents that act on myocardial, pulmonary, and vascular receptor sites (Table 21.8). These sites include cardiac β_1 adrenergic, peripheral β_2 adrenergic, peripheral α_1 adrenergic, and peripheral dopaminergic (dopa$_1$ and dopa$_2$) receptors. These naturally occurring catecholamines are synthesized primarily in sympathetic nerve endings, the chromafin tissue of the adrenal medullae, and the brain. All are initially derived from tyrosine with subsequent conversion to dopa as the rate-limiting step via tyrosine hydroxylase in the cytoplasm of adrenergic cells. Dopa is converted to dopamine and on to norepinephrine (primarily in adrenergic nerve granules), which is converted to epinephrine (primarily in the adrenal medullae) [28]. Norepinephrine is released into the sympathetic nerve ending gap and the others are released and circulated intravenously.

β_1 receptor stimulation works via the G protein to increase cAMP and intracellular Ca^{2+} for muscle contraction and causes the release of myocardial adrenergic norepinephrine stores. β_2 receptor stimulation also increases peripheral cAMP with associated smooth muscle vasodilation (skeletal muscle, renal, splanchnic). α receptor stimulation decreases cAMP with associated vasoconstriction in the peripheral skeletal smooth muscle. Dopa$_1$ receptor stimulation in the postsynaptic splanchnic bed decreases the cAMP levels with associated selective renal, splanchnic, and coronary vasodilation. Dopa$_2$ receptor stimulation in the postganglionic sympathetic nerves inhibits both the sympathetic response and the release of norepinephrine to further increase renal, splanchnic, and coronary vasodilation. Action on β_1 receptors thus increases contractility, heart rate, and AV node conduction, while action on the β_2 receptors increases skeletal muscle vasodilation and bronchodilation. Action on the dopa$_1$ receptors stimulates vasodilation of the splanchnic bed (intestinal and pancreas) and renal bed, while action on the α_1 receptors stimulates vasoconstriction of skeletal bed. The following naturally occurring and synthetic catecholamines are important for improving ventricular performance.

Dopamine: Dopamine is the precursor to norepinephrine and has effects primarily on dopaminergic, β adrenergic cardiac, and α adrenergic vascular receptors. Low dose is used for vasodilation of the splanchnic and renal vascular beds, intermediate dose is used for inotropic effects, and high dose is used for additional blood pressure support (see Table 21.9).

Norepinephrine: Norepinephrine is the precursor to epinephrine and has effects primarily on β adrenergic cardiac and α adrenergic vascular receptors. This agent is effective in decreased ventricular performance with hypotension (see Table 21.9).

Epinephrine: Epinephrine has effects on β adrenergic cardiac, β_2 adrenergic vascular, and α adrenergic vascular receptors. This agent is effective in decreased ventricular performance with modest hypotension (see Table 21.9).

Dobutamine: Dobutamine has effects on β adrenergic cardiac and slightly on β_2 adrenergic vascular and α_1 adrenergic cardiac receptors. This agent is effective in decreased ventricular performance with no or minimal hypotension (see Table 21.9).

Isoproterenol: Isoproterenol has effects on β adrenergic cardiac and β_2 adrenergic vascular receptors and has a marked chronotropic response (increases HR). This agent is effective in bradycardias without heart block and decreased ventricular performance associated with increased afterL (see Table 21.9).

Noncatecholamines

Phosphodiesterase III (PDE III) Inhibitors: Inhibition of the conversion of cAMP to AMP (catalyzed by PDE III) maintains higher levels of cAMP and increases both inotropy and peripheral vasodilation. The increased inotropy is a result of increased cAMP-mediated transsarcolemmal Ca^{2+} flux. The increased vasodilation is a result of increased cAMP mediated Ca^{2+} uptake and dilates both arterioles and veins. In addition, this increased uptake causes improved relaxation and diastolic function of the myocardium. These agents are bipyridine derivatives and are represented by amrinone and milrinone in clinical practice (Table 21.8). The actions of these two agents combine positive inotropy with afterL reduction. There is modest coronary, pulmonary, and

Table 21.9 Adrenergic Activity of Inotropes.

	Receptor				
Agent	α_1/α_2 vascular	α_1 cardiac	β_2 vascular	β_1/β_2 cardiac	DA cardiac and vascular
Dopamine	$++++$	$++$	$+$	$++++$	$++++$
Dobutamine	$+$	$++$	$++$	$++++$	0
Epinephrine	$++++$	$++$	$+++$	$++++$	0
Norepinephrine	$++++$	$++$	$0/+$	$++++$	0
Isoproterenol	0	0	$+++$	$++++$	0
Milrinone	0	0	0	0	0

peripheral vasodilation. There are no major HR or BP effects. Milrinone does not appear to increase myocardial O_2 consumption in contrast to amrinone. The toxicity of amrinone is primarily fever, hepatotoxicity, and thrombocytopenia in $<3\%$ of patients in contrast with milrinone where toxicity is decreased. In renal failure, renal dose reduction is indicated only with milrinone.

CHF, ventricular performance, and β-blockers

The β- blockers inhibit either β_1 alone (selective) or both (nonselective) β_1 and β_2 receptors. Although uncommonly used in the setting of CHF previously, the emphasis on excessive and detrimental compensatory mechanisms in CHF has changed this practice. These mechanisms include activation of the renin–angiotensin system, increased β adrenergic tone, β_1 adrenergic receptor downregulation, ventricular dilation associated with increased afterL and myocardial O_2 consumption, and increased α adrenergic tone. These mechanisms result physiologically in fluid and sodium (Na) retention with hyponatremia, increased heart rate (HR), decreased sensitivity to β adrenergic stimulation, and decreased ventricular performance with increased end-diastolic pressures. In addition, there is decreased myocardial O_2 reserve and redistribution of cardiac output with decreased flow to the skin, kidneys, and GI tract. The oxyhemaglobin dissociation curve is shifted rightward as a result of increased 2,3-diphosphoglycerate, augmenting peripheral O_2 delivery. These mechanisms are triggered both in high output and primary pump failure. Clinically, the triad of tachycardia, tachypnea, and hepatomegaly are manifestations of the above combined congestive symptoms and compensatory mechanisms.

In the past, standard successful therapy for CHF has included inotropy with digoxin, afterL reduction with various agents, and diuresis. Diuretic therapy remains an import adjunct in therapy by decreasing excessively high preL and possibly a direct affect on the pulmonary vasculature but will not be discussed further here. In some patients, this standard therapy failed with no significant improvement in symptoms. In these patients this lead to trials with β-blockers in addition to standard therapy, in an attempt to show clinical improvement by further

countering the above excessive compensatory mechanisms present in CHF.

β-blockers decrease myocardial O_2 consumption, HR, and excessive β adrenergic tone, improving myocardial performance. A new combination of β-and α-blocker, carvedilol, additionally decreases excessive α adrenergic tone and afterL, resulting in further improved cardiac performance. Carvedilol is a nonselective β-blocker and also is an α_1-adrenergic blocker with no intrinsic sympathomimetic activity that is given orally. The drug is metabolized in the liver via the P450 system (CYP2D6) with a $t_{1/2}$ of 7 h. Peripheral vasodilation is prominent at the start of therapy. With continued use, there is increased LV ejection fraction, decreased end-diastolic and pulmonary pressures, decreased HR, and prevention of progressive enlargement of the LV. It is suggested to start at a minimal dose followed by conservative maintenance b.i.d. dosing. Weekly or biweekly increments are given until the desired effect or target dose is reached [29,30] (see Table 21.10). Labetalol, another combined nonselective β-blocker and α-adrenergic blocker with some intrinsic sympathomimetic activity, has shown utility in hypertension therapy and may be applicable for use in CHF (see Table 21.10).

Recently published studies confirm carvedilol improves cardiac performance in the treatment of CHF. Packer *et al.* enrolled 278 adult patients in a double-blind, placebo controlled multicenter trial. Baseline medications included standard therapy with digoxin, diuretics, and/or an ACE inhibitor. Results showed a significant increase in ejection fraction along with a significant decrease in the combined risk of morbidity and mortality in the carvedilol treatment group. In contrast, there was little effect on improved exercise tolerance or quality of life scores [31]. Bruns *et al.* enrolled 46 pediatric patients in a nonrandomized multicenter trial where each patient received carvedilol in addition to standard CHF therapy. After 3 months on carvedilol, significant improvement was noted in the modified NYHA class in 67% of patients and in the mean shortening fraction, using χ^2 and paired t test, respectively. Side effects, including dizziness, hypotension, and headache, occurred in 54% of patients but were well tolerated [32]. In addition, Azeka *et al.* showed recently the improved ventricular performance has allowed a significant percent of pediatric patients to be "delisted" from cardiac transplantation wait lists

Table 21.10 β-Blockers.

Agent	Dose	Route	Comments
Carvedilol (Coreg)	Start 0.1 mg/kg/day divided bid-only po titrate weekly/every other week to 1 mg/kg/day	ped max 1 mg/kg/day- (divided bid) max (<85 kg) 25 mg bid max (>85 kg) 50 mg bid	Dizziness, hypotension, headache bronchospasm, bradycardia increases digoxin levels by 15% both α-/β- blocker scavenger of free radicals
Labetalol (Normodyne)	0.25 mg/kg every 2 min i.v. increase to max 1 mg/kg i.v. 0.4–3 mg(kg h) cont. infusion Ped 1–4 mg(kg day) (b.i.d. po) Adult 100 mg b.i.d. po	max i.v. dose 20 mg total dose 4 mg/kg i.v. titrate to effect max po dose 40 mg(kg day) increase q 2–3 days- max po 2.4 gm/day	Orthostatic hypotension, fever, hepatotoxicity contraindicated-asthma, pul edema, heart block, hypotension both alpha/beta blocker
Propranolol (nonselective) (Inderal)	i.v. 0.05–0.15 mg/kg q 6h p o 1–5 mg(kg day) (given q 6h) p o sustained release 1–5 mg(kg/day) (given b.i.d.) Adult 10–30 mg/dose x t.i.d.-q.i.d.	max. i.v. 1 mg/dose infant max. i.v. 3 mg/dose child max po dose of 80 mg max po 320 mg/day (divided 3–4x/day)	bradycardia, SN arrest, AV block, bronchospasm, hypoglycemia, depression negative inotropy, CHF β_1/β_2, receptor blocker

[33]. The Children's Hospital of Philadelphia is currently involved in a randomized trial in the use of carvedilol in addition to standard therapy in patients with chronic, symptomatic CHF as a result of ventricular systolic dysfunction. This multicenter trial will attempt to establish if carvedilol therapy results in improved ventricular performance as has been shown in adults [34].

Diastolic function and ventricular performance

Diastolic function of the ventricle is determined by two major properties, relaxation and compliance or stiffness. Although evaluated separately, there is overlap of these processes. Relaxation is an active process, involving uptake of calcium in the sarcoplasmic reticulum (SR), and is therefore slowed by ischemia. In contrast, compliance is a passive process, involving the passive elastic properties of the myocardium. These properties are dependent on wall thickness, ventricular geometry, pericardial constraint, coronary filling, and the amount of scar tissue present in the myocardium or endocardium. Another factor, but less well understood, in diastolic function is elastic recoil of the muscle fibers that create diastolic suction forces. These recoil and suction forces are directly proportional to the amount

of systolic fiber shortening and therefore decreases in systolic performance result in decreased diastolic recoil and suction force performance [35].

Pharmacologic therapy for diastolic dysfunction is aimed at the underlying abnormality or etiology. Often, there is associated systolic dysfunction, elevated preL, and afterL, and by correction of the associated dysfunction, the diastolic function improves. Ischemia is attempted to be relieved and supportive therapy is administered for associated dominant symptoms, for example, diuresis for pulmonary edema, inotropy for systolic dysfunction, and afterL reduction for elevated wall stress. In general, there is evidence when systolic function improves as a result of β_1 stimulation, then diastolic function also improves, especially relaxation.

For decreased myocardial compliance as a result of hypertrophy, remodeling to a more normal myocardial thickness is the final common pathway to improved diastolic function. Stimulation of angiotensin and α- and β-receptors have been shown to increase cardiac myocyte growth. ACE inhibitors and angiotensin (AT) receptor blockers appear to have a beneficial effect on hypertrophy and remodeling through the inhibition of the AT_1 receptor. In addition, inhibition of adrenergic receptors (α_1, β_1, and β_2) also has a beneficial effect on cardiac muscle remodeling [36]. Tumor necrosis factor-alpha

(TNF-α) levels have also been shown to be increased in patients with decreased myocardial performance and causes myocyte hypertrophy. TNF-α inhibition has been studied and shown to be effective in adults for reducing hypertrophy but has no application in pediatrics yet [37].

Fetal ventricular performance and pharmacologic agents

In the fetus, structural lesions with AV valve insufficiency, obligatory shunts (e.g. cranial arteriovenous malformations), or primary pump dysfunction can result in poor ventricular performance, congestive symptoms, hydrops, and fetal demise. In addition, brady and tachy arrhythmias outside of physiologic limits can also result in poor ventricular performance and congestive symptoms. The fetal myocardium responds similarly to pharmacologic agents although there is a higher percentage of non-contractile elements, resulting in decreased ventricular compliance. The fetal myocardium operates at the upper end of the Frank–Starling curve and therefore increases cardiac output primarily by increasing HR.

Three major strategies are used to deliver pharmacologic agents to the fetus. The first strategy is to give the desired agent to the mother, which then diffuses across the placenta and enters the fetal circulation. The second strategy is to give the desired agent directly into the fetal umbilical vein/artery via periumbilical blood sampling (PUBS). The third strategy is to give the desired agent directly to the fetus by either intraperitoneal or intramuscular injection when PUBS is unsuccessful. When rapid therapeutic drug levels are indicated for the fetus (e.g. hydrops is present), loading doses should be initiated via transplacental route or direct fetal injection, followed by maintenance oral maternal transplacental therapy. Adenosine therapy of fetal tachyarrhythmias is administered only via PUBS where an umbilical venous bolus is essential for effect, considering the drug's short half-life. Intraamniotic administration of agents is not recommended because of reduced fetal swallowing and subsequent erratic absorption [38].

The major indication for fetal pharmacologic therapy is for control of pathologic tachyarrhythmias, which result in congestive symptoms, including hydrops, atrioventricular valve insufficiency, and cardiomegaly with decreased ventricular performance. Many agents, either alone or in combination, have been successfully administered via the strategies mentioned above (see Table 21.11) to control or

Table 21.11 Pharmacologic Therapeutic Agents Used in the Fetus For Control of Tachyarrhythmias.

Transplacental	Maternal dosages	Comments
Procainamide (Ia)	6 mg/kg po q 4 h	AV block, proarrhythmia, CHF
Quinidine (Ia)	250–500 mg po q 6 h	AV block, proarrhythmia, CHF
Flecanide (Ic)	100–200 mg po bid	Proarrhythmia, neg inotropy
Propranolol (II)	20–160 mg po q 6–8 h	LBW, hypoglycemia
Amiodarone (III)	5 mg/kg po q 12 h	Hypothyroidism, neurologic delay
Sotalol (III)	80–160 mg po q 8 h	QTc prolongation, torsade
Verapamil (IV)	80–160 mg po q 8 h	Reduce Digoxin, neg inotropy
Digoxin	Load: 1–1.5 mg po/i.v. divided 1/2, 1/4, 1/4 (q 8 h apart) maintenance: 0.25–0.5 mg po bid (may divide tid)	Monitor maternal levels and ECG

PUBS/direct injection	Fetal dosages[a]	Route
Adenosine	100–300 μg/est. kg	i.v. bolus
Digoxin	5–10 μg/est. kg (single dose)	i.v./i.m. thigh
Amiodarone	3 mg/est. kg (single dose)	i.v./i.m. thigh

PUBS: periumbilical blood sampling; neg: negative; est.: estimated; CHF: congestive heart failure; LBW: low birth weight; po: oral; i.m.: intramuscular; i.v.: intravenous.

[a]There are no published dosing, efficacy, or safety data. These are Children's Hospital at Philadelphia dosing guidelines based on consensus between fetal echocardiography and electrophysiology. There has been no morbidity or mortality in a small number of anecdotal cases using these guidelines.

Figure 21.1 The relationship of LV pressure or afterload to LV volume or preload. Time from point A to B represents diastolic filling, B to C isovolumic contraction, C to D ejection, and D to A isovolumic relaxation. Varying the afterload at constant preload and contractility generates the end-systolic line, the slope of which is used as a load-independent index of contractility. A change in the contractile or performance state of the ventricle, generates a new end-systolic line and slope. nl: normal; SV: stroke volume.

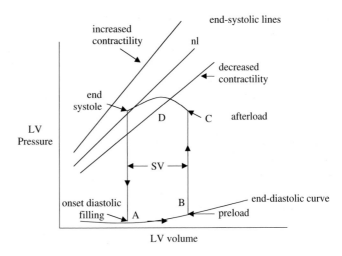

convert fetal tachyarrhythmias to normal sinus rhythm. Single drug therapy with digoxin continues to be the preferred initial therapy and when unsuccessful, an additional agent is added. Combination therapy of digoxin with either flecanide or verapamil have improved results over digoxin alone. One particularly successful combination is digoxin and sotalol for controlling fetal tachyarrhythmias. In one study, this combination therapy resulted in conversion or improvement of 6/7 (86%) fetal tachyarrhythmias, with or without hydrops [39]. Sotalol alone was also very effective in conversion to sinus rhythm in 9/12 (75%) fetuses. Fetal mortality was 4/21 (19%) in this study with 3/4 deaths in the hydropic group (N = 9). Sotalol was speculated to possibly have an increased risk for proarrhythmia in the immature fetal heart. These three successful combination therapies have minimized the therapeutic use of procainamide, quinidine, propranolol, and amiodarone for fetal tachyarrhythmias. Once the arrhythmia is controlled, there is usually rapid return to normal ventricular performance with resolution of the congestive symptoms [38].

To date, there are no published data on the use of inotropy to improve fetal morbidity and mortality when primary pump dysfunction is present. Pedra *et al.* evaluated 22 fetuses with primary pump dysfunction from various causes and found high perinatal mortality. Fetal echocardiographic evidence of ventricular diastolic dysfunction increased the risk of mortality eightfold [40]. This represents an area where further investigation needs to be done.

Ventricular function evaluation

Routine, thorough clinical assessment following medical strategies to improve ventricular systolic and diastolic function remains a cornerstone for medical decision making. With the advent of additional invasive and noninvasive modalities, significant emphasis has been placed on obtaining these additional data to supplement the clinical data.

Occasionally, catheterization data is required for critical decision-making, especially when precise pressures or resistances must be calculated. In addition, angiography remains the gold standard for visualization of the pulmonary vascular tree and coronary arteries. Using specialized catheter measurements, the line of contractility with the generation of pressure/volume loops and dP/dt under multiple conditions can be accurately measured and optimal therapy chosen (see Fig. 21.1).

Magnetic resonance imaging (MRI) is very useful in evaluation of structures that are difficult to image otherwise, for example, complex aortic arch anomalies including vascular rings and the branch pulmonary arteries. The MRI laboratory at Children's Hospital of Philadelphia can additionally evaluate ventricular function with ejection fractions, regurgitant fractions, obstructive flow dynamics and gradients, cardiac output, and pulmonary perfusion percentages. There has also been some success for evaluating coronary flow and perfusion. The increased speed of acquisition has augmented the use of the MRI scanner for obtaining images [41]. The elimination of motion artifact remains a challenge and we routinely sedate any patients younger than 9 years of age for MRI studies. Significant foreign bodies with iron content preclude MRI scanning. Smaller clips and other ferrous objects will cause image artifact.

Echocardiography remains a powerful tool to augment clinical findings and provide information for optimal surgical strategies. The evaluation of ventricular systolic and diastolic function continues to grow as additional Doppler and spectral data are developed, for example, the Tei index [42]. The echocardiographic work by Colan *et al.* to evaluate the relationship of meridional end-systolic wall stress (ESWS), velocity of circumferential fiber shortening (VCFc), and contractility as a load-independent measurement is commonplace for complete ventricular function evaluation [43]. Serial measurements allow medical therapy to be individually tailored (see Fig. 21.2). When significant atrioventricular valve insufficiency is present, accurate mean dP/dt data can be obtained for ventricular systolic (upstroke) and diastolic (downstroke) function. The dynamic, changing shape of left ventricular chamber does not interfere with the dP/dt measurement in contrast to the M mode measurement for shortening fraction

and is particularly useful in evaluating single ventricle function [44]. The most accurate dP/dt systolic echo data is obtained by time interval measurement on the insufficiency envelope from 1 to 3 m/sec and is theoretically afterL independent as this pressure range is before ejection starts, during "isovolumic contraction." Actually, the ventricular volume is changing as a result of the insufficiency and there may be slight changes in afterL the ventricle sees during this time period. The resultant mean dP/dt echo data has been validated at catheterization [45], corresponding closely to peak catheterization dP/dt data.

Diastolic ventricular function can be evaluated with downstroke dP/dt and Doppler tissue imaging (DTI). It has recently been shown that DTI is the optimal choice for distinguishing between identical normal and pseudonormalized inflow patterns, where preL is significantly elevated in the latter [46]. In addition, DTI data evaluating LV dysfunction has shown shortened isovolumic relaxation time and increased lateral mitral valve annulus velocity with low dose Dobutamine (10 mcg/(kg min).

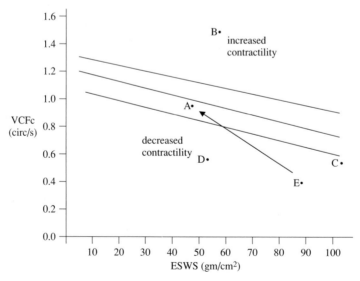

Figure 21.2 The relationship of VCFc/ESWS represents a load-independent ratio to estimate contractility. Examples of contractility changes: A, normal contractility with normal VCFc and ESWS. B, increased contractility resulting in increased VCFc with normal ESWS. C, low normal contractility resulting in low VCFc secondary to elevated ESWS. D, decreased contractility resulting in low VCFc with normal ESWS. E, decreased contractility resulting in very low VCFc with elevated ESWS. To take a patient from point E to point A (arrow) would require decreasing the systemic afterload and augmenting ventricular performance with an inotropic agent. Without the added inotropic support, the patient would end up at point D. ESWS: end-systolic wall stress; VCFc: velocity of circumferential fiber shortening corrected for heart rate. From Colan *et al.* [43] with permission.

This improved diastolic function accompanied the improvement in LV systolic function. Ventricular strain rate evaluation by echo generates useful diastolic data but has limited Pediatric applications at this time. Tsivyan *et al.* utilized echo measurements to generate an end-systolic pressure line and then evaluated the slopes of these lines in 22 asphyxiated full term infants as compared to 32 nonasphyxiated full term infants. They used nonpharmacologic afterL stress to generate the line and showed a decreased LV peak filling rate and an increased LV isovolumic relaxation time, consistent with diastolic dysfunction [47]. Estimating LV preL by echo using pulmonary venous pulse wave sampling and waveform evaluation has been validated at catheterization [48].

Pressure–volume loops and ventricular performance

The use of specialized catheters has allowed the simultaneous measurement of pressure and volume inside the cardiac chambers, especially the LV. The various change points of the generated PV loop are identified in Fig. 21.1. When afterL is varied and ventricular preL and contractility are held constant, an end-systolic pressure line is generated. The slope of this line represents a load-independent index of contractility. Changes in contractility reflect changes in ventricular performance and generate new lines and slopes. The addition of inotropic agents have been shown to generate PV loops with increased contractility. These increases can be directly measured by evaluation of the PV loops in the cardiac catheterization lab. In addition, Tsivyan *et al.* utilized echo measurements to generate an end-systolic pressure line in 22 asphyxiated full term infants as compared to 32 nonasphyxiated full term infants and showed a markedly decreased line slope in the asphyxiated infants [47]. These kinds of evaluations are not yet routinely performed in a typical Pediatric Cardiology patient for assessment of drug therapy.

Velocity of circumferential fiber shortening and meridional end-systolic wall stress relationship and ventricular performance

The VCFc and the meridional ESWS are measurements done routinely in the echo lab. This relationship has been shown to be inversely related and rep-

resents an index of contractility [45] (Fig. 21.2). The echo data needed to calculate these indices include routine M mode, end-systolic M mode, R–R interval, aortic ejection time, and end-systolic BP. This relationship appears to be a load-independent index of contractility and can explain, for example, whether a decrease in VCFc is a result of decreased contractility or an increase in afterL. This etiologic information can be used to direct pharamacological therapy in a patient (see Fig. 21.2). Serial measurements allow tailoring of drug therapy over the long term.

Practical clinical questions

1 *What is the most effective way to treat low cardiac output and decreased ventricular performance after cardiopulmonary bypass?*

The most effective method appears to be initiation of medical therapy in the early postoperative period. Postoperative low cardiac output has a strong association with an increased risk of death, and Wernovsky *et al.* have shown a simultaneous increase in both SVR (25%) and PVR (40%) in postoperative arterial switch repair for d-TGA [49]. To address these important output and resistance issues, a multicenter trial study (PRIMACORP) involving seven pediatric centers established a randomized, double-blind, placebo controlled protocol of prophylactic milrinone postrepair of structural congenital heart disease [50]. Results of the three prophylactic treatment arms (placebo, low dose, and high dose) show a significant reduction in postoperative low cardiac output using high dose milrinone [51]. At the Children's Hospital of Philadelphia, we load postoperative patients with milrinone in the operating room at higher than study doses to take into account the cardiopulmonary bypass circuit. Review of these higher loading doses at our institution is currently underway. Our maintenance dose of milrinone varies from 0.25 to 1 mcg/kg/min, titrating to desired effect and using lower doses in the younger infants.

2 *Are there advantages to using combination therapy in attempting to reduce RV afterL and improve RV performance?*

Initial studies in newborns have shown that combination inhaled therapy with both prostacyclin and milrinone is superior to either agent alone. It is not unreasonable to expect that other combination therapies will also be additive. This would include using inhaled, i.v., and p.o. therapies concurrently in the same patient. Currently at Children's Hospital of Philadelphia we are trying sundry combination strategies in pulm htn patients, which include iO2, iNO, sildenafil (p.o.), milrinone (i.v.), and bosentan (p.o.). The various combinations of supplemental O_2, NO replacement, inhibition of NO metabolism, inhibition of cAMP metabolism, and endothelin receptor blockade we feel offers maximal chance for successful pulmonary vasodilation in patients with normal size pulmonary vascular beds. In newborn patients with limited or fixed pulmonary vascular beds, for example, congenital diaphragmatic hernia patients, we have had limited anecdotal clinical success to combination therapy using iO2, iNO, p.o. sildenafil, and i.v. milrinone.

3 *Does dobutamine cause clinically significant systemic vasodilation/hypotension to preclude use in patients that have modest hypotension on the basis of decreased LV systolic function/contractility?*

In a study looking at 20 preterm infants with hypotension from various causes [52], dobutamine used at a median dose of 20 mcg/(kg min) caused a significant *increase* in the mean BP and cardiac output but not a significant change in SVR (slight *upward* trend). In pediatric studies, no specific studies have evaluated this question. At Children's Hospital of Philadelphia, in the setting of significant hypotension, agents that have additional α activity would be used as first line therapy and then dobutamine added as a second line drug. Anecdotally, no significant BP decreases have been seen in the latter.

4 *Explain the terms downregulation and upregulation of receptors.*

Classically, these terms refer to a decrease of receptor density and an increase of receptor density, respectively. Often, however, these terms are loosely applied to all mechanisms leading to either a decreased and an increased receptor response. Any prolonged β adrenergic stimulation leads to downregulation with increased receptor phosphorylation and subsequent "uncoupling and internalization" of the β_1-receptor. In CHF, there are increased circulating catecholamines, leading to both internalization and downregulation of β_1-receptors. Conversely, the chronic use of β-receptor blockers will increase the density of β-receptors and upregulate the receptors [53].

5 *Does the lung have α- and β-receptors?*

There is evidence in the catheterization and animal labs that routine agents with α and/or β ac-

tivity do affect the PVR but to a lesser degree than the higher receptor concentration in the systemic vascular bed. Therefore, α agonists and β_2-blockers can have deleterious effects on RV performance by increasing RV afterL. In patients that have markedly increased PVR where small further PVR increases would potentially be catastrophic, avoidance of agents in these categories is advised. Use of the above noted successful agents for reduction of RV afterL may avoid the negative effects noted here, although there is no comparison information available.

Conclusions

Pharmacologic manipulation of ventricular performance has advanced tremendously over the last two decades. The use of new agents, the use of combination therapies (e.g., to increase production of an endogenous substance along with decreasing its metabolism), and the use of targeted delivery (e.g. inhalational) has resulted in more effective medical therapy. As new modalities for evaluation of these effects improve with advances in catheterization, echocardiography, and MRI, more effective individualized therapy is possible. Further double-blinded, placebo controlled, multicenter trials will be necessary to guide pharmacologic therapy for improved outcomes both pre- and postoperatively.

References

1. Zile MR, Nappi J. Diastolic heart failure. Curr Treat Options Cardiovasc Med 2000; 2(5):439–450.
2. Morita S. Interdependence of preload, afterload and contractility: Their relation to cardiac function curve. Masui 1992; 41(11):1782–1787.
3. Denfield SW, Gajarski RJ, Towbin JA. Cardiomyopathies. In: The Science and Practice of Pediatric Cardiology, 2nd edn. Williams and Wilkins, Philadelphia, PA, pp. 1863–1864, 1998.
4. Schowengerdt KO, Fisher DJ. Cardiovascular receptors and intracellular signaling. In: The Science and Practice of Pediatric Cardiology, 2nd edn. Williams and Wilkins, Philadelphia, PA, pp. 193–196, 1998.
5. Chen HH, Burnett JC. The natriuretic peptides in heart failure: Diagnostic and therapeutic potentials. Proceed Ass Amer Phys 1999; 111:406–416.
6. Opie LH. Mechanisms of cardiac contraction and relaxation. In: Braunwald, Zipes, Libby, eds., Heart Disease. A Textbook of Cardiovascular Medicine, 6th edn. WB Saunders, Philadelphia, PA, pp. 466–467, 2001.

7. The Medical Letter. Drugs For Hypertension. May 26, 1995, vol 37, 45–58.

8. Bristow MR, Port JD, Kelly RA. Treatment of heart failure: Pharmacological methods. In: Braunwald, Zipes, Libby, edn., Heart Disease. A Textbook of Cardiovascular Medicine, 6th edn. WB Saunders, Philadelphia, PA, pp. 583–584, 2001.

9. Dreyer WJ, Mayer DC, Neish SR. Cardiac contractility and pump function. In: The Science and Practice of Pediatric Cardiology, 2nd edn. Williams and Wilkins, pp. 211–217, 1998.

10. The Medical Letter. A New ACE Inhibitor and Two New Angiotensin Receptor Blockers for Hypertension. Nov 5, 1999, vol 41, 105–106.

11. Chu CC, Lin SM, New SH, et al. Effect of milrinone on postbypass pulmonary hypertension in children after tetralogy of Fallot repair. Zhonghua Yi Xue Za Zhi (Taipei) 2000; 63(4):294–300.

12. Haraldsson SA, Kieler-Jensen N, Ricksten SE. The additive pulmonary vasodilatory effects of inhaled prostacyclin and inhaled milrinone in postcardiac surgical patients with pulmonary hypertension. Anesth Analg 2001; 93(6):1439–1445.

13. Deb B, Bradford K, Pearl RG. Additive effects of inhaled nitric oxide and intravenous milrinone in experimental pulmonary hypertension. Crit Care Med 2000; 28(3):795–799.

14. Schalcher C, Schad K, Brunner-La Rocca HP, et al. Interaction of sildenafil with cAMP-mediated vasodilation in vivo. Hypertension 2002; 40(5):763–767.

15. Goodman LS and Gilman AG. Autacoids: Drug therapy of inflammation. The Pharmacologic Basis of Therapeutics, 9th edn. MacMillan, Indianapolis, IN, pp. 602–610, 1996.

16. Hinderliter AL, Willis PW, Barst RJ, et al. Effects of long-term infusion of prostacyclin (epoprostenol) on echocardiographic measures of right ventricular structure and function in primary pulmonary hypertension. Primary Pulmonary Hypertension Study Group. Circulation 1997; 95(6):1479–1486.

17. Ohnishi M, Oka M, Muramatsu M, Sato K, et al. E4021, a selective phosphodiesterase 5 inhibitor, potentiates the vasodilator effect of inhaled nitric oxide in isolated perfused rat lungs. J Cardiovasc Pharmacol 1999; 33(4):619–624.

18. Fineman JR, Heyman MA, Morin FC. Fetal and postnatal circulations: Pulmonary and persistent pulmonary hypertension of the newborn. In: Moss and Adams' Heart Disease in Infants, Children, and Adolescents, 6th edn. pp. 41–52, 2001.

19. Luscher TF, Barton M. Endothelins and endothelin receptor antagonists. therapeutic considerations for a novel class of cardiovascular drugs. Circulation 2000; 102: 2434–2440.

20. Chen YF, Oparil S. Endothelin and pulmonary hypertension. J Cardiovasc Pharmacol 2000; 35(4, suppl 2):S49–S53.

21. Rondelet B, Kerbaul F, Motte S, et al. Bosentan for the prevention of overcirculation-induced experimental pulmonary arterial hypertension. Circulation 2003; 107(9):1329–1335.

22. Galiè N, Hinderliter AL, Torbicki A, et al. Effects of the oral endothelin-receptor antagonist bosentan on echocardiographic and doppler measures in patients with pulmonary arterial hypertension. J Am Coll Cardiol 2003; 41(8):1380–1386.

23. Sitbon O, Badesch DB, Channick RN, et al. Effects of the dual endothelin receptor antagonist bosentan in patients with pulmonary arterial hypertension: A 1-year follow-up study. Chest 2003; 124(1): 247–254.

24. Barst RJ, Ivy D, Dingemanse J, et al. Pharmacokinetics, safety, and efficacy of bosentan in pediatric patients with pulmonary arterial hypertension. Clin Pharmacol Ther 2003; 73(4): 372–382.

25. Kelly LK, Porta NF, Goodman DM, et al. Inhaled prostacyclin for term infants with persistent pulmonary hypertension refractory to inhaled nitric oxide. J Pediatr 2002; 141(6):830–832.

26. Ivy DD, Griebel JL, Kinsella JP, et al. Acute hemodynamic effects of pulsed delivery of low flow nasal NO in children with pulmonary hypertension. J Peds 1998; 133(3):453–456.

27. Sata M, Sugiura S, Yamashita H, et al. MCI-154 increases Ca++ sensitivity of reconstituted thin filament. A study using a novel in vitro motility assay technique. Circ Res 1995; 76:626–633.

28. Vorhess ML. Adrenal medulla, sympathetic nervous system and multiple endocrine neoplasia syndromes. In: Rudolph's Pediatrics, 20th edn. pp. 1743–1744, 1996.

29. The Medical Letter Carvedilol for Heart Failure. Sept. 26, 1997, Vol 39, pp. 89–91.

30. Laer S, Mir TS, Behn F, et al. Carvedilol therapy in pediatric patients with congestive heart failure: A study investigating clinical and pharmacokinetic parameters. Am Heart J 2002; 143(5):916–922.

31. Packer M, Colucci WS, Sackner-Bernstein JD, et al. Double-blind, placebo-controlled study of the effects of Carvedilol in patients with moderate to severe heart failure. The Precise Trial. Circulation 1996; 94:2793–2799.

32. Bruns LA, Chrisant MK, Lamour JM, et al. Carvedilol as therapy in pediatric heart failure: An initial multicenter experience. J Pediatr 2001; 138:505–511.

33. Azeka E, Franchini Ramires JA, Valler C, et al. Delisting of infants and children from the heart transplantation waiting list after carvedilol treatment. J Am Coll Cardiol 2002; 40(11):2034–2038.

34. Shaddy RE, Curtin El, Sower B, *et al.* The pediatric randomized carvedilol trial in children with heart failure: Rationale and design. Am Heart J 2002; 144(3):383–389.

35. Dreyer WJ, Mayer DC, Neish SR. Cardiac contractility and pump function. In: Geva T ed., Echocardiography and Doppler Ultrasound. The Science and Practice of Pediatric Cardiology, 2nd edn. Williams and Wilkins, pp. 218–219, 834–835, 1998.

36. Bristow MR, Port JD, Kelly RA. Treatment of heart failure: Pharmacological methods. In: Heart Disease. A Textbook of Cardiovascular Medicine, 6th edn. W. B. Saunders, pp. 581–589, 2001.

37. Greenberg B. Treatment of heart failure: State of the art and prospectives. J Cardiovasc Pharmacol 2002; 38(suppl 2):S59–S63.

38. Ayres NA. Fetal cardiology. In: The Science and Practice of Pediatric Cardiology 2nd edn. Williams and Wilkins, pp. 2290–2292, 1998.

39. Oudijk MA, Michon MM, Kleinman CS, *et al.* Sotalol in the treatment of fetal dysrhythmias. Circulation 2000; 101:2721–2726.

40. Pedra SR, Smallhorn JF, Ryan G, *et al.* Fetal cardiomyopathies: Pathogenic mechanisms, hemodynamic findings, and clinical outcome. Circulation 2002;106(5): 585–591.

41. Fogel MA. Assessment of cardiac function by magnetic resonance imaging. Pediatr Cardiol 2000; 21(1): 59–69.

42. Tei C. New non-invasive index for combined systolic and diastolic ventricular function. J Card 1995; 26:135–136.

43. Colon SD, Borow KM, Neumann A. Left ventricular end systolic wall stress—Velocity of fiber shortening relation. A load Independent index of myocardial contractility. JACC 1984; 4:715–724.

44. Michelfelder EC, Vermilion RP, Ludomirshy A, *et al.* Comparison of simultaneous doppler and catheter derived right ventricular dP/dt in hypoplastic left heart syndrome. AJC 1996; 77(2):212–214.

45. Bargiggia GS, Bertucci C, Recusani F, *et al.* A new method for estimating left ventricular dP/dt by continuous wave doppler echocardiography. Validation studies at cardiac catheterization. Circulation 1989; 80:1287–1292.

46. Ommen SR, Nishimura RA, Appleton CP, *et al.* Clinical utility of doppler echocardiography and tissue doppler imaging in the estimation of left ventricular filling pressures. A comparative simultaneous Doppler-catheterzation study. Circualtion 2000; 102:1788–1794.

47. Tsivyan PB, Vasenina AD. Left ventricular systolic and diastolic function in term neonates after mild perinatal asphyxia. Eur J Obstet Gynecol Reprod Biol 1991; 40(2):105–110.

48. Kuecherer HF, Muhiudeen IA, Kusumoto FM, *et al.* Estimation of mean left atrial pressure from transesophageal pulsed doppler echocardiography of pulmonary venous flow. Circualtion 1990; 82:1127–1139.

49. Wernovsky G, Wypij D, Jonas RA, *et al.* Postoperative course and hemodynamic profile after the arterial switch operation in neonates and infants: A comparison of low-flow cardiopulmonary bypass and circulatory arrest. Circulation 1995; 92:2226–2235.

50. Hoffman TM, Wernovsky G, Atz AM, *et al.* Prophylactic intravenous use of milrinone after cardiac operation in pediatrics (PRIMACORP) study. Am Heart J 2002; 143:15–21.

51. Hoffman TM, Wernovsky G, Atz AM, *et al.* Efficacy and safety of milrinone in preventing low cardiac output syndrome in infants and children after corrective surgery for congenital heart disease. Circualtion 2003; 107:996–1002.

52. Roze JC, Tohier C, Maingueneau C, *et al.* Response to dobutamine and dopamine in the hypotensive very preterm infant. Arch Dis Child 1993; 69:59–63.

53. Opie LH, Yusuf S. Beta-blocking agents. In: Drugs for the Heart, 5th edn. W.B. Saunders, Philadelphia, PA, pp. 1–7, 2001.

Index